Lecture Notes in Computer Science   9902

Commenced Publication in 1973
Founding and Former Series Editors:
Gerhard Goos, Juris Hartmanis, and Jan van Leeuwen

More information about this series at http://www.springer.com/series/7412

Sebastien Ourselin · Leo Joskowicz
Mert R. Sabuncu · Gozde Unal
William Wells (Eds.)

Medical Image Computing and Computer-Assisted Intervention – MICCAI 2016

19th International Conference
Athens, Greece, October 17–21, 2016
Proceedings, Part III

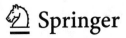 Springer

Editors
Sebastien Ourselin
University College London
London
UK

Leo Joskowicz
The Hebrew University of Jerusalem
Jerusalem
Israel

Mert R. Sabuncu
Harvard Medical School
Boston, MA
USA

Gozde Unal
Istanbul Technical University
Istanbul
Turkey

William Wells
Harvard Medical School
Boston, MA
USA

ISSN 0302-9743   ISSN 1611-3349   (electronic)
Lecture Notes in Computer Science
ISBN 978-3-319-46725-2   ISBN 978-3-319-46726-9   (eBook)
DOI 10.1007/978-3-319-46726-9

Library of Congress Control Number: 2016952513

LNCS Sublibrary: SL6 – Image Processing, Computer Vision, Pattern Recognition, and Graphics

This Springer imprint is published by the registered company Springer Nature Switzerland AG
The registered company address is: Gewerbestrasse 11, 6330 Cham, Switzerland

Preface

In 2016, the 19th International Conference on Medical Image Computing and Computer-Assisted Intervention (MICCAI 2016) was held in Athens, Greece. It was organized by Harvard Medical School, The Hebrew University of Jerusalem, University College London, Sabancı University, Bogazici University, and Istanbul Technical University.

The meeting took place at the Intercontinental Athenaeum Hotel in Athens, Greece, during October 18–20. Satellite events associated with MICCAI 2016 were held on October 19 and October 21. MICCAI 2016 and its satellite events attracted word-leading scientists, engineers, and clinicians, who presented high-standard papers, aiming at uniting the fields of medical image processing, medical image formation, and medical robotics.

This year the triple anonymous review process was organized in several phases. In total, 756 submissions were received. The review process was handled by one primary and two secondary Program Committee members for each paper. It was initiated by the primary Program Committee member, who assigned exactly three expert reviewers, who were blinded to the authors of the paper. Based on these initial anonymous reviews, 82 papers were directly accepted and 189 papers were rejected. Next, the remaining papers went to the rebuttal phase, in which the authors had the chance to respond to the concerns raised by reviewers. The reviewers were then given a chance to revise their reviews based on the rebuttals. After this stage, 51 papers were accepted and 147 papers were rejected based on a consensus reached among reviewers. Finally, the reviews and associated rebuttals were subsequently discussed in person among the Program Committee members during the MICCAI 2016 Program Committee meeting that took place in London, UK, during May 28–29, 2016, with 28 Program Committee members out of 55, the four Program Chairs, and the General Chair. The process led to the acceptance of another 95 papers and the rejection of 192 papers. In total, 228 papers of the 756 submitted papers were accepted, which corresponds to an acceptance rate of 30.1%.

For these proceedings, the 228 papers are organized in 18 groups as follows. The first volume includes Brain Analysis (12), Brain Analysis: Connectivity (12), Brain Analysis: Cortical Morphology (6), Alzheimer Disease (10), Surgical Guidance and Tracking (15), Computer Aided Interventions (10), Ultrasound Image Analysis (5), and Cancer Image Analysis (7). The second volume includes Machine Learning and Feature Selection (12), Deep Learning in Medical Imaging (13), Applications of Machine Learning (14), Segmentation (33), and Cell Image Analysis (7). The third volume includes Registration and Deformation Estimation (16), Shape Modeling (11), Cardiac and Vascular Image Analysis (19), Image Reconstruction (10), and MRI Image Analysis (16).

We thank Dekon, who did an excellent job in the organization of the conference. We thank the MICCAI society for provision of support and insightful comments, the Program Committee for their diligent work in helping to prepare the technical program, as well as the reviewers for their support during the review process. We also thank Andreas Maier for his support in editorial tasks. Last but not least, we thank our sponsors for the financial support that made the conference possible.

We look forward to seeing you in Quebec City, Canada, in 2017!

August 2016   Sebastien Ourselin
                                                                                William Wells
                                                                                Leo Joskowicz
                                                                                Mert Sabuncu
                                                                                Gozde Unal

---

The original version of the book was revised: For detailed information see correction chapter. The correction to the book is available at https://doi.org/10.1007/978-3-319-46726-9_73

Organization

General Chair

Sebastien Ourselin   University College London, London, UK

General Co-chair

Aytül Erçil   Sabanci University, Istanbul, Turkey

Program Chair

William Wells   Harvard Medical School, Boston, MA, USA

Program Co-chairs

Mert R. Sabuncu   A.A. Martinos Center for Biomedical Imaging,
           Charlestown, MA, USA
Leo Joskowicz   The Hebrew University of Jerusalem, Israel
Gozde Unal   Istanbul Technical University, Istanbul, Turkey

Local Organization Chair

Bülent Sankur   Bogazici University, Istanbul, Turkey

Satellite Events Chair

Burak Acar   Bogazici University, Istanbul, Turkey

Satellite Events Co-chairs

Evren Özarslan   Harvard Medical School, Boston, MA, USA
Devrim Ünay   Izmir University of Economics, Izmir, Turkey
Tom Vercauteren   University College London, UK

Industrial Liaison

Tanveer Syeda-Mahmood IBM Almaden Research Center, San Jose, CA, USA

Publication Chair

Andreas Maier   Friedrich-Alexander-Universität Erlangen-Nürnberg,
                              Erlangen, Germany

MICCAI Society Board of Directors

Stephen Aylward   Kitware, Inc., NY, USA
  (Treasurer)
Hervé Delinguette   Inria, Sophia Antipolis, France
Simon Duchesne   Université Laval, Quebéc, QC, Canada
Gabor Fichtinger   Queen's University, Kingston, ON, Canada
  (Secretary)
Alejandro Frangi   University of Sheffield, UK
Pierre Jannin   INSERM/Inria, Rennes, France
Leo Joskowicz   The Hebrew University of Jerusalem, Israel
Shuo Li   Digital Imaging Group, Western University, London,
                                ON, Canada
Wiro Niessen (President   Erasmus MC - University Medical Centre, Rotterdam,
  and Board Chair)   The Netherlands
Nassir Navab   Technical University of Munich, Germany
Alison Noble (Past   University of Oxford, UK
  President - Non Voting)
Sebastien Ourselin   University College London, UK
Josien Pluim   Eindhoven University of Technology, The Netherlands
Li Shen (Executive   Indiana University, IN, USA
  Director)

MICCAI Society Consultants to the Board

Alan Colchester   University of Kent, Canterbury, UK
Terry Peters   University of Western Ontario, London, ON, Canada
Richard Robb   Mayo Clinic College of Medicine, MN, USA

Executive Officers

President and Board Chair   Wiro Niessen
Executive Director   Li Shen
  (Managing Educational
  Affairs)
Secretary (Coordinating   Gabor Fichtinger
  MICCAI Awards)
Treasurer   Stephen Aylward
Elections Officer   Rich Robb

Non-Executive Officers

Society Secretariat	Janette Wallace, Canada
Recording Secretary and Web Maintenance	Jackie Williams, Canada
Fellows Nomination Coordinator	Terry Peters, Canada

Student Board Members

President	Lena Filatova
Professional Student Events officer	Danielle Pace
Public Relations Officer	Duygu Sarikaya
Social Events Officer	Mathias Unberath

Program Committee

Arbel, Tal	McGill University, Canada
Cardoso, Manuel Jorge	University College London, UK
Castellani, Umberto	University of Verona, Italy
Cattin, Philippe C.	University of Basel, Switzerland
Chung, Albert C.S.	Hong Kong University of Science and Technology, Hong Kong
Cukur, Tolga	Bilkent University, Turkey
Delingette, Herve	Inria, France
Feragen, Aasa	University of Copenhagen, Denmark
Freiman, Moti	Philips Healthcare, Israel
Glocker, Ben	Imperial College London, UK
Goksel, Orcun	ETH Zurich, Switzerland
Gonzalez Ballester, Miguel Angel	Universitat Pompeu Fabra, Spain
Grady, Leo	HeartFlow, USA
Greenspan, Hayit	Tel Aviv University, Israel
Howe, Robert	Harvard University, USA
Isgum, Ivana	University Medical Center Utrecht, The Netherlands
Jain, Ameet	Philips Research North America, USA
Jannin, Pierre	University of Rennes, France
Joshi, Sarang	University of Utah, USA
Kalpathy-Cramer, Jayashree	Harvard Medical School, USA
Kamen, Ali	Siemens Corporate Technology, USA
Knutsson, Hans	Linkoping University, Sweden
Konukoglu, Ender	Harvard Medical School, USA
Landman, Bennett	Vanderbilt University, USA
Langs, Georg	University of Vienna, Austria

Lee, Su-Lin	Imperial College London, UK
Liao, Hongen	Tsinghua University, China
Linguraru, Marius George	Children's National Health System, USA
Liu, Huafeng	Zhejiang University, China
Lu, Le	National Institutes of Health, USA
Maier-Hein, Lena	German Cancer Research Center, Germany
Martel, Anne	University of Toronto, Canada
Masamune, Ken	The University of Tokyo, Japan
Menze, Bjoern	Technische Universitat München, Germany
Modat, Marc	Imperial College, London, UK
Moradi, Mehdi	IBM Almaden Research Center, USA
Nielsen, Poul	The University of Auckland, New Zealand
Niethammer, Marc	UNC Chapel Hill, USA
O'Donnell, Lauren	Harvard Medical School, USA
Padoy, Nicolas	University of Strasbourg, France
Pohl, Kilian	SRI International, USA
Prince, Jerry	Johns Hopkins University, USA
Reyes, Mauricio	University of Bern, Bern, Switzerland
Sakuma, Ichiro	The University of Tokyo, Japan
Sato, Yoshinobu	Nara Institute of Science and Technology, Japan
Shen, Li	Indiana University School of Medicine, USA
Stoyanov, Danail	University College London, UK
Van Leemput, Koen	Technical University of Denmark, Denmark
Vrtovec, Tomaz	University of Ljubljana, Slovenia
Wassermann, Demian	Inria, France
Wein, Wolfgang	ImFusion GmbH, Germany
Yang, Guang-Zhong	Imperial College London, UK
Young, Alistair	The University of Auckland, New Zealand
Zheng, Guoyan	University of Bern, Switzerland

Reviewers

Abbott, Jake	Alexander, Daniel	Bai, Ying
Abolmaesumi, Purang	Aljabar, Paul	Bao, Siqi
Acosta-Tamayo, Oscar	Allan, Maximilian	Barbu, Adrian
Adeli, Ehsan	Altmann, Andre	Batmanghelich, Kayhan
Afacan, Onur	Andras, Jakab	Bauer, Stefan
Aganj, Iman	Angelini, Elsa	Bazin, Pierre-Louis
Ahmadi, Seyed-Ahmad	Antony, Bhavna	Beier, Susann
Aichert, Andre	Ashburner, John	Bello, Fernando
Akhondi-Asl, Alireza	Auvray, Vincent	Ben Ayed, Ismail
Albarqouni, Shadi	Awate, Suyash P.	Bergeles, Christos
Alberola-López, Carlos	Bagci, Ulas	Berger, Marie-Odile
Alberts, Esther	Bai, Wenjia	Bhalerao, Abhir

Bhatia, Kanwal
Bieth, Marie
Bilgic, Berkin
Birkfellner, Wolfgang
Bloch, Isabelle
Bogunovic, Hrvoje
Bouget, David
Bouix, Sylvain
Brady, Michael
Bron, Esther
Brost, Alexander
Buerger, Christian
Burgos, Ninon
Cahill, Nathan
Cai, Weidong
Cao, Yu
Carass, Aaron
Cardoso, Manuel Jorge
Carmichael, Owen
Carneiro, Gustavo
Caruyer, Emmanuel
Cash, David
Cerrolaza, Juan
Cetin, Suheyla
Cetingul, Hasan Ertan
Chakravarty, M. Mallar
Chatelain, Pierre
Chen, Elvis C.S.
Chen, Hanbo
Chen, Hao
Chen, Ting
Cheng, Jian
Cheng, Jun
Cheplygina, Veronika
Chowdhury, Ananda
Christensen, Gary
Chui, Chee Kong
Côté, Marc-Alexandre
Ciompi, Francesco
Clancy, Neil T.
Claridge, Ela
Clarysse, Patrick
Cobzas, Dana
Comaniciu, Dorin
Commowick, Olivier
Compas, Colin

Conjeti, Sailesh
Cootes, Tim
Coupe, Pierrick
Crum, William
Dalca, Adrian
Darkner, Sune
Das Gupta, Mithun
Dawant, Benoit
de Bruijne, Marleen
De Craene, Mathieu
Degirmenci, Alperen
Dehghan, Ehsan
Demirci, Stefanie
Depeursinge, Adrien
Descoteaux, Maxime
Despinoy, Fabien
Dijkstra, Jouke
Ding, Xiaowei
Dojat, Michel
Dong, Xiao
Dorfer, Matthias
Du, Xiaofei
Duchateau, Nicolas
Duchesne, Simon
Duncan, James S.
Ebrahimi, Mehran
Ehrhardt, Jan
Eklund, Anders
El-Baz, Ayman
Elliott, Colm
Ellis, Randy
Elson, Daniel
El-Zehiry, Noha
Erdt, Marius
Essert, Caroline
Fallavollita, Pascal
Fang, Ruogu
Fenster, Aaron
Ferrante, Enzo
Fick, Rutger
Figl, Michael
Fischer, Peter
Fishbaugh, James
Fletcher, P. Thomas
Forestier, Germain
Foroughi, Pezhman

Foroughi, Pezhman
Forsberg, Daniel
Franz, Alfred
Freysinger, Wolfgang
Fripp, Jurgen
Frisch, Benjamin
Fritscher, Karl
Funka-Lea, Gareth
Gabrani, Maria
Gallardo Diez,
    Guillermo Alejandro
Gangeh, Mehrdad
Ganz, Melanie
Gao, Fei
Gao, Mingchen
Gao, Yaozong
Gao, Yue
Garvin, Mona
Gaser, Christian
Gass, Tobias
Georgescu, Bogdan
Gerig, Guido
Ghesu, Florin-Cristian
Gholipour, Ali
Ghosh, Aurobrata
Giachetti, Andrea
Giannarou, Stamatia
Gibaud, Bernard
Ginsburg, Shoshana
Girard, Gabriel
Giusti, Alessandro
Golemati, Spyretta
Golland, Polina
Gong, Yuanhao
Good, Benjamin
Gooya, Ali
Grisan, Enrico
Gu, Xianfeng
Gu, Xuan
Gubern-Mérida, Albert
Guetter, Christoph
Guo, Peifang B.
Guo, Yanrong
Gur, Yaniv
Gutman, Boris
Hacihaliloglu, Ilker

Mewes, Philip
Meyer, Chuck
Miller, Karol
Misra, Sarthak
Misra, Vinith
Mlürup, Morten
Moeskops, Pim
Moghari, Mehdi
Mohamed, Ashraf
Mohareri, Omid
Moore, John
Moreno, Rodrigo
Mori, Kensaku
Mountney, Peter
Mukhopadhyay, Anirban
Müller, Henning
Nakamura, Ryoichi
Nambu, Kyojiro
Nasiriavanaki,
    Mohammadreza
Negahdar,
    Mohammadreza
Nenning, Karl-Heinz
Neumann, Dominik
Neumuth, Thomas
Ng, Bernard
Ni, Dong
Näppi, Janne
Niazi, Muhammad
    Khalid Khan
Ning, Lipeng
Noble, Alison
Noble, Jack
Noblet, Vincent
Nouranian, Saman
Oda, Masahiro
O'Donnell, Thomas
Okada, Toshiyuki
Oktay, Ozan
Oliver, Arnau
Onofrey, John
Onogi, Shinya
Orihuela-Espina, Felipe
Otake, Yoshito
Ou, Yangming
Özarslan, Evren

Pace, Danielle
Panayiotou, Maria
Panse, Ashish
Papa, Joao
Papademetris, Xenios
Papadopoulo, Theo
Papie, Bartâomiej W.
Parisot, Sarah
Park, Sang hyun
Paulsen, Rasmus
Peng, Tingying
Pennec, Xavier
Peressutti, Devis
Pernus, Franjo
Peruzzo, Denis
Peter, Loic
Peterlik, Igor
Petersen, Jens
Petersen, Kersten
Petitjean, Caroline
Pham, Dzung
Pheiffer, Thomas
Piechnik, Stefan
Pitiot, Alain
Pizzolato, Marco
Plenge, Esben
Pluim, Josien
Polimeni, Jonathan R.
Poline, Jean-Baptiste
Pont-Tuset, Jordi
Popovic, Aleksandra
Porras, Antonio R.
Prasad, Gautam
Prastawa, Marcel
Pratt, Philip
Preim, Bernhard
Preston, Joseph
Prevost, Raphael
Pszczolkowski, Stefan
Qazi, Arish A.
Qi, Xin
Qian, Zhen
Qiu, Wu
Quellec, Gwenole
Raj, Ashish
Rajpoot, Nasir

Randles, Amanda
Rathi, Yogesh
Reinertsen, Ingerid
Reiter, Austin
Rekik, Islem
Reuter, Martin
Riklin Raviv, Tammy
Risser, Laurent
Rit, Simon
Rivaz, Hassan
Robinson, Emma
Rohling, Robert
Rohr, Karl
Ronneberger, Olaf
Roth, Holger
Rottman, Caleb
Rousseau, François
Roy, Snehashis
Rueckert, Daniel
Rueda Olarte, Andrea
Ruijters, Daniel
Salcudean, Tim
Salvado, Olivier
Sanabria, Sergio
Saritas, Emine
Sarry, Laurent
Scherrer, Benoit
Schirmer, Markus D.
Schnabel, Julia A.
Schultz, Thomas
Schumann, Christian
Schumann, Steffen
Schwartz, Ernst
Sechopoulos, Ioannis
Seeboeck, Philipp
Seiler, Christof
Seitel, Alexander
sepasian, neda
Sermesant, Maxime
Sethuraman, Shriram
Shahzad, Rahil
Shamir, Reuben R.
Shi, Kuangyu
Shi, Wenzhe
Shi, Yonggang
Shin, Hoo-Chang

Siddiqi, Kaleem
Silva, Carlos Alberto
Simpson, Amber
Singh, Vikas
Sivaswamy, Jayanthi
Sjölund, Jens
Skalski, Andrzej
Slabaugh, Greg
Smeets, Dirk
Sommer, Stefan
Sona, Diego
Song, Gang
Song, Qi
Song, Yang
Sotiras, Aristeidis
Speidel, Stefanie
Špiclin, Žiga
Sporring, Jon
Staib, Lawrence
Stamm, Aymeric
Staring, Marius
Stauder, Ralf
Stewart, James
Studholme, Colin
Styles, Iain
Styner, Martin
Sudre, Carole H.
Suinesiaputra, Avan
Suk, Heung-Il
Summers, Ronald
Sun, Shanhui
Sundar, Hari
Sushkov, Mikhail
Suzuki, Takashi
Szczepankiewicz, Filip
Sznitman, Raphael
Taha, Abdel Aziz
Tahmasebi, Amir
Talbot, Hugues
Tam, Roger
Tamaki, Toru
Tamura, Manabu
Tanaka, Yoshihiro
Tang, Hui
Tang, Xiaoying
Tanner, Christine

Tasdizen, Tolga
Taylor, Russell
Thirion, Bertrand
Tie, Yanmei
Tiwari, Pallavi
Toews, Matthew
Tokuda, Junichi
Tong, Tong
Tournier, J. Donald
Toussaint, Nicolas
Tsaftaris, Sotirios
Tustison, Nicholas
Twinanda, Andru Putra
Twining, Carole
Uhl, Andreas
Ukwatta, Eranga
Umadevi Venkataraju,
    Kannan
Unay, Devrim
Urschler, Martin
Vaillant, Régis
van Assen, Hans
van Ginneken, Bram
van Tulder, Gijs
van Walsum, Theo
Vandini, Alessandro
Vasileios, Vavourakis
Vegas-Sanchez-Ferrero,
    Gonzalo
Vemuri, Anant Suraj
Venkataraman, Archana
Vercauteren, Tom
Veta, Mtiko
Vidal, Rene
Villard, Pierre-Frederic
Visentini-Scarzanella,
    Marco
Viswanath, Satish
Vitanovski, Dime
Vogl, Wolf-Dieter
von Berg, Jens
Vrooman, Henri
Wang, Defeng
Wang, Hongzhi
Wang, Junchen
Wang, Li

Wang, Liansheng
Wang, Linwei
Wang, Qiu
Wang, Song
Wang, Yalin
Warfield, Simon
Weese, Jürgen
Wegner, Ingmar
Wei, Liu
Wels, Michael
Werner, Rene
Westin, Carl-Fredrik
Whitaker, Ross
Wörz, Stefan
Wiles, Andrew
Wittek, Adam
Wolf, Ivo
Wolterink,
    Jelmer Maarten
Wright, Graham
Wu, Guorong
Wu, Meng
Wu, Xiaodong
Xie, Saining
Xie, Yuchen
Xing, Fuyong
Xu, Qiuping
Xu, Yanwu
Xu, Ziyue
Yamashita, Hiromasa
Yan, Jingwen
Yan, Pingkun
Yan, Zhennan
Yang, Lin
Yao, Jianhua
Yap, Pew-Thian
Yaqub, Mohammad
Ye, Dong Hye
Ye, Menglong
Yin, Zhaozheng
Yokota, Futoshi
Zelmann, Rina
Zeng, Wei
Zhan, Yiqiang
Zhang, Daoqiang
Zhang, Fan

Zhang, Le
Zhang, Ling
Zhang, Miaomiao
Zhang, Pei
Zhang, Qing
Zhang, Tianhao
Zhang, Tuo

Zhang, Yong
Zhen, Xiantong
Zheng, Yefeng
Zhijun, Zhang
Zhou, Jinghao
Zhou, Luping
Zhou, S. Kevin

Zhu, Hongtu
Zhu, Yuemin
Zhuang, Xiahai
Zollei, Lilla
Zuluaga, Maria A.

Contents – Part III

Registration and Deformation Estimation

Learning-Based Multimodal Image Registration for Prostate Cancer
Radiation Therapy. 1
    *Xiaohuan Cao, Yaozong Gao, Jianhua Yang, Guorong Wu,
    and Dinggang Shen*

A Deep Metric for Multimodal Registration 10
    *Martin Simonovsky, Benjamín Gutiérrez-Becker, Diana Mateus,
    Nassir Navab, and Nikos Komodakis*

Learning Optimization Updates for Multimodal Registration. 19
    *Benjamín Gutiérrez-Becker, Diana Mateus, Loïc Peter,
    and Nassir Navab*

Memory Efficient LDDMM for Lung CT. 28
    *Thomas Polzin, Marc Niethammer, Mattias P. Heinrich, Heinz Handels,
    and Jan Modersitzki*

Inertial Demons: A Momentum-Based Diffeomorphic
Registration Framework. 37
    Andre Santos-Ribeiro, David J. Nutt, and John McGonigle

Diffeomorphic Density Registration in Thoracic Computed Tomography 46
    *Caleb Rottman, Ben Larson, Pouya Sabouri, Amit Sawant,
    and Sarang Joshi*

Temporal Registration in In-Utero Volumetric MRI Time Series. 54
    *Ruizhi Liao, Esra A. Turk, Miaomiao Zhang, Jie Luo, P. Ellen Grant,
    Elfar Adalsteinsson, and Polina Golland*

Probabilistic Atlas of the Human Hippocampus Combining Ex Vivo
MRI and Histology 63
    *Daniel H. Adler, Ranjit Ittyerah, John Pluta, Stephen Pickup,
    Weixia Liu, David A. Wolk, and Paul A. Yushkevich*

Deformation Estimation with Automatic Sliding Boundary Computation 72
    Joseph Samuel Preston, Sarang Joshi, and Ross Whitaker

Bilateral Weighted Adaptive Local Similarity Measure for Registration
in Neurosurgery 81
    *Martin Kochan, Marc Modat, Tom Vercauteren, Mark White, Laura Mancini,
    Gavin P. Winston, Andrew W. McEvoy, John S. Thornton, Tarek Yousry,
    John S. Duncan, Sébastien Ourselin, and Danail Stoyanov*

Model-Based Regularisation for Respiratory Motion Estimation
with Sparse Features in Image-Guided Interventions 89
  Matthias Wilms, In Young Ha, Heinz Handels,
  and Mattias Paul Heinrich

Carotid Artery Wall Motion Estimated from Ultrasound Imaging Sequences
Using a Nonlinear State Space Approach 98
  Zhifan Gao, Yuanyuan Sun, Heye Zhang, Dhanjoo Ghista, Yanjie Li,
  Huahua Xiong, Xin Liu, Yaoqin Xie, Wanqing Wu, and Shuo Li

Accuracy Estimation for Medical Image Registration
Using Regression Forests 107
  Hessam Sokooti, Gorkem Saygili, Ben Glocker,
  Boudewijn P.F. Lelieveldt, and Marius Staring

Embedding Segmented Volume in Finite Element Mesh
with Topology Preservation 116
  Kazuya Sase, Teppei Tsujita, and Atsushi Konno

Deformable 3D-2D Registration of Known Components
for Image Guidance in Spine Surgery 124
  A. Uneri, J. Goerres, T. De Silva, M.W. Jacobson, M.D. Ketcha,
  S. Reaungamornrat, G. Kleinszig, S. Vogt, A.J. Khanna, J.-P. Wolinsky,
  and J.H. Siewerdsen

Anatomically Constrained Video-CT Registration
via the V-IMLOP Algorithm 133
  Seth D. Billings, Ayushi Sinha, Austin Reiter, Simon Leonard,
  Masaru Ishii, Gregory D. Hager, and Russell H. Taylor

Shape Modeling

A Multi-resolution T-Mixture Model Approach to Robust Group-Wise
Alignment of Shapes 142
  Nishant Ravikumar, Ali Gooya, Serkan Çimen, Alejandro F. Frangi,
  and Zeike A. Taylor

Quantifying Shape Deformations by Variation of Geometric Spectrum 150
  Hajar Hamidian, Jiaxi Hu, Zichun Zhong, and Jing Hua

Myocardial Segmentation of Contrast Echocardiograms
Using Random Forests Guided by Shape Model 158
  Yuanwei Li, Chin Pang Ho, Navtej Chahal, Roxy Senior,
  and Meng-Xing Tang

Low-Dimensional Statistics of Anatomical Variability via Compact
Representation of Image Deformations 166
  Miaomiao Zhang, William M. Wells III, and Polina Golland

A Multiscale Cardiac Model for Fast Personalisation and Exploitation   174
Roch Mollero, Xavier Pennec, Hervé Delingette, Nicholas Ayache,
and Maxime Sermesant

Transfer Shape Modeling Towards High-Throughput Microscopy
Image Segmentation   183
Fuyong Xing, Xiaoshuang Shi, Zizhao Zhang, JinZheng Cai,
Yuanpu Xie, and Lin Yang

Hierarchical Generative Modeling and Monte-Carlo EM in Riemannian
Shape Space for Hypothesis Testing   191
Saurabh J. Shigwan and Suyash P. Awate

Direct Estimation of Wall Shear Stress from Aneurysmal Morphology:
A Statistical Approach   201
Ali Sarrami-Foroushani, Toni Lassila, Jose M. Pozo, Ali Gooya,
and Alejandro F. Frangi

Multi-task Shape Regression for Medical Image Segmentation   210
Xiantong Zhen, Yilong Yin, Mousumi Bhaduri, Ilanit Ben Nachum,
David Laidley, and Shuo Li

Soft Multi-organ Shape Models via Generalized PCA: A General
Framework   219
Juan J. Cerrolaza, Ronald M. Summers, and Marius George Linguraru

An Artificial Agent for Anatomical Landmark Detection in Medical Images . . .   229
Florin C. Ghesu, Bogdan Georgescu, Tommaso Mansi,
Dominik Neumann, Joachim Hornegger, and Dorin Comaniciu

Cardiac and Vascular Image Analysis

Identifying Patients at Risk for Aortic Stenosis Through Learning
from Multimodal Data   238
Tanveer Syeda-Mahmood, Yufan Guo, Mehdi Moradi, D. Beymer,
D. Rajan, Yu Cao, Yaniv Gur, and Mohammadreza Negahdar

Multi-input Cardiac Image Super-Resolution Using Convolutional
Neural Networks   246
Ozan Oktay, Wenjia Bai, Matthew Lee, Ricardo Guerrero,
Konstantinos Kamnitsas, Jose Caballero, Antonio de Marvao,
Stuart Cook, Declan O'Regan, and Daniel Rueckert

GPNLPerf: Robust 4d Non-rigid Motion Correction for Myocardial
Perfusion Analysis   255
S. Thiruvenkadam, K.S. Shriram, B. Patil, G. Nicolas, M. Teisseire,
C. Cardon, J. Knoplioch, N. Subramanian, S. Kaushik, and R. Mullick

Recognizing End-Diastole and End-Systole Frames via Deep Temporal
Regression Network   264
    Bin Kong, Yiqiang Zhan, Min Shin, Thomas Denny, and Shaoting Zhang

Basal Slice Detection Using Long-Axis Segmentation for Cardiac Analysis . . .   273
    Mahsa Paknezhad, Michael S. Brown, and Stephanie Marchesseau

Spatially-Adaptive Multi-scale Optimization for Local Parameter
Estimation: Application in Cardiac Electrophysiological Models   282
    Jwala Dhamala, John L. Sapp, Milan Horacek, and Linwei Wang

Reconstruction of Coronary Artery Centrelines from X-Ray Angiography
Using a Mixture of Student's t-Distributions.   291
    *Serkan Çimen, Ali Gooya, Nishant Ravikumar, Zeike A. Taylor,
    and Alejandro F. Frangi*

Barycentric Subspace Analysis: A New Symmetric Group-Wise
Paradigm for Cardiac Motion Tracking   300
    Marc-Michel Rohé, Maxime Sermesant, and Xavier Pennec

Extraction of Coronary Vessels in Fluoroscopic X-Ray Sequences
Using Vessel Correspondence Optimization   308
    *Seung Yeon Shin, Soochahn Lee, Kyoung Jin Noh, Il Dong Yun,
    and Kyoung Mu Lee*

Coronary Centerline Extraction via Optimal Flow Paths and CNN
Path Pruning.   317
    *Mehmet A. Gülsün, Gareth Funka-Lea, Puneet Sharma,
    Saikiran Rapaka, and Yefeng Zheng*

Vascular Registration in Photoacoustic Imaging by Low-Rank Alignment
via Foreground, Background and Complement Decomposition   326
    Ryoma Bise, Yingqiang Zheng, Imari Sato, and Masakazu Toi

From Real MRA to Virtual MRA: Towards an Open-Source Framework   335
    *N. Passat, S. Salmon, J.-P. Armspach, B. Naegel, C. Prud'homme,
    H. Talbot, A. Fortin, S. Garnotel, O. Merveille, O. Miraucourt,
    R. Tarabay, V. Chabannes, A. Dufour, A. Jezierska, O. Balédent,
    E. Durand, L. Najman, M. Szopos, A. Ancel, J. Baruthio, M. Delbany,
    S. Fall, G. Pagé, O. Génevaux, M. Ismail, P. Loureiro de Sousa,
    M. Thiriet, and J. Jomier*

Improved Diagnosis of Systemic Sclerosis Using Nailfold Capillary Flow . . .   344
    *Michael Berks, Graham Dinsdale, Andrea Murray, Tonia Moore,
    Ariane Herrick, and Chris Taylor*

Tensor-Based Graph-Cut in Riemannian Metric Space and Its Application
to Renal Artery Segmentation.   353
Chenglong Wang, Masahiro Oda, Yuichiro Hayashi, Yasushi Yoshino,
Tokunori Yamamoto, Alejandro F. Frangi, and Kensaku Mori

Automatic, Robust, and Globally Optimal Segmentation
of Tubular Structures.   362
Simon Pezold, Antal Horváth, Ketut Fundana, Charidimos Tsagkas,
Michaela Andělová, Katrin Weier, Michael Amann,
and Philippe C. Cattin

Dense Volume-to-Volume Vascular Boundary Detection   371
Jameson Merkow, Alison Marsden, David Kriegman, and Zhuowen Tu

HALE: Healthy Area of Lumen Estimation for Vessel
Stenosis Quantification   380
Sethuraman Sankaran, Michiel Schaap, Stanley C. Hunley,
James K. Min, Charles A. Taylor, and Leo Grady

3D Near Infrared and Ultrasound Imaging of Peripheral Blood Vessels
for Real-Time Localization and Needle Guidance   388
Alvin I. Chen, Max L. Balter, Timothy J. Maguire,
and Martin L. Yarmush

The Minimum Cost Connected Subgraph Problem in Medical
Image Analysis.   397
Markus Rempfler, Bjoern Andres, and Bjoern H. Menze

Image Reconstruction

ASL-incorporated Pharmacokinetic Modelling of PET Data With Reduced
Acquisition Time: Application to Amyloid Imaging.   406
Catherine J. Scott, Jieqing Jiao, Andrew Melbourne,
Jonathan M. Schott, Brian F. Hutton, and Sébastien Ourselin

Probe-Based Rapid Hybrid Hyperspectral and Tissue Surface Imaging
Aided by Fully Convolutional Networks   414
Jianyu Lin, Neil T. Clancy, Xueqing Sun, Ji Qi, Mirek Janatka,
Danail Stoyanov, and Daniel S. Elson

Efficient Low-Dose CT Denoising by Locally-Consistent Non-Local
Means (LC-NLM).   423
Michael Green, Edith M. Marom, Nahum Kiryati, Eli Konen,
and Arnaldo Mayer

Deep Learning Computed Tomography   432
Tobias Würfl, Florin C. Ghesu, Vincent Christlein, and Andreas Maier

Axial Alignment for Anterior Segment Swept Source Optical Coherence
Tomography via Robust Low-Rank Tensor Recovery   441
  Yanwu Xu, Lixin Duan, Huazhu Fu, Xiaoqin Zhang,
  Damon Wing Kee Wong, Baskaran Mani, Tin Aung, and Jiang Liu

3D Imaging from Video and Planar Radiography   450
  Julien Pansiot and Edmond Boyer

Semantic Reconstruction-Based Nuclear Cataract Grading
from Slit-Lamp Lens Images   458
  Yanwu Xu, Lixin Duan, Damon Wing Kee Wong, Tien Yin Wong,
  and Jiang Liu

Vessel Orientation Constrained Quantitative Susceptibility Mapping
(QSM) Reconstruction   467
  Suheyla Cetin, Berkin Bilgic, Audrey Fan, Samantha Holdsworth,
  and Gozde Unal

Spatial-Angular Sparse Coding for HARDI   475
  Evan Schwab, René Vidal, and Nicolas Charon

Compressed Sensing Dynamic MRI Reconstruction Using GPU-accelerated
3D Convolutional Sparse Coding   484
  Tran Minh Quan and Won-Ki Jeong

MRI Image Analysis

Dynamic Volume Reconstruction from Multi-slice Abdominal MRI
Using Manifold Alignment.   493
  Xin Chen, Muhammad Usman, Daniel R. Balfour, Paul K. Marsden,
  Andrew J. Reader, Claudia Prieto, and Andrew P. King

Fast and Accurate Multi-tissue Deconvolution Using SHORE
and H-psd Tensors   502
  Michael Ankele, Lek-Heng Lim, Samuel Groeschel, and Thomas Schultz

Optimisation of Arterial Spin Labelling Using Bayesian Experimental
Design.   511
  David Owen, Andrew Melbourne, David Thomas, Enrico De Vita,
  Jonathan Rohrer, and Sebastien Ourselin

4D Phase-Contrast Magnetic Resonance CardioAngiography
(4D PC-MRCA) Creation from 4D Flow MRI   519
  Mariana Bustamante, Vikas Gupta, Carl-Johan Carlhäll,
  and Tino Ebbers

Joint Estimation of Cardiac Motion and T_1^* Maps for Magnetic Resonance
Late Gadolinium Enhancement Imaging.......................... 527
    Jens Wetzl, Aurélien F. Stalder, Michaela Schmidt, Yigit H. Akgök,
    Christoph Tillmanns, Felix Lugauer, Christoph Forman,
    Joachim Hornegger, and Andreas Maier

Correction of Fat-Water Swaps in Dixon MRI 536
    Ben Glocker, Ender Konukoglu, Ioannis Lavdas, Juan Eugenio Iglesias,
    Eric O. Aboagye, Andrea G. Rockall, and Daniel Rueckert

Motion-Robust Reconstruction Based on Simultaneous Multi-slice
Registration for Diffusion-Weighted MRI of Moving Subjects 544
    Bahram Marami, Benoit Scherrer, Onur Afacan, Simon K. Warfield,
    and Ali Gholipour

Self Super-Resolution for Magnetic Resonance Images 553
    Amod Jog, Aaron Carass, and Jerry L. Prince

Tight Graph Framelets for Sparse Diffusion MRI q-Space Representation ... 561
    Pew-Thian Yap, Bin Dong, Yong Zhang, and Dinggang Shen

A Bayesian Model to Assess T_2 Values and Their Changes Over Time
in Quantitative MRI 570
    Benoit Combès, Anne Kerbrat, Olivier Commowick,
    and Christian Barillot

Simultaneous Parameter Mapping, Modality Synthesis, and Anatomical
Labeling of the Brain with MR Fingerprinting 579
    Pedro A. Gómez, Miguel Molina-Romero, Cagdas Ulas,
    Guido Bounincontri, Jonathan I. Sperl, Derek K. Jones,
    Marion I. Menzel, and Bjoern H. Menze

XQ-NLM: Denoising Diffusion MRI Data via x-q Space Non-local
Patch Matching.. 587
    Geng Chen, Yafeng Wu, Dinggang Shen, and Pew-Thian Yap

Spatially Adaptive Spectral Denoising for MR Spectroscopic Imaging
using Frequency-Phase Non-local Means 596
    Dhritiman Das, Eduardo Coello, Rolf F. Schulte, and Bjoern H. Menze

Beyond the Resolution Limit: Diffusion Parameter Estimation
in Partial Volume 605
    Zach Eaton-Rosen, Andrew Melbourne, M. Jorge Cardoso,
    Neil Marlow, and Sebastien Ourselin

A Promising Non-invasive CAD System for Kidney Function Assessment . . .   613
    M. Shehata, F. Khalifa, A. Soliman, M. Abou El-Ghar, A. Dwyer,
    G. Gimel'farb, R. Keynton, and A. El-Baz

Comprehensive Maximum Likelihood Estimation of Diffusion
Compartment Models Towards Reliable Mapping of Brain Microstructure . . .   622
    Aymeric Stamm, Olivier Commowick, Simon K. Warfield, and S. Vantini

Erratum to: Medical Image Computing and Computer-Assisted
Intervention – MICCAI 2016 . . . .   E1
    Sebastien Ourselin, Leo Joskowicz, Mert R. Sabuncu, Gozde Unal,
    and William Wells

Author Index   631

Learning-Based Multimodal Image Registration for Prostate Cancer Radiation Therapy

Xiaohuan Cao[1,2], Yaozong Gao[2,3], Jianhua Yang[1], Guorong Wu[2],
and Dinggang Shen[2(✉)]

[1] School of Automation, Northwestern Polytechnical University, Xi'an, China
[2] Department of Radiology and BRIC, University of North Carolina
at Chapel Hill, Chapel Hill, NC, USA
dgshen@med.unc.edu
[3] Department of Computer Science, University of North Carolina at Chapel Hill,
Chapel Hill, NC, USA

Abstract. Computed tomography (CT) is widely used for dose planning in the radiotherapy of prostate cancer. However, CT has low tissue contrast, thus making manual contouring difficult. In contrast, magnetic resonance (MR) image provides high tissue contrast and is thus ideal for manual contouring. If MR image can be registered to CT image of the same patient, the contouring accuracy of CT could be substantially improved, which could eventually lead to high treatment efficacy. In this paper, we propose a learning-based approach for multimodal image registration. First, to fill the appearance gap between modalities, a structured random forest with auto-context model is learnt to synthesize MRI from CT and vice versa. Then, MRI-to-CT registration is steered in a dual manner of registering images with same appearances, i.e., (1) registering the synthesized CT with CT, and (2) also registering MRI with the synthesized MRI. Next, a dual-core deformation fusion framework is developed to iteratively and effectively combine these two registration results. Experiments on pelvic CT and MR images have shown the improved registration performance by our proposed method, compared with the existing non-learning based registration methods.

1 Introduction

Prostate cancer is a common cancer worldwide. In clinical treatments, external beam radiation therapy (EBRT) is one of the most efficient methods. In EBRT, computed tomography (CT) is acquired for dose planning since it can provide electron density information. However, due to low tissue contrast, it is difficult to contour major pelvic organs from CT images, such as prostate, bladder and rectum. Also, the low contouring accuracy largely limits the efficacy of prostate cancer treatment. Nowadays, magnetic resonance (MR) image is often used together with CT in the EBRT. MR image provides high tissue contrast, which makes it ideal for manual organ contouring. Therefore, it is clinically desired to register the pelvic MR image to the CT image of the same patient for effective manual contouring.

© Springer International Publishing AG 2016
S. Ourselin et al. (Eds.): MICCAI 2016, Part III, LNCS 9902, pp. 1–9, 2016.
DOI: 10.1007/978-3-319-46726-9_1

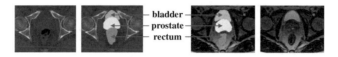

Fig. 1. Pelvic CT and MRI. From left to right: CT, labeled CT, labeled MRI and MRI.

However, there are two main challenges for accurate pelvic MRI-to-CT registration. The first one comes from local anatomical deformation. This is because CT and MRI of the same patient are always scanned at different time points, thus the positions, shapes and appearances of pelvic organs could change dramatically due to possible bladder filling and emptying, bowel gas and irregular rectal movement. This necessitates the use of non-rigid image registration to correct the local deformations.

The second challenge comes from the appearance dissimilarities between CT and MRI. For example, there are no obvious intensity differences among the regions of prostate, bladder and rectum in CT image. But, in MR image, the bladder has brighter intensity than the prostate and rectum, as shown in Fig. 1. Moreover, the texture patterns of prostate in MRI are much more complex. These appearance dissimilarities make it difficult to design a universal similarity metric for MRI-to-CT registration.

To date, many approaches have been developed for multimodal image registration. They fall into two categories [1]. The first category is using mutual information (MI) [2] as similarity metric for registration. However, MI is a global similarity metric, thus has limited power to capture local anatomical details. Although it is technically feasible to compute MI between local patches, the insufficient number of voxels in the patch makes the intensity distribution less robust to compute MI.

The second category is based on image synthesis for registration. In these methods, one modality (e.g., CT) is synthesized from the other modality (e.g., MRI) to reduce large appearance gap between different modalities. Afterwards, the multimodal image registration problem is simplified to unimodal image registration, where most existing methods can be applied. Currently, the synthesis process is often applied to synthesizing the image with simple appearance from the image with rich and complex appearance, i.e., synthesizing CT from MRI [3]. However, such complex-to-simple image synthesis offers limited benefit to the pelvic MRI-to-CT registration. This is because the alignment at soft tissues such as prostate can hardly get improved due to low image contrast in CT. To alleviate this issue, we argue that image synthesis should be performed in bi-directions, and also the estimated deformations from both synthesized modalities should be effectively combined to improve multimodal image registration.

In this paper, we propose a learning-based multimodal image registration method based on our novel bi-directional image synthesis. The contributions of our work can be summarized as follows:

(1) To reduce the large appearance gap between MRI and CT, we propose to use structured random forest and auto-context model for bi-directional image synthesis, i.e., synthesizing MRI from CT and also synthesizing CT from MRI.

(2) To fully utilize the complementary image information from both modalities, we propose a dual-core registration method to effectively estimate the deformation

pathway from MRI to CT space, by iteratively fusing two deformation pathways: (a) from the synthesized CT of MRI to CT, and (b) from MRI to the synthesized MRI of CT. Experimental results show that the registration accuracy could be boosted under this dual-core registration framework.

2 Method

As shown in Fig. 2, the proposed multimodal image registration method consists of the following two major steps.

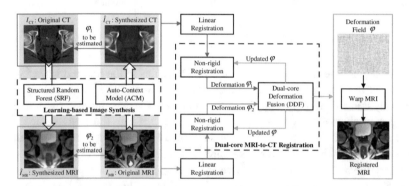

Fig. 2. The framework of proposed learning-based MRI-to-CT image registration.

Learning-Based Image Synthesis. A learning-based image synthesis method is proposed to fill the appearance gap between CT and MRI. Since MRI synthesis is more challenging, our method will introduce in the context of CT-to-MRI synthesis. The same method can be applied to MRI-to-CT synthesis. In our method, a structured random forest is first used to predict the entire MRI patch from the corresponding CT patch. Then we further adopt an auto-context model [4] to iteratively refine the synthesized MRI. The details of this step are described in Sect. 2.1.

Dual-Core MRI-to-CT Image Registration. In the beginning of image registration, a synthesized MRI $\hat{I}_{MR}$ is obtained from CT I_{CT}, and also a synthesized CT $\hat{I}_{CT}$ is obtained from MRI I_{MR}. Then, the deformation between MRI and CT is estimated in two ways: (a) registering $\hat{I}_{CT}$ to I_{CT}, and (b) registering I_{MR} to $\hat{I}_{MR}$, as shown in Fig. 2. Eventually, the MRI is warped to the CT space by following the iterative dual-core deformation fusion framework. The details of this step are described in Sect. 2.2.

2.1 Learning-Based Image Synthesis

Random Forest Regression. Random forest is a general machine learning technique, which can be used for non-linear regression. It can be used to regress MRI intensity from the corresponding CT patch. In the training of random forest, the input is N feature vectors $X = [x_1, x_2, \cdots, x_N]$ and the corresponding N target MRI values $y = [y_1, y_2, \cdots, y_N]$, where each x corresponds to appearance features extracted from a single CT patch, and each y is the MRI value corresponding to the center of the CT patch. Random forest consists of multiple binary decision trees, and each one is trained independently. For a given tree, the training is conducted by learning a set of split nodes to recursively partition the training set. Specifically, in each split node, for a feature indexed by k, its optimal threshold τ is found to best split the training set into left and right subsets S_L and S_R with consistent target MRI values. Mathematically, it is to maximize the variance reduction by a split:

$$\mathrm{argmax}_{k,\tau} V(S) - \frac{|S_L|}{|S|} V(S_L) - \frac{|S_R|}{|S|} V(S_R) \tag{1}$$

$$S_L = \left\{ (x,y) \in S | x^k < \tau \right\}, S_R = \left\{ (x,y) \in S | x^k \geq \tau \right\} \tag{2}$$

where $V(\cdot)$ computes the variance of target MRI values in the training set, x^k indicates the value of the k-th feature, and S indicates a training set. The same split operation is recursively conducted on S_L and S_R, until (a) the tree reaches the maximum tree depth, or (b) the number of training samples is too few to split. In the testing stage, given a testing sample with feature vector x_{new}, it is pushed to the root split node of each tree in the forest. Under the guidance of the split node (i.e., go left if $x^k_{\mathrm{new}} < \tau$, and go right otherwise), the testing sample will arrive at a leaf node of each tree, where the averaged target MRI values of training samples in that leaf is used as the prediction of the tree. The final output is the average of predictions from all trees.

Structured Random Forest (SRF). In our MRI synthesis, structured random forest is adopted for prediction. The main difference between classic random forest and structured random forest is illustrated in Fig. 3. Instead of regressing a single MRI voxel intensity, the whole MRI intensity patch is concatenated as a vector and used as the regression target. Variance $V(\cdot)$ in Eq. (1) is then computed as the average variance across each dimension of the regression target vector. Through predicting a whole MRI patch, the neighborhood information can be preserved during patch-wise prediction and eventually will lead to better image synthesis performance, which is crucial for the subsequent registration. In the testing stage, the prediction is a vector, which can be constructed as a patch. The final prediction of each voxel is obtained by averaging values from all patches containing this voxel.

Feature Extraction. In this paper, we extract Haar-like features [5] from CT patch to serve as appearance features for random forest. Specifically, a Haar-like feature describes (a) an average intensity within a sub-block, or (b) the average intensity difference between two sub-blocks, in the patch. To generate more Haar-like features, we randomly sample information within the patch. To capture both local and global appearances of the

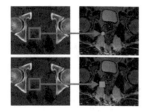

Fig. 3. Classic random forest (*top*) and SRF (*bottom*).

underlying voxel, Haar-like features are extracted from coarse, medium and fine resolutions, respectively.

Auto-Context Model (ACM). To incorporate the neighboring prediction results, an auto-context model [4] is adopted to iteratively refine the synthesized MRI. In this paper, we use three layers as illustrated in Fig. 4. In the first layer, appearance features (Haar-like features) from CT are extracted to train a SRF. Then, the trained forest can be used to provide an initial synthesized MRI. In the second layer, additional features (context features, also Haar-like features) are also extracted from the initial synthesized MRI to capture the information about neighborhood predictions. By combining the context features with appearance features, a second SRF can be trained. Similarly, with this new trained forest, the synthesized MRI and context features can be updated. This process iterates until reaching the maximum number of layers.

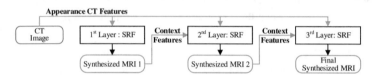

Fig. 4. Iterative refinement of synthesized MRI by the auto-context model.

2.2 Dual-Core MRI-to-CT Image Registration

Intensity-based Non-rigid Registration. After CT and MRI are synthesized from MRI and CT, respectively, we can utilize the existing non-rigid registration methods to estimate the deformation (a) from synthesized CT to CT, and (b) from MRI to synthesized MRI. Here, we choose two popular methods for evaluation: (1) Diffeomorphic Demons (D. Demons) [6] and (2) Symmetric Normalization (SyN) [7].

Dual-Core Deformation Fusion (DDF) for MRI-to-CT Registration. Based on bi-directional image synthesis, both synthesized CT and MRI are utilized in registration. Let I_{CT}, $\hat{I}_{CT}$, I_{MR} and $\hat{I}_{MR}$ denote the CT, synthesized CT, MRI and synthesized MRI, respectively. The goal is to estimate the deformation pathway φ from MRI to CT space. The objective function for MRI-to-CT non-rigid registration can be given as:

$$\mathrm{argmin}_\varphi E(\varphi) = \mathrm{argmin}_\varphi \frac{1}{2}\mathcal{M}(I_{CT}, \mathcal{D}(\hat{I}_{CT}, \varphi)) + \frac{1}{2}\mathcal{M}(\hat{I}_{MR}, \mathcal{D}(I_{MR}, \varphi)) + \lambda\mathcal{R}(\varphi) \quad (3)$$

where $\mathcal{M}$ is a dissimilarity metric, $\mathcal{D}$ is an operator that deforms the image by deformation field φ, and $\mathcal{R}$ is a regularization term to constrain the smoothness of φ.

To solve Eq. (3) and reuse the existing registration tools, we apply an alternative optimization method, by decomposing Eq. (3) into three steps:

$$\mathrm{argmin}_{\varphi_1} \frac{1}{2}\mathcal{M}(I_{CT}, \mathcal{D}(\hat{I}_{CT}, \varphi_1)) + \frac{\lambda}{2}\mathcal{R}(\varphi_1) \quad (4)$$

$$\text{argmin}_{\varphi_2} \frac{1}{2} \mathcal{M}(\hat{I}_{\text{MR}}, \mathcal{D}(I_{\text{MR}}, \varphi_2)) + \frac{\lambda}{2} \mathcal{R}(\varphi_2) \qquad (5)$$

$$\text{argmin}_{\varphi} \frac{1}{2} ||\varphi - \varphi_1||_2^2 + \frac{1}{2} ||\varphi - \varphi_2||_2^2 \qquad (6)$$

The first and second steps (Eqs. (4) and (5)) are used to minimize the image difference (a) between CT modality pair and (b) between MRI modality pair, respectively. The third step (Eq. (6)) is used to ensure that the final deformation pathway φ is close to both separately estimated φ_1 and φ_2.

Both φ_1 and φ_2 can be solved by using either D. Demons or SyN, although the objective functions are slightly different in Eqs. (4) and (5). After fixing φ_1 and φ_2, the final deformation φ can be efficiently solved by letting the gradient of Eq. (6) equals to zero, which brings to $\varphi = \frac{1}{2}(\varphi_1 + \varphi_2)$. To approximate the optimal solution of Eq. (3), we alternate these three steps until convergence, as summarized in Algorithm 1.

In each iteration i, the tentatively deformed images $\hat{I}_{\text{CT}}^{i-1}$ and I_{MR}^{i-1} are used to estimate a next set of deformations φ_1^i and φ_2^i. The estimated deformations are then merged to form a combined deformation φ^i, which is used to update the currently estimated deformation $\varphi = \varphi \circ \varphi^i$. Here, "$\circ$" means deformation field composing. This procedure iterates until the incremental deformation φ^i is small enough.

Algorithm 1. Alternating Optimization of Eq. (3) in the i-th iteration

Result: φ – the final deformation field and approximated solution of Eq. (3)

$i = 0; \hat{I}_{\text{CT}}^0 = \hat{I}_{\text{CT}}; I_{\text{MR}}^0 = I_{\text{MR}}; \varphi = \mathbf{0};$

do {

$\quad i = i + 1; \varphi_1^i = \text{Register}(\hat{I}_{\text{CT}}^{i-1}, I_{\text{CT}}); \varphi_2^i = \text{Register}(I_{\text{MR}}^{i-1}, \hat{I}_{\text{MR}});$

$\quad \varphi^i = \frac{1}{2}(\varphi_1^i + \varphi_2^i); \varphi = \varphi \circ \varphi^i; \hat{I}_{\text{CT}}^i = \mathcal{D}(\hat{I}_{\text{CT}}, \varphi); I_{\text{MR}}^i = \mathcal{D}(I_{\text{MR}}, \varphi);$

} **while** ($\left\| \varphi^i \right\|_2 > \varepsilon$);

---

3 Experiments

The experimental dataset consists of 20 pairs CT and MRI acquired from 20 prostate cancer patients. Three pelvic organs, including prostate, bladder and rectum, are manually labeled by physicians. We use them as the ground-truth. All the images are resampled and cropped to the same size (200*180*80) and resolution (1*1*1 mm^3). The cropped image is sufficiently large to include prostate, bladder and rectum.

In the training step, the CT and MRI of the same patient are pre-aligned to train our image synthesis models and we use manual labels to guide accurate pre-alignment. Specifically, linear (FLIRT [8]) and non-linear (SyN [7]) registrations are first performed to register the CT and MRI of same patient. Then D. Demons [6] is applied to register the manual labels of prostate, bladder and rectum to refine the pre-alignment. Finally, all the subjects are linearly aligned to a common space. Note that, the well-aligned CT and MR image dataset are only used in image synthesis training step.

2-layer ACM and 10-fold cross validation (leave-2-out) are applied. For SRF, the input patch size is 15*15*15 and the target patch size is 3*3*3. We use 25 trees to synthesize MRI from CT, while 20 trees to synthesize CT from MRI. The reason of using more trees in the former case is because CT-to-MRI synthesis is more difficult.

Dice similarity coefficient (DSC), symmetric average surface distance (SASD) and Hausdorff distance (HAUS) between manual segmentations on CT and aligned MRI are used to measure the registration performance.

3.1   Registration Results

Figure 5 illustrates MRI-to-CT registration results from the whole dataset under different layers of ACM in image synthesis (Fig. 5-(a)) and different DDF iterations in image registration (Fig. 5-(b)). As shown in Fig. 5-(a), more layers of ACM lead to better registration accuracy due to better quality of synthesized images. The synthesized CT (S-CT) and synthesized MRI (S-MRI) are also visualized in Fig. 6. Figure 5-(b) demonstrates that the DDF framework improves registration performance of both D. Demons and SyN iteratively. In practice, we found that the use of 2-layer ACM in image synthesis and 3 iterations (3-iter) in DDF often leads to convergence, as shown in Fig. 5, the 3-layer ACM and 4-iter DDF do not have significant improvement.

Table 1 provides the mean and standard deviation of DSC for the three organs. It can be observed that, for D. Demons, which is not applicable for multimodal registration, can now work well by introducing the synthesized image. For SyN, using MI as similarity metric can get reasonable registration results on the original CT and MRI. However, better performance can be obtained using the synthesized image. This demonstrates that using synthesized image can enhance the performance of multimodal registration method. Moreover, the best performance is achieved under our dual-core deformation fusion algorithm as both demonstrated in Tables 1 and 2. The consistently higher DSC and lower SASD and HAUS by our proposed method demonstrate both its robustness and accuracy in multimodal image registration. Also, from those SyN-based registration results shown in Fig. 6, our proposed method can (a) better preserve structures during the registration than the direct registration of MRI to CT with MI, and (b) achieve more accurate results as shown by the overlaps of the label contours and indicated by arrows in the figure.

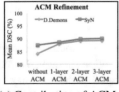
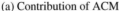

(a) Contribution of ACM

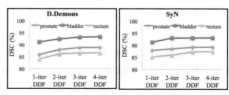

(b) Contribution of iterative DDF

Fig. 5. Comparison of MRI-to-CT non-rigid registration results. (a) The mean DSC of prostate, bladder and rectum by different number of ACM layers in image synthesis. (b) Registration results of D. Demons (*left*) and SyN (*right*) with respect to different DDF iterations in Algorithm 1. Note that, 3-iter DDF is applied in (a), and 2-layer ACM is used in (b).

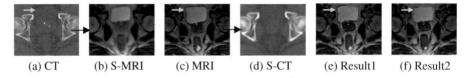

(a) CT   (b) S-MRI   (c) MRI   (d) S-CT   (e) Result1   (f) Result2

Fig. 6. Demonstration of synthesized images and SyN registration results. (e) Result 1: direct registration of MRI to CT using MI; (f) Result 2: registration with our proposed method. Yellow contours: original CT labels of 3 organs. Red contours: warped MRI labels of 3 organs. (Color figure online)

Table 1. Comparison of **DSC** (%) values (with standard deviation of total 20 subjects) of three organs after non-rigid registration through original CT and MRI (**CT & MRI**), single-directional image synthesis (**CT & S-CT, S-MRI & MRI**), and our proposed bi-directional image synthesis under 3-iter DDF (**Proposed**).

Method	Region	CT & MRI	CT & S-CT	S-MRI & MRI	Proposed
D. Demons	Prostate	N/A	86.3 ± 5.0	87.4 ± 6.9	**88.9 ± 4.3**
	Bladder	N/A	91.0 ± 1.1	91.5 ± 0.9	**93.2 ± 0.5**
	Rectum	N/A	84.2 ± 3.1	84.1 ± 6.2	**86.6 ± 2.5**
SyN (MI)	Prostate	86.8 ± 3.5	87.9 ± 2.9	87.3 ± 3.4	**89.2 ± 2.8**
	Bladder	90.4 ± 0.4	91.3 ± 0.5	91.5 ± 0.7	**93.0 ± 0.3**
	Rectum	83.7 ± 4.7	85.0 ± 4.2	85.2 ± 5.4	**87.2 ± 3.2**

Table 2. Comparison of mean **SASD(mm)** and **HAUS(mm)** values (with standard deviation of total 20 subjects) of three pelvic organs after non-rigid registration based on single-directional image synthesis and our proposed bi-directional image synthesis under 3-iter DDF.

Metric	Method	Single-directional		Bi-directional
		CT & S-CT	S-MRI & MRI	Proposed
SASD	D. Demons	1.3 ± 0.7	1.7 ± 0.8	**1.0 ± 0.6**
	ANTs-SyN	1.4 ± 0.8	1.3 ± 0.7	**1.1 ± 0.7**
HAUS	D. Demons	8.9 ± 2.7	8.6 ± 3.0	**6.7 ± 2.3**
	ANTs-SyN	7.6 ± 2.7	7.2 ± 2.0	**6.7 ± 1.9**

4   Conclusion

In this paper, we propose a learning-based multimodal registration method to register pelvic MR and CT images for facilitating prostate cancer radiation therapy. To reduce the appearance gap between two modalities, the structured random forest and auto-context model are used to synthesize CT from MRI, and also synthesize MRI from CT. Furthermore, we propose the dual-core image registration method to drive the deformation pathway from MR image to CT image by fully utilizing the complementary information in multiple modalities. Experimental results show that our method has higher registration accuracy than the compared conventional methods.

References

1. Sotiras, A., Davatzikos, C., Paragios, N.: Deformable medical image registration: a survey. IEEE Trans. Med. Imaging **32**(7), 1153–1190 (2013)
2. Pluim, J.P., Maintz, J.A., Viergever, M.A.: Mutual-information-based registration of medical images: a survey. IEEE Trans. Med. Imaging **22**(8), 986–1004 (2003)
3. Huynh, T., et al.: Estimating CT image from MRI data using structured random forest and auto-context model. IEEE Trans. Med. Imaging **35**(1), 174–183 (2015)
4. Tu, Z., Bai, X.: Auto-context and its application to high-level vision tasks and 3d brain image segmentation. IEEE Trans. Pattern Anal. Mach. Intell. **32**(10), 1744–1757 (2010)
5. Viola, P., Jones, M.J.: Robust real-time face detection. Int. J. Comput. Vision **57**(2), 137–154 (2004)
6. Vercauteren, T., et al.: Diffeomorphic demons: efficient non-parametric image registration. NeuroImage **45**(1), S61–S72 (2009)
7. Avants, B.B., et al.: Symmetric diffeomorphic image registration with cross-correlation: evaluating automated labeling of elderly and neurodegenerative brain. Med. Image Anal. **12**(1), 26–41 (2008)
8. Jenkinson, M., Smith, S.: A global optimisation method for robust affine registration of brain images. Med. Image Anal. **5**(2), 143–156 (2001)

A Deep Metric for Multimodal Registration

Martin Simonovsky[1]([✉]), Benjamín Gutiérrez-Becker[2], Diana Mateus[2],
Nassir Navab[2], and Nikos Komodakis[1]

[1] Imagine, Université Paris Est/École des Ponts ParisTech,
Champs-sur-Marne, France
{martin.simonovsky,nikos.komodakis}@enpc.fr
[2] Computer Aided Medical Procedures, Technische Universität München,
Munich, Germany
gutierrez.becker@tum.de, {mateus,navab}@in.tum.de

Abstract. Multimodal registration is a challenging problem due the
high variability of tissue appearance under different imaging modalities.
The crucial component here is the choice of the right similarity measure.
We make a step towards a general learning-based solution that can be
adapted to specific situations and present a metric based on a convolutional neural network. Our network can be trained from scratch even
from a few aligned image pairs. The metric is validated on intersubject deformable registration on a dataset different from the one used for
training, demonstrating good generalization. In this task, we outperform
mutual information by a significant margin.

1 Introduction

Multimodal registration is a very challenging problem commonly faced during
image-guided interventions and data fusion [12]. The main difficulty of the multimodal registration task comes from the great variability of tissue or organ
appearance when imaged by different physical principles, which translates in the
lack of a general rule to compare such images. Therefore, efforts to tackle this
problem focus mainly on the design of multimodal similarity metrics.

Recent works have explored the use of supervised methods to learn similarity
metrics from a set of aligned examples [2,7,10], showing potential to outperform
hand-crafted metrics in particular applications. However, a general method to
learn similarity between any two modalities calls for higher capacity models.

Inspired by their success in computer vision, we propose to learn such general
similarity metric based on Convolutional Neural Networks (CNNs). The problem
is modelled as a classification task, where the goal is to discriminate between
aligned and misaligned patches from different modalities. To the best of our
knowledge, this is the first time that CNNs are used in the context of multimodal
medical image registration.

The ability of our metric to obtain reliable registrations is demonstrated on
the ALBERTs database of neonatal images [5], where we outperform Mutual
Information [9]. Importantly, we train on a separate dataset (IXI database of

© Springer International Publishing AG 2016
S. Ourselin et al. (Eds.): MICCAI 2016, Part III, LNCS 9902, pp. 10–18, 2016.
DOI: 10.1007/978-3-319-46726-9_2

adults [1]), demonstrating the capability to generalize to data acquired with different scanners and with demographic differences in the subjects. We also show that our method is able to learn reliable multimodal similarities even with a small training set, as is often the case in medical imaging applications.

1.1 Related Work

The idea of using supervised learning to build a similarity metric for multimodal images has been explored in a number of works. On one side, there are probabilistic approaches which rely on modelling the joint-image distribution. For instance, Guetter *et al.* propose a generative method based on Kullback-Leibler Divergence [6]. Our work is closer to the discriminative concept proposed by Lee *et al.* [7] and Michel *et al.* [10], where the problem of learning a similarity metric is posed as binary classification. Here the goal is to discriminate between aligned and misaligned patches given pairs of aligned images. Lee *et al.* propose the use of a Structured Support Vector Machine while Michel *et al.* use a method based on Adaboost. Different to these approaches we rely on CNN as our learning method of choice as the suitable set of characteristics for each type of modality combinations can be directly learned from the training data.

The power of CNNs to capture complex relationships between multimodal medical images has been shown in the problem of modality synthesis [11], where CNNs are used to map MRI-T2 images to MRI-T1 images using jointly the appearance of a small patch together with its localization. Our work is arguably most similar to the approach of Cheng *et al.* [3] who train a multilayer fully-connected network pretrained with autoencoder for estimating similarity of 2D CT-MR patch pairs. Our network is a CNN, which enables us to scale to 3D due to weight sharing and train from scratch. Moreover, we evaluate our metric on the actual task of registration, unlike Cheng *et al.*

2 Method

Image registration is the task of estimating the best spatial transformation $\mathcal{T}$: $\Omega_f \mapsto \mathbb{R}^d$ between a *fixed image* $I_f : \Omega_f \subset \mathbb{R}^d \mapsto \mathbb{R}$ and a *moving image* $I_m : \Omega_m \subset \mathbb{R}^d \mapsto \mathbb{R}$. In our setting $d = 3$ and the images come each from a different modality. The problem is often solved by minimizing the energy

$$E(\theta) = M(I_f, I_m(\mathcal{T}(\theta))) + R(\mathcal{T}(\theta)) \tag{1}$$

where the first term M is a metric quantifying the cost of the alignment by transformation $\mathcal{T}$ parameterized by θ and the second term R is a regularization constraining the mapping. We denote the moving image resampled into Ω_f by $\mathcal{T}$ as the *warped image* $I'_m = I_m(\mathcal{T}(\theta)) : \Omega_f \subset \mathbb{R}^d \mapsto \mathbb{R}$. The minimization is commonly solved in a continuous or discrete optimization framework [12], depending on the nature of θ.

In this work we explore formulating M as a convolutional neural network. To this end we rely on network $N(P_f, P_m)$ which outputs a scalar value estimating the dissimilarity between two image patches $P_f \subset I_f$ and $P_m \subset I'_m$ of the same size. Its incorporation into a continuous optimization framework is explained in Subsect. 2.1. The architecture and training of N is described in Subsect. 2.2.

2.1   Continuous Optimization

Continuous optimization methods iteratively update parameters θ based on the gradient of the objective function $E(\theta)$. We restrict ourselves to first-order methods and use gradient descent in particular. Our metric is defined to aggregate local patch comparisons as

$$M(I_f, I'_m) = \sum_{P \in \mathcal{P}} N(I_f(P), I'_m(P)) \tag{2}$$

where $\mathcal{P}$ is the set of patch domains $P \subset \Omega_f$ sampled on a dense uniform grid with significant overlaps.

Its gradient $\nabla M(\theta)$, which is required for $\nabla E(\theta)$, can be computed by applying chain rule as follows:

$$\frac{\partial \sum_{P \in \mathcal{P}} N(I_f(P), I'_m(P))}{\partial \theta} = \sum_{\mathbf{x} \in \Omega_f} \sum_{P \in \mathcal{P}_{\mathbf{x}}} \frac{\partial N(I_f(P), I'_m(P))}{\partial I'_m(\mathbf{x})} \frac{\partial I'_m(\mathbf{x})}{\partial \theta} \tag{3}$$

$$= \sum_{\mathbf{x} \in \Omega_f} \sum_{P \in \mathcal{P}_{\mathbf{x}}} \frac{\partial N(I_f(P), I'_m(P))}{\partial I'_m(\mathbf{x})} \frac{\partial I_m(\mathcal{T}(\theta, \mathbf{x}))}{\partial \mathcal{T}(\theta, \mathbf{x})} \frac{\partial \mathcal{T}(\theta, \mathbf{x})}{\partial \theta} \tag{4}$$

$$= \sum_{\mathbf{x} \in \Omega_f} \frac{\partial N(I_f, I'_m)}{\partial I'_m(\mathbf{x})} \nabla I_m(\mathcal{T}(\theta, \mathbf{x})) J_{\mathcal{T}}(\mathbf{x}) \tag{5}$$

Equation (3) shows that the derivative of N w.r.t. the intensity of an input pixel $\mathbf{x}$ depends on all patches containing it, denoted as $\mathcal{P}_{\mathbf{x}}$. Thus, high overlap of neighboring patches leads to smoother, more stable derivatives. We found that registration quality drops considerably unless the grid stride s of $\mathcal{P}$ is small. On the other hand, subsampling Ω_f to obtain a sparser set of samples $\mathbf{x}$ has a minor impact on performance.

In the transition from Eqs. (4) to (5), patch-wise evaluation of N is replaced by fully convolutional evaluation over the whole domain Ω_f. This makes the computation very efficient, as results in intermediate network layers can be shared among neighboring patches [8].

Ultimately, the contribution of each pixel $\mathbf{x}$ to $\nabla M(\theta)$ is a product of three terms, c.f. Eq. (5): the derivative $\partial N / \partial I'_m(\mathbf{x})$ of the estimated dissimilarity of patches around $\mathbf{x}$ w.r.t. its intensity in the warped image, which can be readily computed by standard backpropagation, the gradient of the moving image ∇I_m, which can be precomputed, and the local Jacobian matrix $J_{\mathcal{T}}$ of transformation $\mathcal{T}$. Note that the choice of a particular transformation type is decoupled from the network, therefore a single network will work with any transformation.

Computing one iteration thus requires resampling of the moving image and one forward and one backward pass in the network. All operations can be efficiently computed on a GPU.

2.2   Network Architecture and Training

Architecture. A feed-forward convolutional neural network N is used to estimate the dissimilarity of two cubic patches of the same size of $p \times p \times p$ pixels. The architecture is based on recent works on learning to compare patches, notably the 2-channel network of Zagoruyko and Komodakis [13]. The two patches are considered as a 2-channel 3D image (each channel represents a different modality), which is fed to the first layer of the network. The network consists of a series of volumetric convolutional layers with ReLU non-linearities finalized by a convolutional layer without any non-linearity, which produces a scalar score.

To gradually subsample the spatial domain within the network and increase spatial context (perceptive field), we prefer convolutions with non-unit output stride to pooling used in [13], as it has led to better performance. We hypothesize that too much spatial invariance might be detrimental in our case of learning cross-modal identity, unlike aiming for robustness to distortions such as perspective deformation. The product of convolutional strides determines the overall network stride s used in the fully-convolutional mode.

The 2-channel architecture is powerful as it considers both patches jointly from the beginning. However, its evaluation does not exploit the fact that the fixed image I_f does not change during optimization and its deep representation could be precomputed in the form of descriptors and cached. We have therefore experimented on architectures with two independent input branches, such as the pseudo-siamese network in [13]. Unfortunately, we have observed consistent decrease in registration performance.

Training. We suppose to have a set of k aligned pairs of training images $\{(A_j, B_j)\}_{j=1}^k$ with $A_j, B_j : \Omega_j \subset \mathbb{R}^d \mapsto \mathbb{R}$. We sample transformations $\mathcal{T}_{i,A_j}$, $\mathcal{T}_{i,B_j} : \Omega_j \mapsto \Omega_j$ for j-th image pair for data augmentation by varying position, scale, rotation, and mirroring. Patch pairs $X_i = (A_j(\mathcal{T}_{i,A_j}(P)), B_j(\mathcal{T}_{i,B_j}(P)))$ with fixed-size domain P are used for training the network. Sample X_i is defined to be positive (labeled $y_i = -1$) if $\mathcal{T}_{i,A_j} = \mathcal{T}_{i,B_j}$ and negative ($y_i = 1$) otherwise. Positive and negative samples are mined with equal probability. Imposing restrictions on negatives (such as minimum or maximum overlap of source patch domains) or on patch content (such as minimum contrast [7]) were experimentally shown detrimental to the registration quality.

The network is trained to classify training samples X_i by minimizing hinge loss $L = \sum_i \max(0, 1 - y_i N(X_i))$, which we found to perform better than cross-entropy. We observed that softmax leads to overly flat gradients in continuous optimization, as shown in the bottom plots in Fig. 2. SGD with learning rate 0.01, momentum 0.9 and batch size 128 is used to optimize the network.

Instead of preparing a fixed dataset of patches like in [3], we sample X_i online. This, together with the augmentations described above, allows us to feed the network with practically unlimited amount of training data. Even for small k we observed no overfitting in learning (see also Subsect. 3.2).

Implementation. We use Torch with cuDNN library for deep learning, elastix for GPU-based image resampling, and ITK for registration[1] Our network has 5 layers, 2M parameters, patch size $p = 17$, and stride $s = 4$. We plan to open source our implementation and the trained network.

3   Experiments and Results

We evaluate the effectiveness of the learned metric in registration experiments on a set of clinical brain images in Subsect. 3.1 and conduct further experiments to demonstrate its interesting properties in Subsects. 3.2 and 3.3.

3.1   Deformable Registration of Neonatal Brain MRI Images

Datasets. We conducted intersubject deformable registration experiments on a set of neonatal brain image volumes taken from the publicly available brain atlases ALBERTs [5]. This database consists of T1 and T2-weighted MRI scans of 20 newborns. Each T1-T2 pair is aligned and annotated with a segmentation map of 50 anatomical regions, which allows us to evaluate registration quality in terms of overlap measures; we compute average Dice and Jaccard coefficients.

To make the experiment challenging and demonstrate good generalization of our learned metric (denoted CNN), we train on IXI [1], a completely independent dataset of adult brain images. Let us remark that there are structural differences between the brains of neonates and adults. The dataset contains about 600 approximately aligned T1–T2 image pairs and we use $k = 557$ for training and the rest for validation, although in Subsect. 3.2 we demonstrate that much less is actually needed. Image intensities in both datasets are normalized to $[0, 1]$.

Baseline. Our baseline is mutual information (MI) [9], the standard metric for multimodal registration. We observed that MI perform better when image domains are restricted to the head region, thus we use a fixed intensity threshold of 0.01 for masking the background and denote this variant MI+M. Such masking made nearly no difference to our metric. Unfortunately, we could not compare to other learning-based metrics [7, 10] as their implementation was not available.

Protocol. We test on 18 subjects in ALBERTs and perform 68 intersubject registrations, half of them aligning T1 to T2 and half of them the other way round. We reserve the remaining 2 subjects for validating registration parameters and model selection. Both metrics are evaluated in exactly the same registration pipeline with the same transformation model and optimizer. The pipeline consists of multiresolution similarity transform registration followed by multiresolution B-spline registration (2 scales, 1000 control points on the fine scale, 200 k image sampling points), optimized by gradient descent with regular step and 500 iterations per scale. MI is used with 75 histogram bins (validated optimum). An explicit regularization term R in Eq. (1) was used neither for MI

---

[1] www.torch.ch, developer.nvidia.com/cudnn, elastix.isi.uu.nl, www.itk.org.

Table 1. Overlap scores (mean ± SD) after registration using the proposed metric (CNN) and mutual information with (MI+M) or without masking (MI)

	MI+M	MI	CNN $k = 557$	CNN $k = 11$	CNN $k = 6$	CNN $k = 3$
Dice	0.665 ± 0.096	0.497 ± 0.180	0.703 ± 0.037	0.704 ± 0.037	0.701 ± 0.040	0.675 ± 0.093
Jaccard	0.519 ± 0.091	0.369 ± 0.151	0.555 ± 0.041	0.556 ± 0.041	0.554 ± 0.044	0.527 ± 0.081

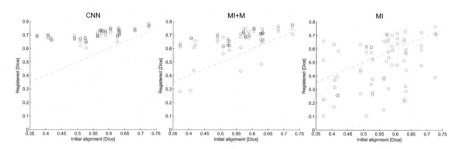

Fig. 1. Improvement in average Dice score due to registration using the proposed metric (CNN) and mutual information with (MI+M) or without masking (MI). Each data point represents a registration run. Dashed line denotes identity transformation.

nor for CNN. Instead, we regularize implicitly by the design of the pipeline and the choice of its hyperparameters.

Results. The results are listed in Table 1 and demonstrate statistically significant improvement of registration quality due to CNN by about 4 points in both coefficients (as by one-sided t-test with significance $\alpha = 0.01$). Figure 1 exhibits scatter plots of initial and final Dice scores for each registration run (Jaccard scores follow similar trend). We can see that while CNN has improved on the alignment in all runs, this is not the case for MI+M and especially MI, showing rather low precision. The highest accuracies achieved by both methods are rather similar (up to 0.8) and seem nearly independent on the initial level of misalignment. Furthermore, the registration using CNN is only about 2x slower than using MI (on Nvidia Titan Black), the difference mostly due to expensive resampling of moving image.

3.2   Influence of Training Set Size

The huge number of aligned volumes in IXI dataset is rather exceptional in medical domain. We are therefore interested in how much we can decrease the training set size k without noticeable impact on the quality. To this end, we train networks with only $k = 11$, 6, and 3 random image pairs under the same setting as above. Table 1 shows that even with little training data the results are very good and only for $k = 3$ our metric does not significantly outperform MI+M. On one hand, this suggests that our online sampling and data augmentation methodology works well. On the other hand, either the inherent variability in the dataset is very low (especially compared to natural image recognition problems, where more data typically improves performance) or our network is not able to exploit it. We expect that the amount of necessary data will be higher for more challenging modalities, such as ultrasound.

3.3   Plausibility of Metric and Its Derivatives

To investigate the behavior of metric value and its actual derivatives used for continuous optimization, we visualize these quantities by manually perturbing a single parameter of a transformation initialized to identity on an aligned validation image pair in IXI. Figure 2 suggests that the metric behaves reasonably as its curves are smooth with the correct local minima. The analytic derivatives, as in Eq. (5), have the correct sign over a large range, albeit their magnitude is slightly noisy. Nevertheless, this was shown not to prevent the metric from obtaining good registration results.

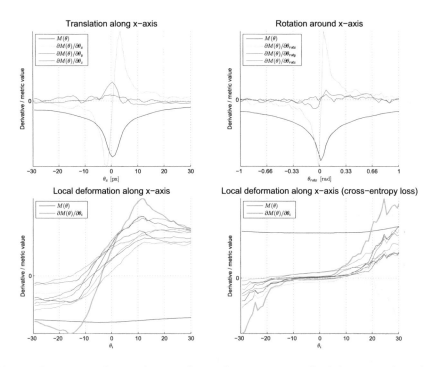

Fig. 2. The impact of perturbation of a single parameter in Euclidean transform (top) and B-spline transform (bottom) on metric value M and its derivatives as per Eq. (5). The curve of M is not up to scale. Curves without legend correspond to other parameters strongly affected due to overlapping patches.

4   Conclusion

We have presented a similarity metric for multimodal 3D image registration based on a convolutional neural network. The network can be trained from scratch even from a few aligned image pairs, mostly due to our data sampling scheme. We have described the incorporation of this metric into first-order continuous optimization frameworks. The experimetal evaluation was performed on the task of intersubject T1–T2 deformable registration on a dataset different from the one used for training, demonstrating good generalization. In this task, we outperform mutual information by a significant margin.

We envision incorporating our network into a discrete optimization framework as an easy extension. In a MRF-based formulation, the local alignment cost is expressed by unary potentials over nodes in a graph [4]. In particular, a unary potential $g_n(\mathbf{u}_n)$ related to the cost of assigning a label/translation $\mathbf{u}_n$ to node n might be defined as $g_n(\mathbf{u}_n) = N(I_f(P_n), I_m(\mathcal{T}(\theta, P_n) + \mathbf{u}_n))$, where $P_n \subset \Omega_f$ is a patch domain centered at the control point of transformation $\mathcal{T}$ corresponding to node n. As such an optimization is derivative-free, only the forward pass in the network would be necessary.

We also plan to apply our method to more modalities, such as ultrasound.

Acknowledgments. We gratefully acknowledge NVIDIA Corporation for the donated GPU used in this research. ALBERTs atlases are copyrighted by Imperial College of Science, Technology and Medicine and Ioannis S. Gousias 2013. B. Gutiérrez-Becker thanks the financial support of CONACYT and the DAAD.

References

1. IXI - Information eXtraction from images. www.brain-development.org
2. Cao, T., Jojic, V., Modla, S., Powell, D., Czymmek, K., Niethammer, M.: Robust multimodal dictionary learning. In: Mori, K., Sakuma, I., Sato, Y., Barillot, C., Navab, N. (eds.) MICCAI 2013. LNCS, vol. 8149, pp. 259–266. Springer, Heidelberg (2013). doi:10.1007/978-3-642-40811-3_33
3. Cheng, X., Zhang, L., Zheng, Y.: Deep similarity learning for multimodal medical images. In: Computer Methods in Biomechanics and Biomedical Engineering: Imaging and Visualization, pp. 1–5 (2015)
4. Glocker, B., Sotiras, A., Komodakis, N., Paragios, N.: Deformable medical image registration: setting the state of the art with discrete methods. Ann. Rev. Biomed. Eng. **13**, 219–244 (2011)
5. Gousias, I., Edwards, A., Rutherford, M., Counsell, S., Hajnal, J., Rueckert, D., Hammers, A.: Magnetic resonance imaging of the newborn brain: manual segmentation of labelled atlases in term-born and preterm infants. Neuroimage **62**, 1499–1509 (2012). www.brain-development.org
6. Guetter, C., Xu, C., Sauer, F., Hornegger, J.: Learning based non-rigid multi-modal image registration using kullback-leibler divergence. In: Duncan, J.S., Gerig, G. (eds.) MICCAI 2005. LNCS, vol. 3750, pp. 255–262. Springer, Heidelberg (2005). doi:10.1007/11566489_32

7. Lee, D., Hofmann, M., Steinke, F., Altun, Y., Cahill, N., Scholkopf, B.: Learning similarity measure for multi-modal 3D image registration. In: CVPR, pp. 186–193 (2009)

8. Long, J., Shelhamer, E., Darrell, T.: Fully convolutional networks for semantic segmentation. In: CVPR, pp. 3431–3440 (2015)

9. Mattes, D., Haynor, D.R., Vesselle, H., Lewellyn, T.K., Eubank, W.: Nonrigid multimodality image registration. In: SPIE, vol. 4322, pp. 1609–1620 (2001)

10. Michel, F., Bronstein, M., Bronstein, A., Paragios, N.: Boosted metric learning for 3D multi-modal deformable registration. In: ISBI, pp. 1209–1214 (2011)

11. Nguyen, H., Zhou, K., Vemulapalli, R.: Cross-domain synthesis of medical images using efficient location-sensitive deep network. In: Navab, N., Hornegger, J., Wells, W.M., Frangi, A.F. (eds.) MICCAI 2015. LNCS, vol. 9349, pp. 677–684. Springer, Heidelberg (2015). doi:10.1007/978-3-319-24553-9_83

12. Sotiras, A., Davatzikos, C., Paragios, N.: Deformable medical image registration: a survey. TMI **32**(7), 1153–1190 (2013)

13. Zagoruyko, S., Komodakis, N.: Learning to compare image patches via convolutional neural networks. In: CVPR, pp. 4353–4361 (2015)

Learning Optimization Updates
for Multimodal Registration

Benjamín Gutiérrez-Becker$^{(\boxtimes)}$, Diana Mateus, Loïc Peter, and Nassir Navab

Computer Aided Medical Procedures, Technische Universität München,
Munich, Germany
gutierrez.becker@tum.de, {mateus,peter,navab}@in.tum.de

Abstract. We address the problem of multimodal image registration
using a supervised learning approach. We pose the problem as a regression task, whose goal is to estimate the unknown geometric transformation from the joint appearance of the fixed and moving images. Our
method is based on (i) context-aware features, which allow us to guide
the registration using not only local, but also global structural information, and (ii) regression forests to map the very large contextual feature
space to transformation parameters. Our approach improves the capture
range, as we demonstrate on the publicly available IXI dataset. Furthermore, it can also handle difficult settings where other similarity metrics
tend to fail; for instance, we show results on the deformable registration
of Intravascular Ultrasound (IVUS) and Histology images.

1 Introduction

A core difficulty in multimodal registration is the lack of a general law to measure
the alignment between images of the same organ acquired with different physical
principles. The unknown relationship between the image intensities is in general
neither linear nor bijective. Following Sotiras *et al.* [15], there have been three
main approaches to address the problem: (i) *information theoretic* methods [13],
(ii) mapping of the modalities to a *common representation* [3,4], and (iii) *learning*
multimodal similarity measures [10,11]. This paper relates to the latter category,
whose main assumption is that prior knowledge (in the form of examples of
aligned images) can be afforded. This extra effort can be justified both, in cases
where large-scale databases need to be registered, or when the two modalities
are so different that general multi-modal similarity measures do not suffice.

Up to now, the focus of learning based approaches has been on approximating
multimodal similarity measures, independent of the optimization scheme used
during the registration task itself. However, due to the usually complex mapping between the intensities of the two modalities, non-linearities and ambigui-
ties tend to shape local-optima and plateaus in the energy landscape. Thereby,
the optimizer plays an important role in the success of the registration. In this
work we explore a combined view of the problem, where we take the optimizer
into account. In particular, we restrict ourselves to gradient-based methods, and
focus on directly inferring the motion parameters from changes in the joint visual

© Springer International Publishing AG 2016
S. Ourselin et al. (Eds.): MICCAI 2016, Part III, LNCS 9902, pp. 19–27, 2016.
DOI: 10.1007/978-3-319-46726-9_3

content of the images. We model the problem as a regression approach, where for a given pair of misaligned images the goal is to retrieve the global direction towards which the motion parameters should be updated for correct alignment. In order to ensure that the direction of the update points towards a globally optimal solution, we describe the images taking into account both their local appearance and their long-range context, by means of Haar-like features [2]. In order to efficiency handle the resultant very high-dimensional feature space, we use regression forests [2], also known for their fast training and testing. The main contribution of our work is twofold: (1) this is the first time a regression method is used to predict registration updates in the multimodal setting; (2) the use of long-range context-aware features instead of local structural features is novel for the problem of multimodal registration. We demonstrate the advantages of our method in the difficult case of 2-D deformable registration of histological to intravascular ultrasound images (IVUS). We also perform a quantitative evaluation for the 3-D registration of T1-T2 MR images showing an advantageous increase in the capture range.

1.1   Related Work

There have been two trends in learning based methods for multimodal registration. *Generative* approaches [14], approximate the joint intensity distribution between the images to be registered and minimize the difference of a new test pair of images to the learned distribution. *Discriminative* methods, on the other hand, model the similarity learning problem as the classification of positive (aligned) and negative (misaligned) examples, typically at patch level [5,10,11]. Different learning strategies have been explored to approximate such patch-wise similarities, including margin-based approaches [10] and boosting [11]. In contrast to the discriminative approaches above, which aim at discerning between aligned and misaligned patches, we focus on learning a motion predictor that guides the registration process towards alignment.

There have been prior attempts of using motion prediction for monomodal tracking and registration. For instance, Jurie *et al.* [6] proposed a linear predictor for template tracking, which related the difference between the compared images to variations in template position. In the medical domain, Chou *et al.* [1] present an approach to learn updates of the transformation parameters in the context of 2D-3D registration. Similarly, in [9], Kim *et al.* proposed the prediction of a deformation-field for registration initialization, achieved by modeling the statistical correlation between image appearances and deformation fields with Support Vector Regression. The work presented here is, to the best of our knowledge, the first approach for motion prediction in the multimodal case.

2   Method

Multimodal registration aims to find the transformation $\mathcal{W}(\mathbf{p})$ that optimally aligns two images of different modalities, namely, a fixed image $\mathbf{I} : \Omega \subset \mathbb{R}^3 \rightarrow \mathbb{R}$

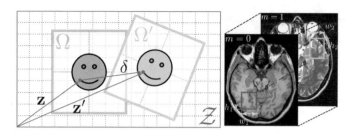

Fig. 1. Left: Learned displacement under a given transformation. Right: long-range Haar-like features to encode local and long range context.

and a moving image $\mathbf{I}' : \Omega' \subset \mathbb{R}^3 \to \mathbb{R}$. A common method to find the optimal parameters $\mathbf{p} \in \mathbb{R}^{N_p}$ that define $\mathcal{W}$ is by maximizing a similarity function $S(\mathbf{I}, \mathbf{I}')$ between the two images. Denoting by $\mathbf{I}'_{\mathbf{p}}$ the moving image resampled in the fix domain Ω according to parameters $\mathbf{p}$, we have:

$$\mathbf{p}^* = \max_{\mathbf{p}} S(\mathbf{I}, \mathbf{I}'_{\mathbf{p}}). \tag{1}$$

The maximization of Eq. 1 can be done either by gradient-free (usually preferred for discriminatively learned implicit similarities) or gradient-based optimization approaches. In the latter, the gradient of S is computed to iteratively estimate the parameter update $\varDelta_k \in \mathbb{R}^{N_p}$, such that $\mathbf{p}_k = \mathbf{p}_{k-1} + \varDelta_k$, where k is the iteration index. In a typical steepest-ascent-like strategy, the update direction is determined in terms of the similarity gradient as $\varDelta_k = -\frac{\partial S/\partial \mathbf{p}}{\|\partial S/\partial \mathbf{p}\|}$, which is in turn obtained based on the *local* approximation of this gradient. Depending on the similarity such local approximations may be poor and lead to local optima or slow convergence rates.

Here, we reformulate the multimodal registration problem as that of learning a motion predictor, *i.e.* a function that directly maps the intensity configuration of the two images in the fixed space to the corresponding motion update:

$$\widehat{\varDelta_k} = F(\mathbf{I}, \mathbf{I}'_{\mathbf{p}}). \tag{2}$$

We learn F from labeled examples (images with a known misalignment), which allows us to enforce desirable properties for the optimization, namely: a parameter update pointing in the direction of the global maximum and a smooth gradient. In analogy to the steepest ascent approach, our update may be seen as a *global* approximation of the gradient $\frac{\partial S}{\partial \mathbf{p}}$. We explain next how to approximate F from a training set of images by means of regression.

2.1   Learning Multimodal Motion Predictors

We choose to model the motion predictor at the image level, F, as the aggregation of local motion predictors f. We consider that the input to these local predictors are not patch intensities but rather a joint feature representation

$\Theta(\mathbf{z}, \mathbf{I}, \mathbf{I}'_\mathbf{p}) \in \mathbb{R}^H$, which describes the local appearance of $\mathbf{I}$ and $\mathbf{I}'_\mathbf{p}$ relative to a point $\mathbf{z} \in \mathbb{R}^3$. Hereafter, we denote the feature vector $\Theta(\mathbf{z})$ for simplicity. Given a number N_{im} of aligned multimodal images $\{\mathbf{I}_i, \mathbf{I}'_i\}_{i=1}^{N_{\mathrm{im}}}$ our aim is to approximate a function $f(\mathbf{z}) : \Theta(\mathbf{z}) \mapsto \boldsymbol{\delta}$ capable of predicting a local displacement $\boldsymbol{\delta} \in \mathbb{R}^3$ towards alignment. The approximation of f is done by means of a learning-based regression approach. In the following, we describe the details of our method.

Generating a Set of Training Labels. To generate examples with known misalignment, we apply multiple known transformations $\{\mathcal{W}_j, \mathcal{W}'_j\}_{j=1}^{N_{\mathrm{transfo}}}$ to the initially aligned images, mapping the coordinates of two originally corresponding points $\mathbf{x} \in \Omega$ and $\mathbf{x}' \in \Omega'$ to distinct locations in a common image domain $\mathbf{z}, \mathbf{z}' \in \mathcal{Z} \subset \mathbb{R}^3$ (see Fig. 1). Because the applied transformations are known, we can determine the ground truth displacement $\boldsymbol{\delta}_n \in \mathbb{R}^3$ needed to find the originally corresponding point $\mathbf{z}'_n$ in the moving image, and bring it into alignment with $\mathbf{z}$, $i.e.\boldsymbol{\delta}_n = \mathbf{z}'_n - \mathbf{z}_n$. With this information we build the training set $\mathcal{X} = \{\Theta(\mathbf{z}_n), \boldsymbol{\delta}_n\}_{n=1}^{N_{\mathrm{points}}}$. Notice that we have chosen to use $\boldsymbol{\delta}_n$ as the regression targets instead of the transformation parameters. In this way the learning stage is independent of the motion parametrization. In fact, these displacements play the role of the similarity gradients $\frac{\partial S}{\partial \mathbf{z}}$, which can be then related to a given parametrization using the chain rule $\frac{\partial S}{\partial \mathbf{p}} = \frac{\partial S}{\partial \mathbf{z}} J$, by means of the Jacobian $J = \frac{\partial \mathbf{z}}{\partial \mathbf{p}}$.

Context Aware Features. We characterize the cross-modal appearance of each point $\mathbf{z}_n$ in the training set, by a variation of the context-aware Haar-like features [2]. These features effectively capture how the joint-appearance variations in the vicinity of each point relate to different transformation parameters. The feature vector $\Theta(\mathbf{z}_n)$ is a collection of H features $[\theta_1, \ldots, \theta_h, \ldots, \theta_H]^\top$; where each θ_h is computed as a simple operation on a pair of boxes located at given offsets locations relative to point $\mathbf{z}_n$. More formally, θ_h is characterized by two boxes $\mathbf{b_1}, \mathbf{b_2}$ (c.f. Fig. 1), parametrized by their location $(\mathbf{v}_1, \mathbf{v}_2 \in \mathbb{R}^3)$, size $(w_1, h_1, w_2, h_2, d_1, d_2 \in \mathbb{R})$, modality $m_1 = \{0, 1\}$ and an *operation* between boxes: $\{ \overline{\mathbf{b_1}}, \overline{\mathbf{b_2}}, \overline{\mathbf{b_1}} + \overline{\mathbf{b_2}}, \overline{\mathbf{b_1}} - \overline{\mathbf{b_2}}, |\overline{\mathbf{b_1}} - \overline{\mathbf{b_2}}|, \overline{\mathbf{b_1}} > \overline{\mathbf{b_2}}\}$, where the overline denotes the mean over the box intensities. These operations are efficiently calculated with precomputed integral volumes [2]. The binary *modality* parameters m_1 and m_2 determine whether the two boxes are taken from the same modality or across modalities, thereby modeling the spatial context of each image as well as the functional relation between the two modalities. Using different offsets and box sizes enables capturing the visual context of each point without explicitly determining the scale. If we consider the combinatorial nature of the box parameters we face a very-large feature space $\mathbb{R}^H$. To deal with it, we use regression forests, which among other advantages do not require the pre-computation of features.

Regression Forest. Using the features described above, we characterize each point $\mathbf{z}_i$ in the training set $\mathcal{X}$ by its corresponding feature vector $\Theta_i(\mathbf{z}_n)$. We then use regression forests to approximate the function $f : \Theta(\mathbf{z}_n) \mapsto \boldsymbol{\delta}_n$ mapping

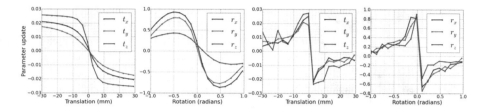

Fig. 2. Left side: parameter updates obtained using our motion estimation method. Right side: parameter updates obtained using the gradient of normalized mutual information. Our estimated parameter updates are smoother over a larger range.

these feature vectors to an estimation of the target displacements. We train our regression forest in a standard setting, using as splitting criteria the reduction of the covariance trace associated to the target values in a particular node. Once the forest has grown, we store the Gaussian distribution (mean $\mu_{t(l)}$ and covariance $\Sigma_{t(l)}$) of the target displacements vectors falling in each leaf l. At test time, a new feature vector $\theta(\mathbf{z}_{\text{test}})$ is passed down through the forest. Every tree assigns an estimate of the predicted motion $\hat{\boldsymbol{\delta}}_t$ (given by the mean vector $\mu_{t(l)}$ stored in the leaf) along with its covariance $\Sigma_{t(l)}$. We then rank and select the $\tilde{N}_{\text{trees}}$ with the smaller values of covariance trace. The predicted displacement at point $\mathbf{z}_{\text{test}}$ is obtained as the average over the prediction of the selected trees.

2.2 Using Multimodal Motion Predictors for Registration

To register a pair of images $\mathbf{I}$ and $\mathbf{I}'$ we define a set of testing points on a grid $\{\mathbf{z}_m\}_{m=1}^{N_{\text{test}}} \in \mathcal{Z}$, extract their feature vectors $\{\Theta(\mathbf{z}_m)\}_{m=1}^{N_{\text{test}}}$, and pass them through the forest to obtain the local displacement estimates $\{\hat{\boldsymbol{\delta}}_m\}_{m=1}^{N_{\text{test}}}$. We then compute the global update (*c.f.* Eq. 2) by adding the contributions of each local displacement to the transformation parameters: $\hat{\Delta} = \sum_{m=1}^{N_{\text{test}}} \hat{\boldsymbol{\delta}}_m J$ where J corresponds to the Jacobian of the transformation.

3 Experiments and Results

To evaluate the performance of our method in comparison to previous registration approaches we performed two series of experiments. In the first we evaluate the performance of our method in a challenging multimodal setting: the registration of IVUS-Histology images, using the dataset from [7]. In the second, we use T1-T2 images from the IXI Dataset[1] to evaluate the capture range of our method, where we measure the registration accuracy for varying initial displacements between the fixed and moving image. This experiment shows the robustness of our method to different initial conditions.

---

[1] Available at: http://brain-development.org/ixi-dataset/.

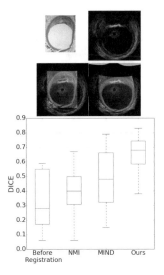

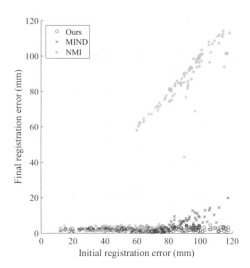

Fig. 3. Top left: registration results on an IVUS-Histology pair. The initial unregistered images are shown as well as the overlay between the images before and after registration. Bottom left: DICE scores on the overlap between stenosis regions before and after registration. Right: final registration error given different starting initial conditions on the T1-T2 image pairs of the IXI dataset.

In both cases, we compare our method to the widely used Normalized Mutual Information (NMI) [16] optimized using a gradient descent optimizer and with the Modality Independent Neighborhood Descriptor (MIND) [3] coupled with the Gauss-Newton optimization suggested by the authors.

In all the experiments we used forests consisting of 40 trees, keeping the top 10 best trees during testing. We evaluated 1000 possible splits per node and grew the trees to a maximum depth of 15, stopping earlier if not enough samples reached one of the child nodes. We limited the size of the offsets and the boxes in the feature space to half of the image size. To optimise the scale of these features we used the scale adaptive forest training approach presented in [12].

3.1   IVUS-Histology Deformable Registration

In this experiment we tackled the registration between 10 Intravascular Ultrasound images (IVUS) and histological slices. We used the method in [7] [8] to obtain the initial set of aligned images needed for training. For evaluation we performed deformable registrations using our method and we compare to MI and MIND by measuring the overlap (DICE) of segmented stenosis regions both in IVUS and the histology images. For all methods we use the same 3rd-order b-spline parametrization with 5 nodes per dimension.

During training we split the dataset in 2 groups of 5 images and perform cross validation. The final registration results are shown in Fig. 3. This dataset is particularly challenging because the underlying assumptions of most similarity metrics, like local structural similarities or relationships between statistics on the intensities of the images, are not verified. The methods we used for comparison therefore presented high registration errors for the IVUS-Histology pairs. Our supervised approach, on the other hand, was capable to register the images thanks to prior knowledge and the non-local context of each point.

3.2   Capture Range

To test the capture range, we take a set of 10 prealigned T1-T2 image pairs from the IXI dataset splitting them in 2 groups of 5 images for cross validation. For each image pair we apply a rigid transformation to one of the images and then we find the transformation that brings it back into alignment. The applied transformations were in the range of ±100 mm for translations along each axis and $\pm\pi/2$ radians for rotations. We repeat this procedure 20 times per image with different transformations for a total of 200 registration evaluations.

The results of this experiment can be seen in Fig. 3. Each point in the plot corresponds to the registration of a pair of images. We can clearly observe that our method presents a larger capture range than the metrics we compared with. Note that there is a breaking point where MIND and MI start to fail, as these metrics tend to underperform when the overlap between images is small and no local structure can be used to evaluate the metrics reliably. Our method on the other hand, was able to register the images even when they had no overlap, thanks to the prior knowledge and the use of context aware features which together to pull the optimizer in the right direction. Additionally, our method was able to converge in a smaller number of iterations (5) compared to NMI ($\sim$ 250 gradient ascent iterations) and MIND (16 iterations). In terms of computational time our method performed each registration in an average of $\sim$10 s compared to $\sim$200 s for NMI and $\sim$35 s for MIND. The faster convergence can be attributed to the smoothness of our parameter updates in comparison to the updates estimated using the derivative of NMI (see Fig. 2). In this way, we are entitled to use a more aggressive step size without a decrease on the final registration error and depend less on the initial misalignment between images.

4   Conclusions

We present a novel approach to the problem of multimodal registration, which combines supervised regression with simple gradient-based optimizers. Supervised regression let us infer motion from changes in the visual appearance of the images to be registered. In this way, it is no longer necessary to rely on prior assumptions about local appearance correlations. Although our method requires the use of aligned images for training, we have observed that the required amount of training images to achieve good results is reasonably small (not more than 5 images in each case). Building datasets with aligned multimodal images requires additional effort, but this extra effort can be justified in cases where other metrics are not sufficient or when a large dataset of similar images has to be registered. For more common scenarios (such as multimodal MR registration), our method produces registrations with comparable accuracy to other similarities but with faster convergence and a larger capture range.

Acknowledgements. Benjamin Gutierrez thanks CONACYT and the DAAD for their financial support.

References

1. Chou, C.-R., Frederick, B., Mageras, G., Chang, S., Pizer, S.: 2D/3D image registration using regression learning. Comput. Vis. Image Underst. **117**(9), 1095–1106 (2013)
2. Criminisi, A., Shotton, J., Bucciarelli, S.: Decision forests with long-range spatial context for organ localization in CT volumes. In: Medical Image Computing and Computer-Assisted Intervention (MICCAI), pp. 69–80. Citeseer (2009)
3. Heinrich, M., Jenkinson, M., Bhushan, M., Matin, T., Gleeson, F.V., Brady, M., Schnabel, J.: MIND: Modality independent neighbourhood descriptor for multimodal deformable registration. Med. Image Anal. **16**, 1423–1435 (2012)
4. Heinrich, M.P., Jenkinson, M., Papież, B.W., Brady, S.M., Schnabel, J.A.: Towards realtime multimodal fusion for image-guided interventions using self-similarities. In: Mori, K., Sakuma, I., Sato, Y., Barillot, C., Navab, N. (eds.) MICCAI 2013. LNCS, vol. 8149, pp. 187–194. Springer, Heidelberg (2013). doi:10.1007/978-3-642-40811-3_24
5. Jiang, J., Zheng, S., Toga, A., Tu, Z.: Learning based coarse-to-fine image registration. In: CVPR, pp. 1–7, June 2008
6. Jurie, F., Dhome, M.: Hyperplane approximation for template matching. TPAMI **24**(7), 996–1000 (2002)
7. Katouzian, A., Karamalis, A., Lisauskas, J., Eslami, A., Navab, N.: IVUS-histology image registration. In: Dawant, B.M., Christensen, G.E., Fitzpatrick, J.M., Rueckert, D. (eds.) WBIR 2012. LNCS, vol. 7359, pp. 141–149. Springer, Heidelberg (2012). doi:10.1007/978-3-642-31340-0_15
8. Katouzian, A., Sathyanarayana, S., Li, W., Thomas, T., Carlier, S.: Challenges in tissue characterization from backscattered intravascular ultrasound signals. In: Medical Imaging, p. 6513. International Society for Optics and Photonics (2007)
9. Kim, M., Wu, G., Yap, P.T., Shen, D.: A general fast registration framework by learning deformation appearance correlation. IEEE Trans. Image Process. **21**(4), 1823–1833 (2012)
10. Lee, D., Hofmann, M., Steinke, F., Altun, Y., Cahill, N.D., Scholkopf, B.: Learning similarity measure for multi-modal 3D image registration. In: CVPR (2009)
11. Michel, F., Bronstein, M., Bronstein, A., Paragios, N.: Boosted metric learning for 3D multi-modal deformable registration. In: ISBI, pp. 1209–1214. IEEE (2011)
12. Peter, L., Pauly, O., Chatelain, P., Mateus, D., Navab, N.: Scale-adaptive forest training via an efficient feature sampling scheme. In: Navab, N., Hornegger, J., Wells, W.M., Frangi, A.F. (eds.) MICCAI 2015. LNCS, vol. 9349, pp. 637–644. Springer, Heidelberg (2015). doi:10.1007/978-3-319-24553-9_78
13. Pluim, J., Maintz, J., Viergever, M.: f-information measures in medical image registration. TMI **23**(12), 1508–1516 (2004)

14. Sabuncu, M.R., Ramadge, P.: Using spanning graphs for efficient image registration. TMI **17**(5), 788–797 (2008)
15. Sotiras, A., Davatzikos, C., Paragios, N.: Deformable medical image registration: a survey. TMI **32**(7), 1153–1190 (2013)
16. Viola, P., Wells III, W.M.: Alignment by maximization of mutual information. In: IEEE International Conference on Computer Vision (ICCV), pp. 16–23, June 1995

Memory Efficient LDDMM for Lung CT

Thomas Polzin[1][(✉)], Marc Niethammer[2], Mattias P. Heinrich[3], Heinz Handels[3], and Jan Modersitzki[1,4]

[1] Institute of Mathematics and Image Computing,
University of Lübeck, Lübeck, Germany
polzin@mic.uni-luebeck.de

[2] Department of Computer Science and Biomedical Research Imaging Center,
University of North Carolina at Chapel Hill, Chapel Hill, USA

[3] Institute of Medical Informatics, University of Lübeck, Lübeck, Germany

[4] Fraunhofer MEVIS, Lübeck, Germany

Abstract. In this paper a novel Large Deformation Diffeomorphic Metric Mapping (LDDMM) scheme is presented which has significantly lower computational and memory demands than standard LDDMM but achieves the same accuracy. We exploit the smoothness of velocities and transformations by using a coarser discretization compared to the image resolution. This reduces required memory and accelerates numerical optimization as well as solution of transport equations. Accuracy is essentially unchanged as the mismatch of transformed moving and fixed image is incorporated into the model at high resolution. Reductions in memory consumption and runtime are demonstrated for registration of lung CT images. State-of-the-art accuracy is shown for the challenging DIR-Lab chronic obstructive pulmonary disease (COPD) lung CT data sets obtaining a mean landmark distance after registration of 1.03 mm and the best average results so far.

1 Introduction

COPD is the fourth leading cause of death and 24 million people are afflicted in the US alone [14]. Lung registration could support assessment of COPD phenotypes as well as disease progression [6] and improved treatment of patients and speedups in clinical workflows are expected if registration is used for follow-up inspection and/or motion estimation in treatment planning [12,14]. Hence, registration of inhale/exhale and longitudinal data is critical, but also challenging due to the presence of large non-linear deformations, which should be diffeomorphic [12]. LDDMM can address these difficulties [2]. However, its drawbacks are large memory use and high computational costs: e.g. run times of up to three hours are reported in [17] for moderately sized data of $256 \times 192 \times 180$ voxels using 32 CPUs and 128 GB RAM. We present a new variant of LDDMM which

---

Electronic supplementary material The online version of this chapter (doi:10. 1007/978-3-319-46726-9_4) contains supplementary material, which is available to authorized users.

S. Ourselin et al. (Eds.): MICCAI 2016, Part III, LNCS 9902, pp. 28–36, 2016.
DOI: 10.1007/978-3-319-46726-9_4

– has significantly lower computational and memory demands,
– employs the well-suited distance measure Normalized Gradient Fields [11],
– and is as accurate as standard LDDMM and state-of-the-art algorithms.

Lung registration faces severe challenges. Diffeomorphic modeling of large lung motion (for inhale/exhale in the order of 50 mm [5]) is necessary [12]. Lung volume changes are large: a doubling of lung capacity is not unusual during inspiration [5]. Additionally, acquisitions with limited dose deteriorate CT quality [14].

Related Work: Sakamoto et al. [17] applied LDDMM in pulmonary computer-aided diagnosis (CAD) to analyze and detect growing or shrinking nodules in follow-up CT scans with encouraging results, but at high computational cost. A finite dimensional Lie algebra was introduced and integrated into a geodesic shooting approach by Zhang and Fletcher [19] to considerably speed up computations. Their experiments on 3D brain MRI data showed no loss of accuracy. Risser et al. [15] used appropriate kernels for LDDMM to cope with sliding motion occurring at the interface between lungs and the ribcage as this motion is not diffeomorphic. Our focus is on the registration of inner lung structures, hence we use lung segmentations as in [16] and thereby avoid sliding issues.

Contributions: We focus on the relaxation formulation of LDDMM [2], but the approach could easily be generalized to shooting formulations [1,18]. Our scheme is based on the smoothness of transformations and velocities computed with LDDMM allowing discretizations at lower spatial resolution and consequentially substantially reduced memory requirements. The image match is computed at the original resolution thereby maintaining accurate results. Furthermore, we employ the Normalized Gradient Fields (NGF) image similarity measure [11] that aligns edges, e.g. vessels. We use NGF to cope with large volume changes influencing tissue densities and thus absorption of X-rays. The resulting gray values of the parenchyma are quite different for inhale and exhale scans. Hence, sum of squared differences might not be an appropriate similarity measure.

Outline: In Sect. 2 the optimization problem, including the energy with NGF distance measure, and the memory efficient implementation of LDDMM are described. We evaluate our method on 20 3D lung CT scan pairs in Sect. 3, compare the results to the state of the art and show that a coarser discretization of velocities and transformations is sufficient for an accurate registration. In Sect. 4 results and possible extensions are discussed.

2 Methods

2.1 Continuous Model and LDDMM Background

Let I_0, $I_1 \colon \mathbb{R}^d \supset \Omega \to \mathbb{R}$ denote the moving and fixed images with domain Ω. LDDMM uses space- and time-dependent velocity ($v \colon \Omega \times [0,1] \to \mathbb{R}^d$) and transformation ($\varphi\colon \Omega \times [0,1] \to \mathbb{R}^d$) fields and seeks the minimizer (v^*, φ^*) of the following energy subject to a transport constraint [2,7]:

$$E(v,\varphi) := \int_0^1 \langle Lv(\cdot,t), Lv(\cdot,t)\rangle \mathrm{d}t + \tfrac{1}{\sigma^2} D(\varphi(\cdot,1); I_0, I_1) \to \min, \atop \text{s.t.}\quad \varphi_t + J_\varphi v = \mathbf{0}, \quad \varphi(\boldsymbol{x},0) = \boldsymbol{x} \text{ for all } \boldsymbol{x} \in \Omega, \ t \in [0,1] \Bigg\} \tag{1}$$

We denote the partial time derivative as $\varphi_t(\boldsymbol{x},t) \in \mathbb{R}^d$ and the Jacobian with respect to the spatial coordinates as $J_\varphi(\boldsymbol{x},t) \in \mathbb{R}^{d\times d}$. L is a suitable differential operator enforcing smoothness of v. In our method the Helmholtz operator $Lv := \gamma v - \alpha \Delta v$ with $\alpha, \gamma > 0$ was used, which is a standard choice for LDDMM registration, cf., e.g., [2,7]. In all experiments we fixed $\gamma = 1$. D is a general distance measure and $\sigma > 0$ its weighting parameter. As motivated in Sect. 1 we use the Normalized Gradient Fields (NGF) distance measure [11]. NGF was successfully applied to lung CT registration [9,16] in the following adaption of the original formulation:

$$D(\varphi_1; I_0, I_1) := \int_\Omega 1 - \left(\frac{\langle \nabla I_0(\varphi_1(\boldsymbol{x})), \nabla I_1(\boldsymbol{x})\rangle_\eta}{\|\nabla I_0(\varphi_1(\boldsymbol{x}))\|_\eta \, \|\nabla I_1(\boldsymbol{x})\|_\eta} \right)^2 \mathrm{d}\boldsymbol{x}, \tag{2}$$

with $\varphi_1 := \varphi(\cdot,1)$, $\langle \boldsymbol{u}, \boldsymbol{v}\rangle_\eta := \eta^2 + \sum_{i=1}^d u_i v_i$ and $\|\boldsymbol{u}\|_\eta^2 := \langle \boldsymbol{u}, \boldsymbol{u}\rangle_\eta$ for $\boldsymbol{u}, \boldsymbol{v} \in \mathbb{R}^d$. The parameter $\eta > 0$ is used to decide if a gradient is considered noise or edge [11]. Throughout this paper $\eta = 100$ is used as proposed in [16].

Following the steps of [7] we add the transport equation constraint of (1) into the objective functional employing Lagrange multipliers $\lambda\colon \Omega \times [0,1] \to \mathbb{R}^d$. After some straightforward calculations we obtain the necessary conditions as

$$L^\dagger L v + J_\varphi^\top \lambda = 0, \tag{3}$$

$$\varphi_t + J_\varphi v = \mathbf{0}, \ \varphi(\boldsymbol{x},0) = \boldsymbol{x}, \tag{4}$$

$$\lambda_t + J_\lambda v + \mathrm{div}(v)\lambda = \mathbf{0}, \quad \lambda(\boldsymbol{x},1) = -(1/\sigma^2)\nabla_\varphi D(\varphi_1(\boldsymbol{x}); I_0, I_1) \tag{5}$$

for all $\boldsymbol{x} \in \Omega$, $t \in [0,1]$ and a differentiable D. Solving (4) means transporting the transformation maps according to the velocities whereas solving (5) is the flow of the image mismatch (given by the derivative of the distance measure) backward in time, cf. [7]. As in [7] we apply the smoothing kernel $(L^\dagger L)^{-1}$ before updating the velocities in (3) to improve numerical optimization:

$$p := v + (L^\dagger L)^{-1}(J_\varphi^\top \lambda). \tag{6}$$

2.2 Discretization and Algorithm

From now on we use $d = 3$. Velocities v and transformations φ were discretized on a nodal grid in 4D (3D + t) [11]. The number of time points was set to $n_4 = 11$. The number of points in space varied during the multi-level optimization but was chosen equal for all spatial directions, i.e. $n_1 = n_2 = n_3$. Defining $\bar{n} := n_1 n_2 n_3$ and using linear ordering in space yields arrays $\boldsymbol{v}, \boldsymbol{\varphi} \in \mathbb{R}^{3\bar{n} \times n_4}$.

Algorithm 1. 3D multi-level LDDMM

Data: $I_0^i, I_1^i \in \mathbb{R}^{m_1^i \times m_2^i \times m_3^i}$, $i = 1, \ldots, F$; $\alpha, \gamma, \sigma > 0$, $\boldsymbol{n} \in \mathbb{N}^4$
Optional Data: $\boldsymbol{\psi} \in \mathbb{R}^{3\bar{n}}$
Result: $\boldsymbol{v}, \boldsymbol{\varphi} \in \mathbb{R}^{3\bar{n} \times n_4}$

Initialize $\boldsymbol{v} \leftarrow \boldsymbol{0} \in \mathbb{R}^{3\bar{n} \times n_4}$, $\boldsymbol{\varphi}_{:,1} \in \mathbb{R}^{3\bar{n}}$ as regular nodal grid on Ω or $\boldsymbol{\varphi}_{:,1} \leftarrow \boldsymbol{\psi}$
for $i \in \{1, 2, ..., F\}$ **do**
    if $i > 1$ **then**
        // Interpolate solution of level $i-1$ to level i
        $\boldsymbol{v} \leftarrow$ Prolongate($\boldsymbol{v},\boldsymbol{n}$); $\boldsymbol{\varphi}_{:,1} \leftarrow$ Prolongate($\boldsymbol{\varphi}_{:,1},\boldsymbol{n}$)
    while *stopping criteria not satisfied* **do**
        for $j \in \{1, 2, \ldots, n_4 - 1\}$ **do**
            Compute $\boldsymbol{\varphi}_{:,j+1}$ from $\boldsymbol{\varphi}_{:,j}$ and $\boldsymbol{v}_{:,j}$ according to (4)
        $\boldsymbol{\lambda}_{:,n_4} \leftarrow -(1/\sigma^2)\nabla_\varphi D(\boldsymbol{P}\boldsymbol{\varphi}_{:,n_4}; \boldsymbol{I}_0^i, \boldsymbol{I}_1^i)$
        for $k \in \{n_4 - 1, n_4 - 2, \ldots, 1\}$ **do**
            Compute $\boldsymbol{\lambda}_{:,k}$ from $\boldsymbol{\lambda}_{:,k+1}$ and $\boldsymbol{P}\boldsymbol{v}_{:,k}$ using (5). Save only $\boldsymbol{P}^\top\boldsymbol{\lambda}$.
        $\boldsymbol{p} \leftarrow \boldsymbol{v} + (\boldsymbol{L}_{\alpha,\gamma}^\top\boldsymbol{L}_{\alpha,\gamma})^{-1}(J_\varphi^\top\boldsymbol{P}^T\boldsymbol{\lambda})$
        $\boldsymbol{v} \leftarrow \boldsymbol{v} - \beta\boldsymbol{H}\boldsymbol{p}$ // β is computed by line search, $\boldsymbol{H}$ by L-BFGS
    $n_l \leftarrow 2n_l - 1$, $l = 1, 2, 3$
return $\boldsymbol{v}, \boldsymbol{\varphi}$

We use central differences and Neumann boundary conditions for the discretization of div, L, $L^\dagger$ and J_φ. NGF and its derivative were implemented according to [11]. Equations (4) and (5) were solved with a fourth order Runge-Kutta scheme. Given images $\boldsymbol{I}_0, \boldsymbol{I}_1 \in \mathbb{R}^{m_1 \times m_2 \times m_3}$ with $\bar{m} := m_1 m_2 m_3$ voxels, smoothed and downsampled versions $\boldsymbol{I}_0^i, \boldsymbol{I}_1^i \in \mathbb{R}^{m_1^i \times m_2^i \times m_3^i}$ with $m_j^i = \lfloor m_j \cdot 2^{-F+i} \rfloor$ were computed for $j = 1, 2, 3$ and $i = 1, \ldots, F$ [11]. Problem (1) was then solved using a coarse-to-fine resolution multi-level strategy with $F \in \mathbb{N}$ levels.

Choosing $n_i = m_i$ exceeds common memory limitations and results in an extremely expensive solution of (4) and (6). As v and φ are assumed to be smooth functions it is usually not necessary to use a high resolution for v and φ. This motivates our choice of $n_i < m_i$. Nevertheless, we use image information at the highest resolution. Hence v and φ have to be prolongated to image resolution to solve (5). This can be done gradually, i.e. for only one time point at once and reduces memory consumption substantially. Following [9], we use a prolongation matrix $\boldsymbol{P} \in \mathbb{R}^{3\bar{m} \times 3\bar{n}}$ that linearly interpolates v and φ on the cell-centered grid points of the images. $\boldsymbol{P}$ is sparse but large and does not need to be kept in memory [9]. We use matrix *notation*, but *implemented* a matrix-free operator.

After (5) is solved, the adjoint $\boldsymbol{\lambda} \in \mathbb{R}^{3\bar{m} \times n_4}$ has to be brought back to grid resolution by computation of $\boldsymbol{P}^\top\boldsymbol{\lambda}$ which is then used to solve (3). A memory efficient way to do this is storing $\boldsymbol{P}^\top\boldsymbol{\lambda}$ instead of $\boldsymbol{\lambda}$ and doing computations gradually again. The numerical solution of Eqs. (3) to (6) is performed in the multi-level registration described in Algorithm 1. It is useful to start Algorithm 1 with the result of a pre-registration $\boldsymbol{\psi} \in \mathbb{R}^{3\bar{n}}$. Given a (preferably diffeomorphic) ψ only the initial condition of (4) has to be adapted: $\varphi(\cdot, 0) = \psi(\cdot)$.

The discretized objective function was optimized with a L-BFGS approach [13] saving the last $M = 5$ iterate vectors for approximation of the inverse Hessian. The maximum number of iterations was set to $k_{\max} = 50$. Additional stopping criteria proposed in [11] were used to terminate the while loop in Algorithm 1. During the optimization an Armijo line search with parameters $\beta_k = 0.5^{k-1}$, $k_{\max}^{\mathrm{LS}} = 30$ and $c_1 = 10^{-6}$ was used to guarantee a decrease of the objective function.

3 Experiments and Results

The proposed method was applied to the DIR-Lab 4DCT [4] (see Sect. 3.1) and COPD [5] (see Sect. 3.2) data sets, as they are a well-known benchmark for lung CT registration. In total 20 inhale/exhale scan pairs are available that include 300 expert annotated landmarks each. The scans were masked with a lung segmentation obtained using [10]. For all experiments a PC with 3.4 GHz Intel i7-2600 quad-core CPU was used. We implemented Algorithm 1 with Matlab and employed C++ code for computations of D, L and P.

3.1 Experiments for Varying n

Since we assume smooth velocities and transformations, we investigated the influence of a coarse grid on registration accuracy. The 4DCT data sets were affinely pre-registered to obtain ψ and Algorithm 1 was used with $\alpha = 200$, $\sigma = 0.01$ and $F = 4$ for all registrations. Initially we set $\bar{n} = 5^3$, $\bar{n} = 9^3$ and $\bar{n} = 17^3$ respectively. The final number of grid points in space for the registration on full image resolution was 33^3, 65^3 and 129^3 accordingly. We compared the performance for different n parameters using the mean distance of expert annotated landmarks, runtime and memory consumption. See Table 1 for results. One-sided paired t-tests with significance level 0.05 were used to identify improvements in mean landmark error compared to the 65^3 method. Registrations were repeated without the finest image pyramid level to see if a reduction in image data influences accuracy. Again paired t-tests were used to compare to the methods with the same number of grid points that were registered with all levels.

Using 129^3 grid points does not provide the best results, which could be explained by the fact that the optimization is prone to local minima because more degrees of freedom are given. This is visible for case 7, where 129^3 is the fastest method but yields the worst results. Using 65^3 grid points results in significantly better accuracy compared to both 33^3 and 129^3 although improvements with respect to 33^3 are small. For memory consumption and runtime 33^3 is clearly the best choice while 129^3 requires most resources. However, memory requirements do not grow with factor 8 as there is an overhead for saving images and computing λ, therefore 65^3 offers the best compromise. Omitting the last image pyramid level results in a mean memory consumption of 0.80, 1.98 and 10.91 GB for 33^3, 65^3 and 129^3 grid points respectively. Using the full image data is beneficial for the registration accuracy which is also confirmed by the significance tests.

Table 1. Mean landmark distance per DIR-Lab 4DCT data set, necessary memory and runtime. Rounding to the next regular grid voxel was performed prior to computing the distance. Best values are printed bold. Significant differences to 65^3 are indicated by $*$ and to the respective method with full image information by $+$.

Case	Mean (mm)			Mean, omitted last image level (mm)			Memory (GB)			Runtime (h:min)		
	33^3	65^3	129^3	33^3	65^3	129^3	33^3	65^3	129^3	33^3	65^3	129^3
4DCT1	**0.81**	0.86	0.96	1.24	1.16	1.18	**0.97**	2.15	11.36	**0:17**	0:36	0:49
4DCT2	0.80	**0.79**	0.92	1.04	0.87	1.68	**1.12**	2.30	11.52	**0:20**	0:32	0:53
4DCT3	**0.96**	**0.96**	1.23	1.25	1.20	2.29	**1.05**	2.23	11.45	**0:15**	0:29	0:50
4DCT4	1.37	**1.23**	1.45	1.59	1.44	2.70	**1.01**	2.19	10.45	**0:10**	0:25	0:41
4DCT5	1.29	**1.20**	1.57	1.55	1.53	2.70	**1.07**	2.25	10.50	**0:11**	0:29	0:43
4DCT6	1.05	**1.03**	1.04	1.41	1.20	1.18	**4.50**	5.67	13.93	0:56	**0:55**	3:43
4DCT7	1.06	**0.98**	1.42	1.40	1.37	1.99	**4.77**	5.94	14.20	1:15	1:13	**0:42**
4DCT8	1.23	**1.13**	1.41	1.38	1.32	2.15	**4.50**	5.67	13.93	1:01	0:55	**0:54**
4DCT9	1.11	**1.06**	1.37	1.39	1.25	1.25	**4.50**	5.67	13.93	**0:37**	0:55	1:08
4DCT10	1.00	**0.98**	1.19	1.25	1.23	1.21	**4.23**	5.40	13.66	0:57	1:05	**0:44**
Avg	1.07*	**1.02**	1.26*	1.35+	1.26+	1.83+	**2.77**	3.95	12.49	**0:36**	0:45	1:07

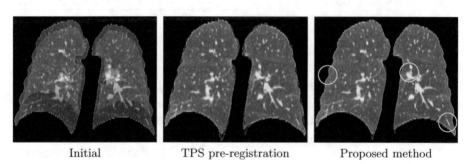

| Initial | TPS pre-registration | Proposed method |

Fig. 1. Overlay of a coronal slice of the fixed (blue) and (transformed) moving image (orange) of data set 10 of the DIR-Lab COPD data [5]. Aligned structures are displayed in gray or white due to addition of RGB values. Yellow circles highlight improvements. (Color figure online)

3.2   Comparison to State-of-the-Art Algorithms

In the following experiments we used a thin-plate spline (TPS) pre-registration with keypoints [8] to provide a very accurate initial estimate on the COPD data sets [5]. We ensured that ψ is diffeomorphic by removal of keypoints whose set of six nearest neighbors changes after TPS computation by more than one point, which indicates a violation of topology preservation. This procedure reduced the number of keypoints to approximately one quarter of the original number. Parameters were fixed to $\sigma = 0.1$, $\alpha = 85$ and $F = 5$. Motivated by the

Table 2. Mean and standard deviation of the distances of the 300 expert annotated landmarks per DIR-Lab COPD data set. All values are given in mm. Rounding to the next regular grid voxel was performed prior to computing the distances. Results for state-of-the-art methods are the reported ones from [3,8,16]. The p-values were computed performing paired t-tests with the hypothesis that the respective method is better than the proposed one. Best values are printed bold.

Case	Mean ± Standard deviation					
	Initial	MILO [3]	MRF [8]	NLR [16]	Prereg.	Proposed
COPD1	26.34 ± 11.43	0.93 ± 0.92	1.00 ± 0.93	1.33 ± 1.55	1.15 ± 1.00	**0.90 ± 0.93**
COPD2	21.79 ± 6.47	1.77 ± 1.92	1.62 ± 1.78	2.34 ± 2.88	2.18 ± 2.10	**1.56 ± 1.67**
COPD3	12.64 ± 6.39	**0.99 ± 0.91**	1.00 ± 1.06	1.12 ± 1.07	1.19 ± 1.03	1.03 ± 0.99
COPD4	29.58 ± 12.95	1.14 ± 1.04	1.08 ± 1.05	1.54 ± 1.61	1.32 ± 1.12	**0.94 ± 0.98**
COPD5	30.08 ± 13.36	1.02 ± 1.23	0.96 ± 1.13	1.39 ± 1.38	1.18 ± 1.21	**0.85 ± 0.90**
COPD6	28.46 ± 9.17	0.99 ± 1.08	1.01 ± 1.25	2.08 ± 3.01	1.27 ± 1.45	**0.94 ± 1.12**
COPD7	21.60 ± 7.74	1.03 ± 1.08	1.05 ± 1.07	1.10 ± 1.28	1.32 ± 1.45	**0.94 ± 1.25**
COPD8	26.46 ± 13.24	1.31 ± 1.76	**1.08 ± 1.24**	1.57 ± 2.08	1.47 ± 1.94	1.12 ± 1.56
COPD9	14.86 ± 9.82	0.86 ± 1.06	**0.79 ± 0.80**	0.99 ± 1.29	1.02 ± 1.10	0.88 ± 0.98
COPD10	21.81 ± 10.51	1.23 ± 1.27	1.18 ± 1.31	1.42 ± 1.44	1.51 ± 1.39	**1.17 ± 1.28**
Average	23.36 ± 10.11	1.13 ± 1.23	1.08 ± 1.16	1.49 ± 1.76	1.36 ± 1.38	**1.03 ± 1.16**
p-value	$4.8 \cdot 10^{-7}$	$5.5 \cdot 10^{-3}$	0.054	$9.5 \cdot 10^{-4}$	$1.5 \cdot 10^{-5}$	–

results of Sect. 3.1 we used $n = (65, 65, 65, 11)$ on the finest level. Resulting mean and standard deviations of landmark distances and p-values of one-sided paired t-tests are given in Table 2. The filtering of the keypoints results in a diffeomorphic pre-registration with worse mean landmark distances as visible by comparing the columns MRF and Prereg. respectively.

We compared the proposed method to the MILO [3] and MRF [8] algorithms, which are the two best ranked methods for registration of DIR-Lab COPD data sets. Results of the NLR [16] algorithm are reported because it also uses the NGF distance measure. The proposed registration achieves in most cases the best result and performed significantly better than the pre-registration, MILO [3] and NLR [16]. Mostly it is also better than MRF, which may have singularities while our method is diffeomorphic. The registrations took on average 46 min and used at most 5.9 GB of RAM. Figure 1 shows an exemplary central coronal slice of data set 10 without registration, after TPS pre-registration and after the proposed LDDMM registration. The TPS pre-registration captures the large motion and aligns most of the vessels. The subsequent LDDMM registration improves the alignment of lung boundaries and nearby vessels as well as small vessels as highlighted by the yellow circles.

4   Discussion

In this paper a memory efficient LDDMM scheme was introduced that employs the well-suited NGF distance measure for the registration of pulmonary CT data. Although the method was tested only for lung CT images it is applicable for other anatomical sites or modalities. We accomplish at least a 25-fold reduction of memory requirements (cf. supplementary material) compared to full resolution LDDMM and obtain diffeomorphic mappings without impairment of registration quality. The proposed method achieves the currently lowest average landmark error (1.03 mm) and advances the state of the art on challenging lung CT data [5]. A trustworthy registration is vital for clinical applications such as COPD classification or CAD of lung nodule evolution [6,14]. A possible extension of our method would be a lung mask similarity term as described in [16] to improve the lung boundary alignment. Another option is the integration of sliding motion into the model as in [15]. We also plan to submit results to the EMPIRE10 challenge [12] for additional evaluation of our method.

Acknowledgments. This work was supported by a fellowship of the German Academic Exchange Service (DAAD) and NSF grant ECCS-1148870.

References

1. Ashburner, J., Friston, K.J.: Diffeomorphic registration using geodesic shooting and Gauss-Newton optimisation. NeuroImage **55**(3), 954–967 (2011)
2. Beg, M.F., Miller, M.I., Trouvé, A., Younes, L.: Computing large deformation metric mappings via geodesic flows of diffeomorphisms. IJCV **61**(2), 139–157 (2005)
3. Castillo, E., Castillo, R., Fuentes, D., Guerrero, T.: Computing global minimizers to a constrained B-spline image registration problem from optimal l1 perturbations to block match data. Med. Phys. **41**(4), 041904 (2014)
4. Castillo, E., Castillo, R., Martinez, J., Shenoy, M., Guerrero, T.: Four-dimensional deformable image registration using trajectory modeling. Phys. Med. Biol. **55**(1), 305–327 (2010)
5. Castillo, R., Castillo, E., Fuentes, D., Ahmad, M., Wood, A.M., et al.: A reference dataset for deformable image registration spatial accuracy evaluation using the COPDgene study archive. Phys. Med. Biol. **58**(9), 2861–2877 (2013)
6. Galbán, C.J., Han, M.K., Boes, J.L., Chughtai, K., Meyer, C.R., et al.: Computed tomography-based biomarker provides unique signature for diagnosis of COPD phenotypes and disease progression. Nat. Med. **18**, 1711–1715 (2012)
7. Hart, G.L., Zach, C., Niethammer, M.: An optimal control approach for deformable registration. In: IEEE CVPR Workshops, pp. 9–16 (2009)
8. Heinrich, M.P., Handels, H., Simpson, I.J.A.: Estimating large lung motion in COPD patients by symmetric regularised correspondence fields. In: Navab, N., Hornegger, J., Wells, W.M., Frangi, A.F. (eds.) MICCAI 2015. LNCS, vol. 9350, pp. 338–345. Springer, Heidelberg (2015). doi:10.1007/978-3-319-24571-3_41
9. König, L., Rühaak, J.: A fast and accurate parallel algorithm for non-linear image registration using normalized gradient fields. In: IEEE ISBI, pp. 580–583 (2014)

10. Lassen, B., Kuhnigk, J.M., Schmidt, M., Krass, S., Peitgen, H.O.: Lung and lung lobe segmentation methods at Fraunhofer MEVIS. In: Proceedings of the Fourth International Workshop on Pulmonary Image Analysis, pp. 185–199 (2011)

11. Modersitzki, J.: FAIR: Flexible Algorithms for Image Registration. SIAM (2009)

12. Murphy, K., van Ginneken, B., Reinhardt, J.M., Kabus, S., Ding, K., et al.: Evaluation of registration methods on thoracic CT: the EMPIRE10 challenge. IEEE Trans. Med. Imaging **30**(11), 1901–1920 (2011)

13. Nocedal, J., Wright, S.: Numerical Optimization. Springer, New York (2006)

14. Regan, E.A., Hokanson, J.E., Murphy, J.R., Lynch, D.A., Beaty, T.H., et al.: Genetic Epidemiology of COPD (COPDGene) study design. COPD **7**, 32–43 (2011)

15. Risser, L., Vialard, F.X., Baluwala, H.Y., Schnabel, J.A.: Piecewise-diffeomorphic image registration: application to the motion estimation between 3D CT lung images with sliding conditions. Med. Image Anal. **17**(2), 182–193 (2013)

16. Rühaak, J., Heldmann, S., Kipshagen, T., Fischer, B.: Highly accurate fast lung CT registration. In: SPIE 2013, Medical Imaging, p. 86690Y-1-9 (2013)

17. Sakamoto, R., Mori, S., Miller, M.I., Okada, T., Togashi, K.: Detection of time-varying structures by large deformation diffeomorphic metric mapping to aid reading of high-resolution CT images of the lung. PLoS ONE **9**(1), 1–11 (2014)

18. Vialard, F.X., Risser, L., Rueckert, D., Cotter, C.J.: Diffeomorphic 3D image registration via geodesic shooting using an efficient adjoint calculation. IJCV **97**(2), 229–241 (2012)

19. Zhang, M., Fletcher, P.T.: Finite-dimensional Lie Algebras for fast diffeomorphic image registration. In: Ourselin, S., Alexander, D.C., Westin, C.-F., Cardoso, M.J. (eds.) IPMI 2015. LNCS, vol. 9123, pp. 249–260. Springer, Heidelberg (2015). doi:10.1007/978-3-319-19992-4_19

Inertial Demons: A Momentum-Based Diffeomorphic Registration Framework

Andre Santos-Ribeiro[✉], David J. Nutt, and John McGonigle

Centre for Neuropsychopharmacology, Division of Brain Sciences,
Department of Medicine, Imperial College London, London, UK
afs13@imperial.ac.uk

Abstract. Non-linear registration is an essential part of modern neu-roimaging analysis, from morphometrics to functional studies. To be practical, non-linear registration methods must be precise and computational efficient. Current algorithms based on Thirion's demons achieve high accuracies while having desirable properties such as diffeomorphic deformation fields. However, the increased complexity of these methods lead to a decrease in their efficiency. Here we propose a modification of the demons algorithm that both improves the accuracy and convergence speed, while maintaining the characteristics of a diffeomorphic registration. Our method outperforms all the analysed demons approaches in terms of speed and accuracy. Furthermore, this improvement is not limited to the demons algorithm, but applicable in most typical deformable registration algorithms.

1   Introduction

In any modern neuroimaging study non-linear registration is an essential step, allowing for the quantitative analysis of form, such as detecting changes in brain shape and size, or the precise alignment of the anatomy required for functional group studies. To be useful, non-linear registration methods must be both accurate and computationally efficient [1]. The former reduces the inter-subject anatomical variability allowing identification of small anatomical or functional changes between groups, while the latter is required to enable timely analysis of large datasets [7]. Additionally, non-linear registration should generate well-behaved spatial transformations that best align two images [16]. To achieve this, most typical algorithms [2,3,12,16] constrain the displacement fields to diffeomorphic deformations (i.e. deformations fields which have an inverse, and both the field and its inverse are differentiable).

The demons algorithm, as originally introduced by Thirion [14], presented a step forward in both speed and accuracy. He proposed a method that alternates between the computation of the demons forces (inspired from Maxwell's Demons, and optical flow equations) and a Gaussian smoothing regularization. This allowed dense correspondences within a computationally efficient algorithm.

Due to its success and implementation simplicity further developments were proposed to improve convergence speed and precision, such as the introduction

© Springer International Publishing AG 2016
S. Ourselin et al. (Eds.): MICCAI 2016, Part III, LNCS 9902, pp. 37–45, 2016.
DOI: 10.1007/978-3-319-46726-9_5

of a normalization factor α [5] bounding the step size, and the addition of an "active" force [17] based in the moving image gradient. To extend the classical demons algorithm to provide diffeomorphic transformations, Vercauteren et al. [15] proposed looking for an update step u on the Lie algebra and then mapping it to the space of diffeomorphisms through the exponential map; and later [16] suggested an extension of the demons algorithm to work completely in the log domain, showing improvements over the diffeomorphic-demons. To improve the demons algorithm to intensity inhomogeneities and contrast changes other similarity metrics such as the local cross correlation (LCC [4,7]) or the point-wise mutual information (PMI [8]) were further proposed.

While subsequent extensions of the demons algorithm showed better total accuracy and higher accuracy per iteration, they also increased the computational cost at each iteration.

Here we propose an adaptation of the demons algorithm to improve total convergence speed of all demon-like variants without compromising on accuracy. The remainder of this paper is organized as follows: the demons framework is presented in Sect. 2 followed by the introduction of the Inertial Demons; both the original and proposed demons are evaluated in Sect. 3; final remarks regarding the applicability of this extension to other non-linear registration approaches are presented in Sect. 4.

2   Demons Framework

2.1   Demons as a Minimization Problem

In non-linear registration, the transformation $T(x)$ that best aligns a source image $I_0(x)$ to a reference image $I_1(x)$ is obtained by the optimization of a similarity function $Sim(I_1(x), I_0(T(x))$. Classically, in intensity-based methods the sum of square differences (SSD) is used as the similarity metric, Eq. 1:

$$Sim = \sum (I_1(x) - I_0(T(x)))^2 \tag{1}$$

Since the optimization of the Sim term alone is ill-posed, a regularization term $Reg(T(x))$ is usually added to the global energy function E, Eq. 2:

$$E(T(x)) = Sim(I_1(x), I_0(T(x)) + Reg(T(x)) \tag{2}$$

The demons algorithm can then be seen as the optimization of Eq. 2 with the addition of a hidden correspondences $C(x)$ variable [4] that allows the alternate optimization of the similarity and regularization terms, Eq. 3.

$$E(C(x), T(x)) = Sim(I_1(x), I_0(C(x)) + \sigma \|C(x) - T(x)\|^2 + Reg(T(x)) \tag{3}$$

One first optimizes $Sim(I_1(x), I_0(C(x)) + \sigma \|C(x) - T(x)\|^2$ with respect to $C(x)$ and with $T(x)$ fixed, and then optimizes $\sigma \|C(x) - T(x)\|^2 + Reg(T(x))$ with respect to $T(x)$ with $C(x)$ fixed. The minimization of the second term is usually obtained by the convolution of the global transformation with a Gaussian kernel, yet more complex approaches such as the use of edge preserving filters have also been proposed [6].

2.2   Demons Forces

In the classical demons the minimization of the first term is performed through the computation of Thirion's "fixed" demons force, Eq. 4, which was shown to be equivalent to the second order gradient descendent with the SSD as the similarity term [11].

$$u(x) = (I_1(x) - I_0(T(x))) \frac{\nabla I_1(x)}{\|\nabla I_1(x)\|^2 + \alpha^2 (I_1(x) - I_0(T(x)))^2} \tag{4}$$

Following this framework one can instead derive different demons forces through different minimization procedures. Of particular interest in this work are the symmetric Sym forces, Eq. 5, obtained through the Efficient Second-order Minimization (ESM) [9].

$$u(x) = 2(I_1(x) - I_0(T(x))) \frac{\nabla I_1(x) + \nabla I_0(T(x))}{\|\nabla I_1(x) + \nabla I_0(T(x))\|^2 + \alpha^2 (I_1(x) - I_0(T(x)))^2} \tag{5}$$

2.3   Demons Composition

As non-linear registration should present desirable properties such as diffeomorphism, Vercauteren et al. [15] proposed looking for an update step $u(x)$ on the Lie algebra and then mapping it to the space of diffeomorphisms through the exponential map, Eq. 6,

$$T(x) \leftarrow T(x) \circ exp\,(u(x)) \tag{6}$$

and later [16] suggested to work completely in the log-domain, by considering the spatial transformations as exponentials of smooth velocity fields, Eq. 7, with the advantage of having access to the true inverse transformation.

$$\begin{cases} v(x) \leftarrow v(x) \circ u(x) \\[2mm] T(x) = exp\,(v(x)) \end{cases} \tag{7}$$

Although both these approaches are particularly attractive (since the exponential map can be efficiently approximated by the scaling and squaring approach [10]), it can still be computationally demanding if the magnitudes of the velocity field (in the case of the log-demons) or the update field (in the diffeomorphic-demons) are large. On the other hand, diffeomorphic registration can also be achieved by composing $u(x)$ to $T(x)$ while constraining $u(x)$ to small optimization steps (by treating the voxels as B-Spline control points, it can be shown that a maximal displacement of 0.4 leads to a diffeomorphic field [12,18]), Eq. 8.

$$\begin{cases} \|u(x)\| \leqslant 0.4 \\[2mm] T(x) \leftarrow T(x) \circ u(x) \end{cases} \tag{8}$$

2.4   Demons Momentum

Although computationally efficient, the demons framework relies on forces derived from the images' gradients (e.g. Eqs. 4 and 5). This fundamentally limits the ability of demons algorithms to converge quickly where gradients are scarce or non-existent (such as homogeneous regions or texture-less images).

To overcome this deficiency, multilevel frameworks are typically employed. Such approaches attempt to retrieve large deformations by sub-sampling the space of deformations, and progressively increasing the resolution to resolve local deformations. However, they do not solve the intrinsic problem of gradient-based methods within each level. Other approaches such as using preconditioning schemes have also been proposed [19].

Here we propose to use the previous update field $u(x)^{[n-1]}$, Eq. 9, as a predictive update step for the subsequent iteration $[n]$.

$$p(x)^{[n]} \leftarrow \alpha \times u(x)^{[n-1]} \tag{9}$$

The momentum term $p(x)$ simply adds a fraction of the previous update field to the current one $u(x)^{[n]}$, controlled by a constant α between $[0,1]^1$, Eq. 10.

$$u(x)^{[n]} \leftarrow u(x)^{[n]} \circ \alpha \times p(x)^{[n]} \tag{10}$$

Here the system is seen as having an inertia preventing sudden changes in $u(x)$. When the image gradient and the momentum have the same direction, this leads to an increase in step size towards the minimum. When they have different directions this approach leads to smoother updates. Since it is also desirable for $T(x)$ to be part of a diffeomorphic group $\mathscr{D}$, the inclusion of the momentum term should not change the behaviour of each approach presented in Sect. 2.3. Here we show that these conditions still apply with the use of momentum.

Diffeomorphic-demons: Since $(exp(u(x)/A)^A \subseteq \mathscr{D})$ if $(\|u(x)/A\| \leqslant 0.4)$, through the scaling and squaring approach, then $(exp(u(x)/B)^B \subseteq \mathscr{D})$ if $(\|u(x)\circ p(x)/B\| \leqslant 0.4)$, with $\{A, B\} \in \mathbb{N}$. Note A and B will often be different. Also, although $u(x)$ is updated through composition with $p(x)$, the update through addition is also possible.

Log-demons: Similarly to the diffeomorphic demons $(T(x) \subseteq \mathscr{D})$ if $(exp(v(x)/A)^A \subseteq \mathscr{D})$, with the latter true if $(\|v(x)/A\| \leqslant 0.4)$. Therefore, the above logic can be applied here to show that $(T(x) \subseteq \mathscr{D})$, when $(u(x)^{[n]} \leftarrow u(x)^{[n]} \circ \alpha \times p(x)^{[n]})$.

Restricted-demons: In this approach $(T(x) \subseteq \mathscr{D})$ if $(\|u(x)\| \leqslant 0.4)$. We can also observe that, $(T(x) \subseteq \mathscr{D})$ if $(u(x) \subseteq \mathscr{D})$ since $(\|u(x)\| \leqslant 0.4) \Rightarrow (u(x) \subseteq \mathscr{D})$. This way we can see that, since $(u(x)^{[n]} \leftarrow u(x)^{[n]} \circ \alpha \times p(x)^{[n]})$ and $(p(x)^{[n]} \leftarrow \alpha \times u(x)^{[n-1]})$ with $\alpha = [0, 1]$, $(p(x) \subseteq \mathscr{D}) \Rightarrow (u(x) \subseteq \mathscr{D}) \Rightarrow (T(x) \subseteq \mathscr{D})$.

---

[1] A value higher than 1 leads to instability of the registration process as the magnitude of the update field $\|u(x)\|$ keeps increasing at each iteration.

2.5   Demons Iterative Process

We can now define the whole demons framework (at each level) with the addition of the momentum term:

Algorithm 1. Inertial Demons

1. Calculate the update field through the demon forces (e.g. Eq. 5).
2. Add the momentum term to the update field through Eq. 10.
3. Convolve the update field with a Gaussian kernel (fluid-like regularization).
4. Choose one diffeomorphic approach:
   (a) Diffeomorphic-demons:
       i. Calculate $exp(u(x))$ and update $T(x)$ through Eq. 6.
       ii. Convolve $T(x)$ with a Gaussian kernel (diffusion-like regularization).
   (b) Log-demons:
       i. Calculate $exp(v(x))$ through Eq. 7.
       ii. Convolve $v(x)$ with a Gaussian kernel (diffusion-like regularization).
       iii. Calculate $T(x)$ through Eq. 7.
   (c) Restricted-demons:
       i. Calculate $T(x)$ through Eq. 8.
       ii. Convolve $T(x)$ with a Gaussian kernel (diffusion-like regularization).
5. Update $p(x)$ through Eq. 9.
6. Repeat from 1. to 5. until convergence.

---

3   Experiments

3.1   Circle to C

To first test the convergence speed improvement of the proposed methodology we applied the original and proposed diffeomorphic-demons, log-demons, and restricted-demons to register the classic "circle to C".

Since in this example the emphasis is on the comparison of the different methods with and without momentum, all methods use the symmetric demons force (Eq. 5), a single-resolution framework, and a 1 voxel FWHM Gaussian kernel for both the fluid-like and diffusion-like regularizers. Since the restricted-demons can only guarantee diffeomorphic deformations for small optimization steps, the maximal step was set as 0.4 voxels, and 2 voxels for the diffeomorphic and log -demons. For all momentum-based approaches an $\alpha = 0.9$ was used.

As shown in Fig. 1 all the original demons were unable to fully deform the native "circle" to the target "C", while all the proposed variations are visually identical to the target image (note that all registrations were limited to the same computation time, since time per iteration differs for the different approaches). Regarding topology, all methods presented invertible fields with positive Jacobian determinants, with the proposed methods visually more symmetric than their counterparts (i.e. more symmetric deformation grids).

Globally, the proposed diffeomorphic-demons achieved the quickest convergence, followed by the proposed restricted-demons. The proposed log-demons was unable to achieve the same convergence within the maximum allowed computation time.

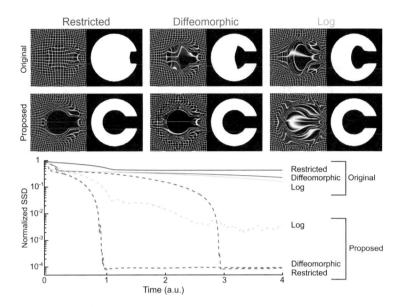

Fig. 1. Non-linear registration of the classical "circle to C". Top - Deformation fields and registered images; Bottom - Normalized SSD against time. Full lines: original methods; Dashed lines: proposed variation. For all cases lower is better.

3.2   Anatomical MRI

To further study the precision of each of the original demons approaches against our methodology we used the simulation framework presented in [13]. In this framework, 20 individual healthy T1-weighted brain images along with cortical and sub-cortical manual segmentation were used to generate a total of 400 ground truth deformations. For each simulation the different demons approaches were used to register the native to the simulated images. In this example, the same parameters used in Sec. 3.1 were applied within a multi-resolution framework with 3 levels, and 50 iterations at the highest resolution. The registration accuracy of each method was obtained by comparing the generated deformation fields and corresponding Jacobian map with the ground truth.

As shown in Fig. 2 (Top) for all approaches the proposed methodology achieved visually closer Jacobian maps to the ground truth, than the original framework. Further quantitative analysis, Fig. 2 (Bottom), show that the deformation field error and Jacobian error scores are significantly lower for the proposed methods (dark shade) comparatively with the original framework (light shade), but similar within them[2]. From all methods here, the proposed restricted-demons achieved the best scores, and showed the largest improvement relative to the original framework (DFE $= 55\%$, JE $= 38\%$).

---

[2] The statistical comparison between each original and proposed methods was performed through a Mann-Whitney U test. Although not shown here a significant improvement is also seen if $\|u(x)\| \leq 0.4$ for all methods.

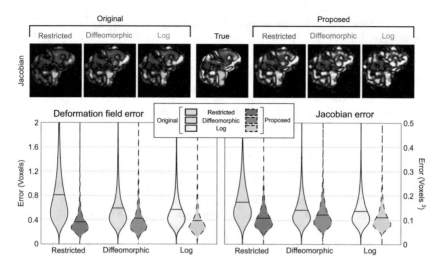

Fig. 2. Anatomical MRI. Top - Jacobian map comparison between the original and proposed methods, and the ground truth; Warmer colors refer to contractions, cooler colors to expansions. Bottom - Violin plot comparison between the original (light shade) and proposed (dark shade) frameworks for the restricted (blue), diffeomorphic (magenta), and log (cyan) -demons approaches; Lower is better for both evaluation metrics. (Color figure online)

4   Conclusion

Although computationally efficient, the demons framework relies on forces derived from the images' gradients, fundamentally limiting its ability to converge quickly where gradients are scarce or non-existent. Here we proposed an extension of the demons framework to improve the convergence speed through the addition of a momentum term, without compromising on accuracy.

Our experiments showed that the proposed methodology achieves faster and more accurate results for the restricted, diffeomorphic and log -demons for the classical "circle to C" registration, and closer results to the ground truth for the anatomical MRI non-linear registration. While in the classical "circle to C" the proposed log-demons was less accurate than the two other proposed approaches (for the allowed computational time), it showed similar results for the anatomical MRI dataset (where the number of iterations were fixed). Regarding computation time, the original diffeomorphic and log -demons took longer (by approximately 40 % and 90 % more time respectively) than the original restricted-demons. For each approach, the proposed methodology only increased the computation time by less than a third.

In this paper, we considered only the SSD similarity criteria, yet this extension can be conveniently applied to other similarity metrics such as the LCC or PMI. Furthermore, it is easily applicable to other non-linear registration frameworks (e.g. free-form deformations), or group-wise non-linear registration and atlas construction.

References

1. Arbel, T., De Nigris, D.: Fast and efficient image registration based on gradient orientations of minimal uncertainty. In: International Symposium on Biomed Imaging, pp. 1163–1166 (2015)
2. Ashburner, J.: A fast diffeomorphic image registration algorithm. Neuroimage **38**, 95–113 (2007)
3. Avants, B., Epstein, C., Grossman, M., Gee, J.: Symmetric diffeomorphic image registration with cross-correlation: evaluating automated labeling of elderly and neurodegenerative brain. Med. Image Anal. **12**, 26–41 (2008)
4. Cachier, P., Bardinet, E., Dormont, D., Pennec, X., Ayache, N.: Iconic feature based nonrigid registration: the PASHA algorithm. Comput. Vis. Image Und. **89**, 272–298 (2003)
5. Cachier, P., Pennec, X., Ayache, N.: Fast non-rigid matching by gradient descent: study and improvement of the demons algorithm. INRIA RR-3706 (1999)
6. Demirovic, D., Serifovic-Trbalic, A., Prljaca, N., Cattin, P.: Bilateral filter regularized accelerated demons for improved discontinuity preserving registration. Comput. Med. Imaging Graph. **40**, 94–99 (2015)
7. Lorenzi, M., Ayache, N., Frisoni, G., Pennec, X.: LCC-Demons: a robust and accurate symmetric diffeomorphic registration algorithm. Neuroimage **81**, 470–483 (2013)
8. Lu, H., Reyes, M., Serifovi, A., Weber, S., Sakurai, Y., Yamagata, H., Cattin, P.: Multi-modal diffeomorphic demons registration based on point-wise mutual information. In: International Symposium on Biomed Imaging, pp. 372–375 (2010)
9. Malis, E.: Improving vision-based control using efficient second-order minimization techniques. IEEE Int. Conf. Robot. **2**, 1843–1848 (2004)
10. Moler, C., Van Loan, C.: Nineteen dubious ways to compute the exponential of a matrix, twenty-five years later. SIAM J. Appl. Math. **45**(1), 3–49 (2003)
11. Pennec, X., Cachier, P., Ayache, N.: Understanding the "Demon's Algorithm": 3D non-rigid registration by gradient descent. In: Taylor, C., Colchester, A. (eds.) MICCAI 1999. LNCS, vol. 1679, pp. 597–605. Springer, Heidelberg (1999). doi:10. 1007/10704282_64
12. Rueckert, D., Aljabar, P., Heckemann, R.A., Hajnal, J.V., Hammers, A.: Diffeomorphic registration using B-splines. In: Larsen, R., Nielsen, M., Sporring, J. (eds.) MICCAI 2006. LNCS, vol. 4191, pp. 702–709. Springer, Heidelberg (2006). doi:10. 1007/11866763_86
13. Ribeiro, A.S., Nutt, D.J., McGonigle, J.: Which metrics should be used in nonlinear registration evaluation? In: Navab, N., Hornegger, J., Wells, W.M., Frangi, A.F. (eds.) MICCAI 2015. LNCS, vol. 9350, pp. 388–395. Springer, Heidelberg (2015). doi:10.1007/978-3-319-24571-3_47
14. Thirion, J.: Image matching as a diffusion process: an analogy with maxwells demons. Med. Image Anal. **2**(3), 243–260 (1998)
15. Vercauteren, T., Pennec, X., Perchant, A., Ayache, N.: Non-parametric diffeomorphic image registration with the demons algorithm. In: Ayache, N., Ourselin, S., Maeder, A. (eds.) MICCAI 2007. LNCS, vol. 4792, pp. 319–326. Springer, Heidelberg (2007). doi:10.1007/978-3-540-75759-7_39

16. Vercauteren, T., Pennec, X., Perchant, A., Ayache, N.: Symmetric log-domain diffeomorphic registration: a demons-based approach. In: Metaxas, D., Axel, L., Fichtinger, G., Székely, G. (eds.) MICCAI 2008. LNCS, vol. 5241, pp. 754–761. Springer, Heidelberg (2008). doi:10.1007/978-3-540-85988-8_90
17. Wang, H., Dong, L., O'Daniel, J., Mohan, R., Garden, A., Ang, K., Kuban, D., Bonnen, M., Chang, J., Cheung, R.: Validation of an accelerated 'demons' algorithm for deformable image registration in radiation therapy. Phys. Med. Biol. **50**(12), 2887–2905 (2005)
18. Yang, D., Li, H., Low, D., Deasy, J., Naqa, I.: A fast inverse consistent deformable image registration method based on symmetric optical flow computation. Phys. Med. Biol. **53**(21), 6143–6165 (2008)
19. Zikic, D., Baust, M., Kamen, A., Navab, N.: Natural gradients for deformable registration. In: Proceedings of the CVPR, pp. 2847–2854. IEEE (2010)

Diffeomorphic Density Registration in Thoracic Computed Tomography

Caleb Rottman$^{1(\boxtimes)}$, Ben Larson^1, Pouya Sabouri^2, Amit Sawant^2,
and Sarang Joshi^1

^{1} Scientific Computing and Imaging Institute, Department of Bioengineering,
University of Utah, Salt Lake City, USA
crottman@sci.utah.edu
^{2} University of Maryland School of Medicine, Baltimore, MD, USA

Abstract. Accurate motion estimation in thoracic computed tomography (CT) plays a crucial role in the diagnosis and treatment planning of lung cancer. This paper provides two key contributions to this motion estimation. First, we show we can effectively transform a CT image of effective linear attenuation coefficients to act as a density, i.e. exhibiting conservation of mass while undergoing a deformation. Second, we propose a method for diffeomorphic density registration for thoracic CT images. This algorithm uses the appropriate density action of the diffeomorphism group while offering a weighted penalty on local tissue compressibility. This algorithm appropriately models highly compressible areas of the body (such as the lungs) and incompressible areas (such as surrounding soft tissue and bones).

Keywords: Diffeomorphisms · Thoracic motion estimation · Density action · Image registration

1 Introduction

According to the Centers for Disease Control and Prevention, lung cancer is the leading cause of cancer death, accounting for 27 % of all cancer deaths in the United States [1]. Accurate modeling of the motion and biomechanics of the lungs under respiration is essential for the diagnosis and treatment of this disease. In particular, accurate estimation of organ movement and deformations plays a crucial role in dose calculations and treatment decisions in radiation therapy of lung cancer [8,11].

Essential to our method of motion estimation is that CT images act similar to densities: i.e. they exhibit some conservation of mass properties while undergoing deformations. The relationship between CT images and densities can be clearly seen by viewing a single patient thoracic CT throughout the breathing cycle. During inhalation, lung volume increases and lung CT intensities decrease,

S. Joshi—This work was partially supported through research funding from the National Institute of Health (R01CA169102).

S. Ourselin et al. (Eds.): MICCAI 2016, Part III, LNCS 9902, pp. 46–53, 2016.
DOI: 10.1007/978-3-319-46726-9_6

and during exhalation, lung volume decreases and lung CT intensities increase. Because of these changing image intensities, the L^2 image action of a diffeomorphism does not accurately reflect motion in CT imaging. Most state-of-the-art methods deal with these changing intensities by not using the L^2 metric between images but to instead use either mutual information or normalized cross correlation [2]. We incorporate these intensity changes into our deformation model by treating these images as densities. Some mass-preserving registration methods using cubic B-splines have also been introduced [9,12]. In contrast, we use the full space of diffeomorphisms equipped with an H^1 metric, and use the recently discovered link between densities and diffeomorphisms [4]. Furthermore, we show experimentally that CT images are not inherently mass preserving and must be transformed to become mass preserving.

We will first introduce the mathematical definition of a density and then describe how it relates to material density and CT images. Mathematically, a 3D density $I(x) \, dx$ is a volume form on a domain $\Omega \subseteq \mathbb{R}^3$ where $I(x)$ is a non-negative function on Ω and $dx = dx^1 \wedge dx^2 \wedge dx^3$ is the standard volume element on $\mathbb{R}^3$. The key difference between a density and a function is how a diffeomorphism $\varphi \in \text{Diff}(\Omega)$ acts on them. The left action of φ on a *function* $g(x)$ (called the L^2 action) is simply function composition:

$$\varphi_* g(x) = g \circ \varphi^{-1}(x). \tag{1}$$

The left action of φ on a *density* $I(x) \, dx$ is:

$$\varphi_*(I(x) \, dx) = I \circ \varphi^{-1}(x) |D\varphi^{-1}(x)| \, dx, \tag{2}$$

where $|D\varphi^{-1}|$ is the Jacobian determinant of the diffeomorphism.

A unique property of a density is that the total mass is conserved under the action of a diffeomorphism, where here the total mass is defined as the integral of the density over Ω:

$$\int_\Omega I \circ \varphi^{-1}(x) |D\varphi^{-1}(x)| \, dx = \int_\Omega I(y) \, dy. \tag{3}$$

This equality holds by performing a change of variables: $x = \varphi(y)$, $dx = |D\varphi(y)| dy$, and using the identity $|D\varphi^{-1}(x)| = \frac{1}{|D\varphi(y)|}$.

This conservation of mass property extends to its traditional meaning in a physical mass density $\rho(x)$ (units g/cm^3). Physical mass density integrated over a domain becomes physical mass (units g). Similarly, the narrow beam X-ray linear attenuation coefficient (LAC) for a single material (units cm^{-1}) is defined as $\mu(x) = m\rho(x)$, where m is a material-specific property called the mass attenuation coefficient (units cm^2/g) that depends on the energy of the X-ray beam. In a mixture of materials, the total linear attenuation coefficient is $\mu(x) = \sum_i m_i \rho_i(x)$. Integrating $\mu(x)$ over a domain gives us the total LAC, which we will call the LAC mass (units cm^2). Therefore, conservation of physical mass implies conservation of LAC mass in a closed system.

During respiration, we assume that the change in physical lung mass due to air in the lungs is negligible. We then expect conservation of LAC mass in the lungs.

2   CT Images as Densities

We have shown that LAC mass is theoretically conserved. Unfortunately, CT image intensities do not represent true narrow beam linear attenuation coefficients. Instead, modern CT scanners use wide beams that yield secondary photon effects at the detector. CT image intensities reflect *effective* linear attenuation coefficients as opposed to the true narrow beam linear attenuation coefficient.

To see the relationship between effective LAC and true narrow beam LAC, we ran a Monte Carlo simulation using an X-ray spectrum and geometry from a Philips CT scanner at various densities of water (since lung tissue is very similar to a mixture between water and air) [6]. The nonlinear relationship between effective LAC and narrow beam LAC relationship is clear (see Fig. 1).

If we have conservation of mass within a single subject in a closed system, we expect an inverse relationship between average density in a region Ω and volume of that region: $D_t = \frac{M}{V_t}$. Here $V_t = \int_{\Omega_t} 1 dx$, $D_t = \int_{\Omega_t} I_t(x) dx / V_t$, Ω_t is the domain of the closed system (that moves over time), and t is a phase of the breathing cycle. This relationship becomes linear in log space with a slope of -1:

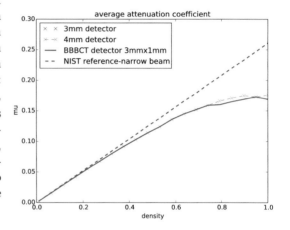

Fig. 1. Effective LAC from Monte Carlo simulation (solid line) and NIST reference narrow beam LAC (dashed line). The true relationship between effective LAC and narrow beam LAC is nonlinear.

$$\ln(D_t) = \ln(M) - \ln(V_t) \quad (4)$$

Our experimental results confirm the Monte Carlo simulation in that lungs imaged under CT do not follow this inverse relationship. Rather, the slope found in these datasets in log space is consistently greater than -1 (see Fig. 3). Because of this, we seek a nonlinear intensity transformation for CT images such that CT mass is preserved under deformation.

In this paper, we model this intensity transformation as an exponential function, i.e. $I(x) \mapsto I(x)^\alpha$, and we solve for the α that yields the best mass preservation. We chose an exponential model because it is a single parameter monotonic function that preserves the density of air at zero. Furthermore, using an exponential function makes our analysis invariant to image scaling. That is, if $I_t(x)^\alpha$ exhibits conservation of mass, so does $(cI_t(x))^\alpha$, for $c \in \mathbb{R}^+$.

Note that the field of view of the CT scanner is not a closed system, as portions of the body leave and enter the field of view during respiration. We therefore evaluate the accuracy of this intensity transformation inside the lungs, which is essentially a closed system. We evaluate our methods using the Deformable

Image Registration (DIR) Laboratory dataset (http://www.dir-lab.com/) [7], which consists of ten subjects with ten 4DCT timepoints each. Second, we evaluate on a set of 30 subjects with ten 4DCT timepoints each procured at UT Southwestern Medical Center. The lungs for each patient at each timepoint are segmented with active contours using ITK-SNAP [13] (http://www.itksnap. org/) combined with an intensity based segmentation to remove high-density regions in the lungs and around the lung border due to imperfect initial segmentations.

For each subject, we perform a linear regression of the measured LAC density and calculated volume in log space. Let $\mathbf{d}(\alpha) = \log\left(\int_{\Omega_t} I_t(x)^\alpha dx / \int_{\Omega_t} 1 dx\right)$ (the log density) and $v = \log(\int_{\Omega_t} 1 dx)$ (the log volume), where again t is a breathing cycle timepoint. The linear regression then models the relationship in log space as $\mathbf{d}(\alpha) \approx av + b$. Let $a_j(\alpha)$ be the slope solved for in this linear regression for the jth subject. To find the optimal α for the entire dataset, we solve

$$\alpha = \arg\min_{\alpha'} \sum_j (a_j(\alpha') + 1)^2, \tag{5}$$

which finds the value of α that gives us an average slope closest to -1. We solve for α using a brute force search.

Applying this exponential function to the CT data allows us to perform our density matching algorithm described in the next section.

3   Weighted Diffeomorphic Density Matching

Mathematically, our problem is to find a diffeomorphic (bijective and smooth) transformation between two densities I_0 and I_1, using our exponentially transformed CT images defined in the previous section as our densities. We use the Fisher-Rao metric on densities which has the unique property that it is the only metric between densities that is invariant to the action of a diffeomorphism [3]. When vol(Ω) is infinite, the Fisher-Rao metric between two densities becomes the Hellinger distance:

$$d_F^2(I_0 dx, I_1 dx) = \int_\Omega (\sqrt{I_0} - \sqrt{I_1})^2 dx. \tag{6}$$

The Riemannian geometry of the diffeomorphism group with a Sobolev H^1 metric is intimately linked to the geometry of the space of densities with the Fisher-Rao metric. In particular, there are Sobolev H^1 metrics on the diffeomorphism group that descend to the Fisher-Rao metric on the space of densities [4]. This descending property from $\text{Diff}(\Omega)$ to $\text{Dens}(\Omega)$ allows us to compute the distance on $\text{Diff}(\Omega)$ by using the Fisher-Rao metric. Since the space of densities is flat, we can solve for the distance in $\text{Diff}(\Omega)$ in closed form: we do not need to time-integrate velocity fields or solve for adjoint equations as is necessary in LDDMM [5].

We therefore seek to minimize the following energy functional:

$$E(\varphi) = d_F^2(\varphi_*(f\,dx), (f \circ \varphi^{-1})dx) + d_F^2(\varphi_*(I_0\,dx), I_1\,dx)) \tag{7}$$

$$= \underbrace{\int_\Omega (\sqrt{|D\varphi^{-1}|} - 1)^2 f \circ \varphi^{-1}\,dx}_{E_1(\varphi)} + \underbrace{\int_\Omega \left(\sqrt{|D\varphi^{-1}|I_0 \circ \varphi^{-1}} - \sqrt{I_1} \right)^2 dx}_{E_2(\varphi)}.$$

$$\tag{8}$$

To better understand this energy functional, we describe its two terms. The first term $E_1(\varphi)$ is the metric on the regularity of the deformation, descended from the Sobolev H^1 metric. This penalizes φ as it becomes non volume preserving: a unitary Jacobian determinant at a location indicates that the transformation is volume preserving. Furthermore, the density $f(x)\,dx$ is a positive weighting on the domain Ω: regions where $f(x)$ is high have a higher penalty on non-volume preserving deformations and regions where $f(x)$ is low have a lower penalty on non-volume preserving deformations.

Physiologically, we know the lungs are quite compressible as air enters and leaves. Surrounding tissue including bones and soft tissue, on the other hand, is essentially incompressible. Therefore, our penalty function $f(x)$ is low inside the lungs and outside the body and high elsewhere. For our penalty function, we simply implement a sigmoid function of the original CT image: $f(x) = \text{sig}(I_0(x))$.

The second term $E_2(\varphi)$ is the Fisher-Rao distance between the deformed density and the target density.

We take the Sobolev gradient with respect to the energy functional which is given by

$$\delta E = -\Delta^{-1}\Big(-\nabla\big(f \circ \varphi^{-1}(1 - \sqrt{|D\varphi^{-1}|})\big)$$

$$- \sqrt{|D\varphi^{-1}|\,I_0 \circ \varphi^{-1}}\nabla\big(\sqrt{I_1}\big) + \nabla\big(\sqrt{|D\varphi^{-1}|\,I_0 \circ \varphi^{-1}}\big)\sqrt{I_1}\Big). \tag{9}$$

Then, the current estimate of φ^{-1} is updated directly via a Euler integration of the gradient flow [10]:

$$\varphi_{j+1}^{-1}(x) = \varphi_j^{-1}(x + \epsilon\delta E) \tag{10}$$

for some step size ϵ. Since we take the Sobolev gradient the resulting deformation is guaranteed to be invertable with a sufficiently small ϵ.

4 Results

For the DIR dataset, we used the method from Sect. 2 to solve for the exponent that yields conservation of mass. We solved for $\alpha = 1.64$ that gives us the best fit. Without using the exponential fit, the average slope of log density log volume plot was -0.66 (SD 0.048). After applying the exponential to the CT intensities, the average slope is -1.0 (SD 0.054). The log-log plots of all ten patients in the DIR dataset as well as box plots of the slope is shown in Fig. 2.

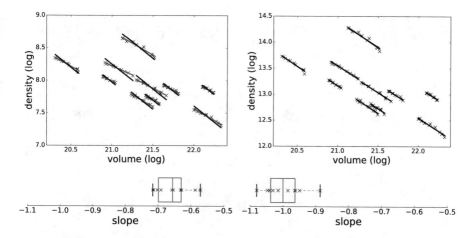

Fig. 2. Density and volume log-log plots. Upper left: log-log plots without applying the exponential correction for all ten DIR subjects. The best fit line to each dataset is in red and the mass-preserving line (slope $= -1$) is in black. Upper right: log-log plots after applying the exponential correction $I(x)^\alpha$ to the CT images. In this plot, the best fit line matches very closely to the mass-preserving line. Bottom row: corresponding box plots of the slopes found in the regression. (Color figure online)

For the 30 subject dataset, we solved for $\alpha = 1.90$ that gives us conservation of mass. Without using the exponential fit, the average slope of the log-log plot was -0.59 (SD 0.11).

We applied our proposed weighted density matching algorithm to the first subject from the DIR dataset. This subject has images at 10 timepoints and has a set of 300 corresponding landmarks between the full inhale image and the full exhale image. These landmarks were manually chosen by three independent observers. Without any deformation, the landmark error is 4.01 mm (SD 2.91 mm). Using our method, the landmark error is reduced to 0.88 mm (SD 0.94 mm), which is only slightly higher than the observer repeat registration error of 0.85 mm (SD 1.24 mm).

We implement our algorithm on the GPU and plot the energy as well as the Fisher-Rao metric with and without applying the deformation. These results are shown in Fig. 3. In this figure, we show that we have excellent data match, while the deformation remains physiologically realistic: inside the lungs there is substantial volume change due to respiration, but the deformation outside the lungs is volume preserving. With a $256 \times 256 \times 94$ voxel dataset, our algorithm takes approximately nine minutes running for four thousand iterations on a single nVidia Titan Z GPU.

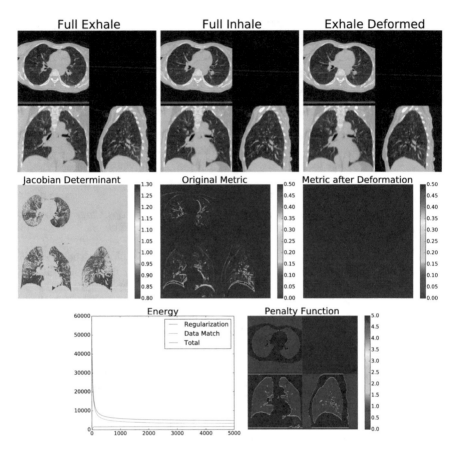

Fig. 3. Registration results. Top row: full inhale, full exhale, and the deformed exhale density estimated using our method. Middle row: Jacobian determinant of the transformation, initial Fisher-Rao metric, and Fisher-Rao metric after applying the density action. Notice that outside the lungs the estimated deformation is volume preserving. Bottom row: Energy as a function of iterations, and penalty function.

5   Discussion

In this paper, we have shown that although the narrow beam linear attenuation acts as a density, the effective linear attenuation coefficient found in CT does not act as a density. However, applying a simple exponential function transforms the CT dataset into a set of images that exhibit conservation of mass. This simple non-linear approximation yields excellent results even when using the same exponential function for multiple subjects in a single dataset.

We suspect that the biggest cause of the nonlinearity between true linear attenuation and effective attenuation is the presence of X-ray scatter and secondary photons, which are dependent on the scanner geometry and the energy spectrum. Therefore, we do not necessarily expect that the same α parameter of the exponential functions works across different CT scanners; however we found that the same α parameter accurately corrects the nonlinearity across multiple subjects on the same scanner.

We have also shown that we can use these corrected images as densities with a great deal of accurately. Our method uses the appropriate density action when dealing with CT images, and our weighting function on the domain constrains the deformation to be physiologically realistic.

References

1. CDC - basic information about lung cancer. http://www.cdc.gov/cancer/lung/basic_info/index.htm. Accessed 06 Mar 2016
2. Avants, B.B., Tustison, N.J., Song, G., Cook, P.A., Klein, A., Gee, J.C.: A reproducible evaluation of ANTs similarity metric performance in brain image registration. NeuroImage **54**(3), 2033–2044 (2011)
3. Bauer, M., Bruveris, M., Michor, P.W.: Uniqueness of the Fisher-Rao metric on the space of smooth densities. submitted (2015)
4. Bauer, M., Joshi, S., Modin, K.: Diffeomorphic density matching by optimal information transport, pp. 1–35 (2015)
5. Beg, M.F., Miller, M.I., Trouvé, A., Younes, L.: Computing large deformation metric mappings via geodesic flows of diffeomorphisms. Int. J. Comput. Vis. **61**(2), 139–157 (2005)
6. Boone, J.M., Seibert, J.A.: An accurate method for computer-generating tungsten anode x-ray spectra from 30 to 140 kv. Med. phys. **24**(11), 1661–1670 (1997)
7. Castillo, R., Castillo, E., Guerra, R., Johnson, V.E., McPhail, T., Garg, A.K., Guerrero, T.: A framework for evaluation of deformable image registration spatial accuracy using large landmark point sets. Phys. Med. Biol. **54**(7), 1849–1870 (2009)
8. Geneser, S.E., Hinkle, J.D., Kirby, R.M., Wang, B., Salter, B., Joshi, S.: Quantifying variability in radiation dose due to respiratory-induced tumor motion. Med. Image Anal. **15**(4), 640–649 (2011)
9. Gorbunova, V., Sporring, J., Lo, P., Loeve, M., Tiddens, H.A., Nielsen, M., Dirksen, A., de Bruijne, M.: Mass preserving image registration for lung CT. Med. Image Anal. **16**(4), 786–795 (2012)
10. Rottman, C., Bauer, M., Modin, K., Joshi, S.C.: Weighted diffeomorphic density matching with applications to thoracic image registration. In: 5th MICCAI Workshop on Mathematical Foundations of Computational Anatomy (MFCA 2015), pp. 1–12 (2015)
11. Sawant, A., Keall, P., Pauly, K.B., Alley, M., Vasanawala, S., Loo, B.W., Hinkle, J., Joshi, S.: Investigating the feasibility of rapid MRI for image-guided motion management in lung cancer radiotherapy. BioMed. Res. Int. 2014 (2014)
12. Yin, Y., Hoffman, E.A., Lin, C.L.: Mass preserving nonrigid registration of CT lung images using cubic B-spline. Med. Phys. **36**(9), 4213–4222 (2009)
13. Yushkevich, P.A., Piven, J., Hazlett, H.C., Smith, R.G., Ho, S., Gee, J.C., Gerig, G.: User-guided 3D active contour segmentation of anatomical structures: Significantly improved efficiency and reliability. Neuroimage **31**(3), 1116–1128 (2006)

Temporal Registration in In-Utero Volumetric MRI Time Series

Ruizhi Liao[1]([⊠]), Esra A. Turk[1,2], Miaomiao Zhang[1], Jie Luo[1,2],
P. Ellen Grant[2], Elfar Adalsteinsson[1], and Polina Golland[1]

[1] Massachusetts Institute of Technology, Cambridge, MA, USA
ruizhi@mit.edu
[2] Harvard Medical School, Boston Children's Hospital, Boston, MA, USA

Abstract. We present a robust method to correct for motion and deformations in in-utero volumetric MRI time series. Spatio-temporal analysis of dynamic MRI requires robust alignment across time in the presence of substantial and unpredictable motion. We make a Markov assumption on the nature of deformations to take advantage of the temporal structure in the image data. Forward message passing in the corresponding hidden Markov model (HMM) yields an estimation algorithm that only has to account for relatively small motion between consecutive frames. We demonstrate the utility of the temporal model by showing that its use improves the accuracy of the segmentation propagation through temporal registration. Our results suggest that the proposed model captures accurately the temporal dynamics of deformations in in-utero MRI time series.

1 Introduction

In this paper, we present a robust method for image registration in temporal series of in-utero blood oxygenation level dependent (BOLD) MRI. BOLD MRI is a promising imaging tool for studying functional dynamics of the placenta and fetal brain [1–3]. It has been shown that changes in fetal and placental oxygenation levels with maternal hyperoxygenation can be used to detect and characterize placental dysfunction, and therefore hold promise for monitoring maternal and fetal well-being [4]. Investigating hemodynamics of the placenta and fetal organs necessitates robust estimation of correspondences and motion correction across different volumes in the dynamic MRI series. Temporal MRI data suffers from serious motion artifacts due to maternal respiration, unpredictable fetal movements and signal non-uniformities [5], as illustrated in Fig. 1. Our approach exploits the temporal nature of the data to achieve robust registration in this challenging setup.

Prior work in in-utero MRI has focused on the fetal brain and demonstrated that rigid transformations capture brain motion accurately [6,7]. The rigid model, however, fails to fully account for movement and deformation of the placenta. Recently, B-spline transformations have been employed for tracking of regions-of-interest (ROIs) in placental images by registering all volumes to

© Springer International Publishing AG 2016
S. Ourselin et al. (Eds.): MICCAI 2016, Part III, LNCS 9902, pp. 54–62, 2016.
DOI: 10.1007/978-3-319-46726-9_7

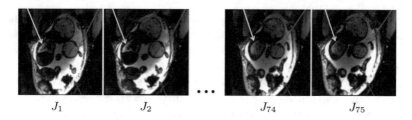

Fig. 1. Example twin pregnancy case from the study. The same cross-section from frames J_1, J_2, J_{74}, and J_{75} is shown. Arrows indicate areas of substantial motion of the placenta (red), fetal head (green), and fetal body (yellow). (Color figure online)

a reference frame [8]. This approach ignores the temporal nature of the data and yields a substantial number of outlier volumes that fail registration due to significant motion. In this paper, we demonstrate that a temporal model of movement improves the quality of alignment.

Beyond the specific application to in-utero MRI time series, the problem of temporal alignment has been investigated in longitudinal [9,10], cardiac [11–14] and lung imaging [14–18]. Longitudinal studies often involve subtle changes, and the algorithms are fine-tuned to detect small deformations [9]. Both cardiac and lung motion patterns are somewhat regular and smooth across time, and lend themselves to biomechanical modeling [12,13,15]. In contrast to these applications, in-utero volumetric MRI time series contain a combination of subtle non-rigid deformation of the placenta and large-scale unpredictable motion of the fetus. At the same time, consecutive frames in a series are quite close to each other in time, which is the property we exploit in our modeling.

Existing methods for temporal registration in image series can be categorized into three distinct groups. The first group applies a variant of groupwise registration to this problem. This approach relies on a group template – estimated or selected from the image set – that yields acceptable registration results for all frames [10,14,16,18]. Unfortunately, large motion present in in-utero MRI makes some frames to be substantially different from the template, leading to registration failures. The second group aligns consecutive frames and concatenates resulting deformations to estimate alignment of all frames in the series [17]. In application to long image series (BOLD MRI series contain hundreds of volumes), this approach leads to substantial errors after several concatenation steps. The third approach formulates the objective function in terms of pairwise differences between consecutive frames, leading to algorithms that perform pairwise registration of consecutive frames iteratively until the entire series comes into alignment [14]. Our method is also related to filtering approaches in respiratory motion modeling [15]. Since in-utero motion is much more complex than respiratory motion, we do not attempt to explicitly model motion but rather capture it through deformations of the latent template image.

In this paper, we construct the so called filtered estimates of the deformations by making a Markov assumption on the temporal series. We derive a sequential procedure to determine the non-rigid transformation of the template to each frame in the series. This work represents a first step towards efficient and robust temporal alignment in this challenging novel application, and provides a flexible framework that can be augmented in the future with clinically relevant estimation of MRI intensity dynamics in organs of interest. We demonstrate the method on real in-utero MRI time series, and report robust improvements in alignment of placenta, fetal brains, and fetal livers.

2   HMM and Filtered Estimates

In this section, we briefly review inference in HMMs [19,20], and introduce our notation in the context of temporal registration. We assume existence of a latent (hidden) state whose temporal dynamics is governed by a Markov structure, i.e., the future state depends on the history only through the current state. In our application, we assume that template I deforms at each time point to describe the anatomical arrangement at that time. Deformation φ_n defines the latent state at time $n \in \{1, ..., N\}$, where N is the number of images in the series. The observed image J_n at time n is generated by applying φ_n to template I independently of all other time points.

We aim to estimate the latent variables $\{\varphi_n\}$ from observations $\{J_n\}$. Formally, we construct and then maximize posterior distribution $p(\varphi_n | J_{1:n}; I)$, where we use $J_{k:m}$ to denote sub-series $\{J_k, J_{k+1}, ..., J_m\}$ of the volumetric time series $\{J_1, J_2, ..., J_N\}$. This distribution, referred to as a filtered estimate of the state, can be efficiently constructed using forward message passing [19,20], also known as sequential estimation. The message $m_{(n-1)\to(n)}(\varphi_n)$ from node $n-1$ to node n is determined through forward recursion that integrates a previous message $m_{(n-2)\to(n-1)}(\varphi_{n-1})$ with the data likelihood $p(J_n | \varphi_n; I)$ and dynamics $p(\varphi_n | \varphi_{n-1})$:

$$m_{(n-1)\to(n)}(\varphi_n) \triangleq p(\varphi_n | J_{1:n}; I) \propto p(J_n | \varphi_n; I)\, p(\varphi_n | J_{1:n-1}; I) \qquad (1)$$

$$= p(J_n | \varphi_n; I) \int_{\varphi_{n-1}} p(\varphi_n | \varphi_{n-1})\, m_{(n-2)\to(n-1)}(\varphi_{n-1})\, d\varphi_{n-1}, \quad (2)$$

where $m_{0\to1}(\varphi_1) = p(\varphi_1)$ and $n = \{1, ..., N\}$. The forward pass produces the posterior distribution $p(\varphi_n | J_{1:n}; I)$ for each time point n in the number of steps that is linear with n. Similarly, efficient backward pass enables computation of posterior distribution $p(\varphi_n | J_{1:N}; I)$ based on all data, often referred to as smoothing. In this paper, we investigate advantages of the temporal model in the context of filtering and leave the development of a smoothing algorithm for future work.

3 Modeling Temporal Deformations Using HMM

The likelihood term $p(J_n|\varphi_n; I)$ in Eq. (2) is determined by the model of image noise:

$$p(J_n|\varphi_n; I) \propto \exp\left(-\text{Dist}\left(J_n, I\left(\varphi_n^{-1}\right)\right)\right), \tag{3}$$

where $\text{Dist}(\cdot, \cdot)$ is a measure of dissimilarity between images. The transition probability $p(\varphi_n|\varphi_{n-1})$ encourages temporal and spatial smoothness:

$$p(\varphi_n|\varphi_{n-1}) \propto \exp\left(-\lambda_1 \text{Reg}(\varphi_n) - \lambda_2\|\varphi_n \circ \varphi_{n-1}^{-1}\|^2\right), \tag{4}$$

where $\text{Reg}(\cdot)$ is the regularization term that encourages spatial smoothness of the deformation, $\|\cdot\|$ is the appropriate norm that encourages φ_n to be close to φ_{n-1}, and λ_1 and λ_2 are regularization parameters.

Since the integration over all possible deformation fields is intractable, we resort to a commonly used approximation of evaluating the point estimate that maximizes the integrand. In particular, if φ_{n-1}^* is the best deformation estimated by the method for time point $n-1$, the message passing can be viewed as passing the optimal deformation φ_{n-1}^* to node n:

$$m_{(n-1)\to(n)}(\varphi_n) \propto p(J_n|\varphi_n; I) \int_{\varphi_{n-1}} p(\varphi_n|\varphi_{n-1}) \mathbb{1}\{\varphi_{n-1} = \varphi_{n-1}^*\} d\varphi_{n-1} \tag{5}$$

$$= p(J_n|\varphi_n; I) p(\varphi_n|\varphi_{n-1}^*), \tag{6}$$

and the estimate for time point n is recursively estimated as

$$\varphi_n^* = \arg\max_{\varphi_n} p(J_n|\varphi_n; I) p(\varphi_n|\varphi_{n-1}^*). \tag{7}$$

This estimate is then used to determine φ_{n+1}^*, and so on until we reach the end of the series.

4 Implementation

In this work, we choose the first image J_1 as the reference template I and focus on exploring the advantages of the Markov structure. The model can be readily augmented to include a model of a bias field and a latent reference template that is estimated jointly with the deformations, similar to prior work in groupwise registration [10, 14, 16, 18]. We manipulate Eq. (7) to obtain

$$\varphi_n^* = \arg\max_{\varphi_n} p(J_n|\varphi_n; I) p(\varphi_n|\varphi_{n-1}^*) \tag{8}$$

$$= \arg\min_{\varphi_n} \text{Dist}\left(J_n, I\left(\varphi_n^{-1}\right)\right) + \lambda_1 \text{Reg}(\varphi_n) + \lambda_2\|\varphi_n \circ (\varphi_{n-1}^*)^{-1}\|^2, \tag{9}$$

and observe that this optimization problem reduces to pairwise image registration of the template I and the observed image J_n. The algorithm proceeds as follow. Given the estimate φ^*_{n-1} of the template deformation to represent image J_{n-1}, we apply the registration algorithm to I and J_n while using φ^*_{n-1} as an initialization, resulting in the estimate φ^*_n.

We implemented our method using symmetric diffeomorphic registration with cross-correlation [21]. Diffeomorphic registration ensures that the estimated deformation is differentiable bijective with differentiable inverse. We employ cross-correlation to define the measure of image dissimilarity $\text{Dist}(\cdot, \cdot)$, because cross-correlation adapts naturally to the image data with signal non-uniformities. We set the size of the local window for computing cross-correlation to be 5 voxels. We use the state-of-the-art implementation provided in the ANTS software package [21]. Following the common practice in the field, ANTS implements spatial regularization via Gaussian smoothing.

5   Experiments and Results

Data. Ten pregnant women were consented and scanned on a 3T Skyra Siemens scanner (single-shot GRE-EPI, $3 \times 3\text{mm}^2$ in-plane resolution, 3mm slice thickness, interleaved slice acquisition, TR $= 5.8 - 8$s, TE $= 32 - 36$ms, FA $= 90^o$) using 18-channel body and 12-channel spine receive arrays. Each series contains around 300 volumes. To eliminate the effects of slice interleaving, we resampled odd and even slices of each volume onto a common isotropic $3\,\text{mm}^3$ image grid. This study included three singleton pregnancies, six twin pregnancies, and one triplet pregnancy, between 28 and 37 weeks of gestational age. A hyperoxia task paradigm was used during the scans, comprising three consecutive ten-minute episodes of initial normoxic episode ($21\,\%\text{O}_2$), hyperoxic episode ($100\,\%\text{O}_2$), and a final normoxic episode ($21\,\%\text{O}_2$). To enable quantitative evaluation, we manually delineated the placentae (total of 10), fetal brains (total of 18), and fetal livers (total of 18), in the reference template $I = J_1$ and in five additional randomly chosen volumes in each series.

Experiments. To evaluate the advantages of the temporal model, we compare it to a variant of our algorithm that does not assume temporal structure and instead aligns each image in the series to the reference frame using the same registration algorithm used by our method. Algorithmically, this corresponds to setting λ_2 in Eq. (9) to be 0, and initializing the registration step with an identity transformation instead of the previously estimated transformation φ^*_{n-1}. To quantify the accuracy of the alignment, we transform the manual segmentations in the reference template to the five segmented frames in each series using the estimated deformations. We employed Dice coefficient [22] to quantify volume overlap between the transferred and the manual segmentations. In our application, the goal is to study average temporal signals for each ROI, and therefore delineation of an ROI provides an appropriate evaluation target.

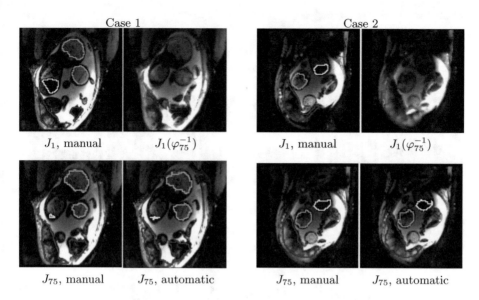

Fig. 2. Two example cases from the study. For each case, we display the reference frame J_1 with manual segmentations, the reference frame $J_1(\varphi_{75}^{-1})$ transformed into the coordinate system of frame J_{75}, frame J_{75} with manual segmentations, and frame J_{75} with segmentations transferred from the reference frame J_1 via φ_{75}. Both cases are twin pregnancies. Segmentations of the placentae (pink), fetal brains (green), and fetal livers (yellow) are shown. Two-dimensional cross-sections are used for visualization purposes only; all computations are performed in 3D. (Color figure online)

Experimental Results. Fig. 2 illustrates results for two example cases from the study. We observe that the reference frame was warped accurately by the algorithm to represent a frame in the series that is substantially different in the regions of the placenta and the fetal liver. The delineations achieved by transferring manual segmentations from the reference frame to the coordinate system of the current frame (J_{75} in the figure) are in good alignment with the manual segmentations for the current frame. Figure 3 reports volume overlap statistics for the placentae, fetal brains, and fetal livers, for each case in the study. We observe that temporal alignment improves volume overlap in important ROIs and offers consistent improvement for all cases over pairwise registration to the reference frame. We also note that temporal alignment offers particularly substantial gains in cases with a lot of motion, i.e., low original volume overlap.

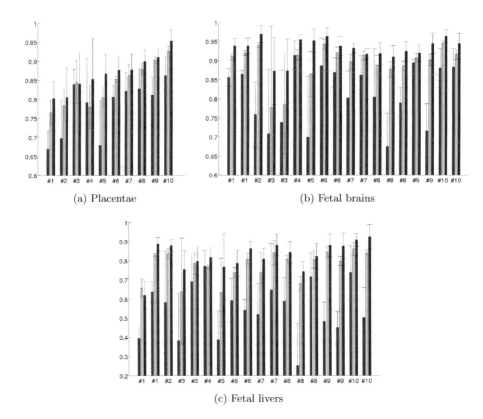

Fig. 3. Volume overlap between transferred and manual segmentations: (a) placentae (b) fetal brains, and (c) fetal livers. The cases in the study are reported in the increasing order of placental volume overlap for our method. Duplicate case numbers correspond to twin and triplet pregnancies. Statistics are reported for our method (red), pairwise registration to the template frame (green), and no alignment (blue). (Color figure online)

6   Conclusions

We presented a HMM-based registration method to align images in in-utero volumetric MRI time series. Forward message passing incorporates the temporal model of motion into the estimation procedure. The filtered estimates are therefore based on not only the present volume frame and the template, but also on the previous frames in the series. The experimental results demonstrate the promise of our approach in a novel, challenging application of in-utero BOLD MRI analysis. Future work will focus on obtaining robust estimates of the MRI signal time courses by augmenting the method with a backward pass and a model of ROI-specific intensity changes.

Acknowledgments. This work was supported in part by NIH NIBIB NAC P41EB015902, NIH NICHD U01HD087211, NIH NIBIB R01EB017337, Wistron Corporation, and Merrill Lynch Fellowship.

References

1. Schöpf, V., Kasprian, G., Brugger, P., Prayer, D.: Watching the fetal brain at rest. Int. J. Dev. Neurosci. **30**(1), 11–17 (2012)
2. Sørensen, A., Peters, D., Simonsen, C., Pedersen, M., Stausbøl-Grøn, B., Christiansen, O.B., Lingman, G., Uldbjerg, N.: Changes in human fetal oxygenation during maternal hyperoxia as estimated by BOLD MRI. Prenat. Diagn. **33**(2), 141–145 (2013)
3. Luo, J., Turk, E.A., Hahn, T., Teulon Gonzalez, M., Gagoski, B., Bibbo, C., Palanisamy, A., Tempany, C., Torrado-Carvajal, A., Malpica, N., Martnez Gonzlez, J., Robinson, J.N., Hernandez-Tamames, J.A., Adalsteinsson, E., Grant, P.E.: Human placental and fetal response to maternal hyperoxygenation in IUGR pregnancy as measured by BOLD MRI. In: Proceedings of the 23rd Annual Meeting of ISMRM, Toronto, Ontario, Canada, 2015, International Society of Magnetic Resonance in Medicine (ISMRM), p. 633 (2015)
4. Aimot-Macron, S., Salomon, L., Deloison, B., Thiam, R., Cuenod, C., Clement, O., Siauve, N.: In vivo MRI assessment of placental and fetal oxygenation changes in a rat model of growth restriction using blood oxygen level-dependent (bold) magnetic resonance imaging. Eur. Radiol. **23**(5), 1335–1342 (2013)
5. Studholme, C.: Mapping fetal brain development in utero using MRI: the big bang of brain mapping. Ann. Rev. Biomed. Eng. **13**, 345 (2011)
6. Ferrazzi, G., Murgasova, M.K., Arichi, T., Malamateniou, C., Fox, M.J., Makropoulos, A., Allsop, J., Rutherford, M., Malik, S., Aljabar, P., et al.: Resting state fMRI in the moving fetus: a robust framework for motion, bias field and spin history correction. Neuroimage **101**, 555–568 (2014)
7. You, W., Serag, A., Evangelou, I.E., Andescavage, N., Limperopoulos, C.: Robust motion correction and outlier rejection of in vivo functional MR images of the fetal brain and placenta during maternal hyperoxia. In: SPIE Medical Imaging, International Society for Optics and Photonics, pp. 941700–941700 (2015)
8. Turk, E.A., Luo, J., Torrado-Carvajal, A., Hahn, T., Teulon Gonzalez, M., Gagoski, B., Bibbo, C., Robinson, J.N., Hernandez-Tamames, J.A., Grant, P.E., Adalsteinsson, E., Pascau, J., Malpica, N.: Automated roi extraction of placental and fetal regions for 30 minutes of EPI BOLD acquisition with different maternal oxygenation episodes. In: Proceedings of the 23rd Annual Meeting of ISMRM, Toronto, Ontario, Canada, 2015, International Society of Magnetic Resonance in Medicine (ISMRM), p. 639 (2015)
9. Reuter, M., Fischl, B.: Avoiding asymmetry-induced bias in longitudinal image processing. Neuroimage **57**(1), 19–21 (2011)
10. Durrleman, S., Pennec, X., Trouvé, A., Braga, J., Gerig, G., Ayache, N.: Toward a comprehensive framework for the spatiotemporal statistical analysis of longitudinal shape data. Int. J. Comput. Vis. **103**(1), 22–59 (2013)
11. Chandrashekara, R., Rao, A., Sanchez-Ortiz, G.I., Mohiaddin, R.H., Rueckert, D.: Construction of a statistical model for cardiac motion analysis using nonrigid image registration. In: Taylor, C., Noble, J.A. (eds.) IPMI 2003. LNCS, vol. 2732, pp. 599–610. Springer, Heidelberg (2003). doi:10.1007/978-3-540-45087-0_50

12. Sundar, H., Davatzikos, C., Biros, G.: Biomechanically-constrained 4D estimation of myocardial motion. In: Yang, G.-Z., Hawkes, D., Rueckert, D., Noble, A., Taylor, C. (eds.) MICCAI 2009. LNCS, vol. 5762, pp. 257–265. Springer, Heidelberg (2009). doi:10.1007/978-3-642-04271-3_32

13. Park, J., Metaxas, D., Young, A.A., Axel, L.: Deformable models with parameter functions for cardiac motion analysis from tagged MRI data. IEEE Trans. Med. Imaging 15(3), 278–289 (1996)

14. Metz, C., Klein, S., Schaap, M., van Walsum, T., Niessen, W.J.: Nonrigid registration of dynamic medical imaging data using nD+t B-splines and a groupwise optimization approach. Med. Image Anal. 15(2), 238–249 (2011)

15. McClelland, J.R., Hawkes, D.J., Schaeffter, T., King, A.P.: Respiratory motion models: a review. Med. Image Anal. 17(1), 19–42 (2013)

16. Rietzel, E., Chen, G.T.: Deformable registration of 4D computed tomography data. Med. Phys. 33(11), 4423–4430 (2006)

17. Reinhardt, J.M., Ding, K., Cao, K., Christensen, G.E., Hoffman, E.A., Bodas, S.V.: Registration-based estimates of local lung tissue expansion compared to xenon CT measures of specific ventilation. Med. Image Anal. 12(6), 752–763 (2008)

18. Singh, N., Hinkle, J., Joshi, S., Fletcher, P.T.: Hierarchical geodesic models in diffeomorphisms. Int. J. Comput. Vis. 117(1), 70–92 (2016)

19. Baum, L.E., Petrie, T.: Statistical inference for probabilistic functions of finite state markov chains. Ann. Math. Stat. 37(6), 1554–1563 (1966)

20. Bishop, C.M.: Pattern recognition. Machine Learning (2006)

21. Avants, B.B., Epstein, C.L., Grossman, M., Gee, J.C.: Symmetric diffeomorphic image registration with cross-correlation: evaluating automated labeling of elderly and neurodegenerative brain. Medical Image Anal. 12(1), 26–41 (2008)

22. Dice, L.R.: Measures of the amount of ecologic association between species. Ecology 26(3), 297–302 (1945)

Probabilistic Atlas of the Human Hippocampus Combining Ex Vivo MRI and Histology

Daniel H. Adler[3], Ranjit Ittyerah[1], John Pluta[1], Stephen Pickup[1], Weixia Liu[1], David A. Wolk[2], and Paul A. Yushkevich[1(✉)]

[1] Department of Radiology, University of Pennsylvania, Philadelphia, PA, USA
pauly2@upenn.edu
[2] Department of Neurology, University of Pennsylvania, Philadelphia, PA, USA
[3] Departments of Radiology and Bioengineering, University of Pennsylvania, Philadelphia, PA, USA

Abstract. The human hippocampus is a complex structure consisting of multiple anatomically and functionally distinct subfields. Obtaining subfield-specific measures from in vivo MRI is challenging, and can benefit from a detailed 3D anatomical reference. This paper builds a computational atlas of the hippocampus from high-resolution ex vivo MRI of 26 specimens using groupwise deformable registration. A surface-based approach based on the explicit segmentation and geometric modeling of hippocampal layers is used to initialize deformable registration of ex vivo MRI scans. This initialization improves of groupwise registration quality, as measured in terms of similarity metrics and qualitatively. The resulting atlas, which also includes annotations mapped from histology, is a unique resource for describing variability in hippocampal anatomy.

1 Introduction

The hippocampus, located in the medial temporal lobe (MTL), is a major component of the declarative memory system, and is of acute interest in many brain disorders. It is a complex anatomical structure formed by multiple layers in a "swiss roll" configuration. The outer layers include subfields Cornu Ammonis (CA) 1–3 and subiculum, and the inner layer includes the dentate gyrus (DG), divided into the inner hilus region and the outer DG proper. Hippocampal subfields are hypothesized to be selectively affected by Alzheimer's disease, aging, epilepsy, and other disorders [10], and to play different roles in normal memory.

Given their differential involvement in disease and memory, there has been increased interest in using in vivo MRI to interrogate hippocampal subfields [5]. However, even with highly optimized parameters, in vivo MRI provides only limited ability to distinguish hippocampal subfields. For instance, T2-weighted MRI with high resolution in the plane parallel to the main axis of the hippocampus makes it possible to see a dark layers separating the CA and subiculum from

This work is supported by NIH grants R01 AG037376, R01 EB017255, and R01 AG040271. Specimens obtained from NDRI and UPenn brain banks.

S. Ourselin et al. (Eds.): MICCAI 2016, Part III, LNCS 9902, pp. 63–71, 2016.
DOI: 10.1007/978-3-319-46726-9_8

the DG; but boundaries between CA subfields, CA3 and DG, and CA1 and subiculum have to be inferred, typically based on heuristic rules [5].

Some authors have proposed to use ex vivo MRI, which can provide dramatically better resolution and contrast, to inform and guide the analysis of in vivo MRI. In [15], an atlas of the hippocampus was created from five specimens using groupwise image registration, and subfield distributions from the atlas were mapped into the in vivo MRI space using shape-based interpolation. More recently, in [7], an atlas was constructed by applying groupwise registration to multi-label manual segmentations of 15 ex vivo MRI scans, and used as a shape and intensity prior for in vivo MRI segmentation.

In addition to MRI, ex vivo specimens can be processed histologically, and rich information from histology can be mapped into the MRI space. This makes it possible to define anatomical boundaries in the MRI space based on the cytoarchitectural features used by anatomists to define subfields, rather than based on heuristic rules used in the MRI literature [1]. Furthermore, histology can be used to quantify pathology, e.g., tau neurofibrillary tangles in Alzheimer's disease. Mapping such pathological information into an atlas of the hippocampal region can provide a statistical characterization of the distribution of pathology in this region, and in turn, serve as valuable resource for analysis and interpretation of in vivo MRI (or PET) studies.

The current paper develops the largest ex vivo computational atlas of the hippocampus to date, and the first such atlas to combine information from high-resolution MRI and dense serial histology. The algorithmic contribution of the paper lies in the use of a surface-based registration scheme to initialize pairwise registration of ex vivo MRI scans, leading to improved groupwise registration.

2   Methods and Results

2.1   Ex Vivo Imaging

Intact ex vivo brain bank specimens of the hippocampus (n = 26, 14 left / 12 right, 10 left/right pairs from same subject) were scanned after >21 days formalin fixation at 9.4 tesla at $0.2 \times 0.2 \times 0.2\,\text{mm}^3$ or similar resolution using a multi-slice spin echo sequence described in [15] (see Fig. 1 for example). A subset of specimens (n = 8) was processed histologically, by cutting tissue into 1 cm blocks, paraffin embedding, slicing at $\sim 200\,\mu\text{m}$ intervals, staining using the Kluver-Barrera method, and optical scanning at $0.5 \times 0.5\,\mu\text{m}^2$ resolution.

2.2   Overview of the Two-Stage Registration Approach

As shown below in Fig. 3, direct image registration between specimens does not align structures in the hippocampus well. The proposed two-stage approach is based on the segmentation of two anatomical structures: the whole hippocampus, and the myelinated layers of CA and DG (strata radiatum and lacunosomolecular; SRLM) that separate these two structures and appear dark in MRI. Laying

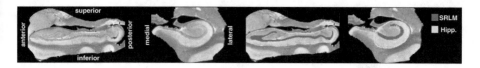

Fig. 1. Sagittal and coronal views of ex vivo MRI of the hippocampus, with pseudo-manual segmentation of SRLM and hippocampus overlaid. Note: for this atlas, medial portion of subiculum is excluded from the hippocampus.

between CA and DG, and spanning the whole length of the hippocampus, the SRLM forms a natural "skeleton" of the structure (figuratively speaking, distinct from the medial axis of the hippocampus). To make our atlas, SRLM and whole hippocampus were segmented manually, but we show that semi-automatic segmentation is feasible. For each specimen, we solve the Laplace equation to obtain a half-way surface between the hippocampal boundary and SRLM. Surface correspondences between half-way surfaces of different specimens are obtained by solving the Laplace equation between each half-way surface and the tightest fitting ellipsoid. These correspondences are then propagated to the entire image volume and used to initialize groupwise volumetric image registration between specimens. The sections below detail the different steps in this approach.

2.3 Ex Vivo MRI Segmentation

One author segmented the hippocampus and SRLM in all specimens (Fig. 1). Given the size of data, fully manual segmentation was impractical, and instead we manually edited segmentations generated semi-automatically (hippocampus: multi-atlas segmentation [13] using "rough" segmentations drawn in earlier work; SRLM: random forest [3] classifier applied to intensity processed with sheetness filter [6]). Overall, manual editing was extensive – over 8 h per specimen.

To establish the feasibility of automating segmentation in future work, we implemented a multi-atlas automatic pipeline for hippocampus and SRLM segmentation. This pipeline requires the user to label the outer hippocampal boundary every 20th coronal slice of the target image, which is interpolated and used for initial affine registration. Then each atlas is registered to the target image using diffeomorphic deformable registration with the normalized cross-correlation metric [2]. Consensus hippocampus and SRLM labels are obtained using the joint label fusion (JLF) algorithm [13]. This is repeated 5 times, with each iteration's affine atlas-target registrations bootstrapped by the results of the previous iteration's joint label fusion. This pipeline was applied in a leave-one-out framework. The average Dice coefficient between the (pseudo) manual segmentation and JLF segmentation was 0.80 ± 0.08 for SRLM and 0.94 ± 0.02 for the hippocampus. Unfortunately, there is no prior data on the reliability of manual or automatic segmentation of SRLM in ex vivo MRI to put these numbers into context. The most comparable high-resolution in vivo MRI study [14] reports intra-rater Dice coefficient 0.71 for SRLM and 0.91 for whole hippocampus. Overall, our Dice

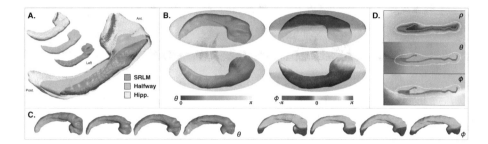

Fig. 2. Surface-based correspondence approach. **A.** Hippocampal and SRLM boundaries and the halfway (mid-potential) surface L_i^0 of one subject. **B.** Superior and inferior views of halfway surface L_i^0, rendered within its minimum volume enclosing ellipsoid (MVEE), and colored by its spherical parameterization angles θ and ϕ. **C.** Spherical coordinate parameterization of the halfway surface in 4 specimens. **D.** Parameterization of the image domain by potential ρ and spherical coordinates θ and ϕ. (Color figure online)

coefficients can be considered high, particularly since SRLM is a thin structure. This suggests that semi-automatic segmentation may be used in place of extensive manual workup in the future, as new specimens are added to the atlas.

2.4   Initial Shape-Based Normalization

The hippocampus occupies a different location in each specimen, and before intensity-based image registration can be performed, initial alignment of the hippocampi is required. In [15], a strategy based on the continuous medial representation (cm-rep) was proposed. The cm-rep is a deformable model that approximates the hippocampus and imposes a shape-based coordinate system on its interior (the coordinate system follows the medial axis of the deformable model). Each MRI scan can then be warped into the space of the cm-rep template, such that the outer boundaries and the medial axes of the hippocampi in different specimens approximately align. This step is not necessary per se for the proposed surface-initialized registration strategy, but to facilitate its comparison with [15], cm-rep normalization was applied as a preprocessing step.

2.5   Surface Registration

Surface registration in our method leverages special properties of harmonic functions, and is closely related to prior work on cortical thickness estimation [8]. For subject i, let $\mathcal{S}_i$ and $\mathcal{H}_i$ denote the SRLM and hippocampus segmentation, respectively. Let Ω be the image domain after initial normalization. Since SRLM is fully contained in the hippocampus label, $\mathcal{S}_i \subset \mathcal{H}_i \subset \Omega$. Surface registration begins with solving the Laplace equation on Ω, with the boundaries of $\mathcal{S}_i$, $\mathcal{H}_i$ and Ω modeled as equipotential surfaces. We find $\rho : \Omega \to \mathbb{R}$ that solves

$$\nabla^2 \rho = 0 \quad \text{subj. to} \quad \rho|_{\partial \mathcal{S}_i} = -1; \quad \rho|_{\partial \mathcal{H}_i} = 1; \quad \rho|_{\partial \Omega} = 2 \tag{1}$$

Assuming ∂S_i and $\partial \mathcal{H}_i$ have spherical topology, the shells $L_i^t = \{x : \rho(x) = t\}$ for $t \in (-1, 1)$ are a family of nested spherical surfaces that smoothly span the region between ∂S_i and $\partial \mathcal{H}_i$. We define the mid-potential surface L_i^0 as the "halfway surface" between SRLM and hippocampus for subject i. Shown in Fig. 2A, this surface captures the geometric characteristics of both SRLM and overall hippocampus, which, we believe, makes it the ideal target for finding geometric correspondences between specimens.

To establish such correspondences, for each subject i, we construct a bijective mapping $f : L_i^0 \rightarrow S^2$ from the halfway surface to the unit sphere S^2, based on diffeomorphic potential gradient flow mapping between L_i^0 and its minimum volume enclosing ellipsoid (MVEE), denoted E_i. E_i is the tri-axial ellipsoid of minimum volume and arbitrary spatial orientation that entirely encloses L_i^0. It is uniquely defined and may be seen as a tight, quadric approximation of L_i^0 that, being the affine image of S^2, has a trivial spherical parameterization. The MVEE is computed using Khachiyan's method [12]. Next, we solve the Laplace equation on the image domain, with L_i^0 and E_i as equipotential surfaces:

$$\nabla^2 \tau = 0 \quad \text{subj. to} \quad \tau|_{L_i^0} = 0; \quad \tau|_{E_i} = 1 \tag{2}$$

The field $\nabla \tau(x)$ is then integrated along its non-intersecting gradient field lines (or streamlines) from L_i^0 to E_i. Each point $x \in L_i^0$ is assigned the spherical coordinate (θ, ϕ) of the point in E_i at which the streamline traced at x terminates. This yields a coordinate map $\theta(x), \phi(x)$ on L_i^0 (Fig. 2B). We note that this approach is analogous to the spherical shape parameterization strategy in [4], except that [4] used a spherical enclosing boundary (rather than ellipsoid).

Correspondences obtained using gradient flow to the MVEE do not take into account local surface features like curvature, but rather the overall hippocampal shape. As shown for four specimens in Fig. 2C, they appear sensible upon visual inspection. Since our method does not "lock in" these correspondences but uses them as an initial point for groupwise intensity registration (see Sect. 2.6), such approximate correspondence is suitable for our purposes.

Lastly, the spherical coordinates (θ, ϕ) for each subject i are propagated from L_i^0 to the entire image volume Ω. This is done by tracing the streamlines of $\nabla \rho$ from each voxel center $y \in \Omega$ to the endpoint $x_y \in L_i^0$. Voxel y is then assigned a triple of coordinates $\{\rho(y), \theta(x_y), \phi(x_y)\}$, where $\rho(y)$ can be interpreted as the "depth" coordinate (e.g. $0 < \rho < 1$ means y is between L_i^0 and $\mathcal{H}_i$). An example of the resulting image of ρ, θ, ϕ coordinates is plotted in Fig. 2D.

2.6   Groupwise Intensity Registration

Deformable image registration [2] was performed in a groupwise unbiased framework proposed in [9]. Given input images $Z_1 \ldots Z_k$ and initial groupwise template T_0 (initialized as the voxel-wise average of $Z_1 \ldots Z_k$), this iterative approach alternates between performing diffeomorphic registration between $Z_1 \ldots Z_k$ and T_p and updating T_{p+1} as the average of images $Z_1 \ldots Z_k$ warped to T_p. Groupwise registration was applied in three settings:(1) directly to the MRI intensity of

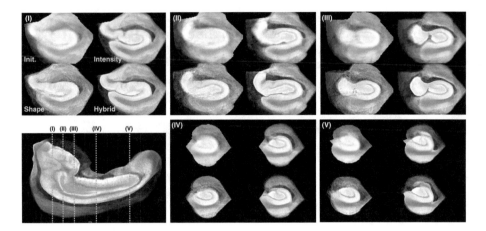

Fig. 3. Coronal slices through the voxel-wise average of ex vivo MRI after initial normalization (labeled Init), and templates created by the intensity-only, shape-only, and hybrid groupwise registration methods.

the ex vivo scans after initial cm-rep normalization; (2) to the coordinate maps ρ, θ, ϕ; (3) to the MRI intensity of ex vivo scans after applying warps obtained by groupwise registration of coordinate maps ρ, θ, ϕ in Method 2. Method 1 is the "reference" intensity-based approach used in [15]. Method 2 is a shape-based method that disregards MRI intensity. Method 3 is the proposed "hybrid" method. The normalized cross-correlation (NCC) metric was used for MRI registration, and the mean square difference metric was used for coordinate map registration; otherwise registration parameters were the same. Template-building ran for 5 iterations. Fig. 3 shows the templates obtained by these three methods. The hybrid method yields the sharpest template.

Table 1 reports mean pairwise agreement between specimens warped into the space of the three templates. Average Dice coefficient for SRLM and hippocampus masks is highest for the shape-based method, followed closely by the hybrid method. This is to be expected, since ρ, θ, ϕ maps are derived directly from SRLM and hippocampus segmentations. The key observation in

Table 1. Metrics of mean pairwise agreement between specimens after groupwise registration with Methods 1–3.

	Hipp Dice	SRLM Dice	MRI NCC
Initial alignment	0.863	0.370	0.169
Intensity (1)	0.884	0.590	0.485
Shape (2)	0.938	0.862	0.351
Hybrid (3)	0.924	0.776	0.552

Table 1 is that *the template created with the hybrid method has greater average intensity similarity between pairs of MRI scans,* as measured by the NCC metric. This suggests that *initialization by surface correspondences yields a better groupwise MRI registration result, although further confirmation of this using expert-placed anatomical landmarks is needed.*

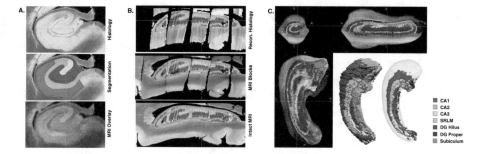

Fig. 4. A. Example histology slice, with manual segmentation, and overlay on the corresponding MRI slice. **B.** Serial histology stacks, reconstructed and aligned to the intact specimen MRI, through the intermediate stage of aligning to 1 cm tissue block MRI. **C.** Distribution of histologically-derived subfield labels in MRI template space obtained by averaging aligned annotations from 8 specimens.

2.7 Mapping Histology to Atlas Space

Interactive software HistoloZee was used to manually label hippocampal subfields in individual histology slices (Fig. 4A) and to reconstruct histology stacks in 3D with MRI as a reference (Fig. 4B). The software tool allows interactive in-plane translation, rotation, scaling, shearing of histology slices, adjustment of histology slice z-spacing, and 3D rigid transformation of the MRI volume. Histology slices were matched in this way to intermediate ex vivo MRI scans of the 1 cm blocks sectioned for histology. The intermediate block MRI scans were registered to the intact specimen MRI scans. These transformations were composed with the transformations from groupwise registration to map histology segmentations of 8 specimens into MRI template space. Figure 4C shows the mean distribution of histologically-derived subfield labels in the MRI template space.

3 Discussion

Contribution. Our ex vivo hippocampus atlas, constructed from 26 MRI specimen scans and 8 dense serial histology datasets, is the largest and most complex such atlas, to our knowledge. In contrast to the large (n = 15) atlas in [7], our atlas incorporates histology, which, according to [11], is the most accurate way to identify subfield boundaries. There are many potential uses of this atlas, including as a prior for in vivo segmentation [7], as an anatomical reference space for analysis of functional MRI data [15], and as a way to relate cytoarchitectonic aspects of hippocampal anatomy to MRI-observable macroscopic features.

Limitations. The surface-volume registration approach was built and evaluated using pseudo-manual segmentation, which is acceptable for the one-time purpose of creating this unique atlas, but problematic for extending the atlas to new specimens. The accuracy of automatic segmentation of SRLM and hippocampus reported in Sect. 2.3 is encouraging, but it remains to be shown that the gains from the surface-based initialization will persist when applied to automatic segmentations. Relatedly, the evaluation of templates in Table 1 is biased in the sense that Dice agreement in same structures that are used to establish correspondence is reported. This does not preclude us from reaching the main conclusion – that leveraging shape helps improve intensity match (NCC metric), but in the future, the use of expert-placed landmarks could help evaluate the method more extensively. Lastly, the proposed groupwise registration strategy did not combine matching of (ρ, θ, ϕ) maps and MRI intensity in the same optimization, but rather performed the two types of registration sequentially. Joint optimization of shape and intensity matching may lead to even better templates.

References

1. Adler, D.H., Pluta, J., Kadivar, S., Craige, C., Gee, J.C., Avants, B.B., Yushkevich, P.A.: Histology-derived volumetric annotation of the human hippocampal subfields in postmortem MRI. Neuroimage **84**, 505–523 (2014)
2. Avants, B., Epstein, C., Grossman, M., Gee, J.: Symmetric diffeomorphic image registration with cross-correlation: evaluating automated labeling of elderly and neurodegenerative brain. Med. Image Anal. **12**, 26–41 (2008)
3. Breiman, L.: Random forests. Mach. Learn. **45**(1), 5–32 (2001)
4. Chung, M.K., Worsley, K.J., Nacewicz, B.M., Dalton, K.M., Davidson, R.J.: General multivariate linear modeling of surface shapes using surfstat. Neuroimage **53**(2), 491–505 (2010)
5. de Flores, R., La Joie, R., Chételat, G.: Structural imaging of hippocampal subfields in healthy aging and Alzheimer's disease. Neuroscience **309**, 29–50 (2015)
6. Frangi, A.F., Niessen, W.J., Vincken, K.L., Viergever, M.A.: Multiscale vessel enhancement filtering. In: Wells, W.M., Colchester, A., Delp, S. (eds.) MICCAI 1998. LNCS, vol. 1496, pp. 130–137. Springer, Heidelberg (1998). doi:10.1007/BFb0056195
7. Iglesias, J.E., Augustinack, J.C., Nguyen, K., Player, C.M., Player, A., Wright, M., Roy, N., Frosch, M.P., McKee, A.C., Wald, L.L., Fischl, B., Van Leemput, K.: Alzheimer's disease neuroimaging initiative: a computational atlas of the hippocampal formation using ex vivo, ultra-high resolution MRI: Application to adaptive segmentation of in vivo MRI. Neuroimage **115**, 117–137 (2015)
8. Jones, S.E., Buchbinder, B.R., Aharon, I.: Three-dimensional mapping of cortical thickness using laplace's equation. Hum. Brain Mapp. **11**(1), 12–32 (2000)
9. Joshi, S., Davis, B., Jomier, M., Gerig, G.: Unbiased diffeomorphic atlas construction for computational anatomy. Neuroimage **23**(Suppl 1), S151–S160 (2004)
10. Small, S., Schobel, S., Buxton, R., Witter, M., Barnes, C.: A pathophysiological framework of hippocampal dysfunction in ageing and disease. Nat. Rev. Neurosci. **12**(10), 585–601 (2011)
11. van Strien, N.M., Widerøe, M., van de Berg, W.D.J., Uylings, H.B.M.: Imaging hippocampal subregions with in vivo MRI: advances and limitations. Nat. Rev. Neurosci. **13**(1), 70 (2012)
12. Todd, M.J., Yıldırım, E.A.: On khachiyan's algorithm for the computation of minimum-volume enclosing ellipsoids. Discrete Appl. Math. **155**(13), 1731–1744 (2007)

13. Wang, H., Suh, J.W., Das, S.R., Pluta, J., Craige, C., Yushkevich, P.A.: Multi-atlas segmentation with joint label fusion. IEEE Trans. Pattern Anal. Mach. Intell. **35**(3), 611–623 (2013)
14. Winterburn, J.L., Pruessner, J.C., Chavez, S., Schira, M.M., Lobaugh, N.J., Voineskos, A.N., Chakravarty, M.M.: A novel in vivo atlas of human hippocampal subfields using high-resolution 3 T magnetic resonance imaging. Neuroimage **74**, 254–265 (2013)
15. Yushkevich, P.A., Avants, B.B., Pluta, J., Das, S., Minkoff, D., Mechanic-Hamilton, D., Glynn, S., Pickup, S., Liu, W., Gee, J.C., Grossman, M., Detre, J.A.: A high-resolution computational atlas of the human hippocampus from postmortem magnetic resonance imaging at 9.4 t. Neuroimage **44**(2), 385–398 (2009)

Deformation Estimation with Automatic Sliding Boundary Computation

Joseph Samuel Preston[3(✉)], Sarang Joshi[1,3], and Ross Whitaker[2,3]

[1] Deptartment of Bioengineering, University of Utah, Salt Lake City, USA
[2] School of Computing, University of Utah, Salt Lake City, USA
[3] Scientific Computing and Imaging (SCI) Institute, University of Utah,
Salt Lake City, USA
{jsam,sjoshi,whitaker}@sci.utah.edu

Abstract. We present a novel method for image registration via a piecewise diffeomorphic deformation which accommodates sliding motion, such as that encountered at organ boundaries. Our method jointly computes the deformation as well as a coherent sliding boundary, represented by a segmentation of the domain into regions of smooth motion. Discontinuities are allowed only at the boundaries of these regions, while invertibility of the total deformation is enforced by disallowing separation or overlap between regions. Optimization alternates between discrete segmentation estimation and continuous deformation estimation. We demonstrate our method on chest 4DCT data showing sliding motion of the lungs against the thoracic cage during breathing.

Keywords: Image registration · Sliding motion · Motion segmentation

1 Introduction

Dense image registration driven by a pointwise dissimilarity term is an ill-posed problem, requiring regularization to produce meaningful results. For medical images, smoothness and invertibility of the resulting deformations have become the standard requirements used to define regularization penalties. This represents assumptions regarding the physical system being modeled – that objects should not appear or disappear, and that nearby points should remain nearby. However, certain anatomical motions violate these assumptions. In particular, many organs are not directly attached to adjacent anatomical structures, but are able to slide freely along a boundary. Most notable in CT imaging is the sliding of the lower lungs against the thoracic cage.

We propose a method for jointly computing a segmentation representing regions of smooth motion, and a set of deformations modeling the motion in each region. Driven by a novel formulation of the sliding constraint as a discrete pairwise penalty, optimization alternates between a graph-cut based estimation of the motion segmentation and a continuous optimization of the constituent deformations. The resulting composite deformation is globally invertible and

© Springer International Publishing AG 2016
S. Ourselin et al. (Eds.): MICCAI 2016, Part III, LNCS 9902, pp. 72–80, 2016.
DOI: 10.1007/978-3-319-46726-9_9

piecewise-smooth. The motion segmentation guarantees that discontinuities due to sliding occur only along coherent boundaries in the image, and the joint estimation of mask and deformations allows anatomical structures to be automatically grouped based on the similarity of their motion.

Previous work has attempted to address the errors caused by using globally smooth deformations to represent lung motion. Wu et al. [11] segment regions and separately register them, while adding a penalty to avoid 'gaps' (or overlaps) in the resulting deformation. Recent work in this area has either required a precomputed segmentation of the sliding boundary (e.g. [2,6]) or used a discontinuity preserving regularization on the deformation (such as Total Variation [10] or Bilateral Filtering [5]), which may introduce spurious discontinuities and does not guarantee the invertibility of the deformation. Vandemeulebroucke et al. [9] give an automated method for creating a 'motion mask' of the anatomy defining the sliding boundaries, but base this on anatomical features, and not the observed motion. Schmidt-Richberg et al. [7] propose a diffusion-based regularization which allows sliding along organ boundaries. Boundaries are either precomputed or estimated based on an ad-hoc measure of deformation discontinuity at precomputed image edge locations. Work from computer vision has also considered motion-based segmentation (e.g. [8]), but the modalities dictate that deformations model occlusion instead of invertibility/sliding. The most similar to our work is [2], which also formulates the sliding conditions in terms of a region segmentation, but assumes a predefined segmentation on one of the images.

2   Methods

We first formulate or registration problem and constraints for a piecewise diffeomorphic deformation $\bar{\phi}$. Given two D-dimensional scalar-valued images $f_0 : \Omega_0 \to \mathbb{R}$ and $f_t : \Omega_t \to \mathbb{R}$ (assigned artificial time indices 0 and t) where $\Omega_0, \Omega_t \subset \mathbb{R}^D$, we attempt to find a deformation $\bar{\phi} : \Omega_t \to \Omega_0$ such that $f_0 \circ \bar{\phi} \approx f_t$, where the dissimilarity is measured by a functional of the form

$$E_{\text{data}}(f_0 \circ \bar{\phi}, f_t) := \int_{\Omega_t} D(f_0(\bar{\phi}(\boldsymbol{x})), f_t(\boldsymbol{x})) \, d\boldsymbol{x}, \tag{1}$$

where $D : \mathbb{R} \times \mathbb{R} \to \mathbb{R}$ is a pointwise dissimilarity term.

Our method formulates piecewise-diffeomorphic deformation $\bar{\phi}$ via K diffeomorphic deformations, $\phi := \{\phi^k\}_{k=1...K}$, $\phi^k : \Omega_t \to \Omega_0$ (where we assume identical codomains Ω_0 for simplicity), and a segmentation $\ell_0 : \Omega_0 \to \{1...K\}$ defining the region over which each deformation has effect.

We define indicator functions of each label as

$$\chi_0^k(\boldsymbol{y}) := \begin{cases} 1 & \text{if } \ell_0(\boldsymbol{y}) = k \\ 0 & \text{otherwise} \end{cases} \tag{2}$$

and the indicator function deformed by the corresponding deformation as

$$\chi_t^k := \chi_0^k \circ \phi^k.$$

We assume that each ϕ^k is diffeomorphic, and therefore invertible. In order to maintain invertibility of the composite deformation we require that it does not result in 'tearing' or 'overlap' between regions. This can be expressed as a pointwise constraint on the sum of indicator functions

$$\sum_{k=1}^{K} \chi_t^k(\boldsymbol{x}) = 1 \quad \forall \, \boldsymbol{x} \in \Omega_t. \tag{3}$$

Intuitively, $\chi_t^k = 1$ asserts that deformation ϕ^k is in effect at point $\boldsymbol{x}$. The constraint stated in terms of the labeling is then *at each* $\boldsymbol{x}$, $\ell_0\left(\phi^k(\boldsymbol{x})\right) = k$ *should be true for exactly one* k. If the statement is not true for any label k, then we have tearing in the deformation at time t, and if it is true for two or more labels we have overlap at this point.

We can now define the segmentation at time t

$$\ell_t(\boldsymbol{x}) := k \;\; s.t. \;\; \chi_t^k(\boldsymbol{x}) = 1 \tag{4}$$

which, for $\boldsymbol{x} \in \Omega_t$, is guaranteed to exist and be unique by (3). We can then define a single piecewise-smooth deformation as

$$\bar{\phi}(\boldsymbol{x}) := \phi^{\ell_t(\boldsymbol{x})}(\boldsymbol{x}). \tag{5}$$

It is easy to verify that $\bar{\phi}(\boldsymbol{x})$ is invertible. It is surjective since each point $\boldsymbol{y} \in \Omega_0$ can be mapped to a point $\boldsymbol{x} \in \Omega_t$ via $\boldsymbol{x} = (\phi^{\ell_0(\boldsymbol{y})})^{-1}(\boldsymbol{y})$ via the invertibility of the constituent deformations, and injective because $\bar{\phi}(\boldsymbol{x})$ s.t. $\boldsymbol{x} \in \chi_t^k$ is a unique mapping among $\hat{\boldsymbol{x}} \in \chi_t^k$ via the invertibility of the constituent deformations, and unique among $\hat{\boldsymbol{x}} \notin \chi_t^k$ as $\hat{\boldsymbol{x}} \notin \chi_t^k$ implies $\chi_0^k(\bar{\phi}(\hat{\boldsymbol{x}})) \neq k$, contradicting $\boldsymbol{x} \in \chi_t^k$.

2.1 Optimization Criteria

We have now given constraints on the labeling ℓ_0 and deformations $\boldsymbol{\phi}$ guaranteeing a piecewise-diffeomorphic deformation, and we choose among these valid deformations by optimizing over a composite objective function that balance the tradeoff between data matching and the regularity of the deformation and labeling

$$\mathrm{E}(\boldsymbol{\phi}, \ell_0) := \mathrm{E}_{\mathrm{data}}(\boldsymbol{\phi}, \ell_0) + \lambda_{\mathrm{per}}\mathrm{E}_{\mathrm{per}}(\ell_0) + \lambda_{\mathrm{pdf}}\mathrm{E}_{\mathrm{pdf}}(\ell_0) + \lambda_{\mathrm{reg}} \sum_{k=1}^{K} \mathrm{E}_{\mathrm{reg}}(\phi^k), \tag{6}$$

where we reformulate the data term (1) as a function of $\boldsymbol{\phi}$ and ℓ_0

$$\mathrm{E}_{\mathrm{data}}(\boldsymbol{\phi}, \ell_0) := \sum_{k=1}^{K} \int_{\Omega_t} \chi_t^k(\boldsymbol{x}) \, \mathrm{D}(\mathrm{f}_0\left(\phi^k(\boldsymbol{x})\right), \mathrm{f}_t(\boldsymbol{x})) \, \mathrm{d}\boldsymbol{x}, \tag{7}$$

and the regularization is taken over each constituent deformation (the form of the deformation regularization $\mathrm{E}_{\mathrm{reg}}$ is dependent on the registration method used).

The term E_{per} is a 'perimeter' penalty on the size of the segmentation boundaries, enforcing the notion that discontinuity should be allowed at a limited set of points. In addition, the penalty E_{pdf} is a region-based intensity segmentation penalty, encouraging the labeling ℓ_0 to segment regions of similar intensity. This helps produce 'anatomically reasonable' results (where segmentations follow organ boundaries) in regions such as the top of the lungs, where no sliding is observed and therefore motion segmentation is ambiguous.

The problem we wish to solve can then be stated as

$$\operatorname*{argmin}_{\phi,\ell_0} E(\phi,\ell_0) \quad s.t. \quad \sum_{k=1}^{K} \chi_t^k(x) = 1 \quad \forall x \in \Omega_t. \tag{8}$$

This is clearly a challenging nonconvex optimization problem. In order to achieve an approximate solution, the hard constraint (3) is relaxed to a penalty,

$$E_{sum}(\phi,\ell_0) := \left\| \sum_{k=1}^{K} \chi_t^k - 1 \right\|_1, \tag{9}$$

We write the relaxed version of (8) as

$$\operatorname*{argmin}_{\phi,\ell_0} E(\phi,\ell_0) + \lambda_{sum} E_{sum}(\phi,\ell_0), \tag{10}$$

and optimization alternates between finding an optimal labeling ℓ_0 for a fixed set of deformations ϕ, and optimizing over ϕ while keeping ℓ_0 fixed. This alternating optimizations do not increase the objective (10) at each step, guaranteeing convergence.

2.2 Segmentation Estimation

In the segmentation estimation step we hold the deformations ϕ fixed and optimize (10) over ℓ_0

$$\operatorname*{argmin}_{\ell_0} E_{data}(\phi,\ell_0) + \lambda_{per} E_{per}(\ell_0) + \lambda_{pdf} E_{pdf}(\ell_0) + \lambda_{sum} E_{sum}(\phi,\ell_0). \tag{11}$$

Note that for a large enough value of λ_{sum}, this becomes a hard constraint; since a single-label segmentation $\mathbf{k}$ s.t. $\mathbf{k}(x) = k \ \forall x$ is guaranteed to satisfy the constraints and also have zero boundary cost ($E_{per}(\mathbf{k}) = 0$), setting $\lambda_{sum} = \min_{\mathbf{k}} (E_{data}(\phi,\mathbf{k})) + \epsilon$ guarantees that the optimal solution satisfies the constraint.

As the segmentation ℓ_0 takes discrete values, we propose a discrete optimization formulation for its estimation. We discretize our problem by defining f_0 and ℓ_0 only on a discrete set of points arranged on a regular grid, $\{y_n\}_{n=1}^{N} \subset \Omega_0$, and similarly define f_t, ℓ_0, ϕ^k, etc. on $\{x_n\}_{n=1}^{N} \subset \Omega_t$. For simplicity we will assume equal numbers of points indexed by n. For interpolation of images linear interpolation is used, and for label images nearest-neighbor interpolation is used. The objective is written as a discrete set of unary and pairwise functions of node labelings which can be solved exactly for binary labelings (K=2), and approximately otherwise, via graph-cut algorithms [3].

The data matching term E_{data} (7) can be written discretely as a unary point-wise penalty on the labeling ℓ_0, as can E_{pdf}. We write E_{pdf} as a negative log likelihood penalty on ℓ_0

$$E_{\text{pdf}}(\ell_0) := -\log(p(f_t|\ell_0)) = -\sum_{n=1}^{N} p(f_t(\boldsymbol{y}_n)|\ell_0(\boldsymbol{y}_n)), \tag{12}$$

where $p(f_t(\boldsymbol{y}_n)|\ell_0(\boldsymbol{y}_n) = k)$ is a kernel density estimate of the distribution of $\{f_t(\boldsymbol{y}_n) \ s.t. \ (\ell_0)^-(\boldsymbol{y}_n) = k\}$, and $(\ell_0)^-$ is the segmentation from the previous iteration. As this penalty is intended only to resolve ambiguous situations, and not lead to an intensity based segmentation, its influence is kept relatively weak.

We now formulate E_{per} and E_{sum} discretely as sums of pairwise terms. For ease of notation when working with label values, we define the functions q : $\{1 \ldots K\} \rightarrow \{0, 1\}$ (and similarly ¬q) for indicating equality (or inequality) of labelings (q for equals):

$$q(i,j) := \begin{cases} 1 & \text{if } i = j \\ 0 & \text{otherwise} \end{cases} \qquad \neg q(i,j) := \begin{cases} 1 & \text{if } i \neq j \\ 0 & \text{otherwise} \end{cases} \tag{13}$$

Our 'perimeter' penalty E_{per} is written as a simple Potts model smoothness term on ℓ_0,

$$E_{\text{per}}(\ell_0) := \sum_{n=1}^{N} \sum_{\boldsymbol{y}_m \in \mathcal{N}(\boldsymbol{y}_n)} \neg q\left(\ell_0(\boldsymbol{y}_n), \ell_0(\boldsymbol{y}_m)\right), \tag{14}$$

where $\mathcal{N}(\boldsymbol{y}_n)$ is a set containing the neighbors of $\boldsymbol{y}_n$, in our case a 4- or 6-connected neighborhood in 2D or 3D, respectively.

We can directly write the discretized version of $E_{\text{sum}}(\boldsymbol{\phi}, \ell_0)$ (9) as the sum of N terms (one associated with each $\boldsymbol{x}_n$), term n taking as inputs the labelings $\{\ell_0\left(\phi^k(\boldsymbol{x}_n)\right)\}_{k=1}^{K}$

$$E_{\text{sum}}(\boldsymbol{\phi}, \ell_0) := \sum_{n=1}^{N} \left| \left(\sum_{k=1}^{K} q\left(\ell_0\left(\phi^k(\boldsymbol{x}_n)\right), k\right) \right) - 1 \right|. \tag{15}$$

Due to nearest-neighbor interpolation of the labeling, each $\ell_0\left(\phi^k(\boldsymbol{x}_n)\right)$ is equivalent to $\ell_0(\boldsymbol{y}_n)$ for some $n \in \{1 \ldots N\}$. However, the K-input terms associated with each point are difficult and costly to optimize over. Instead, we introduce auxiliary variables representing the labeling ℓ_t, and optimize over both ℓ_0 and ℓ_t. Under the sum constraint (9), ℓ_t is uniquely determined via ℓ_0 and $\boldsymbol{\phi}$, so we have not introduced any additional unknowns. However it allows us to rewrite each K-input term in (15) as the sum of K pairwise terms

$$E_{\text{sum}}(\boldsymbol{\phi}, \ell_0, \ell_t) := \sum_{n=1}^{N} \sum_{k=1}^{K} c^k\left(\ell_0\left(\phi^k(\boldsymbol{x}_n)\right), \ell_t(\boldsymbol{x}_n)\right), \tag{16}$$

where $c^k(i,j) := \neg q(q(i,k), q(j,k))$. The function $c^k \left(\ell_0 \left(\phi^k(\boldsymbol{x}_n) \right), \ell_t(\boldsymbol{x}_n) \right)$ indicates whether labels $\ell_0 \left(\phi^k(\boldsymbol{x}_n) \right)$ and $\ell_t(\boldsymbol{x}_n)$ agree that deformation k is (or is not) in effect at $\phi^k(\boldsymbol{x}_n)$. It takes value zero if $\ell_0 \left(\phi^k(\boldsymbol{x}_n) \right) = \ell_t(\boldsymbol{x}_n) = k$ (the labelings agree that $\bar{\phi}(\boldsymbol{x}_n) = \phi^k(\boldsymbol{x}_n)$) or if $\ell_0 \left(\phi^k(\boldsymbol{x}_n) \right) \neq k$ and $\ell_t(\boldsymbol{x}_n) \neq k$ (the labelings agree that $\bar{\phi}(\boldsymbol{x}_n) \neq \phi^k(\boldsymbol{x}_n)$), but takes value 1 if the labelings are in disagreement.

We now have the objective function (11) written as unary (E_{data} and E_{pdf}) and pairwise (E_{per} and E_{sum}) terms on the label values $\ell_0(\boldsymbol{y}_n)$ and $\ell_t(\boldsymbol{x}_n)$, which can be optimized by efficient discrete methods [3].

In practice, the effects of discretization mean that enforcing hard constraints give unsatisfactory results, even if the true deformations are known. Instead, λ_{sum} is chosen to allow some constraint violations. In locations of constraint violation the labeling of ℓ_t is ambiguous, but the given optimization chooses among ambiguous labels by minimizing the data energy.

2.3   Deformation Estimation

In the deformations estimation step, we hold the labeling ℓ_0 fixed and optimize (10) over the deformations ϕ

$$\underset{\phi}{\operatorname{argmin}} \, E_{data}(\phi, \ell_0) + \lambda_{reg} \sum_{k=1}^{K} E_{reg}(\phi^k) + \lambda_{sum} E_{sum}(\phi, \ell_0), \qquad (17)$$

We represent each ϕ^k via a b-spline control grid, and impose additional regularization via $E_{reg}(\phi^k) := \|\nabla \phi^k\|^2$. While invertibility is not guaranteed by this regularization, it can be easily verified. In practice the regularization is significant (as allowed by the piecewise formulation) and the deformations are sufficiently well-behaved that we do not observe noninvertibility during optimization. However, the optimization is agnostic towards the deformation model, and in particular a flow-based diffeomorphic model could be substituted without additional changes.

The L^1 norm in E_{sum} (9) is replaced by a differentiable approximation, and optimization is performed via gradient descent.

2.4   Segmentation Initialization

As we are optimizing a highly nonconvex function, a reasonable initialization is needed. As the goal is to segment deformations along regions of motion discontinuity, we automatically create an initial segmentation which separates regions showing different motion. We first generate a deformation on downsampled versions of the input data enforcing only the anisotropic TV penalty

$$\underset{\nu}{\operatorname{argmin}} \int_{\Omega_t} D(f_0(\boldsymbol{x} + \nu(\boldsymbol{x})), f_t) + \sum_{d=1}^{D} |\nabla_d \nu(\boldsymbol{x})| \, d\boldsymbol{x}, \qquad (18)$$

where ∇_d is the gradient along dimension d.

This penalty results in a discontinuous motion field containing piecewise-constant regions. The elements of ν are then grouped into K clusters using the k-means algorithm, and the cluster labels are then mapped back to the corresponding spatial locations creating an initial segmentation.

3 Results

We test our method on the publicly available DIR-lab dataset [1], which consists of ten 4DCT datasets as well as landmark correspondences. Resolution (voxel size) is $\approx 1 \times 1 \times 2.5$ mm. Datasets 6–10 contain a large volume of empty space around the patient, and were cropped to a region of interest around the patient body. We use a binary motion segmentation ($K = 2$) to represent the breathing motion. A multiscale optimization was used, both on the image resolution and the b-spline grid resolution (two image resolutions, with a total of three b-spline grid refinements for cases 1–5 and four for cases 6–10). Other parameters for both the initialization and optimization steps were empirically chosen, but fixed across all datasets. In order to better register fine features and overcome intensity differences due to density changes in the lung during breathing, we chose a Normalized Gradient Field (NGF) dissimilarity [4] as the pointwise image dissimilarity measure. Figure 1 shows the computed motion segmentation for each dataset. The segmented region includes the lungs as well as regions of visible motion continuing into the organs of the abdominal cavity, while excluding structures such as bone which show little motion. Table 1 gives the landmark errors on these datasets, showing similar results to methods which rely on a precomputed segmentation, or do not guarantee the invertibility of the deformation (average correspondence error of 1.07 mm across all ten datasets, compared to 1.00 mm for method NGF(b) of [4] and 1.01 mm for method pTV of [10]). Figure 2 compares the effect of the piecewise-smooth deformation to that of a single smooth deformation run with the same parameters.

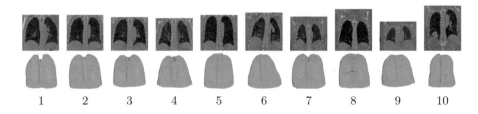

1 2 3 4 5 6 7 8 9 10

Fig. 1. Motion segmentation results for all datasets. Top row shows a coronal slice near the spine with motion mask region highlighted in red. Bottom row shows transparent 3D rendering of this region. Bottom number indicates the dataset. (Color figure online)

Table 1. landmark errors (in millimeters) for the $n = 300$ landmarks defined at the extreme breathing phases for each dataset

dataset	1	2	3	4	5	6	7	8	9	10	ttl
err mean (mm)	0.79	0.79	0.87	1.35	1.25	1.05	1.12	1.22	1.12	1.12	1.07
err std (mm)	0.90	0.95	1.04	1.28	1.53	1.04	1.18	1.26	1.03	1.38	1.17

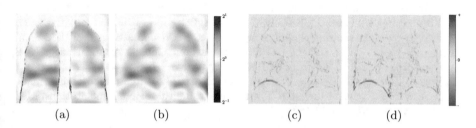

(a)   (b)   (c)   (d)

Fig. 2. Comparison of our piecewise-smooth deformation ((a) and (c)), and a single globally smooth deformation ((b) and (d)), on the DIR-lab dataset 1. The figures on the left show the jacobian determinant of the deformation on a log-scale colormap. Note the clear sliding boundary (dark/red colors where the jacobian is undefined along the tearing boundary) in (a), and the nonphysical deformation of the spine region in (b). On the right are difference images between exhale and deformed inhale for the two methods. Again notice the motion of the spine with a single deformation. (Color figure online)

Acknowledgements. This work was supported in part by NIH R01 CA169102-01A13 and a grant from GE Medical Systems.

References

1. Castillo, R., Castillo, E., Guerra, R., Johnson, V.E., McPhail, T., Garg, A.K., Guerrero, T.: A framework for evaluation of deformable image registration spatial accuracy using large landmark point sets. Phys. Med. Biol. **54**(7), 1849 (2009)
2. Heldmann, S., Polzin, T., Derksen, A., Berkels, B.: An image registration framework for sliding motion with piecewise smooth deformations. In: Aujol, J.-F., Nikolova, M., Papadakis, N. (eds.) SSVM 2015. LNCS, vol. 9087, pp. 335–347. Springer, Heidelberg (2015). doi:10.1007/978-3-319-18461-6_27
3. Kolmogorov, V., Zabin, R.: What energy functions can be minimized via graph cuts? IEEE Trans. Pattern Anal. Mach. Intell. **26**(2), 147–159 (2004)
4. Konig, L., Ruhaak, J.: A fast and accurate parallel algorithm for non-linear image registration using normalized gradient fields. In: 2014 IEEE 11th International Symposium on Biomedical Imaging (ISBI), pp. 580–583. IEEE (2014)
5. Papież, B.W., Heinrich, M.P., Fehrenbach, J., Risser, L., Schnabel, J.A.: An implicit sliding-motion preserving regularisation via bilateral filtering for deformable image registration. Med. Image Anal. **18**(8), 1299–1311 (2014)
6. Risser, L., Vialard, F.X., Baluwala, H.Y., Schnabel, J.A.: Piecewise-diffeomorphic image registration: Application to the motion estimation between 3d ct lung images with sliding conditions. Med. Image Anal. **17**(2), 182–193 (2013)

7. Schmidt-Richberg, A., Werner, R., Handels, H., Ehrhardt, J.: Estimation of slipping organ motion by registration with direction-dependent regularization. Med. Image Anal. **16**(1), 150–159 (2012)
8. Sun, D., Sudderth, E.B., Black, M.J.: Layered segmentation and optical flow estimation over time. In: IEEE CVPR, pp. 1768–1775. IEEE (2012)
9. Vandemeulebroucke, J., Bernard, O., Rit, S., Kybic, J., Clarysse, P., Sarrut, D.: Automated segmentation of a motion mask to preserve sliding motion in deformable registration of thoracic ct. Med. Phys. **39**(2), 1006–1015 (2012)
10. Vishnevskiy, V., Gass, T., Székely, G., Goksel, O.: Total variation regularization of displacements in parametric image registration. In: Yoshida, H., Näppi, J.J., Saini, S. (eds.) Abdominal Imaging: Computational and Clinical Applications. LNCS, vol. 8676, pp. 211–220. Springer, Heidelberg (2014)
11. Wu, Z., Rietzel, E., Boldea, V., Sarrut, D., Sharp, G.C.: Evaluation of deformable registration of patient lung 4DCT with subanatomical region segmentations. Med. Phys. **35**(2), 775–781 (2008)

Bilateral Weighted Adaptive Local Similarity Measure for Registration in Neurosurgery

Martin Kochan[1]([✉]), Marc Modat[1,3], Tom Vercauteren[1], Mark White[1,2],
Laura Mancini[2], Gavin P. Winston[4,5], Andrew W. McEvoy[2],
John S. Thornton[2], Tarek Yousry[2], John S. Duncan[4], Sébastien Ourselin[1,3],
and Danail Stoyanov[1]

[1] Centre for Medical Image Computing,
University College London, London, UK
m.kochan.12@ucl.ac.uk
[2] National Hospital for Neurology and Neurosurgery,
UCLH NHS Foundation Trust, London, UK
[3] Dementia Research Centre, Institute of Neurology,
University College London, London, UK
[4] Department of Clinical and Experimental Epilepsy, Institute of Neurology,
University College London, London, UK
[5] Epilepsy Society MRI Unit, Chesham Lane, Chalfont St Peter, UK

Abstract. Image-guided neurosurgery involves the display of MRI-based preoperative plans in an intraoperative reference frame. Interventional MRI (iMRI) can serve as a reference for non-rigid registration based propagation of preoperative MRI. Structural MRI images exhibit spatially varying intensity relationships, which can be captured by a local similarity measure such as the local normalized correlation coefficient (LNCC). However, LNCC weights local neighborhoods using a static spatial kernel and includes voxels from beyond a tissue or resection boundary in a neighborhood centered inside the boundary. We modify LNCC to use locally adaptive weighting inspired by bilateral filtering and evaluate it extensively in a numerical phantom study, a clinical iMRI study and a segmentation propagation study. The modified measure enables increased registration accuracy near tissue and resection boundaries.

Keywords: Non-rigid registration · Similarity measure · Neurosurgery

1 Introduction

Image-guided neurosurgery involves the display of preoperative anatomy and surgical plans in intraoperative reference frame to increase the accuracy of pathological tissue resection and to reduce damage to the surrounding structures. Preoperative MRI can reveal information such as nerve fiber tracts and brain activation areas. Interventional MRI (iMRI) can image intraoperative deformations due to cerebrospinal fluid (CSF) drainage, gravity and edema (collectively,

S. Ourselin et al. (Eds.): MICCAI 2016, Part III, LNCS 9902, pp. 81–88, 2016.
DOI: 10.1007/978-3-319-46726-9_10

brain shift) [9]. Non-rigid registration of preoperative MRI to intraoperative iMRI enables surgical guidance using propagated preoperative plans [2].

Correspondences missing due to resection present a challenge to the registration. Daga *et al.* [2] estimated brain shift intraoperatively by masking out voxels lying outside a brain mask. However, automated brain extraction such as using FSL-BET [11] can be inaccurate near the resection cavity due to fluid accumulation and surgical gauze in the cavity. Another challenge to registration arises from contrast changes due to CSF drainage, bleeding, edema, MRI bias field and low signal to noise ratio (SNR) of iMRI.

We consider registration of a T1-weighted (T1w) image pair. The local normalized correlation coefficient (LNCC, [1]) captures a local affine intensity relationship. LNCC involves smoothing based on convolution with a Gaussian kernel, which includes voxels located outside a tissue or resection boundary in the statistics of a local neighborhood centered inside the boundary. This potentially reduces the matching specificity near the resection margin.

The *bilateral filter* was introduced for edge-preserving image smoothing and weights the voxels in the local neighborhood based on their spatial distance and intensity difference from the central voxel [13]. Bilateral filtering was used for locally adaptive patch-based similarity cost evaluation in a stereo reconstruction problem [14]: as pixels on a surface tended to have similar colors, the estimated disparity map became more accurate. In a T1w image pair, the voxels from the same tissue tend to have similar intensities and we suggest that bilateral weighting can lead to more accurate brain shift estimation.

We propose to introduce adaptive bilateral weighting into LNCC calculation as illustrated in Fig. 1. We evaluated the modified measure in registration experiments on three datasets and found an improvement in registration accuracy.

2   Methods

2.1   Bilateral Adaptively Weighted LNCC Similarity

LNCC was first used in the context of image registration by [1]. Let R be the reference image and F the floating image in the same coordinate space, then LNCC for the local neighborhood of a point v is defined as

$$\mathrm{LNCC}_v(R, F)^2 = \frac{\langle R, F\rangle_v^2}{\langle R, R\rangle_v \cdot \langle F, F\rangle_v}, \tag{1}$$

where the $\langle R, R\rangle_v$ and $\langle F, F\rangle_v$ are the local variances and $\langle R, F\rangle_v$ is the local covariance. The latter is defined as $\langle R, F\rangle_v = \overline{R \cdot F}_v - \overline{R}_v \cdot \overline{F}_v$, where $\overline{R}_v$ and $\overline{F}_v$ are the respective local means. The local variances are defined analogously. The local mean for R is defined as $\overline{R}_v = \frac{1}{N}\sum_x R(v - x)w_v(x)$, where N is the number of voxels in the neighborhood of v, x is the offset relative to v and $w_v(x)$ are the weights, here given by a generic term that depends on v. The local mean for F is defined analogously.

LNCC uses a Gaussian kernel for the local weights, $w_v(\boldsymbol{x}) = G_\beta(\boldsymbol{x}) = \frac{1}{\sqrt{2\pi}\beta}\exp\left(-\frac{|\boldsymbol{x}|^2}{2\beta^2}\right)$, where β controls the neighborhood's size (negligible for $|\boldsymbol{x}| > 3\beta$). Since $G_\beta(\boldsymbol{x})$ does not depend on $\boldsymbol{v}$, the local mean can be implemented using convolution $\bar{I}_v = (G_\beta * I)(\boldsymbol{v})$.

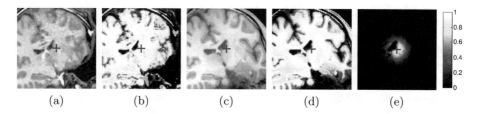

| (a) | (b) | (c) | (d) | (e) |

Fig. 1. (a) T1-weighted reference image and (b) intensity-based weights for a point (blue cross). (c) T1-weighted floating image and (d) intensity-based weights for the point. (e) Final weights based on (b), (d) and distance from the point. (Color figure online)

We introduce bilateral adaptive weighting and refer to the modified measure as LNCC-AW. A bilateral filtered smoothing of an arbitrary image I is

$$\bar{I}_v^{\text{bilat.}} = \frac{1}{N}\sum_{\boldsymbol{x}} I(\boldsymbol{v} - \boldsymbol{x}) \cdot G_\beta(\boldsymbol{x}) \cdot G_\alpha\left(I(\boldsymbol{v} - \boldsymbol{x}) - I(\boldsymbol{v})\right), \tag{2}$$

where $G_\alpha(d)$ is a *range* kernel i.e. a kernel for the intensity difference $d = I(\boldsymbol{v} - \boldsymbol{x}) - I(\boldsymbol{v})$. The edge-preserving property arises as the voxels beyond an intensity rise/drop are excluded. Given images R and F to register, we guide the adaptive weighting by both the images as in [14] by using the composite term

$$w_v(\boldsymbol{x}) = G_\beta(\boldsymbol{x}) \cdot G_\alpha\left(R(\boldsymbol{v} - \boldsymbol{x}) - R(\boldsymbol{v})\right) \cdot G_\alpha\left(F(\boldsymbol{v} - \boldsymbol{x}) - F(\boldsymbol{v})\right) \tag{3}$$

as illustrated in Fig. 1. Since $w_v(\boldsymbol{x})$ vary spatially, we can no longer implement the local mean using convolution nor take advantage of kernel separability.

The low SNR of iMRI can potentially cause the weights of adjacent neighborhoods in homogeneous areas to vary along with the varying intensity of the central voxels. In order to reduce spatial inconsistencies in similarity values, we replace the Gaussian range kernel, as used in [13,14], with a kernel shaped as Student's t-distribution, which down-weights rather than suppresses differing intensities:

$$G_\alpha(d) = \frac{\Gamma(\frac{\nu+1}{2})}{\sqrt{\nu\pi\alpha^2}\Gamma(\frac{\nu}{2})}\left(1 + \frac{d^2}{\nu\alpha^2}\right)^{-\frac{\nu+1}{2}}. \tag{4}$$

We selected $\nu = 2$ as it has a gradual drop-off and provides a trade-off between boundary-preservation and robustness to noise. For $\alpha = \infty$, the weighting reduces to locally non-varying.

2.2   Registration Using a Discrete Optimization Framework

The derivation of analytical gradient of the similarity measure, for instance with respect to a voxel-based deformation field, for use in gradient-based non-rigid registration schemes becomes complicated when using adaptive weighting, because the gradient depends on the local weights which in turn depend on the deformation. However, [4] reformulated non-rigid registration as a discrete Markov Random Field (MRF) optimization problem, for which the similarity measure gradient is not needed. We employ the proposed measure in a related discrete optimization scheme of [6]. A grid $\mathcal{P}$ of B-spline transformation control points $p \in \mathcal{P}$ with positions c_p is overlaid onto the reference image. The control point displacements in the floating image are $u_p = [u_p, v_p, w_p]$ with discrete valued components. For efficiency, a minimum spanning tree $\mathcal{N}$ of the most relevant edges $(p, q) \in \mathcal{N}$ is optimized rather than a full MRF. Displacements are sought minimizing the energy

$$\sum_{p \in \mathcal{P}} \left(1 - \|\text{LNCC}_{c_p}(R(\boldsymbol{\xi}), F(\boldsymbol{\xi} + \boldsymbol{u}_p))\|\right) + \alpha \sum_{(p,q) \in \mathcal{N}} \frac{\|\boldsymbol{u}_p - \boldsymbol{u}_q\|^2}{\|\boldsymbol{x}_p - \boldsymbol{x}_q\|}. \tag{5}$$

3   Experiments

3.1   Patch Matching on 2D Synthetic Phantom

We compare matching accuracy for two 2D synthetic phantoms. We place a fixed patch representing a local neighborhood in the reference image and a moving patch in the floating image to plot the similarity profile of LNCC and LNCC-AW, respectively. We assess two phantoms. A *contrast-enhanced lesion near a resection* phantom is shown in Fig. 2(a–d). The similarity profile for LNCC has a mild maximum at the true zero displacement due to voxels included from the resected area. The similarity profile for LNCC-AW has a clear maximum due voxels down-weighted in the resected area. A phantom of the *medial longitudinal fissure* is shown in Fig. 2(e–h). The reference and floating image are the same axial slice from the BrainWeb database. The patch is centered next to the medial longitudinal fissure that contains dark voxels in the CSF and the falx cerebri. The similarity profile for LNCC has a band of false matches due to voxels included in the fissure. The similarity profile for LNCC-AW has a unique maximum at the true zero displacement due to these voxels being down-weighted.

3.2   Recovery of a 3D Synthetic Deformation

We perform a registration experiment on a BrainWeb dataset. The reference image is made by inserting a synthetic resection cavity in the right temporal lobe. The floating image is resampled using B-spline interpolation from the BrainWeb image using a synthetic sinusoidal deforming field (period 100 mm in all directions, displacement amplitude 4 mm). The voxel intensities are normalized to

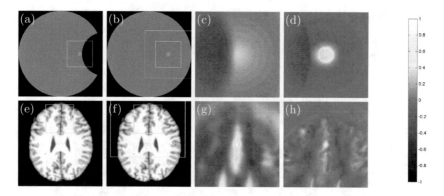

Fig. 2. 2D numerical phantoms. (a–d) A contrast-enhanced lesion near a resection. (e–h) Medial longitudinal fissure. (a, e) Reference image. The outline shows the fixed patch. (b, f) Floating image. The inner and outer outline show the moving patch at zero and maximum displacement, respectively. (c, g) Similarity profile of LNCC as a function of displacement. (d, h) Same for LNCC-AW.

0–1 range. We use 5 discrete registration grid levels with grid spacing (7, 6, 5, 4 and 3 voxels), search radius (6, 5, 4, 3 and 2 control point grid spacings) and discretization step (5, 4, 3, 2 and 1 voxels). The floating image is updated between levels using B-spline interpolation. We run the scheme for LNCC ($\beta = 5\,\mathrm{mm}$) and twice for LNCC-AW ($\beta = 5\,\mathrm{mm}, \alpha = 0.30$ and $\alpha = 0.10$).

We quantify registration accuracy using landmarks found in the reference using 3D-SIFT [12]. We include 43 landmarks from a 2 cm region from the resection margin. We propagate the landmarks using the true and recovered deformations. The target registration error (TRE) is shown in Fig. 3(c). TRE for LNCC-AW is significantly lower (for both $\alpha = 0.30$ and $\alpha = 0.10$) than for LNCC (paired t-tests, $p < 0.001$). The log of Jacobian determinant maps for true and recovered deformations are shown in Fig. 3(d–g). The deformations recovered using LNCC-AW follow the true deformation closer than using LNCC.

3.3   Evaluation on an iMRI Surgical Dataset

We validate the measure on 12 cases of anterior temporal lobe resection. The dataset is described in [2]. We skull-strip the pre- and the intraoperative image, normalize the 1st–99th intensity percentile linearly to the range 0–1, crop the intraoperative image to only contain the brain, resample the intraoperative image to a resolution $1.1 \times 1.1 \times 1.1\,\mathrm{mm}$ and register the preoperative image affinely to the intraoperative reference [8]. We use the bilateral filter as per Eq. 2 on the reference and floating image pair in order to generate a guidance image pair using settings ($\beta = 2.2\,\mathrm{mm}, \alpha = 0.03$) that we found to produce a mild smoothing in homogeneous areas whilst preserving edges. We perform a non-rigid registration for LNCC ($\beta = 5.5\,\mathrm{mm}$) and two non-rigid registrations for LNCC-AW ($\beta = 5.5\,\mathrm{mm}, \alpha = 0.30$ and $\alpha = 0.10$), using the guidance image

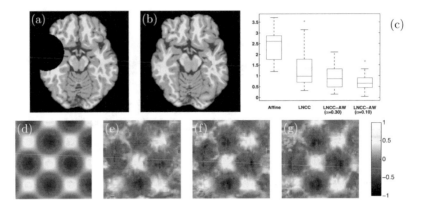

Fig. 3. Axial view of 3D BrainWeb based phantom. (a) Reference image (inserted resection). (b) Floating image (synthetic deformation). (c) Target registration error. (d) Map of log Jacobian determinant for ground truth deformation (forward field). (e) Same map for fields recovered using LNCC, (f) LNCC-AW with $\alpha = 0.30$ and (g) LNCC-AW with $\alpha = 0.10$.

pair to construct the weights in Eq. 3. The discrete optimization parameters are identical as in Sect. 3.2 (in voxels). The registration takes approx. 10 h per subject using 4 threads on a computing cluster node.

For each case, we annotate 50–60 landmarks pairs in the pre/intraoperative image a few cm from the resection margin. We propagate the landmarks using the recovered deformations. The mean TRE for all cases is shown in Fig. 4(a) and is significantly lower for registrations based on LNCC-AW with $\alpha = 0.30$ (paired t-test, $p = 0.0236$) and LNCC-AW with $\alpha = 0.10$ ($p = 0.0054$), respectively, than for registrations based on LNCC. The effect size is below the image resolution, potentially as few reliably identifiable landmark pairs exist near the resection margin. We evaluate the smoothness of the recovered deformations and assess the absolute log Jacobian determinant maps in a region of interest (ROI) in the brain less than 2 cm from the base of the resection cavity (located in iMRI). The means within the ROI are shown in Fig. 4(b) and are significantly lower for LNCC-AW with $\alpha = 0.30$ (paired t-test, $p = 0.0133$) and for LNCC-AW with $\alpha = 0.10$ ($p < 0.001$), respectively, than for LNCC.

3.4   Segmentation Propagation Experiment

We explore how the adaptive weighting affects registration accuracy for brain structures. We use a database of 35 T1w scans with parcellations of 140 key structures provided by Neuromorphometrics for the MICCAI 2012 Grand Challenge and Workshop on Multi-Atlas Labeling[1]. We normalize image intensities and use each image as a reference image and the remaining images as floating images. For

---

[1] https://masi.vuse.vanderbilt.edu/workshop2012/index.php/Challenge_Details.

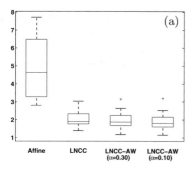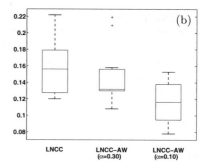

Fig. 4. Registration results for 12 iMRI cases. (a) Target registration error. (b) Mean (in vicinity of the resection) of abs. log Jacobian determinant map.

each of the 1190 image pairs, we perform affine registration and non-rigid registrations using LNCC ($\beta = 5\,\text{mm}$) and LNCC-AW ($\beta = 5\,\text{mm}, \alpha = 0.10$ only) using discrete registration parameters as above. We propagate the floating image segmentations using nearest-neighbor interpolation and calculate Dice score for each label. The average Dice score for 1190 affine registration image pairs is 0.422 ± 0.00187, for LNCC based non-rigid registrations it is 0.517 ± 0.0101 and for LNCC-AW based registrations it is 0.526 ± 0.00947. Average Dice score is significantly higher when using LNCC-AW than LNCC ($p < 10^{-6}$).

4   Discussion and Conclusion

We introduced bilateral adaptive weighting into a local similarity measure (LNCC). The modification facilitated a more accurate landmark localization in several T1w registration experiments. In a study on clinical iMRI data, we recovered a smoother deformation near the resection margin, which is biomechanically more plausible and potentially enables more accurate guidance near the resection margin. The brain shift we assessed arose from CSF leakage and postural drainage, but in principle our approach can improve accuracy near distinct intensity edges at margins of tumors, collapsed cysts or haematomas from bleeding into the brain, which should be confirmed in a future study.

Unoptimized bilateral weighting introduces a time bottleneck that precludes intraoperative application. We note that the discrete optimization steps collectively take approx. one minute. However, powerful options are open toward optimizing the bilateral weighting, such as guided image filtering [5]. The proposed method could be extended to a multi-channel local similarity measure such as LCCA [7]. A related approach to ours is to constrain the deforming field using bilateral filtering [10] and a unified scheme should be investigated. The analytical gradient could potentially be derived using the approach of [3].

Acknowledgments. This work was part funded by the Wellcome Trust (WT101957, WT106882, 201080/Z/16/Z), the Engineering and Physical Sciences Research Council (EPSRC grants EP/N013220/1, EP/N022750/1, EP/N027078/1, NS/A000027/1) and the National Institute for Health Research University College London Hospitals Biomedical Research Centre (NIHR BRC UCLH/UCL High Impact Initiative). MK is supported by the UCL Doctoral Training Programme in Medical and Biomedical Imaging studentship funded by the EPSRC (EP/K502959/1). MM is supported by the UCL Leonard Wolfson Experimental Neurology Centre (PR/ylr/18575) and received further funding from Alzheimer's Society (AS-PG-15-025). GPW is supported by MRC Clinician Scientist Fellowship (MR/M00841X/1). DS receives further funding from the EU-Horizon2020 project EndoVESPA (H2020-ICT-2015-688592).

References

1. Cachier, P., Bardinet, E., Dormont, D., Pennec, X., Ayache, N.: Iconic feature based nonrigid registration: the PASHA algorithm. Comput. Vis. Image Underst. **89**(2), 272–298 (2003)
2. Daga, P., Winston, G., Modat, M., White, M., Mancini, L., Cardoso, M.J., Symms, M., Stretton, J., McEvoy, A.W., Thornton, J., Micallef, C., Yousry, T., Hawkes, D.J., Duncan, J.S., Ourselin, S.: Accurate localization of optic radiation during neurosurgery in an interventional MRI suite. IEEE Trans. Med. Imaging **31**(4), 882–891 (2012)
3. Darkner, S., Sporring, J.: Locally orderless registration. IEEE Trans. Pattern Anal. Mach. Intell. **35**(6), 1437–1450 (2013)
4. Glocker, B., Komodakis, N., Tziritas, G., Navab, N., Paragios, N.: Dense image registration through MRFs and efficient linear programming. Med. Image Anal. **12**(6), 731–741 (2008)
5. He, K., Sun, J., Tang, X.: Guided image filtering. IEEE Trans. Pattern Anal. Mach. Intell. **35**(6), 1397–1409 (2013)
6. Heinrich, H., Jenkinson, M., Brady, M., Schnabel, J.: MRF-based deformable registration and ventilation estimation of lung CT. IEEE Trans. Med. Imaging **32**(7), 1239–1248 (2013)
7. Heinrich, M.P., Papież, B.W., Schnabel, J.A., Handels, H.: Multispectral image registration based on local canonical correlation analysis. In: Golland, P., Hata, N., Barillot, C., Hornegger, J., Howe, R. (eds.) MICCAI 2014. LNCS, vol. 8673, pp. 202–209. Springer, Heidelberg (2014). doi:10.1007/978-3-319-10404-1_26
8. Modat, M., Cash, D.M., Daga, P., Winston, G.P., Duncan, J.S., Ourselin, S.: Global image registration using a symmetric block-matching approach. J. Med. Imaging **1**(2), 024003–024003 (2014)
9. Nimsky, C., Ganslandt, O., Cerny, S., Hastreiter, P., Greiner, G., Fahlbusch, R.: Quantification of, visualization of, and compensation for brain shift using intraoperative magnetic resonance imaging. Neurosurgery **47**(5), 1070–1080 (2000)
10. Papież, B.W., Heinrich, M.P., Fehrenbach, J., Risser, L., Schnabel, J.A.: An implicit sliding-motion preserving regularisation via bilateral filtering for deformable image registration. Med. Image Anal. **18**(8), 1299–1311 (2014)
11. Smith, S.M.: Fast robust automated brain extraction. Hum. Brain Mapp. **17**(3), 143–155 (2002)
12. Toews, M., Wells, W.M.: Efficient and robust model-to-image alignment using 3D scale-invariant features. Med. Image Anal. **17**(3), 271–282 (2013)
13. Tomasi, C., Manduchi, R.: Bilateral filtering for gray and color images. In: Sixth International Conference on Computer Vision, 1998, pp. 839–846. IEEE (1998)
14. Yoon, K.J., Kweon, I.S.: Adaptive support-weight approach for correspondence search. IEEE Trans. Pattern Anal. Mach. Intell. **28**(4), 650–656 (2006)

Model-Based Regularisation for Respiratory Motion Estimation with Sparse Features in Image-Guided Interventions

Matthias Wilms$^{(\boxtimes)}$, In Young Ha, Heinz Handels, and Mattias Paul Heinrich

Institute of Medical Informatics, University of Lübeck, Lübeck, Germany
`wilms@imi.uni-luebeck.de`

Abstract. Intra-interventional respiratory motion estimation has become vital for image-guided interventions, especially radiation therapy. While real-time tracking of highly discriminative landmarks like tumours and markers is possible with classic approaches (e.g. template matching), their robustness decreases when used with non-ionising imaging (4D MRI or US). Furthermore, they ignore the motion of neighbouring structures. We address these challenges by dividing the computation of dense deformable registration in two phases: First, a low-parametric full domain patient-specific motion model is learnt. Second, a sparse subset of feature locations is used to track motion locally, while the global motion patterns are constrained by the learnt model. In contrast to previous work, we optimise both objectives (local similarity and globally smooth motion) jointly using a coupled convex energy minimisation. This improves the tracking robustness and leads to a more accurate global motion estimation. The algorithm is computationally efficient and significantly outperforms classic template matching-based dense field estimation in 12 of 14 challenging 4D MRI and 4D ultrasound sequences.

1 Introduction

Effective respiratory motion compensation is a key factor for successful non-invasive radiotherapy or High Intensity Focused Ultrasound (HIFU) treatments of thoracic and abdominal tumours. Recent advances in imaging technologies have led to the integration of 4D (3D+t) ultrasound (US)- and magnetic resonance imaging (MRI)-guidance into HIFU and radiation therapy [1–3]. Compared to traditional motion management using external breathing signals or X-ray projections, this opens up new possibilities for accurate intra-fraction motion estimation. However, the intra-interventional images need to be processed in real-time to control the treatment beam, which excludes the use of accurate but computationally demanding deformable image registration approaches.

Most published methods for online respiratory motion estimation based on temporal MRI or US have limitations compared to traditional deformable image registration algorithms (see [4] for an overview on US tracking). A common shortcoming is the use of template matching [5–7], which only focuses on a direct

© Springer International Publishing AG 2016
S. Ourselin et al. (Eds.): MICCAI 2016, Part III, LNCS 9902, pp. 89–97, 2016.
DOI: 10.1007/978-3-319-46726-9_11

tracking of the tumour or sparse landmarks (markers, vessels, ...) and ignores the spatial regularity of organ motion. These approaches achieve high computational speed with good accuracy for the specified template location, but do not provide an estimate of the motion of other structures, which requires dense estimation of displacements (e.g. using [8]). Dense displacement fields for the full patient body can then be reconstructed from the sparse motion vectors using trained motion models [7,9–12]. So far, sparse feature point matching and dense motion field reconstruction have been often treated as separate disconnected tasks (see e.g. [7,10]). We, however, think that prior knowledge about respiratory motion should and can be incorporated into the sparse motion estimation step for improved robustness and accuracy without substantially increasing the computation time.

We propose a novel, robust, and efficient model-based method for online respiratory motion estimation in image-guided interventions that jointly combines local similarity-based block matching for sparse feature points with a global patient-specific statistical motion model for regularisation. The resulting minimisation problem is efficiently solved using ideas from discrete coupled convex optimisation for image registration [13]. This enables the use of very sparsely distributed feature vectors and achieves highly accurate dense displacement fields for complex respiratory motion (including a natural handling of sliding motion). Our approach is (to our knowledge) the first non-linear respiratory motion estimation approach that jointly optimises sparse feature point matching and model-based regularisation with computationally fast discrete optimisation techniques. In previous work on the joint use of image data and model-based regularisation, authors either use all the image data available [8,14] instead of sparse features, perform gradient descent-based optimisation [14], only estimate affine transformations [14], and/or only compute 2D motion vectors [8].

2   Method

Although being independent of the imaging modality used, we will describe our method in an MRI-guided radiotherapy scenario for ease of understanding. Modern integrated MRI linear accelerators are able to acquire (multiple) 2D slices of the moving patient anatomy in real-time during the treatment [1].

Given a static 3D reference image $I_R : \Omega \to \Omega$ $(\Omega \subset \mathbb{R}^3)$ depicting the region of interest at a reference time point, our goal is to determine a transformation $\varphi_t = Id + u_t : \Omega \to \Omega$ that describes the deformation of the structures in I_R at treatment time t based on the 2D or 3D moving image frame(s) $I_{M,t} : \Omega \to \mathbb{R}$ provided by the treatment system. Here, u_t represents a dense displacement field.

For computational efficiency, we initially restrict the motion estimation process to a sparse set of N feature points $\Omega_N = \{\mathbf{x}_1, \ldots, \mathbf{x}_N\}$, within the reference image. Our method aims to find an optimal sparse displacement field $\tilde{u}_t$ defined at these feature points, which minimises a cost function $E(\tilde{u}_t)$:

$$E(\tilde{u}_t) = \sum_{\Omega_N} \mathcal{D}(I_R, I_{M,t}, \tilde{u}_t) + \alpha \mathcal{R}(\tilde{u}_t). \tag{1}$$

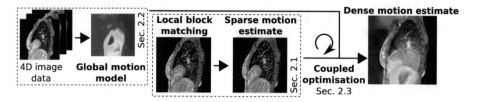

Fig. 1. Graphical overview of the proposed model-based method for respiratory motion estimation that combines local block matching with a global motion model.

Here, $\mathcal{D}$ quantifies the point-wise (dis)similarity between $I_R(\mathbf{x})$ and $I_{R,t}(\mathbf{x} + \tilde{u}_t(\mathbf{x}))$ around locations $\mathbf{x}$ and $\mathcal{R}$ is a regularisation term, which penalises deviations of $\tilde{u}_t$ from plausible solutions and is weighted by α.

In this work, $\mathcal{D}$ is based on the self-similarity context descriptor (SSC, cf. Sec. 2.1) [15] and $\mathcal{R}$ is derived from a patient-specific motion model (cf. Sec. 2.2), which is used both for regularisation and the final reconstruction of the dense displacement field u_t given a sparse estimate $\tilde{u}_t$. Minimising the joint cost function Eq. 1 is difficult due to its non-linear dependency on $\tilde{u}_t$. We, therefore, propose an efficient coupled convex discrete optimisation approach (cf. Sec. 2.3), which alternately optimises over the dissimilarity distribution of the local sparse block-matching and the global model-based regularisation (see Fig. 1 for a graphical overview).

2.1 Sparse Feature Point Detection and Similarity-Driven Block Matching

The feature points Ω_N are automatically selected in the reference image I_R using the Harris/Foerstner corner detector [16] (alternatively, manually defined landmarks could also be employed). The tracking of Ω_N is based on the self-similarity context descriptor (SSC) [15], which has been chosen for its insensitivity to local changes in image contrast and to image noise as these effects regularly degrade the quality of interventional images. Furthermore, based on quantised SSC descriptors SSC_R and $SSC_{M,t}$ it allows the definition of a L_1 metric [15]

$$\mathcal{D}(\mathbf{x}_i, \mathbf{y}_{i,t}) = \frac{1}{|\mathcal{P}|} \sum_{p \in \mathcal{P}} \Xi\{SSC_R(\mathbf{x}_i + p) \oplus SSC_{M,t}(\mathbf{y}_{i,t} + p)\}. \tag{2}$$

$\mathcal{D}$ assesses the similarity of the image contents at feature point $\mathbf{x}_i$ in I_R and its potentially corresponding location $\mathbf{y}_{i,t} = \mathbf{x}_i + \mathbf{d}_{i,t}$ in $I_{M,t}$, which can be efficiently computed in Hamming space using an XOR operator $\oplus$ followed by a bit count Ξ. $\mathbf{d}_{i,t}$ denotes a displacement vector out of a predefined set of 3D displacements $\mathcal{L}$ (chosen according to the expected motion magnitude). Here, $\mathcal{P}$ is a local 3D block around each location $\mathbf{x}_i$ or $\mathbf{y}_i$ for which a block sum is formed. Using an unrestricted block-matching (minimising Eq. 1 with $\alpha = 0$), the optimal displacement $\hat{\mathbf{d}}_{i,t}$ could be directly obtained, resulting in a sparse displacement field $\tilde{u}_t$. This outcome might, however, be highly irregular.

2.2   Patient-Specific Motion Model Building

In addition to the reference image I_R, we expect a patient-specific dynamic 4D MRI data set $\{I_j\}_{j \in \{1,...,M\}}$ covering a small number of breathing cycles to be available prior to the intervention to build a statistical motion model. In practise, this data could be acquired during a short set-up phase.

First, all M images $I_j \in \Omega \to \mathbb{R}$ are nonlinearly registered to the reference image I_R, resulting in a set of displacement fields $\{u_j\}_{j \in \{1,...,M\}}$. While being independent of the registration approach in principle, we chose the fast *deeds* algorithm [17], as it has demonstrated high accuracy in respiratory motion estimation tasks, and is able to correctly handle sliding motion.

Second, a principal components analysis (PCA) is applied to the vectorised displacement fields $\mathbf{u}_j \in \mathbb{R}^{3V}$ (V denotes the number of image voxels) to obtain a low-parametric representation of the space of plausible displacement fields. PCA is a widely used technique for respiratory motion modelling [7,9–11] and can be performed using an eigendecomposition of the sample covariance matrix

$$\mathbf{C} = \frac{1}{M} \sum_{j=1}^{M} (\mathbf{u}_j - \bar{\mathbf{u}})(\mathbf{u}_j - \bar{\mathbf{u}})^T = \mathbf{P}\mathbf{\Lambda}\mathbf{P}^T \quad , \text{ with } \bar{\mathbf{u}} = \frac{1}{M} \sum_{j=1}^{M} \mathbf{u}_j. \qquad (3)$$

The columns of the orthonormal matrix $\mathbf{P} \in \mathbb{R}^{3V \times 3V}$ are the eigenvectors of $\mathbf{C}$ and the diagonal elements of diagonal matrix $\mathbf{\Lambda} = diag(\lambda_1, \ldots, \lambda_{3V}) \in \mathbb{R}^{3V \times 3V}$ are the corresponding eigenvalues in descending order. Aiming at a low-parametric representation of the space of plausible displacement fields, only the eigenvectors with the k largest eigenvalues that explain a certain percentage of variance (here: 95%) are retained. Displacement fields belonging to the space spanned by a reduced $\mathbf{P}_k \in \mathbb{R}^{3V \times k}$ can be generated by $\mathbf{u} = \bar{\mathbf{u}} + \mathbf{P}_k \mathbf{\Sigma}_k \mathbf{b}$, with weights $\mathbf{b} \in \mathbb{R}^k$ and diagonal matrix $\mathbf{\Sigma}_k = diag(\sqrt{\lambda_1}, \ldots, \sqrt{\lambda_k})$. We aim to find an optimal weight vector $\mathbf{b}$ that reconstructs a dense displacement field vector $\mathbf{u}$ based on the sparse (vectorised) displacements $\tilde{\mathbf{u}}_t$. This can be achieved by minimising the ridge regression-like cost function [7,12]:

$$E(\mathbf{b}) = \|\tilde{\mathbf{P}}_k \mathbf{\Sigma}_k \mathbf{b} - (\tilde{\mathbf{u}}_t - \bar{\mathbf{u}})\|_2^2 + \eta \|\mathbf{b}\|_2^2. \qquad (4)$$

Here, matrix $\tilde{\mathbf{P}}_k \in \mathbb{R}^{3N \times k}$ only contains the $3N$ elements of the k eigenvectors that correspond to the elements present in the sparse displacement field $\tilde{u}_t/\tilde{\mathbf{u}}_t$. The regularised least-squares cost (Eq. 4) balances a close estimate of the observed sparse motion and deviations from the mean motion due to noise and has been frequently used to reconstruct dense displacement fields (e.g. in [7,10,11]).

2.3   Coupled Convex Optimisation of Model-Based Regularisation

The displacement vectors $\hat{\mathbf{d}}_{i,t}$ obtained independent of each other using an unconstrained block-matching search (Eq. 1 with $\alpha = 0$) will contain erroneous estimates for challenging data. The ridge regression (Eq. 4 with $\eta > 0$) can dampen these errors but may reduce the overall accuracy of the densely reconstructed field. It will therefore be advantageous to minimise the block-matching dissimilarity and the model-penalty jointly (see Eq. 1). Due to the nonlinear dependency on $\tilde{u}_t$, directly minimising Eq. 1 is difficult. Following [13], a good approximation to the global optimum can be obtained in few iterations by adding a coupling term $\|\tilde{u}_t - \tilde{v}_t\|_2^2$ to Eq. 1 and introducing an auxiliary vector $\tilde{v}_t$:

$$E(\tilde{u}_t, \tilde{v}_t) = \sum_{\Omega_N} \mathcal{D}(I_R, I_{M,t}, \tilde{u}_t) + \theta\|\tilde{u}_t - \tilde{v}_t\|_2^2 + \alpha\mathcal{R}(\tilde{v}_t) \tag{5}$$

The optimisation of Eq. 5 is initialised with results of the unconstrained (here: $\theta{=}0$) block-matching search $\tilde{u}_t$, which is used to estimate a first regularised sparse field $\tilde{v}_t$ by projecting $\tilde{u}_t$ to the space spanned by the model using Eq. 4. The weighting parameter α in Eq. 5 is implicitly set through the number of eigenvectors k used to form $\mathbf{P}_k$. This alternating scheme is iterated using a series of increasing values of θ. During this process, the two objectives are encouraged to converge to a similar optimum, while updated estimates of $\tilde{u}_t$ (including the non-zero coupling term) make use of the full distribution of block-matching dissimilarities $\mathcal{D}$ of Eq. 2 (Eq. 2 only has to be computed once). In contrast to [13], which used an unspecific Gaussian regularisation, our approach elegantly incorporates both local uncertainty information from sparse feature points and a global domain-specific motion model. This enables us to estimate complex dense motion very efficiently and avoid the negative influence of errors from an unconstrained block-matching. Note, that this method will correctly estimate sliding motion, if it was present in the training data. We have used 6 iterations of the optimisation scheme in our experiments with $\theta = \{0.5, 1.5, 2.5, 10, 50, 100\}$.

Furthermore, prior knowledge of temporally smooth motion can be included by adding a second regularisation term $\beta\|\tilde{u}_t - \tilde{u}_{t-1}\|_2^2$ to Eq. 5 that penalises

Table 1. Mean estimation errors with respect to the ground-truth displacement fields obtained for the different approaches applied on the 4D MRI and US data. Results are given as mean ± standard deviation in mm over all patients and frames included in each collection. The first row gives the error for all body voxels while the second row lists only the errors at the feature point locations. For the MRI data, results at voxels with large mean motion (>80th percentile of each case) are given for comparison (3rd row).

Data	Motion	GT recon.	BM $\eta = 0$	BM $\eta > 0$	Model-based	Model & temporal
4D MRI experiments						
All voxels	1.76 ± 0.39	0.74 ± 0.26	1.76 ± 0.38	1.09 ± 0.31	0.87 ± 0.26	**0.87±0.26**
Feature pts.	1.70 ± 0.40	0.57 ± 0.14	1.28 ± 0.31	0.90 ± 0.34	0.69 ± 0.15	**0.69±0.15**
Large mot.	4.48 ± 1.21	1.31 ± 0.56	3.12 ± 0.75	2.01 ± 0.48	1.64 ± 0.66	**1.66±0.67**
4D US experiments						
All voxels	4.22 ± 1.14	1.07 ± 0.27	7.29 ± 1.59	2.82 ± 0.89	2.20 ± 0.81	**1.86±0.64**
Feature pts.	3.82 ± 1.40	0.66 ± 0.28	4.19 ± 1.29	2.48 ± 1.03	1.77 ± 0.84	**1.38±0.57**

deviations of motion vectors compared to the previous frame in the sequence. The weighting parameter β should be chosen according to the expected inter-frame differences of the motion and the image noise level (here: $\beta = \{0, 0, 0, 0, 5, 10\}$).

3   Experiments and Results

Experiments on 5 thoracic/abdominal 4D MRI data sets and 9 liver 4D US data sets are performed to show the benefits of our new model-based respiratory motion estimation approach when compared to separate block matching and dense displacement field reconstruction. The 14 4D data sets are used to mimic the online motion estimation process in MR/US-guided treatment scenarios. A subset of each data set is used to train a patient-specific motion model while the remaining images serve as intra-interventional data.

Data: The 4D MRI data collection contains 3 data sets from our own fund and 2 publicly available data sets [11]. Each sequence consists of 157 – 200 3D images (see Fig. 1 for example slices) acquired with a temporal resolution of 200 – 500 ms, an isotropic in-plane spatial resolution of 1.2 – 3.9 mm, and an inter-slice distance of 5 – 10 mm. The 4D US data collection used here is a subset (data sets SMT-01 – 09) of the CLUST challenge data [4][1]. Each data set consists of 96 – 97 3D frames acquired at 8Hz with an isotropic spatial resolution of 0.70mm.

Experimental Design: The first image in each MRI/US sequence is chosen as the reference image for an inter-sequence registration using *deeds* (cf. Sec. 2.2). The first third (MRI)/half (US) of the resulting displacement fields are used to build the patient-specific motion models. The remaining fields serve as ground-truth data for the quantitative evaluation. Their accuracy was evaluated on a subset of the data with a small number of manually defined landmarks. Landmark errors were in the range of 1mm (MRI, in-plane)/1 – 2mm (US) for landmarks with an average mean motion of 4 mm (MRI)/6 mm (US).

Our model-based algorithm is then employed to estimate the motion between the reference image and each image not used for model formation based on 250 – 300 (MRI)/70 – 80 (US) automatically determined feature points (cf. Sec. 2.1). For the MRI data, feature point selection and block matching are restricted to 5 – 10 equidistantly spaced 2D slices to simulate the sparse data acquired by an MR scanner during the treatment. We quantitatively assess the estimation accuracy by computing mean vector differences between the estimated fields and the ground-truth fields for all inner-body voxels/feature point locations. Due to the large inter-slice distances out-of-plane motion is ignored for MRI data sets.

Results: The results of our experiments are summarised in Table 1. In addition to two versions of our algorithm (model-based regularisation and model-based regularisation + temporal constraint (cf. Sec. 2.3)), Table 1 list results for an unrestricted block matching followed by a dense field reconstruction (BM) with

---

[1] We thank the CLUST challenge organisers for providing the US data.

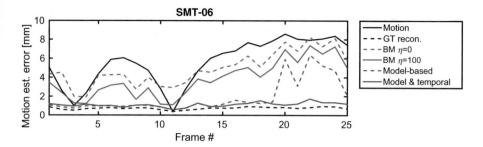

Fig. 2. Mean motion estimation errors obtained for different frames of the SMT-06 US data set at the feature point locations. The advantage of the model-based regularisation with additional temporal constraint is clearly seen starting from frame 20.

$\eta = 0$/optimised $\eta > 0$ (cf. Eq. 4, [7]). The η parameter controls the amount of regularisation during least-squares fitting and was patient-specifically optimised with respect to the mean error over all frames. For comparison, the motion to be compensated and the error obtained by performing an optimal model-based least-squares reconstruction of the dense ground-truth field (GT recon.) is given.

From Table 1 and Fig. 2, it can be seen that the unrestricted BM with $\eta = 0$ leads to unsatisfactory results due to large outliers present in the sparse field. Their effect is substantially reduced by using $\eta > 0$ for dense field reconstruction. Including our proposed coupled optimisation with model-based regularisation outperforms both BM approaches ($\eta = 0$ & $\eta > 0$) in a statistically significant way (paired t-test, $p < 0.05$) in 86 % of the cases (12 of 14). The differences in Table 1 between BM ($\eta = 0$ & $\eta > 0$) and model-based regularisation for the US experiments are also statistically significant, whereas the differences for the MRI experiments and $\eta > 0$ are not. Table 1 and Fig. 2 also show the advantages of incorporating the temporal constraint into the optimisation for the US experiments due to the low image quality that leads to severe inter-frame differences. Computationally, our approach needs 0.5–4 s to process each frame on a six-core Xeon CPU. Most of the time is spent for the BM and the SSC descriptor calculations, which could be easily transferred to the GPU with substantial speed-up, whereas the overhead for the coupled optimisation is minimal.

4   Conclusion

In this work, a novel model-based method for online respiratory motion estimation in image-guided interventions has been presented. The approach combines local similarity-based block matching for sparse feature points and a global motion model for regularisation. The resulting cost function is efficiently minimised by using a coupled convex discrete optimisation scheme. Our experiments show that this approach significantly outperforms decoupled template matching and dense motion field reconstruction methods implemented in the same framework.

The evaluation in this paper serves as a first proof-of-concept and further experiments on additional data would strengthen our findings. However, we expect the relative performances of the different approaches to remain the same. Future work will also include the integration of more sophisticated feature selection approaches, which might further improve the estimation accuracy.

Acknowledgments. This work is partially funded by the German Research Foundation DFG (HE 7364/1)

References

1. Lagendijk, J.J.W., Raaymakers, B.W., den Berg, C.A.T.V., Moerland, M.A., Philippens, M.E., van Vulpen, M.: MR guidance in radiotherapy. Phys. Med. Biol. **59**(21), R349–R369 (2014)
2. de Senneville, B.D., Ries, M., Bartels, L.W., Moonen, C.T.W.: MRI-guided high-intensity focused ultrasound sonication of liver and kidney. In: Kahn, T., Busse, H. (eds.) Interventional Magnetic Resonance Imaging. Medical Radiology, pp. 349–366. Springer, Heidelberg (2012)
3. Fontanarosa, D., van der Meer, S., Bamber, J., Harris, E., OShea, T., Verhaegen, F.: Review of ultrasound image guidance in external beam radiotherapy: I. Treatment planning and inter-fraction motion management. Phys. Med. Biol. **60**(3), R77–R114 (2015)
4. Luca, V.D., Benz, T., Kondo, S., et al.: The 2014 liver ultrasound tracking benchmark. Phys. Med. Biol. **60**(14), 5571–5599 (2015)
5. Cervino, L.I., Du, J., Jiang, S.B.: MRI-guided tumor tracking in lung cancer radiotherapy. Phys. Med. Biol. **56**(13), 3773–3785 (2011)
6. Brix, L., Ringgaard, S., Sorensen, T.S., Poulsen, P.R.: Three-dimensional liver motion tracking using real-time two-dimensional MRI. Med. Phys. **41**(4), 042302 (2014)
7. Preiswerk, F., Luca, V.D., Arnold, P., Celicanin, Z., Petrusca, L., Tanner, C., Bieri, O., Salomir, R., Cattin, P.C.: Model-guided respiratory organ motion prediction of the liver from 2D ultrasound. Med. Image Anal. **18**(5), 740–751 (2014)
8. de Senneville, B.D., Hamidi, A.E., Moonen, C.: A direct PCA-based approach for real-time description of physiological organ deformations. IEEE Trans. Med. Imag. **34**(4), 974–982 (2015)
9. McClelland, J., Hawkes, D., Schaeffter, T., King, A.: Respiratory motion models: A review. Med. Image Anal. **17**(1), 19–42 (2013)
10. Klinder, T., Lorenz, C.: Respiratory motion compensation for image-guided bronchoscopy using a general motion model. In: ISBI 2012, pp. 960–963 (2012)
11. Boye, D., Samei, G., Schmidt, J., Szkely, G., Tanner, C.: Population based modeling of respiratory lung motion and prediction from partial information. In: SPIE Medical Imaging 2013, vol. 8669. p. 86690U–86690U-7 (2013)
12. Wulff, J., Black, M.J.: Efficient sparse-to-dense optical flow estimation using a learned basis and layers. In: CVPR 2015, pp. 120–130 (2015)
13. Heinrich, M.P., Papież, B.W., Schnabel, J.A., Handels, H.: Non-parametric discrete registration with convex optimisation. In: Ourselin, S., Modat, M. (eds.) WBIR 2014. LNCS, vol. 8545, pp. 51–61. Springer, Heidelberg (2014). doi:10.1007/978-3-319-08554-8_6

14. Peressutti, D., Penney, G.P., Housden, R.J., Kolbitsch, C., Gomez, A., Rijkhorst, E.J., Barratt, D.C., Rhode, K.S., King, A.P.: A novel bayesian respiratory motion model to estimate and resolve uncertainty in image-guided cardiac interventions. Med. Image Anal. **17**(4), 488–502 (2013)
15. Heinrich, M.P., Handels, H., Simpson, I.J.A.: Estimating large lung motion in COPD patients by symmetric regularised correspondence fields. In: Navab, N., Hornegger, J., Wells, W.M., Frangi, A.F. (eds.) MICCAI 2015. LNCS, vol. 9350, pp. 338–345. Springer, Heidelberg (2015). doi:10.1007/978-3-319-24571-3_41
16. Rohr, K.: On 3D differential operators for detecting point landmarks. Image Vis. Comput. **15**(3), 219–233 (1997)
17. Heinrich, M.P., Jenkinson, M., Brady, M., Schnabel, J.A.: MRF-based deformable registration and ventilation estimation of lung CT. IEEE Trans. Med. Imag. **32**(7), 1239–1248 (2013)

Carotid Artery Wall Motion Estimated from Ultrasound Imaging Sequences Using a Nonlinear State Space Approach

Zhifan Gao[1,2], Yuanyuan Sun[3], Heye Zhang[1(✉)], Dhanjoo Ghista[4], Yanjie Li[3],
Huahua Xiong[5], Xin Liu[1], Yaoqin Xie[1], Wanqing Wu[1], and Shuo Li[6]

[1] Shenzhen Institutes of Advanced Technology,
Chinese Academy of Sciences, Shenzhen, China
hy.zhang@siat.ac.cn
[2] Shenzhen College of Advanced Technology,
University of Chinese Academy of Sciences, Shenzhen, China
[3] Harbin Institute of Technology Shenzhen Graduate School, Shenzhen, China
[4] University 2020 Foundation, Stanford, USA
[5] Department of Ultrasonography, The Second People's Hospital of Shenzhen,
Shenzhen, China
[6] University of Western Ontario, London, Canada

Abstract. It is very challenge to investigate the motion of the carotid artery wall in ultrasound images, because of the high nonlinear dynamics of this motion. In our study, the nonlinear dynamics of carotid artery wall motion is first approximated by our nonlinear state-space approach driven by a mathematical model of the mechanical deformation of carotid artery wall. Then, the two-dimensional motion of carotid artery wall is computed by solving the nonlinear state-space approach using the unscented Kalman filter. We have then evaluated the performance of our approach by comparing it with the manual tracing method (the correlation coefficient equals 0.9897 for the radial motion and 0.9703 for the longitudinal motion) and three other state-of-the-art methods for 73 subjects. The results indicate the reliable applicability of our approach in tracking the motion of the carotid artery wall and its potential usefulness in routine clinical diagnosis.

Keywords: Vessel wall motion · Carotid ultrasound · Unscented Kalman filter · Block matching method

1 Introduction

Early diagnosis of atherosclerotic disease is very important since it can direct therapies to prevent its complications. Traditional measurements (such as intima-media thickness), however, cannot effectively detect the preclinical and subclinical lesions due to the insignificant morphological changes in the vessel

---

Z. Gao and Y. Sun—Contributed equally to this work.

© Springer International Publishing AG 2016
S. Ourselin et al. (Eds.): MICCAI 2016, Part III, LNCS 9902, pp. 98–106, 2016.
DOI: 10.1007/978-3-319-46726-9_12

during this period. On the other hand, the motion of carotid arteries (Fig. 1) can be used to identify the atherosclerotic disease in the early stage by characterizing the artery stiffness [1]. In particular, it has been recently proved that the longitudinal motion of carotid artery wall is associated with atherosclerotic disease, and could be sensitive to show its early lesions [2]. For instance, the magnitude of longitudinal motion has been shown to be reduced in subjects with carotid plaques, type 2 diabetes and periodontal disease [2]. More importantly, in recent literatures, the longitudinal motion of the carotid artery wall was considered as a potential predictor of cardiovascular events in a large population screening, as it was associated with traditional risk factors while being independent of traditional risk markers [3].

However, manual tracing of the motion trajectories of the carotid artery wall is labor-intensive and time-consuming. Furthermore, it is very challenging to extract the longitudinal motion of the carotid artery wall from ultrasound image because of the poor longitudinal spatial resolution of ultrasound probe. Different block matching (BM) methods have been frequently applied to track the motion of the carotid artery wall. In the previous BM approaches, many similarity measures, including normalized cross correlation [4] and sum of square difference [3], have been proposed to locate the target block in the searching region. However, if those similarity measures are used directly without considering the noises in the reference and targeting images, the conventional BM method might not be able to locate the best-matched block in the targeted image [4]. Therefore, a recent study adopted the Kalman filter to estimate the motion of carotid artery wall by treating the noises as the uncertainties in the state space [3]. However, the movements of the block between two neighboring imaging frames are modeled as a constant process, and this may provide a biased motion of the carotid artery wall because of its nonlinear dynamics.

In order to properly handle the nonlinear arterial wall dynamics, we have developed a nonlinear periodic function with a deterministic input from a mathematic model of the arterial wall deformation, in order to appropriately match the dynamics of the carotid artery wall [5,6]. Then, we have built a nonlinear state-space approach based on this nonlinear periodic function, and solved this problem by combining the BM method and unscented Kalman filter (UKF). We have then validated the performance of our approach by comparing the results of our method with the manual tracing method and three state-of-the-art methods [3,4,6] on monitored ultrasound imaging sequences from 73 subjects.

2 Methodology

In this study, a nonlinear state space approach have been developed to track the two-dimensional (2D) motion of the carotid artery wall. In this state space approach, the nonlinear dynamics of carotid artery wall is approximated by using a nonlinear periodic function [7], and the biased motion trajectories are corrected by means of a mathematical model of carotid artery wall [5]. Then, we have solved the state space problem by combined the UKF and the BM method

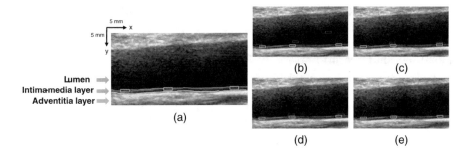

Fig. 1. (a) Sample carotid ultrasound image. The blue curve and the yellow curve are respectively the lumen border and the media-adventitia border of the carotid artery. The green rectangles are user-defined reference blocks, and the red rectangles are the tracked blocks corresponding to the green rectangles. (b), (c), (d) and (e) the examples of the blocks' locations tracked by BM, KBM, OP and our approach in the same ultrasound frame. (Color figure online)

together in this work. In order to reduce the influences from the out-of-plane motion, weak echoes, and motion artifacts during the ultrasound imaging, three user-defined reference blocks were selected in the first frame of each ultrasound sequence before the motion tracking, shown in Fig. 1. The size of these reference blocks were all $0.5\,\mathrm{mm} \times 1.7\,\mathrm{mm}$. Then, three search regions were selected by making their centers the same as the corresponding reference blocks. All search regions were set at $1.3\ \mathrm{mm} \times 2.5\,\mathrm{mm}$.

Prediction model. In tracking the 2D motion of carotid artery wall, the dynamics of the reference block in the ultrasound sequence was described by the discrete-time nonlinear state space equations, as

$$\mathbf{x}_{n+1} = f(\mathbf{x}_n, \mathbf{u}_n) + \mathbf{w}_n, \quad \mathbf{y}_n = \mathbf{x}_n + \mathbf{v}_n \tag{1}$$

where n is the time index or frame index. $\mathbf{w}_n$ and $\mathbf{v}_n$ are the noise obeyed by gaussian distribution with covariance matrices $\mathbf{Q}$ and $\mathbf{R}$, that is $\mathbf{w}_n \sim \mathcal{N}(0, \mathbf{Q})$ and $\mathbf{v}_n \sim \mathcal{N}(0, \mathbf{R})$. $\mathbf{Q} = 0.01\mathbf{I}$ and $\mathbf{R} = 100\mathbf{I}$, where $\mathbf{I}$ is the identity matrix. $\mathbf{x}_n = [x_n^1, x_n^2]^{\mathrm{T}}$ is the center point's location of reference block $\mathcal{B}_n^{ref}$ in the nth frame, and x_n^1, x_n^2 are the y-coordinate and the x-coordinate respectively. Similarly, $\mathbf{x}_{n+1} = [x_{n+1}^1, x_{n+1}^2]^{\mathrm{T}}$ is the center point's location of reference block $\mathcal{B}_{n+1}^{ref}$ in the $n+1$th frame, and $\mathbf{y}_n = [y_n^1, y_n^2]^{\mathrm{T}}$ is the center point's location of reference block $\mathcal{B}_n^{best}$. $\mathbf{u}_n = [u_1, u_2]^{\mathrm{T}}$ is the input signal inspired by a mathematical model of carotid arterial wall's mechanical deformation [5,6]. Therein, T denotes the number of ultrasound frames sampled in a cardiac cycle. $\mathbf{u}_n = \mathbf{g}_1(n)$ when $n \leqslant 0.4T$, and $\mathbf{u}_n = \mathbf{g}_2(n)$ when $0.4T < n \leqslant T$, where

$$\mathbf{g}_1(n) = \begin{bmatrix} 0.25 \tanh(1.22(n - 0.4T))(1 - \tanh(1.22n)) \sin^2 \frac{\pi n}{3.5T} \\ 0.25 \tanh(2.07(n - 0.4T))(1 - \tanh(2.07n)) \sin^2 \frac{\pi n}{0.65T} \end{bmatrix} \tag{2}$$

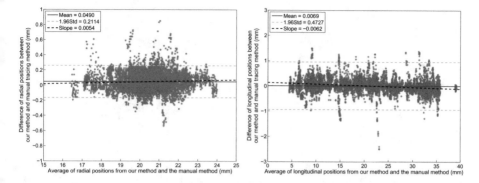

Fig. 2. Bland-Altman plot for the radial motion (left) and the longitudinal motion (right). The x-axis and y-axis represent the average and the difference between the motion positions separately tracked by our approach and manual tracing method. The blue solid line shows the bias between our approach and manual tracing method. The intervals between green dotted lines are the 95 % confidence interval. The black dotted lines are linearly fitting lines of all the scatter points.

and

$$
\mathbf{g}_2(n) = \begin{bmatrix} 0.25(1 + \tanh(1.22(n - T)))(1 + \tanh(1.22(0.39T - n)))(1.15 - 0.4n) \\ 0.25(1 + \tanh(2.07(n - T)))(1 + \tanh(1.22(0.39T - n)))(7 - 0.2n) \end{bmatrix}
\tag{3}
$$

The nonlinear function f in Eq. (1) is defined, based on [7], as below,

$$
\begin{aligned}
x_{n+1}^1 &= x_n^1 - \frac{T}{5}x_n^2 + Tu_1 \\
x_{n+1}^2 &= (1 - \frac{T}{5})x_n^2 + Tx_n^1 - \frac{T}{373}x_n^1 x_n^2 + Tu_2
\end{aligned}
\tag{4}
$$

Then the state space equations in Eq. (1) are solved to obtain the best estimate of $\mathbf{x}_{n+1}$ (denoted by $\hat{\mathbf{x}}_{n+1}$) in the $n + 1$th frame by using the unscented Kalman filter (UKF) [8]. The UKF samples a set of points (called sigma points) around the mean and then approximates the nonlinear transformation by the evolution of the sigma points with time. Thus, it can reduce the error from the linearized transformation of the nonlinear function. The process of UKF can be divided into two steps: state updating and observation updating. In this process, the state of the reference block $\mathbf{x}_n$ in the nth frame and $\mathbf{x}_{n+1}$ in the $n + 1$th frame are respectively considered to be the posterior state $\hat{\mathbf{x}}_n^+$ and $\hat{\mathbf{x}}_{n+1}^+$ in UKF.

State updating. State updating estimates the priori state $\hat{\mathbf{x}}_{n+1}^-$ and priori error covariance $\hat{\mathbf{P}}_{n+1}^-$ of the reference block $\mathcal{B}_{n+1}^{ref}$ in the $n + 1$th frame from the information in the last frame, formulated as

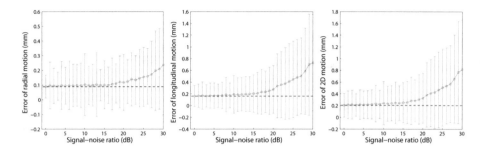

Fig. 3. Errors of our approach for the radial motion (left), the longitudinal motion (middle) and the 2D motion (right) in different noise levels. The x-axis represents the signal-noise ratio of the Rayleigh noise added into the ultrasound dataset. The red lines show the errors without adding the noise. (Color figure online)

$$\hat{\mathbf{x}}_{n+1}^- = \frac{1}{2M}\sum_{s=1}^{2M}\hat{\mathbf{x}}_{n+1}^s, \quad \hat{\mathbf{P}}_{n+1}^- = \frac{1}{2M}\sum_{s=1}^{2M}\left(\hat{\mathbf{x}}_{n+1}^s - \hat{\mathbf{x}}_{n+1}^-\right)\left(\hat{\mathbf{x}}_{n+1}^s - \hat{\mathbf{x}}_{n+1}^-\right)^{\mathrm{T}} + \mathbf{Q}$$

$$(5)$$

where M is the dimension of the state $\mathbf{x}$. $\hat{\mathbf{x}}_{n+1}^s$ are the sigma points in the $n+1$th frame, and can be obtained from the sigma points $\hat{\mathbf{x}}_n^s$ in the nth frame by the nonlinear function f, i.e. $\hat{\mathbf{x}}_{n+1}^s = f(\hat{\mathbf{x}}_n^s, \mathbf{u}_n)$. Therein, $\hat{\mathbf{x}}_n^s$ can be computed by the posterior state $\hat{\mathbf{x}}_n^+$ and posterior error covariance $\hat{\mathbf{P}}_n^+$ in the nth frame

$$\hat{\mathbf{x}}_n^s = \hat{\mathbf{x}}_n^+ + \check{\mathbf{x}}_n^s, \quad s = 1, 2, ..., 2M$$
$$\check{\mathbf{x}}_n^s = \left(\sqrt{M\mathbf{P}_n^+}\right)_s, \quad \check{\mathbf{x}}_n^{M+s} = -\left(\sqrt{M\mathbf{P}_n^+}\right)_s, \quad s = 1, 2, ..., M \tag{6}$$

where $\left(\sqrt{M\mathbf{P}_n^+}\right)_s$ is the ith row of the matrix $\sqrt{M\mathbf{P}_n^+}$.

Observation updating. Observation updating estimates the posterior state $\hat{\mathbf{x}}_{n+1}^+$ and priori error covariance $\hat{\mathbf{P}}_{n+1}^+$ of the reference block $\mathcal{B}_{n+1}^{ref}$ in the $n+1$th frame, formulated as

$$\mathbf{K}_{n+1} = \mathbf{P}_{xy}\mathbf{P}_y^{-1}, \quad \hat{\mathbf{x}}_{n+1}^+ = \hat{\mathbf{x}}_{n+1}^- + \mathbf{K}_{n+1}(\mathbf{y}_{n+1} - \hat{\mathbf{y}}_{n+1})$$
$$\hat{\mathbf{P}}_{n+1}^+ = \hat{\mathbf{P}}_{n+1}^- - \mathbf{K}_{n+1}\mathbf{P}_y\mathbf{K}_{n+1}^{\mathrm{T}} \tag{7}$$

where $\mathbf{P}_y$ is the covariance of the measurement noise, $\mathbf{P}_{xy}$ is the cross covariance between the state variable and the measurement variable and $\hat{\mathbf{y}}_{n+1}$ is the estimate of the measurement variable. They can be obtained as:

$$\hat{\mathbf{y}}_{n+1} = \frac{1}{2M}\sum_{s=1}^{2M}\hat{\mathbf{y}}_{n+1}^s, \quad \hat{\mathbf{y}}_{n+1}^s = \hat{\mathbf{x}}_{n+1}^s$$

$$\mathbf{P}_y = \frac{1}{2M}\sum_{s=1}^{2M}\left(\hat{\mathbf{y}}_{n+1}^s - \hat{\mathbf{y}}_{n+1}\right)\left(\hat{\mathbf{y}}_{n+1}^s - \hat{\mathbf{y}}_{n+1}\right)^{\mathrm{T}} + \mathbf{R} \tag{8}$$

$$\mathbf{P}_{xy} = \frac{1}{2M}\sum_{s=1}^{2M}\left(\hat{\mathbf{x}}_{n+1}^s - \hat{\mathbf{x}}_{n+1}^-\right)\left(\hat{\mathbf{y}}_{n+1}^s - \hat{\mathbf{y}}_{n+1}\right)^{\mathrm{T}}$$

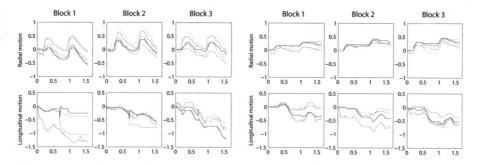

Fig. 4. Example of the motion trajectories of three reference blocks on the carotid artery wall from a healthy subject (left three columns) and an unhealthy subject (right three columns) for manual tracing method (green), as well as for our approach (red), CBM (blue), KBM (black) and OP (magenta). The x-axis of each subfigure represents the time of the ultrasound sequence (second). The y-axis of each subfigure represents the displacement of the block (mm) with respect to its position in the first frame. (Color figure online)

Measurement acquisition. The measurement $\mathbf{y}_{n+1}$ in Eq. (7) is the center point's location of the best-matched block $\mathcal{B}_{n+1}^{best}$ in the $n+1$th frame. Then, $\mathcal{B}_{n+1}^{best}$ can be computed from the reference block $\mathcal{B}_{n+1}^{ref}$ in the $n+1$th frame of the ultrasound sequence, by the block matching (BM) method with normalized cross-correlation [4].

3   Experiments and Results

A total of 14 healthy subjects (7 males, 62.0 ± 8.7 age years; 7 females, 59.7 ± 7.8 age years) and 59 unhealthy subjects (37 males, 59.0 ± 13.6 age years; 22 females, 60.6 ± 12.2 age years) were involved in this study. The inclusion criterion for the unhealthy subjects was the presence of one of the three diseases diagnosed: type 1 or 2 diabetes, hypertension and heart disease. The data collection was implemented by an ultrasound physician with more than 10-year experience by a high-resolution ultrasound system (iU22, Philips Ultrasound, Bothell, WA, USA) and a 7.5 MHz liner array transducer.

Accuracy. The accuracy of our approach was evaluated by comparing the results computed by our approach with those manually performed by an experienced ultrasound physician (considered as the ground truth). The physician identified the center points for each of the three blocks in the first frame and then visually detected the three center points in every single subsequent frame. After the tracking process, two measurements were computed to show the results of our approach: the positions of the radial motion (RP) and the longitudinal motion (LP). The radial motion denotes the dynamics of the best-matched block along the radial direction across the ultrasound sequence, and the longitudinal motion denotes that in the longitudinal direction. The positions of radial/longitudinal

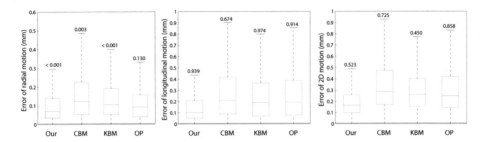

Fig. 5. Comparative results of the tracking error between our approach and the other methods (CBM, KBM and OP) for the radial motion (left), longitudinal motion (middle) and the 2D motion (right). The digits above the boxes in each figure show the p-values of the difference between the computer-aided method and the manual tracing method.

motion show the location of the best-matched block in every frame. Three kinds of errors (defined in [9]) were used to measure the accuracy of our approach: errors of radial motion, longitudinal motion and 2D motion. The results of linear regression showed that our approach was highly correlated with the manual tracing method for different subjects (RP: $r = 0.9897 \pm 0.0140$, p-value < 0.001; LP: $r = 0.9703 \pm 0.0539$, p-value < 0.001). The Bland-Altman plots shown in Fig. 2 illustrate that the bias of our approach with respect to the manual tracing method were 0.049 mm for RP and 0.0069 mm for LP. Then, we linearly fitted the scatter points in the Bland-Altman plots, and the slopes of the fitting straight lines (black dotted lines) were 0.0054 for RP and 0.0062 for LP. In addition, the coefficient of variation (CV) of the difference between our approach and the manual tracing method was 0.8681 for RP and 1.1046 for LP. These results indicate that difference between our approach and the manual tracing method is small, and moreover not much influenced by their averages. Finally, we added different levels of Rayleigh noise (1 dB ∼ 30 dB signal-noise ratio) in the ultrasound dataset and retested the proposed approach. Figure 3 shows that our approach has good performance to resist the noise disturbance.

Comparison with other methods. Our approach was compared with three state-of-the-art methods on all subjects: conventional block matching method (CBM) [4], Kalman-based block matching method (KBM) [3] and optical flow method (OP) [6], with all parameters shown in their own publications except the sizes of the reference block and search region. The values of the two sizes used in the three methods are same as our approach. Figure 4 illustrates the motion trajectories of the carotid artery wall computed by our approach and other methods in a healthy subject and an unhealthy subject; Fig. 1(b)–(e) show examples of the blocks' location obtained by our approach and other methods in the same ultrasound frame. Figure 5 displays the comparative results between our approach and other methods. The results shows that the accuracy of our approach (RP: 0.0895 ± 0.0777 mm, p-value < 0.001; LP: 0.1619 ± 0.1789 mm, p-value $= 0.939$) was higher than those of other methods. This indicates that the use of the nonlinear periodic function and the mathematical model of the mechanical deformation of carotid artery wall in the prediction model was effective. Moreover, we compared the computational cost of our approach with those of other methods. The results showed that our approach (0.0257 ± 0.0046 second per frame) was moderate compared to the other methods (CBM: 0.0249 ± 0.0049 second per frame, KBM: 0.0772 ± 0.0048 second per frame, OP: 0.0101 ± 0.0011 second per frame).

4   Conclusion

In this study, we have developed an approach to automatically track the dynamics of the carotid artery wall. Our methodology involves developing a nonlinear periodic function with input from the mathematic model of mechanical deformation of the carotid artery wall, for the purpose of properly handling the nonlinear components of the dynamics. The performance of our approach was tested on a dataset with 73 carotid ultrasound sequences, and the results were compared with those manually performed by one experienced ultrasound physician and three state-of-the-art methods. The results demonstrated the effectiveness of our approach in the motion tracking of carotid artery wall in ultrasound image sequences.

Acknowledgements. This work was supported in part by Guangdong Image-guided Therapy Innovation Team (2011S013).

References

1. Roger, V., et al.: Heart disease and stroke statistics-2012 upate: a report from the American heart association. Circulation **125**(1), e2–e220 (2012)
2. Zahnd, G., Vray, D., Sérusclat, A., Alibay, D., Bartold, M., Brown, A., Durand, M., Jamieson, L., Kapellas, K., Maple-Brown, L., O'Dea, K., Moulin, P., Celermajer, D., Skilton, M.: Longitudinal displacement of the carotid wall and cardiovascular risk factors: associations with aging, adiposity, blood pressure and periodontal disease independent of cross-sectional distensibility and intima-media thickness. Ultrasound Med. Biol. **38**(10), 1705–1715 (2012)
3. Zahnd, G., Orkisz, M., Sérusclat, A., Moulin, P., Vray, D.: Evaluation of a Kalman-based block matching method to assess the bi-dimensional motion of the carotid artery wall in b-mode ultrasound sequences. Med. Image Anal. **17**(5), 573–585 (2013)
4. Golemati, S., Sassano, A., Lever, M., Bharath, A., Dhanjil, S., Nicolaides, A.: Carotid artery wall motion estimated from B-mode ultrasound using region tracking and block matching. Ultrasound Med. Biol. **29**(3), 387–399 (2003)
5. Stoitsis, J., Golemati, S., Bastouni, E., Nikita, K.: A mathematical model of the mechanical deformation of the carotid artery wall and its application to clinical data. In: Proceedings of the 29th Annual International Conference of the IEEE Engineering in Medicine and Biology Society (EMBS), pp. 2163–2166 (2007)

6. Golemati, S., Stoitsis, J., Gastounioti, A., Dimopoulos, A., Koropouli, V., Nikita, K.: Comparison of block matching and differential methods for motion analysis of the carotid artery wall from ultrasound images. IEEE Trans. Inf. Technol. Biomed. **16**(5), 852–858 (2012)
7. Kandepu, R., Foss, B., Imsland, L.: Applying the unscented Kalman filter for nonlinear state estimation. J. Process Control **18**, 753–768 (2008)
8. Simon, D.: Optimal State Estimation: Kalman, H$_\infty$ and Nonlinear Approaches. Wiley, New York (2006)
9. Gastounioti, A., Golemati, S., Stoitsis, J., Nikita, K.: Kalman-filter-based block matching for arterial wall motion estimation from B-mode ultrasound. In: IEEE International Conference on Imaging Systems and Techniques (IST), pp. 234–239 (2010)

Accuracy Estimation for Medical Image Registration Using Regression Forests

Hessam Sokooti[1]($\boxtimes$), Gorkem Saygili[1], Ben Glocker[2],
Boudewijn P. F. Lelieveldt[1,3], and Marius Staring[1,3]

[1] Leiden University Medical Center, Leiden, The Netherlands
h.sokooti_oskooyi@lumc.nl
[2] Imperial College, London, UK
[3] Delft University of Technology, Delft, The Netherlands

Abstract. This paper reports a new automatic algorithm to estimate the misregistration in a quantitative manner. A random regression forest is constructed, predicting the local registration error. The forest is built using local and modality independent features related to the registration precision, the transformation model and intensity-based similarity after registration. The forest is trained and tested using manually annotated corresponding points between pairs of chest CT scans. The results show that the mean absolute error of regression is 0.72 ± 0.96 mm and the accuracy of classification in three classes (correct, poor and wrong registration) is 93.4 %, comparing favorably to a competing method. In conclusion, a method was proposed that for the first time shows the feasibility of automatic registration assessment by means of regression, and promising results were obtained.

Keywords: Image registration · Registration accuracy · Uncertainty estimation · Regression forests

1 Introduction

Most image registration methods do not provide insights about the quality of their results and devolve this difficult task to human experts, which is very time-consuming. Automatic evaluation of registration reduces the time of manual assessment and can provide information about the registration uncertainty. Having the error of registration is useful to refine the registration, either automatically or with the feedback of human experts. Even if refinement is not possible, information about the registration quality can help decide if subsequent processing is meaningful, and visualizing the error can be helpful in medical applications before making a clinical decision.

Several methods have been suggested to estimate the registration accuracy, such as exploitation of the Bayesian posterior distribution [1] or based on the consistency of multiple registrations [2]. In the stochastic approaches Kybic [3] computed the registration uncertainty by performing multiple registrations with

© Springer International Publishing AG 2016
S. Ourselin et al. (Eds.): MICCAI 2016, Part III, LNCS 9902, pp. 107–115, 2016.
DOI: 10.1007/978-3-319-46726-9_13

bootstrapping on the cost function samples to generate a set of registration solutions. He found a correlation between the variation of the 2D translational parameters and the true registration error but the method is not tested for 3D non-rigid registration with much more transform parameters. Hub *et al.* [4] estimated the uncertainty by perturbing the B-spline grid with random values and check whether or not the local SSD changed. The drawback of this approach is that it is not efficient in homogeneous areas. In 2013, they applied the same perturbation for the Demons algorithm and showed that the variance of the deformation vector field (DVF) is related to the registration error [5]. However, an exhaustive experiment is needed to find large registration errors.

In this paper we turn our attention to methods capable of learning the registration error. This has the advantage that multiple features related to registration uncertainty can be exploited and combined in a single framework. Muenzing *et al.* [6] classified the registration quality into three categories (wrong, poor and correct), and reported that it was not possible to successfully build a regressor. All their features were intensity-based, except for the Jacobian of the transform parameters. In this paper, instead of formulating uncertainty estimation as a classification problem, we formulate it as a regression problem, enabling a continuous prediction of registration accuracy. To the best of our knowledge, there is only one paper that takes a similar approach [7], but it was only tested on synthetically deformed images. We explore several modality independent features (some of them new) related to registration precision, the estimated transformation and the image similarity after registration, and their contribution to the regression performance. The proposed framework can be used in combination with any registration paradigm, i.e. does not depend on specifics such as a Bayesian formulation, and can already be used for pairwise registration.

2   Methods

2.1   System Overview

A block diagram of the proposed algorithm is shown in Fig. 1. The inputs of the system are a fixed I_F and a moving image I_M. We use a limited number of so-called *mother features*, from which much more features are generated using a pooling technique. A regression forest (RF) is then trained from the feature pool to predict local registration error. One class of features is derived from the registration, or from a set of sub-registrations. The other class is derived from the intensities of the fixed and deformed moving images. Details are given in Sect. 2.2.

Mathematically, the registration problems is formulated as an optimization problem in which the cost function $\mathcal{C}$ is minimized with respect to $\boldsymbol{T}$:

$$\widehat{\boldsymbol{T}} = \arg\min_{\boldsymbol{T}} \mathcal{C}\big(\boldsymbol{T}; I_F, I_M\big), \tag{1}$$

where $\boldsymbol{T}$ denotes the transformation. The minimization is solved by an iterative optimization method embedded in a multi-resolution setting. A registration can be initialized by an initial transform $\boldsymbol{T}^{\mathrm{ini}}$.

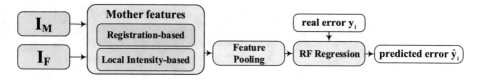

Fig. 1. A block diagram of the proposed algorithm.

2.2   Features and Pooling

Variation of deformation vector field (std T) The initial parameters of an optimization problem can affect the final solution for many registration paradigms, especially in areas where the cost function has multiple local minima or is semi-flat. On the other hand, in cases where the cost function is well-defined, variations in the initial transformation are expected to have much less effect on the final registration result. The variation in the final transformation result is then an intuitive measure for the local registration uncertainty, which is a surrogate for the correctness or at least the precision of the registration. A flow chart of the described feature is given in Fig. 2(a). Consider P randomly generated transformations T_i^{ini} that are used as initializations of the registration algorithm from Eq. (1), resulting in P final transformations $\widehat{T}_i$. The standard deviation of those transformations std T is then used as a mother feature:

$$\overline{T} = \tfrac{1}{P} \sum \widehat{T}_i, \qquad \mathrm{std}\, T = \tfrac{1}{P} \sqrt{ \sum \left\| \widehat{T}_i - \overline{T} \right\|^2 }. \tag{2}$$

The random initializations are generated in this work by adding a uniformly distributed offset to the B-spline coefficients. An example of std T in a manually deformed image is available in Fig. 2(b), for illustration purposes we magnified the imposed deformation field. It is also possible to first perform a registration, resulting in a transformation T^{base}, and then add random offsets to that ($T^{\mathrm{base}} + T_i^{\mathrm{offset}}$), which is approximately similar to Hub's work [5]. Akin to Eq. (2) a mother feature std T^{Hub} is then derived.

Areas with a small std T are still potentially areas of low registration quality, if the difference between $\overline{T}$ and T^{base} is too large. We then consider the bias $\mathcal{E}(T)$ as a complementary feature to std T computed by $\mathcal{E}(T) = \|T^{\mathrm{base}} - \overline{T}\|$. The mother feature $\mathcal{E}(T^{\mathrm{Hub}})$ is computed similarly.

Coefficient of variation of joint histograms (CVH): Based on the multiple registration results we can additionally extract information about the matched intensity patterns of the images. The first step is to calculate the joint histograms $H_i, \forall i$ of the fixed image I_F and the deformed moving image $I_M(T)$. A large variation in the joint histograms implies a large registration error. The scalar CVH is defined as: $\mathrm{CVH} = \mathrm{std}\, H / (\overline{H} + \epsilon)$. The coefficient of variation is used to compensate for large differences between the elements of $\overline{H}$, and the constant ϵ is used to ignore small numbers in the joint histogram. Note that this feature

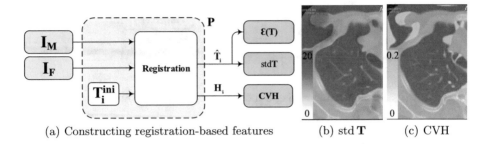

(a) Constructing registration-based features   (b) std **T**   (c) CVH

Fig. 2. The registration-based features require multiple registrations

can also be used in a multi-modality setting, like all our features. An example of the CVH on a manually deformed image is shown in Fig. 2(c).

Determinant of Jacobian (Jac): In addition to previous registration-based features, we also use Jac. Local changes in volume can point to poor registration quality or discontinuous transformations.

Difference of MIND: Heinrich *et al.* [8] introduced the Modality Independent Neighborhood Descriptor (MIND) to register multimodal images by comparing similarities between same patches in the fixed and moving image. The output of this local self-similarity has n features for each voxel, where n is the size of the search region. The n features is aggregated in a single mother feature by using the Euclidean distance between MIND of I_F and that of $I_M(T)$. We calculate MIND with two different search regions, see Sect. 3 for details.

Feature pooling: All features are calculated in a voxel-based fashion. Incorporating local information of each feature can reduce discontinuity and improve interaction with other features. For instance, it is possible to have a high std T in homogeneous regions while the difference of MIND is almost zero. On the other hand, when we have misregistration on the boundaries, the difference of MIND indicates high dissimilarity while std T can have a high value only in the nearby voxels but not exactly on the border. To overcome these problems, the total set of features is largely increased by generating a pool from the mother features by calculating averages and maxima over them using differently sized boxes.

2.3   Regression Forests

Breiman [9] introduced the random forest by extending bagging and making more clever averaging of trees. The general idea is to use some weak learners (trees) and make an efficient combination of them. In contrast to bagging, splitting of each node is done with a random subset of features which speeds up the training phase and reduces correlation between trees in the forest, accordingly decreasing the forest error rate. The reason that we chose the random forest is that it has the ability to handle data without preprocessing such as rescaling data, removing outliers and selecting features. Feature importance is measured over the out-of-bootstrap samples Ω by permuting features, and computing the difference between the mean square error (MSE) before and after permutation:

$$\text{Imp}(x_i) = \frac{1}{N_t} \sum_{t=1}^{N_t} \left(\underset{j \in \Omega}{\text{MSE}}\left(\hat{y}_{\pi_{ij}}, y_j\right) - \underset{j \in \Omega}{\text{MSE}}\left(\hat{y}_j, y_j\right) \right), \tag{3}$$

where y_j is the real value, $\hat{y}_j$ the predicted value after the regression, $\hat{y}_{\pi_{ij}}$ the predicted value when permuting feature i, and N_t the number of trees.

3   Experiments and Results

Materials and ground truth: In this study, the SPREAD database [10] has been used, which has 21 pairs of 3D lung CT images. The dimension of the images is about $446 \times 315 \times 129$ with an average voxel size of $0.781 \times 0.781 \times 2.5\,\text{mm}$. Patients are within the range of 49 to 78 years old and for each patient a baseline image and a follow-up image (after 30 months) are available in which 100 well-distributed corresponding landmarks are selected semi-automatically on distinctive locations [11]. The residual Euclidean distance after registration between the corresponding points can be seen as the accuracy of the registration.

However, 100 training samples for each pair are not enough to reliably train the regression forest. To obtain more training samples, we include voxels in a small local neighborhood of the annotated points. We assume that the registration error is equal to the error at the landmark, which seems reasonable for smooth transformations and within a small region. The neighborhood size is chosen as $10.153 \times 10.153 \times 7.5\,\text{mm}$, which is approximately equivalent to the final grid space of the B-spline registration.

The main programming language is MATLAB 2015a, while feature pooling is implemented in C++ and the regression forest is computed using the scikit-learn package of Python. All registrations are performed by `elastix` [12].

Evaluation and experimental setup: To evaluate the proposed algorithm, the mean absolute error (MAE) between the real registration error y_i and estimated one $\hat{y}_i$ is calculated by $\text{MAE} = \frac{1}{n}\sum_{i=1}^{n}|\hat{y}_i - y_i|$. We also reported the MAE_i in three bins with respect to y_i $[0, 3)$, $[3, 6)$ and $[6, \infty)$ mm, corresponding to correct, poor and wrong registration [6]. It is possible to classify the $\hat{y}_i$ based on these bins and calculate the total accuracy (Acc) and accuracy in each bin (Acc_i). We employ k-fold cross validation, using $k = 10$, splitting the data in 15 image pairs for training and the remaining 6 pairs for testing.

Parameters of features and pooling: The feature std $\boldsymbol{T}$ is computed using $P = 20$ initializations $\boldsymbol{T}_i^{\text{ini}}$, which are constructed randomly using a uniform distribution in the range $[-2, 2]$ mm. P was chosen sufficiently large, such that the overall standard deviation of the resulting transformations did not change considerably, as shown in Fig. 3(a). For the registrations, we used three resolutions of 500 iterations each, with a final B-spline grid spacing of $[10, 10, 10]$ mm. The cost function is mutual information, which is optimized by adaptive stochastic

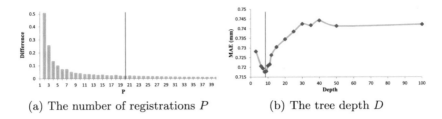

(a) The number of registrations P (b) The tree depth D

Fig. 3. Tuning some of the parameters. The selected ones are indicated by red. (Color figure online)

Table 1. Regression results for the several feature pools

	MAE	MAE$_1$	MAE$_2$	MAE$_3$	Acc	Acc$_1$	Acc$_2$	Acc$_3$
std T	0.76 ± 1.03	0.56 ± 0.47	2.29 ± 1.31	4.29 ± 2.84	93.0	95.1	33.2	65.8
std T^{Hub}	0.84 ± 1.25	0.59 ± 0.53	2.15 ± 1.14	6.28 ± 2.61	91.5	94.0	29.4	54.1
CVH	0.90 ± 1.42	0.61 ± 0.67	2.42 ± 0.94	7.05 ± 2.81	90.8	92.5	21.0	29.4
MIND$_{\mathrm{sp}}$	0.73 ± 1.05	0.54 ± 0.50	1.81 ± 0.99	4.83 ± 2.67	93.0	95.6	40.0	66.0
MIND$_3$	0.74 ± 1.06	0.53 ± 0.43	2.08 ± 1.20	4.83 ± 2.78	93.0	95.5	36.2	62.9
$\mathcal{E}(T)$	0.85 ± 1.25	0.63 ± 0.70	2.13 ± 0.98	5.36 ± 3.08	91.4	94.3	27.7	48.9
$\mathcal{E}(T^{\mathrm{Hub}})$	0.82 ± 1.17	0.58 ± 0.47	2.22 ± 1.13	5.72 ± 2.76	91.9	94.2	29.1	68.2
Jac	0.91 ± 1.43	0.62 ± 0.61	2.26 ± 0.86	7.37 ± 2.86	90.4	92.4	13.8	24.8
All	0.74 ± 1.00	0.55 ± 0.45	2.03 ± 0.98	4.46 ± 2.69	93.1	95.5	34.6	57.1
All-Pooled	0.72 ± 0.96	0.54 ± 0.46	2.00 ± 1.08	4.01 ± 2.66	93.4	95.8	38.9	69.7

gradient descent [12]. In CVH Eq. we set ϵ to 100 in order to ignore small set of voxels. std T^{Hub} is calculated with the same settings except that one resolution is used. The MIND feature is calculated using a $[3 \times 3 \times 3]$ region as suggested by [8] and also compared with a sparse patch including 82 voxels inside a $[7 \times 7 \times 3]$ box, which is physically more isotropic for our data.

After computing the mother features, average and maximum pooling is performed with box sizes of $[2, 4, 6, ..., 60]$ mm. As a result, for each mother feature we obtain a pool of 60 features: 30 from box averages and 30 from box maxima.

Parameters of the regression forest: The RF is trained on 50 trees with a maximum depth of D, while at least 5 samples remain in the leaf nodes. At each splitting node, f features are randomly selected from the pool ($f = 10$ for each single feature; $f = 2$ for 'All'; $f = 20$ for 'All-pooled'). The parameter D is optimized within the range of $[3, 100]$ by comparing the MAE. From the results in Fig. 3(b), we selected $D = 9$ for the remainder of this paper.

Results: RFs are trained for each single mother feature independently and for the combination of all features with or without feature pooling. Table 1 gives the results in terms of regression MAE and classification accuracy. The two MIND-based features have similar regression performance, but the sparse patch shows better classification accuracy in especially the second and third bin. We therefore

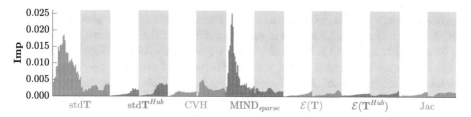

Fig. 4. Feature importance. White areas correspond to box averages, while shaded areas correspond to box maxima.

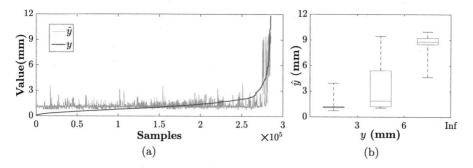

Fig. 5. Real (y) vs predicted ($\hat{y}$) registration error for the combined feature pool.

included the sparse patch MIND in the total feature pool. From Table 1 it can be seen that for the intensity-based features the best performance is obtained from MIND, for the registration-based features from std $\boldsymbol{T}$, and that the joint feature pool performs better than any single feature. The feature importance, see Eq. (3), is displayed in Fig. 4. It confirms that std $\boldsymbol{T}$ and MIND are the features contributing most to the RF performance, followed by CVH. The result of the complete pool is detailed in Fig. 5(a) which shows the real against the predicted error, sorted from small to large. In Fig. 5(b) we grouped the real errors in the three bins, each showing a box plot of the predicted errors. Intuitively, a smaller overlap between the boxes represents a better regression.

4   Conclusion and Discussion

In this paper we proposed a method based on random forests to regress registration accuracy from registration-based as well as intensity-based features. We introduced the variation in registration result from differences in initialization (std $\boldsymbol{T}$) as a feature, which showed higher feature importance and regression and classification performance than an existing variant of it. The proposed feature CVH measuring joint intensity variation also contributed to the regression performance, and can be calculated from the std $\boldsymbol{T}$ results without much additional computation. The combination of those features with several others, using a box-based pooling technique, yielded best overall performance. With a mean overall regression error of 0.72 ± 0.96 mm and a classification accuracy of 93.4 % we conclude that the proposed method is very promising for the a posteriori assessment of local registration error. In future work, we will include additional information such as the variation of $\boldsymbol{T}$ in $[x, y, z]$ separately and estimate the error in each direction. In the current experiment, the number of samples in the second and third bin (poor and wrong) is considerably less than the number of samples in the first bin. We will therefore add poor registration results to the training set, thereby hopefully improving the regression results, especially in the second bin. A post-processing technique such as smoothing or majority voting over a neighborhood potentially also improves regression accuracy. One of the advantages of the proposed method is that all employed features are modality independent, and allow for parallel (GPU) computation. In the future, we will therefore test the algorithm on multi-modality data. Extra advantages are that additional features can be trivially included in the framework, that our method is compatible with any registration method, can already work in pairwise registration.

References

1. Risholm, P., Janoos, F., Norton, I., Golby, A.J., Wells, W.M.: Bayesian characterization of uncertainty in intra-subject non-rigid registration. Med. Image Anal. **17**(5), 538–555 (2013)
2. Datteri, R.D., Dawant, B.M.: Automatic detection of the magnitude and spatial location of error in non-rigid registration. In: Dawant, B.M., Christensen, G.E., Fitzpatrick, J.M., Rueckert, D. (eds.) WBIR 2012. LNCS, vol. 7359, pp. 21–30. Springer, Heidelberg (2012). doi:10.1007/978-3-642-31340-0_3
3. Kybic, J.: Bootstrap resampling for image registration uncertainty estimation without ground truth. IEEE Trans. Image Process. **19**, 64–73 (2010)
4. Hub, M., Kessler, M.L., Karger, C.P.: A stochastic approach to estimate the uncertaintyinvolved in B-spline image registration. IEEE Trans. Med. Imaging **28**(11), 1708–1716 (2009)
5. Hub, M., Karger, C.: Estimation of the uncertainty of elastic image registration with the Demons algorithm. Phys. Med. Biol. **58**(9), 3023 (2013)
6. Muenzing, S.E., van Ginneken, B., Murphy, K., Pluim, J.P.: Supervised quality assessment of medical image registration: application to intra-patient CT lung registration. Med. Image Anal. **16**(8), 1521–1531 (2012)
7. Lotfi, T., Tang, L., Andrews, S., Hamarneh, G.: Improving probabilistic image registration via reinforcement learning and uncertainty evaluation. In: Wu, G., Zhang, D., Shen, D., Yan, P., Suzuki, K., Wang, F. (eds.) MLMI 2013. LNCS, vol. 8184, pp. 187–194. Springer, Heidelberg (2013). doi:10.1007/978-3-319-02267-3_24
8. Heinrich, M.P., Jenkinson, M., Bhushan, M., Matin, T., Gleeson, F.V., Brady, M., Schnabel, J.A.: Mind: modality independent neighbourhood descriptor for multimodal deformable registration. Med. Image Anal. **16**(7), 1423–1435 (2012)
9. Breiman, L.: Random forests. Mach. Learn. **45**(1), 5–32 (2001)
10. Stolk, J., Putter, H., Bakker, E.M., Shaker, S.B., Parr, D.G., Piitulainen, E., Russi, E.W., Grebski, E., Dirksen, A., Stockley, R.A., Reiber, J.H.C., Stoel, B.C.: Progression parameters for emphysema: a clinical investigation. Respir. Med. **101**(9), 1924–1930 (2007)

11. Murphy, K., van Ginneken, B., Klein, S., Staring, M., de Hoop, B.J., Viergever, M.A., Pluim, J.P.: Semi-automatic construction of reference standards for evaluation of image registration. Med. Image Anal. **15**(1), 71–84 (2011)
12. Klein, S., Staring, M., Murphy, K., Viergever, M.A., Pluim, J.P.: Elastix: a toolbox for intensity-based medical image registration. IEEE Trans. Med. Imaging **29**(1), 196–205 (2010)

Embedding Segmented Volume in Finite Element Mesh with Topology Preservation

Kazuya Sase[1], Teppei Tsujita[2], and Atsushi Konno[1(✉)]

[1] Hokkaido University, Sapporo, Japan
sase@scc.ist.hokudai.ac.jp, konno@ssi.ist.hokudai.ac.jp
[2] National Defence Academy, Yokosuka, Japan
tsujita@nda.ac.jp

Abstract. The generation of a patient-specific finite element (FE) model of organs is important for preoperative surgical simulations. Although methods for generating a mesh from a 3D geometric model of organs are well established, the reproduction of complex structures, such as holes, branches, and jaggy boundaries, remains difficult. To approximate the deformation of complex structures, an approach for embedding a fine geometry in a coarse volumetric mesh can be used. In this paper, we introduce a volume embedding method that preserves the topology of a complicated structure on the basis of segmented medical images. Our evaluation shows that the generated FE model precisely reproduces the topology of a human brain according to a segmented medical image.

1 Introduction

The progress in modeling and simulation techniques of soft-tissue deformation has enabled the prediction of the mechanical behaviors of organs before actual surgery in the operation room. One of the problems in applying these techniques to clinical use is the generation of patient-specific biomechanical models including volumetric meshes. In general, the geometry of a patient's organs is obtained using medical imaging and segmentation techniques. To obtain patient-specific volumetric meshes, meshing methods that use segmented medical images as the input have been developed [2,8]. However, preserving the fine geometry in a coarse mesh resolution is still difficult. The left side of Fig. 1 illustrates examples of Delaunay-based meshing of a segmented volume. As shown in this figure, the meshing with feature preservation provides a good volume mesh with boundary conformity. However, the number of vertices tends to become large when the feature constraints are applied. Finer mesh resolutions limit the range of applications becuase of their high computational costs.

In the community of computer graphics, embedding is a popular approach for approximating the deformations of fine geometry. By embedding a fine geometry in a coarse volumetric mesh, the deformation of the fine geometry is interpolated by the deformation of the volumetric mesh. Usually, coarse volumetric meshes are simple grid meshes, and thus, do not meet the boundary conformity. Instead of being limited by the inaccurate boundary conformity, it is easy to reduce

S. Ourselin et al. (Eds.): MICCAI 2016, Part III, LNCS 9902, pp. 116–123, 2016.
DOI: 10.1007/978-3-319-46726-9_14

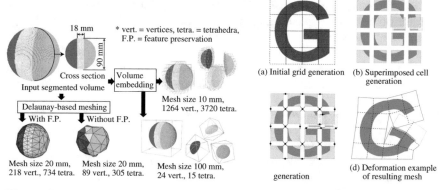

Fig. 1. Comparison between Delaunay-based meshing [2,8] and our volume embedding.

Fig. 2. Algorithm overview.

the computational cost of mechanical simulations by changing the resolution of the grid. The right side of Fig. 1 illustrates examples of the volume embedding approach. They are able to reduce the number of vertices down as far as 24 vertices in this example. One known issue is that a simple grid mesh cannot separate disconnected parts if proximate parts are included in the same cell. Nesme et al. [7] solved this problem by the separation and superposition of elements, but their method was intended for embedding a polygon surface model in a finite element (FE) mesh. In order to apply the method to volume data (medical images), they need to be converted into a surface polygon, which results in loss of volume information. Additionally, the method proposed in [7] did not consider the separation of a completely attached boundary that should be separated.

To solve these problems, we propose an embedding method that directly handles the volume data. Furthermore, we introduce a method of separating completely attached areas on the basis of user-defined segment pairs. The proposed method is evaluated using a brain atlas, and the generated mesh is tested whether it can be used for our interactive surgery simulator [9], which aims to plan the approaching process to the affected area on the insula. The simulator requires a mesh of which the Sylvian fissure is separated, and the fissure is generally completely attached in MR images.

2   Method

2.1   Overview

The proposed method uses superimposed nodes and cells to preserve the topology of the structure. As illustrated in Fig. 2, the degrees of freedom of the deformation are added by superimposing nodes and cells. The topology, i.e., the connections and separations between the local volumetric areas, can be preserved using superimposed nodes and cells. Additionally, we consider the separation of the connection between multiple segments. For example, the "Temporal lobe" segment and the "Parietal lobe" segment should be separated. Such separations are realized by separation label pairs (SLPs), which are explicitly specified by the user. The hexahedral mesh generation is processed according to the segmented volume and SLPs. The definitions of the input and output are given below.

Segmented medical image. A segmented medical image constitutes volume data that contain labels at aligned voxels. A label is an integer value associated with a segment, for example, 0 is empty space, 1 is white matter, and so on. A label at a specific voxel coordinate is denoted by $L(i) \in \mathbb{Z}$, where $i \in \mathbb{Z}^3$ is a voxel coordinate. Voxel coordinate i can be mapped to spatial coordinate $p \in \mathbb{R}^3$ using a vector of volume origin $p_0 \in \mathbb{R}^3$ and a vector of spacing values $s = [s_x, s_y, s_z] \in \mathbb{R}^3$ as $p = p_0 + s \odot i$, where $\odot$ denotes element-wise vector multiplication.

Mesh size. Mesh size $H \in \mathbb{R}$ is the approximate edge length of a hexahedral cell. The actual edge lengths in the x, y, and z directions $h = [h_x, h_y, h_z]$ are determined by multiples of the spacing value of a volume, e.g., $h_x = \mathrm{ceil}(H/s_x)s_x$ for the direction x, where $\mathrm{ceil}(H/s_x)$ is the number of voxels along the x axis.

SLPs. An SLP is a pair of labels $\{L_a, L_b\}$, where L_a and L_b are the labels of segment a and b, respectively. The algorithm for generating a hexahedral mesh is applied to separate the segments that are specified by SLPs. The SLPs need to be generated by users.

Hexahedral mesh. A mesh is represented as nodes and cells. A node has a corresponding position and a cell has references to nodes.

Superimposed nodes and cells. A superimposed node/cell is a node/cell that coexists at the same position as another node/cell. There is no limit to the number of superimposed nodes/cells that can exist at the same position.

2.2   Hexahedral Mesh Generation

First, initial nodes and cells are generated without considering superposition (Fig. 2(a)). The bounding box of the volume is calculated, and an orthogonal lattice is generated, the origin of which is on the corner of the bounding box; the lattice bases are $[h_x, 0, 0]^T$, $[0, h_y, 0]^T$, $[0, 0, h_z]^T$.

Second, a cell that includes multiple regions is divided into multiple cells such that each divided cell includes only one region (Fig. 2(b)). To do so, local segmentation is executed by voxel-level region growing in each cell, as illustrated in Fig. 3. For the region growing, first an initial seed point is arbitrarily selected from voxels inside the cell. Then, it is determined whether the labels of the neighbor are connected to one of the faces of the seed voxel. If the label of a neighbor voxel is not "empty" and is not listed in the SLPs, the voxel is added to the region. These procedures are iterated until no connected voxel is found. After one region is extracted, the region growing procedure is iterated until all non-empty voxels are added to a region. If more than one region is detected, the cell for each region is superimposed. At this time, all cells refer to the same set of nodes. For the subsequent procedure, the set of voxels is stored on the associated region for each superimposed cell. If no region is detected, e.g., all the labels are "empty," the cell is deleted.

Third, nodes shared by superimposed cells are also superimposed (see Figs. 2(c) and 4 for details). At each node, cells that share the node are searched and cell-level region growing is executed. The cell-level region growing is initiated from a seed point (cell), evaluates connectivities with surrounding cells, and finds connecting cells. To determine the cell connectivity, the pairs of neighbor labels on the boundary of two cells are used. If a label pair does not include an empty label and is not listed in the SLPs, the pair is recognized as a connected pair. If at least one connected pair is detected, the two cells are determined to be connected. If more than one region (connected cells) is detected, the node is replicated for each region and the corresponding node references are changed in the cells of the region to the superimposed node. If no region is detected, the node is deleted.

Optionally, floating cells are deleted. In many cases, a segmented medical image includes isolated small segments. Such segments may cause unmeaningful small pieces in mechanical simulation. To avoid this, we count the number of cells for each cell island (a set of connected cells). If the number is smaller than a user-specified threshold, the cells are deleted. From our experience, an adequate threshold is two cells.

2.3   Physics Simulation and Visualization

In this study, the generated meshes were validated by performing finite element method (FEM) simulation based on a corotational formulation and implicit time integration scheme for the calculation of dynamic soft-tissue deformation [6]. Each generated hexahedral cell is divided into five first-order tetrahedral elements and a linear elastic property is applied. The values related to material properties are the same for all elements and we adopts the property of a soft material: Young's modulus 1000 Pa, Poisson's ratio 0.4, density $1.0\,\mathrm{g/cm^3}$.

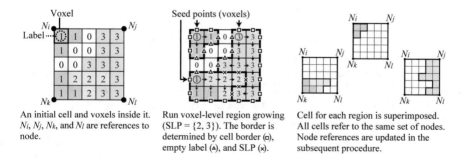

An initial cell and voxels inside it. N_i, N_j, N_k, and N_l are references to node.

Run voxel-level region growing (SLP = {2, 3}). The border is determined by cell border (□), empty label (△), and SLP (×).

Cell for each region is superimposed. All cells refer to the same set of nodes. Node references are updated in the subsequent procedure.

Fig. 3. Superimposed cell generation using voxel-level region growing.

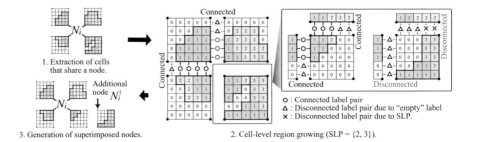

Fig. 4. Superimposed node generation using cell-level region growing.

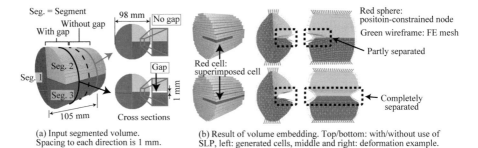

Fig. 5. Evaluation using a cylinder-shaped segmented volume. (Color figure online)

For graphics rendering, the surface polygons of segmented volumes are generated using the marching cubes method. As in [6,7], the polygons are deformed according to the deformed FE mesh obtained by the FEM simulation. In this method, each surface vertex is associated with a tetrahedral element in advance and affine transformation is applied to the vertex to hold the initial barycentric coordinate in the associated tetrahedron. The deformation of volume data is realized by considering voxels as particles. The transformations of the particles are performed in the same way as for surface polygon vertices.

3   Results and Discussions

The proposed method was evaluated using a cylinder-shaped segmented volume and brain atlas dataset published in [4]. All numerical experiments were executed by an implementation on a workstation with an Intel Core i7-3960X (6 cores, overclocked to 4.5 GHz), 64 GB of RAM, and two GPUs, an NVIDIA K20c (2,496 CUDA cores) for the computing of FEM and an NVIDIA Quadro K5000 (1536 CUDA cores) for graphics processing. The proposed meshing algorithms were parallelized using OpenMP.

Cylinder Model. Figure 5 shows the result of the evaluation using a cylinder-shaped segmented volume. As shown in Fig. 5(a), the input volume has three

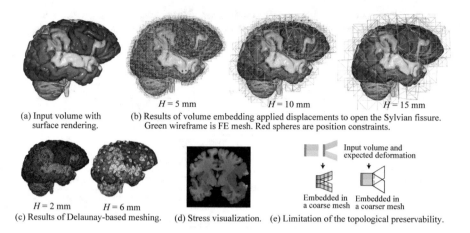

$H = 5$ mm $H = 10$ mm $H = 15$ mm

(a) Input volume with   (b) Results of volume embedding applied displacements to open the Sylvian fissure.
surface rendering.   Green wireframe is FE mesh. Red spheres are position constraints.

$H = 2$ mm $H = 6$ mm

(c) Results of Delaunay-based meshing.   (d) Stress visualization.   (e) Limitation of the topological preservability.

Fig. 6. Evaluation using a brain atlas [4].

segments labeled 1, 2, and 3. In the front-half part of the volume, there is a groove between segments 2 and 3. The width of the groove is equal to the length of a voxel. In the rear-half part, segments 2 and 3 are completely attached without any gap. Figure 5(b) shows the two results of the proposed volume embedding: the top part shows the result without SLP and the bottom part shows the result with SLP $\{2, 3\}$. Both of the results were obtained using a mesh size of $H = 5$ mm. The left part of Fig. 5(b) shows the generated cells. In the figure, gray and red cells indicate normal and superimposed cells, respectively. The right part of Fig. 5(b) shows the deformation examples of the meshes from two different views. In this figure, it is clear that the groove was separated even when the SLP was not used. However, without SLPs, the completely attached boundary of segments 2 and 3 was not separated. In contrast, the separation of the boundary was achieved using the SLP. This result shows that the use of SLPs is effective for separating completely attached segments.

Brain Atlas. Figure 6 shows the results of the evaluation using a brain atlas [4]. Figure 6(b) shows the results of the proposed method. The input SLPs were manually specified by the author to separate the Sylvian fissure in order to utilize the generated mesh in our neurosurgery simulator [9]. The displacements to open the Sylvian fissure was imposed after the FE mesh generation and calculated the shape of the equilibrium. To compare the proposed method with a well-established method, Delaunay-based meshing without feature preservation [8] implemented in CGAL library [1] was also conducted (Fig. 6(c)). The quantitative results are described in Table 1. Note that the measurement of the computational time of the FEM simulation (global matrix assembly and linear system solving with 20 CG iterations [9]) is performed only for our embedding method, and in the case of our method with $H = 2.0$, the simulation was not executed because of out of GPU device memory due to too large mesh.

Table 1. Quantitative results of the evaluation using the brain atlas ($256 \times 256 \times 256$) [4]. N_{vert} and N_{tet} are the number of vertices and tetrahedra, T_{mesh} and T_{fem} are the computational time taken for the mesh generation and a loop of FEM simulation, respectively.

Method	Mesh size (mm)	N_{vert}	N_{tet}	T_{mesh} (s)	T_{fem} (ms)
Pons, et al. [8]	2.0	$149,506$	$799,165$	22.23	–
Pons, et al. [8]	4.0	$44,421$	$95,740$	7.43	–
Pons, et al. [8]	6.0	$6,106$	$29,144$	1.28	–
Ours	2.0	$227,225$	$925,360$	5.78	–
Ours	5.0	$22,999$	$79,650$	0.57	133.3
Ours	10.0	$4,829$	$14,130$	0.19	30.8
Ours	15.0	$2,072$	$5,530$	0.16	11.9

Delaunay-based meshing with a resolution that is too low, as noted in [8], produced a non-manifold mesh that included singular vertices for which the thickness is zero, which leads to instability in FEM. Further, small or thin segments vanished in the resulting mesh. In contrast, the proposed method generated meshes that cover the entire body of the volume and FEM simulation was conducted without instability. Figure 6(c) shows that the frontal and temporal lobes are separated and the topology of the Sylvian fissure is correctly preserved.

Figure 7 shows the parallel scalability of each algorithm stage of the mesh generation by timing the executions with different number of threads. The algorithms for "superimposed cell generation" and "superimposed node generation" were parallelized straightforwardly because they are cell- and node-independent, and their good scalability can be observed. Thanks to this performance, hexahedral mesh generations were finished in several seconds, as shown in Table 1. This enables us to find a balance between accuracy and performance by modifying the mesh size effectively. In our implementation of FEM, a mesh with 5,000 nodes can be calculated in real-time rate (30 fps). Therefore, we were able to determine that a mesh with $H = 10.0\,\text{mm}$ is adequate for interactive simulation.

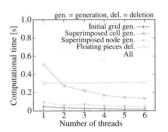

Fig. 7. Parallel scalability.

Figure 6(d) shows a postprocess application example using 3D Slicer [3] that visualizes the stress field inside the brain. This was obtained by exporting a deformed volume with mesh size 5 mm. This is valuable, for example, when objectively assessing the damage of a retraction.

However, there is a limit on the topological preservability. When mesh size H increases, small boundaries with lengths that are smaller than H were connected (Fig. 6(e)). Thus, the mesh size needs to be determined considering the lengths of boundaries that should be preserved.

4   Conclusion and Future Work

In this paper, we proposed a volume embedding method that preserves the topology of a structure according to a segmented medical image and user-defined SLPs. The method was evaluated in terms of its ability to approximate deformations and computational time. The evaluation shows that the proposed method can generate topology-preserved meshes fast and robustly.

There are some problems to address in future. The proposed method ignores the boundary conformity of the FE mesh and decreases in the precision of the mechanical simulations. These issues can be mitigated by modifying the stiffness matrix according to the spatial distribution of labels inside each cell [7]. Furthermore, contact handling can be addressed by placing collision proxy points inside the volumetric mesh [5]. These treatments would enhance the quality of the simulations.

Acknowledgements. This work was supported by the Japan Society for the Promotion of Science (JSPS) through the Grant-in-Aid for Scientific Research (A) (15H01707) and the Grant-in-Aid for JSPS Fellows (15J01452).

References

1. CGAL: Computational Geometry Algorithms Library. http://www.cgal.org/
2. Boltcheva, D., Yvinec, M., Boissonnat, J.-D.: Mesh generation from 3D multi-material images. In: Yang, G.-Z., Hawkes, D., Rueckert, D., Noble, A., Taylor, C. (eds.) MICCAI 2009. LNCS, vol. 5762, pp. 283–290. Springer, Heidelberg (2009). doi:10.1007/978-3-642-04271-3_35
3. Fedorov, A., Beichel, R., Kalpathy-Cramer, J., Finet, J., Fillion-Robin, J.C., Pujol, S., Bauer, C., Jennings, D., Fennessy, F., Sonka, M., Buatti, J., Aylward, S., Miller, J.V., Pieper, S., Kikinis, R.: 3D Slicer as an image computing platform for the quantitative imaging network. Magn. Reson. Imaging **30**(9), 1323–1341 (2012)
4. Halle, M., Talos, I.F., Jakab, M., Makris, N., Meier, D., Wald, L., Fischl, B.,Kikinis, R.: Multi-modality MRI-based atlas of the brain (2015). https://www.spl.harvard.edu/publications/item/view/2037
5. McAdams, A., Zhu, Y., Selle, A., Empey, M., Tamstorf, R., Teran, J., Sifakis, E.: Efficient elasticity for character skinning with contact and collisions. ACM Trans. Graph. **30**(4), 37:1–37:12 (2011)
6. Müller, M., Gross, M.: Interactive virtual materials. In: Proceedings of GraphicsInterface 2004, pp. 239–246 (2004)
7. Nesme, M., Kry, P.G., Jeřábková, L., Faure, F.: Preserving topology and elasticity for embedded deformable models. ACM Trans. Graph. **28**(3), 52:1–52:9 (2009)
8. Pons, J.-P., Ségonne, F., Boissonnat, J.-D., Rineau, L., Yvinec, M., Keriven, R.: High-quality consistent meshing of multi-label datasets. In: Karssemeijer, N., Lelieveldt, B. (eds.) IPMI 2007. LNCS, vol. 4584, pp. 198–210. Springer, Heidelberg (2007). doi:10.1007/978-3-540-73273-0_17
9. Sase, K., Fukuhara, A., Tsujita, T., Konno, A.: GPU-accelerated surgery simulation for opening a brain fissure. ROBOMECH J. **2**(1), 1–16 (2015)

Deformable 3D-2D Registration of Known Components for Image Guidance in Spine Surgery

A. Uneri[1], J. Goerres[2], T. De Silva[2], M.W. Jacobson[2], M.D. Ketcha[2],
S. Reaungamornrat[1], G. Kleinszig[3], S. Vogt[3], A.J. Khanna[4],
J.-P. Wolinsky[5], and J.H. Siewerdsen[1,2,5(✉)]

[1] Computer Science, Johns Hopkins University, Baltimore, MD, USA
[2] Biomedical Engineering, Johns Hopkins University, Baltimore, MD, USA
[3] Siemens Healthcare XP Division, Erlangen, Germany
[4] Orthopaedic Surgery, Johns Hopkins Medical Institute, Baltimore, MD, USA
[5] Neurological Surgery, Johns Hopkins Medical Institute, Baltimore, MD, USA
jeff.siewerdsen@jhu.edu

Abstract. A 3D-2D image registration method is reported for guiding the placement of surgical devices (e.g., K-wires). The solution registers preoperative CT (and planning data therein) to intraoperative radiographs and computes the pose, shape, *and deformation* parameters of devices (termed "components") known to be in the radiographic scene. The deformable known-component registration (dKC-Reg) method was applied in experiments emulating spine surgery to register devices (K-wires and spinal fixation rods) undergoing realistic deformation. A two-stage registration process (i) resolves patient pose from individual radiographs and (ii) registers components represented as polygonal meshes based on a B-spline model. The registration result can be visualized as overlay of the component in CT analogous to surgical navigation but without conventional trackers or fiducials. Target registration error in the tip and orientation of deformable K-wires was (1.5 ± 0.9) mm and $(0.6° \pm 0.2°)$, respectively. For spinal fixation rods, the registered components achieved Hausdorff distance of 3.4 mm. Future work includes testing in cadaver and clinical data and extension to more generalized deformation and component models.

Keywords: 3D-2D registration · Deformable registration · Image-guided surgery · Surgical navigation · Quality assurance · Spine surgery

1 Introduction

Intraoperative x-ray projection images (radiography and fluoroscopy) are commonly used in neurosurgery and orthopaedic surgery for up-to-date visualization of patient anatomy and surgical devices placed therein. However, accurate interpretation of the 3D orientation of devices within complex anatomy can challenge even experienced surgeons – for example, assessing the trajectory of a K-wire within safe margins of a bone corridor in spine or pelvis surgery, which requires accuracies of 1 mm and 5° [1]. Potential solutions include the use of tracking systems and fiducial markers for surgical navigation, but the additional workflow associated with tool calibration and

© Springer International Publishing AG 2016
S. Ourselin et al. (Eds.): MICCAI 2016, Part III, LNCS 9902, pp. 124–132, 2016.
DOI: 10.1007/978-3-319-46726-9_15

patient registration in addition to the requirement for extrinsic fiducials are commonly cited as barriers to ease of use and broad utilization. Furthermore, many classes of trackers are limited to rigid bodies due to the affixed external markers. Electromagnetic trackers offer a potential solution to this problem by embedding markers at the tip of tools within the body (e.g., a flexible endoscope); however such systems tend to exhibit somewhat lower registration accuracy and may suffer from metal interference. Intraoperative 3D imaging systems, such as CT, cone-beam CT (CBCT), and MRI, can provide excellent 3D visualization of anatomy and the surgical product but carry additional expense, patient access, workflow, and (possibly) radiation dose that also challenge broad utilization.

An alternative approach can provide 3D localization from intraoperative 2D radiographic images via 3D-2D registration to preoperative 3D images and planning information therein [2]. Such registration methods can extend the functionality of intraoperative 2D imaging that is already common in the surgical arsenal, integrating more naturally with standard workflow and potentially absolving the aforementioned limitations associated with surgical tracking and intraoperative 3D imaging. These methods have recently been used in the context of spine surgery [3] as well as to solve for the pose of rigid implants [4, 5] as a means of verifying the surgical product. Accurate account of deformation remains a significant challenge, with promising results offered by statistical shape models to solve for interpatient anatomical differences [6].

In this work, we combine a 3D-2D image registration method with deformable models of surgical devices ("known components") to resolve their pose and (deformed) shape within the patient. In a sense, the approach exploits the radiographic imaging system as a "tracker," the patient as their own "reference marker," and surgical components themselves as "tracked tools." The method was applied within the context of spine surgery, using a phantom experiment and mobile C-arm to emulate a spinal fixation procedure. Surgical components (viz., K-wires and spinal fixation rods) were deformably registered based on three intraoperative radiographs. Geometric accuracy was analyzed in terms of target registration error (TRE) as well as concordance with the shape of the deformed component.

2   Methods

2.1   3D-2D Registration Framework

The proposed solution involves a robust, gradient-based 3D-2D registration algorithm composed of two distinct stages that work in tandem to solve for the 3D pose of the patient as well as the components as shown in Fig. 1. In each stage, 2D intraoperative radiographic projections are registered to a particular source of prior information: (i) the patient registration stage (red in Fig. 1) computes the transformation relating one or more radiographs (P_θ) to the preoperative CT (V) acquired for surgical planning; and (ii) the component registration stage (blue in Fig. 1) computes the pose and parameter vector relating two or more radiographs (the same P_θ) to a parametric model ($C(p)$) of surgical devices within the patient (referred to as "known components"). As detailed below, both stages iteratively optimize the gradient similarity between the radiographs (*P*) and digitally reconstructed radiographs (DRRs) of the input 3D information (*V* or *C*). The patient registration stage is based on the method in [3] and can optionally include locally rigid/globally deformable transformation of patient information as in [7]. The component registration is based on the (rigid) "known-component" registration (KC-Reg) method in [5], with the main advance reported below involving a *deformable* transformation model of the known components – e.g., needles, rods, and catheters that would not follow a simple rigid transform.

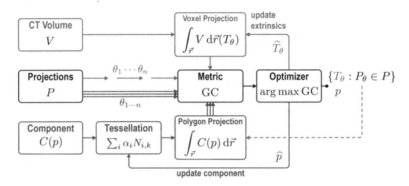

Fig. 1. Flowchart for the deformable known-component registration (dKC-Reg) algorithm. Red: patient registration. Blue: registration of surgical components. The algorithm first solves for the transformation relating one or more radiograph (*P*) to the patient CT (*V*). The pose and deformation parameters of the component are then solved from one or more radiographs (*P_θ*). Note that the system operates free of conventional tracking/navigation systems and fiducial markers and employs simple mobile radiographic imaging systems already common in the operating room. (Color figure online)

The algorithm uses radiographic projections (*P*) (e.g., from a mobile C-arm) as normally acquired within the standard-of-care for anterior-posterior (AP), lateral, and oblique views (*θ*) of patient anatomy. Similarity between the projection and the DRR of the current estimate is then computed using pixel-wise gradient correlation (GC):

$$GC(f, m) = \frac{1}{2}\left\{ NCC\left(\nabla_x f, \nabla_x m\right) + NCC\left(\nabla_y f, \nabla_y m\right)\right\}$$
$$\text{where, } NCC(\nabla f, \nabla m) = \frac{\nabla f \nabla m}{\nabla f \nabla m} \tag{1}$$

and ∇ is the gradient operator applied to the fixed radiograph (*f*) and moving DRR (*m*) images. The similarity metric is iteratively optimized using the covariance matrix adaptation evolution strategy (CMA-ES [8]) with a population of ~200 samples per iteration.

The optimization problem for the first stage uses the preoperative CT volume (*V*) to establish the radiographic pose of a given projection view (*P_θ*), defined as:

$$\hat{T}_\theta = \arg\max_T \ GC\left(P_\theta, \int_{\vec{r}} V d\vec{r}(T_\theta)\right) \tag{2}$$

where T_θ are the rigid extrinsic parameters of projective geometry, governed by 6 degrees-of-freedom (DoF) representing translation and rotation (with extension to a globally deformable model in [7]). This process is repeated for each $P_\theta \in P$ to yield a set of transforms that describe radiographs with respect to the patient coordinate frame in lieu of a predetermined geometric calibration, thereby extending applicability beyond well-calibrated, computer-controlled C-arms and allowing increased DoF in C-arm positioning.

The second stage uses the parameterized component model (C) and optimizes the parameter vector (p) describing the pose, shape (e.g., diameter), and deformation via:

$$\hat{p} = \arg\max_p \sum_\theta GC\left(P_\theta, \int_{\vec{r}} C(p) d\vec{r}(\hat{T}_\theta)\right) \tag{3}$$

Note that the geometric relation established in the previous stage resolves the 3D component within the patient frame of reference and allows simultaneous projection of components and comparison to multiple (2–3) radiographs as expressed by the sum of their similarity. This is important for small, relatively simple surgical device components (unlike large, feature-rich anatomy), since the components have fewer characteristic features and may be ambiguous in certain views (e.g., end on view of a K-wire). This is especially important for deformable components to yield a unique (nondegenerate) solution for $\hat{p}$, and the use of multiple (2 or 3) views provides robustness to such degeneracy and accurate 3D localization.

2.2 Deformable Component Model

The component registration method uses a parametric description of surgical devices represented as polygonal meshes, providing a fairly general framework for modeling various 3D shapes and modes of deformation without manufacturer-specific (often proprietary) knowledge of device design. In this study, as illustrated in Fig. 2, we use a simple B-spline model for the component centerline with a tessellated mesh description of its radial extent, yielding a parametric description suitable to a broad range of devices presenting cylindrical symmetry (e.g., K-wires, needles, rods, shunts, catheters, flexible endoscopes, and some robotic manipulators).

The B-spline model was chosen due to its locality and compatibility with the optimization framework, with individual control points (DoFs) that can be manipulated without changing the shape of the entire curve:

$$C(u) = \sum_{i=0}^{n} \alpha_i N_{i,k}(u) \tag{4}$$

where control points $\alpha_i \in p$ are a subset of the component parameter vector, $\hat{p}$. Cubic splines ($k = 3$) were used for orders $n > 2$ (excepting the first order [$n = 1$] for which

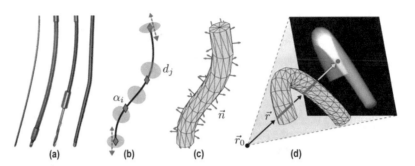

Fig. 2. Deformable component models. (a) Example surgical tools (K-wire, flexible screwdriver, drill, and spinal fixation rod) presenting a cylindrical profile. (b) Parametric B-spline component model showing control points (α_i), attached discs (d_j), and tangent lines at clamped endpoints. (c) Tessellated 3D model with computed surface normals. (d) Non-convex polygon projection with multiple red line segments indicating line integrals through the mesh. (Color figure online)

$k = 1$ and second order [$n = 2$] for which $k = 2$). The spline is clamped by constraining the first and last knots to $u_0 = u_1 \dots = u_k$ and $u_{n+1-k} = \dots = u_n = u_{n+1}$ such that the curve is tangent to the first and the last legs at the first and last control point. Such clamping ensures that the endpoint and approach angle of the device match that of the corresponding control point.

To construct the 3D cylindrical mesh about the centerline, the spline is sampled at locations d_j corresponding to an arbitrary number of discs with radius $r \in p$, where $C(d_j)$ and $C'(d_j)$ define the position and orientation of each disc such that each disc is orthogonal to the spline as shown in Fig. 2. The discs are tessellated using triangles, and the surface normals of the resulting mesh are computed.

A novel polygon projector was defined to compute the DRR for the component model at each iteration of the optimization. The projector handles potential non-convex configurations that may occur (i.e., when the component bends on itself in the radiographic views) as follows:

$$\int_{\vec{r}} C \mathrm{d}\vec{r} \approx \sum_{t=1}^{T} \mathrm{sgn}(\vec{r} \cdot \vec{n}\{C_t\}) ||\psi(\vec{r}, C_t) - \vec{r}_0||_2 \tag{5}$$

which computes the line integral through the mesh by summing the contribution of all triangles (T) for a given ray ($\vec{r}$). The intersection point (ψ) between $\vec{r}$ and any given triangle on the component surface (C_t) is computed using the Möller–Trumbore intersection algorithm. If a triangle is not intersected by $\vec{r}$, then $\psi = \vec{r}_0$ (i.e., ray origin, which in this context is the x-ray source), thereby zeroing its contribution to the DRR. The sgn operation uses the surface normal $\vec{n}$ at C_t to distinguish between and inbound and outbound rays on the mesh such that only the interior of the surface is integrated, thus handling non-convexity.

2.3   Experimental Evaluation

Experiments were conducted to test and evaluate the dKC-Reg algorithm in scenarios emulating the placement of transpedicle K-wires, pedicle screws, and spinal fixation rods in spine surgery. As shown in Fig. 3a, an anthropomorphic spine phantom placed within a soft-tissue holder (Sawbones, Pacific Research Laboratories, WA USA) formed the experimental model, with a CT scan acquired prior to placement of instrumentation (Toshiba Aquilion ONE CT scanner). Projection radiographs were acquired in the course of device placement using a mobile C-arm (Cios Alpha, Siemens, Erlangen Germany) yielding both the 1, 2, or 3 views employed for patient and component registration (Fig. 1) as well as a full orbital scan for CBCT "truth" definition following placement of each device. K-wires were placed in lumbar vertebrae (L1–L5) with the K-wire purposely bent to effect deformation. Device trajectories included medial (L1) and lateral (L2) breaches. Finally, spinal rods were bent to approximate correction of spinal curvature.

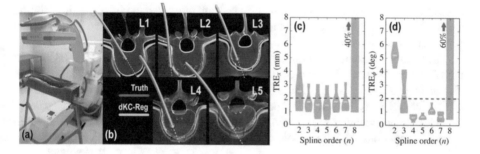

Fig. 3. Deformable registration for K-wire guidance. (a) Experimental setup using a mobile C-arm and spine phantom. (b) Axial views of the pre-op CT showing the registered position of deformed registered components (yellow) in comparison to truth (magenta). (c–d) TRE of the K-wire tip (TRE_x, mm) and trajectory (TRE_ϕ, °) evaluated as a function of B-spline order. The deformable registration is found to be stable over a fairly broad range of spline order ($n = 3$–7) but fails from overfitting for order ≥ 8. (Color figure online)

Geometric accuracy of the registration was quantified in terms of targeting accuracy (at the tip of the K-wire) and proximity to the true shape of the component (for both the K-wire and fixation rods). The true position and shape were defined from thresholding, segmentation, and centerline extraction in a CBCT image acquired using the same C-arm for each device placement. The k-wire tips were conspicuous in these images, despite the usual metal artifacts. For the K-wires, registration accuracy was evaluated in terms of the error in component tip and angular trajectory, quantified using positional and angular variations on TRE:

$$TRE_x = ||C(\alpha_0) - C_{true}(\alpha_0)||_2$$
$$TRE_\phi = \cos^{-1} \frac{C'(\alpha_0) \cdot C'_{true}(\alpha_0)}{||C'(\alpha_0) \cdot C'_{true}(\alpha_0)||} \quad (6)$$

where α_0 is the spline control point for the K-wire tip. For both the K-wires and spinal fixation rods, registration accuracy was also evaluated in terms of the concordance between the true centerline and spline registration result along the entire length of the device. At each point along the component, the distance to the true centerline was computed (Δ_x), as well as Hausdorff distance (HD) used to quantify the degree of overlap of the modeled component:

$$HD = \max_a \left(\min_b ||C(a) - C_{\text{true}}(b)||_2 \right) \tag{7}$$

where C is the model and C_{true} is the segmented medial line.

3   Results

3.1   K-Wires

Registration results for the K-wire guidance task are presented in Fig. 3b, demonstrating successful registration in each vertebral level with overall translational error <2 mm and trajectory angulation error <1° [Fig. 3c–d].

The method also correctly indicated the suboptimal trajectories at L1 (medial breach) and L2 (lateral breach). The non-convex projector correctly handled retrograde curving of tools in generated samples prior to converging at the solution. Analysis of sensitivity to B-spline order (n) showed robust performance for $n = 4$–7; lower-order splines failed to model the deformation of the wire, and higher-order splines ($n \geq 8$) were subject to sporadic excursions from a realistic curve. A nominal spline order $n = 3$ or 4 yielded statistically significant improvement ($p < 0.05$) in TRE_x (1.51 ± 0.90 mm) and TRE_ϕ ($0.58 \pm 0.22°$) compared to a 2nd-order spline.

3.2   Spinal Rods

Applying the dKC-Reg method to curved spinal fixation rods also yielded good agreement with the true curvature of the component as visualized and quantified in Fig. 4. The convergence of the algorithm is illustrated in Fig. 4b, which shows GC similarity increasing monotonically and reaching a stable maximum for >~50 iterations, beyond which performance assessed in terms of Hausdorff distance is better than 5 mm. Analysis of the results with respect to the B-spline order (n) show agreement with the K-wire results. Similar to Fig. 3c–d, the registration results were stable for spline orders in the range $n = 3$–7. For $n = 3$, overall concordance was $\Delta_x = (2.46 \pm 0.72)$ mm, and $HD = 3.35$ mm, which demarks the greatest separation from truth.

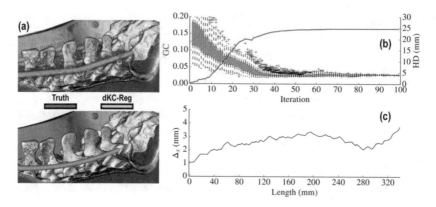

Fig. 4. Deformable registration of spinal fixation rods. (a) Volumetric rendering of the post-op CT with the true component (top, magenta), and the registered component visualized in pre-op CT (bottom, yellow) for spline order $n = 3$. (b) Convergence behavior of the optimizer illustrated in terms of the similarity metric (GC) and the HD measured as a function of iteration number. (c) Mean deviations from true position measured along the length of spinal rod. (Color figure online)

4 Conclusion

A new method for 3D image guidance was presented that utilizes simple mobile radiography/fluoroscopy systems already common in the operating theatre to derive accurate localization and guidance of surgical devices within the body. The algorithm detailed in this work uses low-order parameterization of surgical components and includes deformation of the components (e.g., bending wire) within the solution. Experimental evaluation in a phantom emulating spine surgery yielded registration accuracy better than 2 mm and 2° in the tip and orientation of (deformed) device components. The focus of the experiments were on the deformable component, and while the phantom used is admittedly simple, the patient registration have been shown to be very robust in clinical data that included anatomical deformation [7, 9]. While the system offers the means for navigation without the common workflow limitations of conventional tracking systems and assumption of rigid tools, it does not provide real-time visualization, rather updates with each radiographic view. Future work includes testing in clinical data and application to other clinical applications, such as the placement of catheters, shunts, or stents, where the cylindrical component model described above may be expected to hold. The framework will also be extended to support more general component shapes and modes of deformation, potentially employing more generalized deformation models, such as non-uniform rational basis splines (NURBS), which has shown promise in the field of computer-aided design.

Acknowledgements. Research supported by NIH grant R01-EB-017226 and academic-industry partnership with Siemens Healthcare (XP Division, Erlangen Germany).

References

1. Rampersaud, Y.R., Simon, D.A., Foley, K.T.: Accuracy requirements for image-guided spinal pedicle screw placement. Spine (Phila. Pa. 1976) **26**, 352–359 (2001)
2. Markelj, P., Tomaževič, D., Likar, B., Pernuš, F.: A review of 3D/2D registration methods for image-guided interventions. Med. Image Anal. **16**, 642–661 (2012)
3. Otake, Y., Schafer, S., Stayman, J.W., Zbijewski, W., Kleinszig, G., Graumann, R., Khanna, A.J., Siewerdsen, J.H.: Automatic localization of vertebral levels in x-ray fluoroscopy using 3D-2D registration: a tool to reduce wrong-site surgery. Phys. Med. Biol. **57**, 5485–5508 (2012)
4. Jaramaz, B., Eckman, K.: 2D/3D registration for measurement of implant alignment after total hip replacement. In: Larsen, R., Nielsen, M., Sporring, J. (eds.) MICCAI 2006. LNCS, vol. 4191, pp. 653–661. Springer, Heidelberg (2006)
5. Uneri, A., De Silva, T., Stayman, J.W., Kleinszig, G., Vogt, S., Khanna, A.J., Gokaslan, Z.L., Wolinsky, J.-P., Siewerdsen, J.H.: Known-component 3D–2D registration for quality assurance of spine surgery pedicle screw placement. Phys. Med. Biol. **60**, 8007–8024 (2015)
6. Sadowsky, O., Chintalapani, G., Taylor, R.H.: Deformable 2D-3D registration of the pelvis with a limited field of view, using shape statistics. Med. Image Comput. Comput. Assist. Interv. **10**, 519–526 (2007)
7. Ketcha, M.D., De Silva, T., Uneri, A., Kleinszig, G., Vogt, S., Wolinsky, J.-P., Siewerdsen, J.H.: Automatic masking for robust 3D-2D image registration in image-guided spine surgery. In: SPIE Medical Imaging, San Diego, CA, USA (2016)
8. Hansen, N., Ostermeier, A.: Completely derandomized self-adaptation in evolution strategies. Evol. Comput. **9**, 159–195 (2001)
9. De Silva, T., Lo, S.-F.L., Aygun, N., Aghion, D.M., Boah, A., Petteys, R., Uneri, A., Ketcha, M.D., Yi, T., Vogt, S., Kleinszig, G., Wei, W., Weiten, M., Ye, X., Bydon, A., Sciubba, D.M., Witham, T.F., Wolinsky, J.-P., Siewerdsen, J.H.: Utility of the levelcheck algorithm for decision support in vertebral localization. Spine (Phila. Pa. 1976) (2016)

Anatomically Constrained Video-CT Registration via the V-IMLOP Algorithm

Seth D. Billings[1], Ayushi Sinha[1(✉)], Austin Reiter[1], Simon Leonard[1], Masaru Ishii[2], Gregory D. Hager[1], and Russell H. Taylor[1]

[1] The Johns Hopkins University, Baltimore, USA
asinha8@jhu.edu
[2] Johns Hopkins Medical Institutions, Baltimore, USA

Abstract. Functional endoscopic sinus surgery (FESS) is a surgical procedure used to treat acute cases of sinusitis and other sinus diseases. FESS is fast becoming the preferred choice of treatment due to its minimally invasive nature. However, due to the limited field of view of the endoscope, surgeons rely on navigation systems to guide them within the nasal cavity. State of the art navigation systems report registration accuracy of over 1mm, which is large compared to the size of the nasal airways. We present an anatomically constrained video-CT registration algorithm that incorporates multiple video features. Our algorithm is robust in the presence of outliers. We also test our algorithm on simulated and in-vivo data, and test its accuracy against degrading initializations.

1 Introduction

Sinusitis, a disorder characterized by nasal inflammation, is one of the most commonly diagnosed diseases in the United States, affecting approximately 16 % of the adult population annually [1]. Functional endoscopic sinus surgery (FESS) is a minimally invasive surgical procedure used to relieve symptoms of chronic sinusitis. It is estimated that around 600, 000 endoscopic interventions are performed annually in the United States [2]. The sinuses are small, composed of delicate cartilage and surrounded by critical structures, such as the carotid artery and optic nerves. Approximately 5–7 % of endoscopic sinus procedures result in complications classified as minor, and about 1 % result in major complications [3]. The use of an accurate navigation system during FESS can help reduce the rate of complications, and enhance patient safety, surgical efficiency, and outcome.

The popularity of FESS and its need for enhanced navigation have resulted in several video-CT registration algorithms. Direct methods, such as that described in [4], optimize over a similarity metric to match images obtained from endoscopic video and images rendered from CT data. Tracker-based methods use optical or magnetic trackers to track the position of the endoscope relative to

The original version of the chapter 16 was revised: The acknowledgement text was missing in the initially published paper now acknowledgment text is added. The erratum to this chapter is available at https://doi.org/10.1007/978-3-319-46726-9_73

S. Ourselin et al. (Eds.): MICCAI 2016, Part III, LNCS 9902, pp. 133–141, 2019.
DOI: 10.1007/978-3-319-46726-9_16

the patient. Methods described in [5,6] track image features and reconstruct scaled 3D points from video using structure from motion (SfM). These points are then registered to a pre-operative model shape extracted from CT. The standard algorithm for such registrations is the Iterative Closest Point (ICP) algorithm [7]. ICP is a two-step algorithm, which first finds matches between two sets of points, and then computes the transformation that aligns these matches. These two steps are repeated until convergence. Several variants of ICP have been introduced, such as Trimmed ICP, which improves robustness in the presence of outliers [8]. [9] presents a variant of Trimmed ICP that accounts for scale. Probability-based variants with anisotropic noise models have also been introduced. For instance, the Iterative Most Likely Point (IMLP) algorithm [10] incorporates a generalized noise model into both the registration and the correspondence steps.

However, most of these algorithms are limited by the paucity of reliable, high-accuracy video features, resulting in sparse SfM reconstructions. This can cause registration algorithms to converge to inaccurate solutions. Therefore, state of the art experimental navigation systems report registration errors of over 1 mm, with commercial tracker-based systems reporting errors around 2 mm. This hinders reliable navigation within the sinuses, where the thickness of the boundaries is generally less than 1 mm, going as low as 0.5 mm where the roof of the sinuses separates it from the brain, and 0.2 mm where the lateral lamella separates it from the olfactory system [11]. By comparison, CT images can have resolutions of 0.5 mm or less and, ideally, a navigation system should be as accurate as the underlying CT. We present the Video Iterative Most Likely Oriented Point (V-IMLOP) algorithm, which extends the IMLP framework [10] by registering additional features. More specifically, while most algorithms rely solely on 3D point sets, V-IMLOP also uses oriented 2D contours to compute a registration.

2   Methods

2.1   Video Iterative Most Likely Point (V-IMLOP)

V-IMLOP uses two types of image features for video-CT registration: 3D point features up to scale, and 2D oriented point features representing occluding surface contours. The registration incorporates a probabilistic framework by modeling the uncertainty of these features. The uncertainty of each 3D point is modeled by a 3D anisotropic Gaussian distribution, while the position and orientation uncertainties of a point on a 2D contour are modeled by a 2D anisotropic Gaussian and von Mises distributions [12] respectively. V-IMLOP consists of two main phases, correspondence and registration. In the correspondence phase, a match for each data feature, $\mathbf{x} \in \mathbf{X}$, is computed by selecting the model point, $\mathbf{y} \in \mathbf{Y}$ that maximizes the probability of having generated $\mathbf{x}$. The choice of $\mathbf{y}$ forms the *match likelihood function* (MLF). Assuming zero-mean uncertainty and independence of the features in each measurement, and given a 3D point feature, $\mathbf{x}_{3d}$, and a current registration estimate, $\mathbf{T} = [s, \mathbf{R}, \mathbf{t}]$, the MLF is defined as

$$f_{\text{match\_3d}}(\mathbf{x}_{3d}|\mathbf{y}_{3d}, \mathbf{\Sigma}_{3d}, s, \mathbf{R}, \mathbf{t}) =$$
$$\frac{1}{(2\pi)^{3/2}|\mathbf{\Sigma}_{3d}|^{1/2}} e^{-\frac{1}{2}(\mathbf{y}_{3d}-s\mathbf{R}\mathbf{x}_{3d}-\mathbf{t})^{\mathbf{T}}\mathbf{R}\mathbf{\Sigma}_{3d}^{-1}\mathbf{R}^{\mathbf{T}}(\mathbf{y}_{3d}-s\mathbf{R}\mathbf{x}_{3d}-\mathbf{t})}, \qquad (1)$$

where $\mathbf{T}$ is a similarity transform. $\mathbf{y}_{3d}$ is the 3D position on the model shape that is assumed to be in correspondence with the transformed 3D data point $\mathbf{T}(\mathbf{x}_{3d}) = s\mathbf{R}\mathbf{x}_{3d} + \mathbf{t}$. $\mathbf{\Sigma}_{3d}$ is the covariance matrix of 3D positional uncertainty for the non-transformed 3D data point, and $\mathbf{R}\mathbf{\Sigma}_{3d}\mathbf{R}^{\mathbf{T}}$ is the covariance of the transformed 3D data point. Maximizing Eq. 1 simplifies to computing the model point, $\mathbf{y}_{3d}$, that minimizes the negative log likelihood, simplified as

$$C_{3d} = \frac{1}{2}(\mathbf{y}_{3d} - s\mathbf{R}\mathbf{x}_{3d} - \mathbf{t})^{\mathbf{T}}\mathbf{R}\mathbf{\Sigma}_{3d}^{-1}\mathbf{R}^{\mathbf{T}}(\mathbf{y}_{3d} - s\mathbf{R}\mathbf{x}_{3d} - \mathbf{t}) \qquad (2)$$

Next, we define the MLF for an oriented 2D contour feature, $\mathbf{x}_{2d} = (\mathbf{x}_{2dp}, \hat{\mathbf{x}}_{2dn})$:

$$f_{\text{match\_2d}}(\mathbf{x}_{2d}|\mathbf{y}_{3d}, \mathbf{\Sigma}_{2d}, \kappa, s, \mathbf{R}, \mathbf{t}) =$$
$$\frac{1}{(2\pi)^2|\mathbf{\Sigma}_{2d}|^{1/2}I_0(\kappa)} e^{\kappa\hat{\mathbf{y}}_{2dn}^{\mathbf{T}}\hat{\mathbf{x}}_{2dn}-\frac{1}{2}(\mathbf{y}_{2dp}-\mathbf{x}_{2dp})^{\mathbf{T}}\mathbf{\Sigma}_{2d}^{-1}(\mathbf{y}_{2dp}-\mathbf{x}_{2dp})}, \qquad (3)$$

where $\mathbf{\Sigma}_{2d}$ is the covariance matrix of 2D positional uncertainty for $\mathbf{x}_{2dp}$, and κ is the concentration parameter of 2D orientational uncertainty for $\hat{\mathbf{x}}_{2dn}$. $\mathbf{y}_{2dp}$ is the positional component of the model point, $\mathbf{y}_{3d}$, which has been projected onto the 2D image plane of the video using a perspective projection. The normalized orientation component, $\hat{\mathbf{y}}_{2dn}$, of $\mathbf{y}_{3d}$ is similarly a projection onto the video image plane, but done by orthographic projection to avoid division by zero depth since the 3D model orientations of occluding contours are parallel to the image plane. Both $\mathbf{y}_{2dp}$ and $\hat{\mathbf{y}}_{2dn}$ are scaled to convert from metric to pixel units.

As before, maximizing Eq. 3 with respect to $\mathbf{y}_{3d}$ can be reduced to minimizing a contour match error function. However, we must ensure that only visible model contours are projected onto the video image planes as potential matches. To achieve this, we use the estimated camera positions to compute the occluding contours and render the model. The z-buffers from rendering are then used to determine the subset, $\mathbf{\Psi}$, of occluding contours that are visible to each video image. Therefore, the contour match error for the jth video frame reduces to computing $\mathbf{y}_{2d}$ from the set $\mathbf{\Psi}_j$ that minimizes the projected contour match error function:

$$C_{2d} = \frac{1}{2}(\mathbf{y}_{2dp} - \mathbf{x}_{2dp})^{\mathbf{T}}\mathbf{\Sigma}_{2d}^{-1}(\mathbf{y}_{2dp} - \mathbf{x}_{2dp}) + \kappa(1 - \hat{\mathbf{y}}_{2dn}^{\mathbf{T}}\hat{\mathbf{x}}_{2dn}). \qquad (4)$$

An upper bound on the match orientation error is also imposed to prevent matches of widely differing orientation.

In the registration phase, we determine an updated pose for the data points by computing the similarity transform, $\mathbf{T}$, that minimizes the total match error:

$$\mathbf{T} = \underset{[s,\mathbf{R},\mathbf{t}]}{\text{argmin}} \left(\sum_{i=1}^{n_{3d}} C_{3di} + \sum_{j=1}^{n_{\text{cam}}} \sum_{i=1}^{n_{\text{ctr}j}} C_{2dji} \right), \qquad (5)$$

where n_{3d} is the number of 3D data points, n_{cam} is the number of video images, and n_{ctrj} is the number of contour features in the jth video image. The correspondence and registration phases are repeated until convergence.

Outlier rejection is performed between these phases. A fraction of 3D feature pairs with highest match error are first removed, followed by chi-square tests to identify further outliers satisfying the following inequality:

$$(\mathbf{y}_{3di} - s\mathbf{R}\mathbf{x}_{3di} - \mathbf{t})^{\mathbf{T}}\mathbf{R}(\boldsymbol{\Sigma}_{3di} + \sigma_{in}\mathbf{I})^{-1}\mathbf{R}^{\mathbf{T}}(\mathbf{y}_{3di} - s\mathbf{R}\mathbf{x}_{3di} - \mathbf{t}) > \text{chi2inv}(p, 3),$$

where σ_{in} is the average square match distance of the current 3D inliers and chi2inv$(p, 3)$ is the inverse CDF function of a chi-square distribution with 3 degrees of freedom evaluated at probability p [10]. Similar chi-square tests are used to reject outlying 2D contour features, with independent tests for position and orientation using the normal approximation to the von Mises distribution [12]. An upper limit on the percent of contour outliers per video frame is also enforced.

An anatomical constraint on the optimization prevents the estimated camera positions from leaving the interior feasible region of the sinus cavity. It is enforced by computing the nearest point on the mesh surface to the optical center of each estimated camera. If the surface normal points away from the camera, then the interior boundary has been crossed and the registration is backed up by fractional amounts of the most recent change until a valid pose is re-acquired.

2.2   Implementation

In this section, we explain how we obtain the data required for V-IMLOP. The 3D data points are computed using SfM on endoscopic video sequences of about 30 frames [6]. Our initial scale estimate is obtained by tracking the endoscope using an electromagnetic tracker and scaling the 3D points to match the magnitude of the endoscope trajectory. Since V-IMLOP optimizes over scale, inaccuracies in this estimate do not greatly affect registration accuracy. Our optimization is constrained by user-defined upper and lower bounds on scale to ensure that an unrealistic scale is not computed in the initial iterations when misalignment of $\mathbf{X}$ and $\mathbf{Y}$ may be very large. Each patient also has a pre-operative CT, which is deformably registered to a hand-segmented template CT created from a dataset of 52 head CTs [13]. The model shape is thereby automatically generated by deforming the template meshes to patient space [14].

Occluding contours in video are computed once using the method described in [15], because this method learns boundaries that naturally separate objects, and mimics depth-based occluding contours with high accuracy (Fig. 1(a)). Contour normals are computed by computing gradients on smoothed video frames, and assigning to each contour point the negative gradient at that point. For the model shape, occluding contours relative to each camera pose are computed during every iteration of V-IMLOP by locating all visible edges in the triangular mesh where one face bordering the edge is oriented towards the camera, and the other away from the camera, thereby forming an occluding edge (Fig. 1(a)).

The measurement noise parameters (Σ_{3d}, Σ_{2d}, and κ) are user defined and do not change during registration. Equal influence is granted to the 3D and 2D feature sets regardless of the feature set sizes by normalizing the user-defined 3D covariances (Σ_{3d}) by factor $n_{3d}(1 - p_t)/n_{2d}$, where n_{3d} and n_{2d} are the total number of 3D and 2D features, and p_t is the initial trim ratio for 3D outliers.

2.3   Initialization

We experiment with two approaches to initialize the registration. First, to develop a baseline, we manually set the camera pose by localizing the anatomy near the targeted field-of-view for each image. This allows us to investigate the sensitivity of V-IMLOP to the starting pose towards achieving correct convergence. Next, we relax this constraint by observing in-situ endoscopic trajectories during interventions, and isolating areas-of-interest through which the surgeon commonly inserts the endoscope. Then, we evenly sample *canonical camera poses* throughout these regions, and store them in our template CT space. Through deformable registration of the template to each patient CT [13], we transform each canonical camera pose to serve as a candidate initialization from which we spawn a V-IMLOP registration process. We also slightly vary the initial scale. Finally, we select the solution yielding the minimum contour error. The residual surface error between the data points and model surface after the final transformation does not reflect failures in registration well, since SfM reconstructions are sparse, and therefore do not guarantee a unique registration. ICP and other similar methods suffer from this drawback, which causes them to often converge to solutions regardless of starting pose. Contour error, however, is a better indicator of performance. In a case where the 3D points align well but the camera pose is wrong, the projected mesh contours will not align with the video contours.

3   Results

In order to quantitatively analyze our method, we evaluated our algorithm on simulated data generated in Gazebo [16]. We used images collected from patients

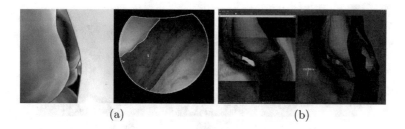

(a)   (b)

Fig. 1. (a) (Left) Mesh contours in red, (right) video contours in white. (b) (Left) Overlay of CT data on the simulated image; (right) red arrows show path of the endoscope with respect to the CT, red dots show registered SfM reconstruction. (Color figure online)

to texture the inside of a sinus mesh extracted from patient CT (Fig. 1(b)). We inserted this model in a simulation with a virtual endoscope, which was navigated within the sinus cavity with physical constraints enforced by enabling collision detection in Gazebo. We computed SfM on a sequence of 30 consecutive simulated endoscopic images, and registered the resulting 2272 data points to the 3D mesh used for simulation (Fig. 1(b)). Using the simulated pose of the endoscope as ground truth, we evaluated the accuracy of the method. The mean positional error for the 30 simulated video frames was 0.5 mm, and orientation error was 0.49°. We also randomly sampled 900 3D points from the mesh visible to the virtual cameras for 6 frames. We added random noise to the 3D points with std. dev. 0.5 mm and 0.3 mm in the parallel and orthogonal directions relative to the virtual optical axes to simulate noisy SfM data, and also to the camera poses with uniform random sampling in $[0, 0.25]$ mm and degrees of translational and rotational errors, respectively, to simulate error in the computed extrinsic parameters. Contour noise was modeled using an isotropic noise model with $\Sigma_{2d} = 9\,\text{pixel}^2$, $\kappa = 200$. The simulated data was randomly misaligned from the mesh in the interval $[2, 3]$ mm and degrees. Registration was assessed using the center points of every mesh triangle visible to the middle virtual camera frame at the ground truth pose to compute a mean TRE. Using V-IMLOP to register this data back to the mesh, we achieved a TRE of 0.2 mm.

We also tested our algorithm on in-vivo data collected from outpatients enrolled in an IRB-approved study. We tested our method with manual initializations on 12 non-overlapping video sequences from two patients, showing differing anatomy. We used an isotropic noise model with $\Sigma_{3d} = 0.25\,\text{mm}^2$, $\Sigma_{2d} = 1\,\text{pixel}^2$, $\kappa = 200$. 11 sequences contained approximately 30 images and 1 sequence contained 68, resulting in a total of 446 images. Results from registration show that V-IMLOP produces better alignment of model contours with the corresponding video frame (Fig. 2). Since it is difficult to isolate a target in in-vivo data, we did not compute TRE. The mean residual error over all sequences is 0.32 mm, and the mean contour error is 16.64 pixels (12.33 pixels for inliers). We also show through an analysis of perturbing our manual initializations that our approach is robust to rough pose and scale initializations, and capable of indicating *failure* when a camera pose initialization is too far away from the

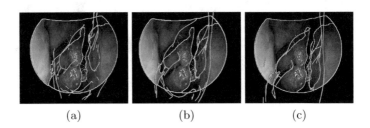

(a)   (b)   (c)

Fig. 2. Alignment between occluding contours from CT mesh projected onto the video frame (green) and occluding contours from video (white) is better using V-IMLOP (c) than both Trimmed ICP (a) and V-IMLOP without contours (b). (Color figure online)

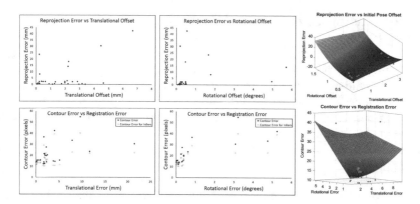

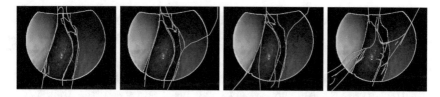

Fig. 3. (Top) Registration accuracy, demonstrated through reprojection error, degrades as the initial pose is offset further from the true pose; (bottom) since contour error increases as registration error worsens, it may be used as an indicator for registration confidence.

Fig. 4. Registration results using V-IMLOP with degrading initializations (left to right) show that the final registration and contour error also degrade, indicated by the alignment of model contours (green) and video contours (white). (Color figure online)

true target anatomy. We ran this test on 31 perturbations from 2 sequences (69 images). The average residual error for the 22 candidate initializations resulting in successful registrations was 0.25 mm. The right-most image in Fig. 4 is a failure case, and corresponds to the data point with the highest contour error in Fig. 3. Therefore, we have constructed an automated initialization procedure combining empirical endoscopic trajectories with CT registration to define realistic starting poses from which registration can succeed, or return failure with confidence.

Finally, under the guidance of a surgeon, we identify sequences with more erectile and less erectile tissue for each patient. This separation is important because structures in the sinuses that contain erectile tissue undergo regular deformation resulting in modified anatomy, and therefore, registration errors. Errors in regions of the sinuses containing more erectile tissue are 0.43 mm for 3D points residual error and 18.07 pixels (12.92 pixels for inliers) contour error. Whereas, errors in regions containing less erectile tissue are 0.28 mm for 3D points residual error and 15.21 pixels (11.74 pixels for inliers) contour error. Overall error is better in less erectile tissue, as expected.

4   Conclusion and Future Work

We present a novel approach for video-CT registration that optimizes over 3D points as well as oriented 2D contours. Our method demonstrates capability to produce sub-millimeter results even with sub-optimal initializations and in the presence of erectile tissue. We are currently working on optimizing our code, and expanding our data set to thoroughly test our method on more outpatients and surgical cases. In the future, we hope to fully automate the initialization, and further improve our method in the presence of erectile tissue by accounting for deformation.

Acknowledgement. This work was funded by NIH R01-EB015530: Enhanced Navigation for Endoscopic Sinus Surgery through Video Analysis and NSF Graduate Research Fellowship Program.

References

1. Slavin, R.G., Spector, S.L., Bernstein, I.L., Kaliner, M.A., Kennedy, D.W., Virant, F.S., Wald, E.R., Khan, D.A., Blessing-Moore, J., Lang, D.M., Nicklas, R.A., Oppenheimer, J.J., Portnoy, J.M., Schuller, D.E., Tilles, S.A., Borish, L., Nathan, R.A., Smart, B.A., Vandewalker, M.L.: The diagnosis and management of sinusitis: a practice parameter update. JACI **116**(6, Suppl.), S13–S47 (2005)
2. Bhattacharyya, N.: Ambulatory sinus and nasal surgery in the United States: demographics and perioperative outcomes. Laryngoscope **120**, 635–638 (2010)
3. Dalziel, K., Stein, K., Round, A., Garside, R., Royle, P.: Endoscopic sinus surgery for the excision of nasal polyps: a systematic review of safety and effectiveness. Am. J. Rhinol. **20**(5), 506–519 (2006)
4. Otake, Y., Leonard, S., Reiter, A., Rajan, P., Siewerdsen, J.H., Gallia, G.L., Ishii, M., Taylor, R.H., Hager, G.D.: Rendering-based video-CT registration with physical constraints for image-guided endoscopic sinus surgery. In: Proceedings of SPIE, vol. 9415, MI, IGPRIM, p. 94150A (2015)
5. Mirota, D.J., Hanzi, W., Taylor, R.H., Ishii, M., Gallia, G.L., Hager, G.D.: A system for video-based navigation for endoscopic endonasal skull base surgery. IEEE TMI **31**(4), 963–976 (2012)
6. Leonard, S., Reiter, A., Sinha, A., Ishii, M., Taylor, R.H., Hager, G.D.: Image-based navigation for functional endoscopic sinus surgery using structure from motion. In: Proceedings of SPIE, vol. 9784, MI, IP, p. 97840V (2016)
7. Besl, P.J., McKay, N.D.: A method for registration of 3-D shapes. IEEE Trans. PAMI **14**, 239–256 (1992)
8. Chetverikov, D., Svirko, D., Stepanov, D., Krsek, P.: The trimmed iterative closest point algorithm. ICPR **3**, 545–548 (2002)
9. Mirota, D., Wang, H., Taylor, R.H., Ishii, M., Hager, G.D.: Toward video-based navigation for endoscopic endonasal skull base surgery. In: Yang, G.-Z., Hawkes, D., Rueckert, D., Noble, A., Taylor, C. (eds.) MICCAI 2009. LNCS, vol. 5761, pp. 91–99. Springer, Heidelberg (2009). doi:10.1007/978-3-642-04268-3_12
10. Billings, S.D., Boctor, E.M., Taylor, R.H.: Iterative most-likely point registration (IMLP): a robust algorithm for computing optimal shape alignment. PLoS ONE **10**(3), e0117688 (2015)

11. Kainz, J., Stammberger, H.: The roof of the anterior ethmoid: A place of least resistance in the skull base. Am. J. Rhinol. **3**(4), 191–199 (1989)
12. Mardia, K.V., Jupp, P.E.: Directional Statistics. Wiley Series in Probability and Statistics. Wiley, West Sussex (2000)
13. Avants, B.B., Tustison, N.J., Song, G., Cook, P.A., Klein, A., Gee, J.C.: A reproducible evaluation of ANTs similarity metric performance in brain image registration. NeuroImage **54**(3), 2033–2044 (2011)
14. Sinha, A., Leonard, S., Reiter, A., Ishii, M., Taylor, R.H., Hager, G.D.: Automatic segmentation and statistical shape modeling of the paranasal sinuses to estimate natural variations. In: Proceedings of SPIE, vol. 9784, MI, IP, p. 97840D (2016)
15. Arbelaez, P., Maire, M., Fowlkes, C., Malik, J.: Contour detection and hierarchical image segmentation. IEEE TPAMI **33**(5), 98–916 (2011)
16. Koenig, N., Howard, A.: Design and use paradigms for Gazebo, an open-source multi-robot simulator. IROS, pp. 2149–2154 (2004)

A Multi-resolution T-Mixture Model Approach to Robust Group-Wise Alignment of Shapes

Nishant Ravikumar[1,2(✉)], Ali Gooya[1,3], Serkan Çimen[1,3],
Alejandro F. Frangi[1,3], and Zeike A. Taylor[1,2]

[1] CISTIB Centre for Computational Engineering
and Simulation Technologies in Biomedicine,
INSIGNEO Institute for in Silico Medicine, Sheffield, UK
mta08nr@shef.ac.uk
[2] Department of Mechanical Engineering, The University of Sheffield, Sheffield, UK
[3] Department of Electronic and Electrical Engineering,
The University of Sheffield, Sheffield, UK

Abstract. A novel probabilistic, group-wise rigid registration framework is proposed in this study, to robustly align and establish correspondence across anatomical shapes represented as unstructured point sets. Student's t-mixture model (TMM) is employed to exploit their inherent robustness to outliers. The primary application for such a framework is the automatic construction of statistical shape models (SSMs) of anatomical structures, from medical images. Tools used for automatic segmentation and landmarking of medical images often result in segmentations with varying proportions of outliers. The proposed approach is able to robustly align shapes and establish valid correspondences in the presence of considerable outliers and large variations in shape. A multi-resolution registration (mrTMM) framework is also formulated, to further improve the performance of the proposed TMM-based registration method. Comparisons with a state-of-the art approach using clinical data show that the mrTMM method in particular, achieves higher alignment accuracy and yields SSMs that generalise better to unseen shapes.

1 Introduction

Generative probabilistic model-based point set registration techniques are used in various medical image analysis applications, such as landmark-based image registration, statistical shape model (SSM) generation, correction of incomplete image segmentations, and 3D shape reconstruction from 2D projection images. Existing probabilistic approaches to rigid [1–3] and non-rigid [4] group-wise point set registration are based on Gaussian mixture models (GMMs) which, while affording efficient solutions for associated model parameters, lack robustness to outliers. An elegant solution to this limitation is to adopt a t-mixture model (TMM) formulation, which is inherently more robust due to TMMs' so-called heavy tails. Such an approach forms the main contribution of this study. Additionally, we propose a novel multinomial distribution-based, multi-resolution

© Springer International Publishing AG 2016
S. Ourselin et al. (Eds.): MICCAI 2016, Part III, LNCS 9902, pp. 142–149, 2016.
DOI: 10.1007/978-3-319-46726-9_17

extension that encapsulates the group-wise TMM registration and involves a process of adaptive sampling from the components of the TMM at each resolution level.

Aligning a group of medical image-derived unstructured point sets is particularly challenging due to the presence of missing information, varying degrees of outliers, and unknown correspondences. Probabilistic approaches offer a solution, by casting the registration problem as one of probability density estimation, where each sample shape in a group is assumed to be a transformed observation of a mixture model, leading to the joint inference of unknown correspondences and desired spatial transformations across the group [3].

Pair-wise point set registration using TMMs has been proposed in two previous studies [5,6]. However, group-wise registration methods are, in general, preferable as they provide an unbiased solution to the registration problem [1]. Use of TMMs in the latter context was recently proposed in [7], wherein rigid transformation parameters were estimated numerically by gradient ascent optimisation. In the present work, closed-form expressions are derived for the transformation parameters, which afford significant improvement in computational efficiency, and a further multi-resolution extension is formulated.

Estimation of valid correspondences and invariance to rigid transformations across a group of shapes are necessary for training SSMs by principal component analysis (PCA). However, the overall process is challenged by the need for cumbersome pre-processing (typically manual) during training set generation. This is prohibitive when learning models from large-scale image databases. We aim to ameliorate this challenge by means of robust methods for jointly establishing correspondence and aligning point sets in the presence of outliers, which are therefore compatible with fully automated segmentation and landmarking tools.

The proposed single- and multi-resolution methods are validated by comparison with a state-of-the-art GMM-based approach [2], based on registration accuracy and quality of SSMs generated.

2 Methods

2.1 Group-Wise Rigid Registration Using TMMs

Student's t-distributions $\mathcal{S}$ are derived as an infinite mixture of scaled Gaussians, where the precision scaling weights, denoted u, are treated as latent variables drawn from a Gamma distribution $\mathcal{G}$:

$$\mathcal{S}(\mathbf{x}|\boldsymbol{\mu}, \Sigma, \nu) = \int_0^\infty \mathcal{N}(\mathbf{x}|\boldsymbol{\mu}, \Sigma/u)\mathcal{G}(u|\nu/2, \nu/2)\mathrm{d}u. \tag{1}$$

t-distributions are a generalisation of Gaussians with heavy tails that result from finite values for the associated degrees of freedom ν [8]. We argue that point set generation from medical images is affected by outliers and, consequently, TMMs are well suited to align and establish correspondence across such point sets.

Optimal TMM and registration parameters are estimated by maximising their posterior probability conditioned on the observed data. A tractable solution to this problem is formulated by maximising the complete data log likelihood, with respect to the unknown parameters Ψ via expectation-maximisation (EM). For a group of K point sets denoted $\mathcal{X}_k \in \mathbf{X}$, to be aligned using an M component mixture model, the complete data log likelihood is expressed as Eq. (2). In Eq. (2), $\mathbb{U} = \{u_{kij}\}, \mathbb{Z} = \{z_{kij}\}$ represent the sets of latent variables associated with each component in the TMM. The former scales the precision of the equivalent Gaussian distribution, while the latter is a binary vector specifying the unique membership of the observed data $(\mathbf{X})$ to components in the mixture model. Subscript $j = 1...M$ is used to represent mixture model components while $i = 1...N_k$ is used to represent N_k data points that belong to the kth shape in the data set.

$$\log p(\mathbf{X}, \mathbb{U}, \mathbb{Z}|\Psi) = \log(p(\mathbb{Z}|\Psi)) + \log(p(\mathbb{U}|\mathbb{Z}, \Psi)) + \log(p(\mathbf{X}|\mathbb{U}, \mathbb{Z}, \Psi)) \qquad (2)$$

This results in an iterative estimation alternating between evaluating the conditional expectation of the latent variables, given an estimate of the M component mixture model parameters $\Theta = \{\boldsymbol{\mu}_j, \sigma^2, \nu_j, \pi_j\}$ and rigid registration parameters $\mathbf{T} = \{\mathcal{T}_{k=1}^K\}$, and updating these parameters $\Psi = \{\Theta, \mathbf{T}\}$. This leads to estimation of the product of the conditional expectations of the two latent variables, $P_{kij}^\star = E(z_{kij}|\mathbf{x}_{ki})E(u_{kij}|\mathbf{x}_{ki}, z_{kij} = 1)$, in the E-step. The posterior probabilities given by $E(z_{kij}|\mathbf{x}_{ki})$ describe the responsibility of the jth mixture component with mean $\boldsymbol{\mu}_j$, variance σ^2, degrees of freedom ν_j and mixing coefficient π_j, in describing the ith point on the kth shape in the group, given by $\mathbf{x}_{ki}$. Subsequently, the M-step maximises the conditional expectation of the complete data log likelihood with respect to each of the unknown parameters, sequentially. M-step equations to update estimates of the model Θ and rigid transformation parameters $\mathcal{T}_k$ are analytically derived. The latter are presented in (3a, b, c):

$$\mathbf{t}_k = [\sum_{i=1}^{N_k}\sum_{j=1}^{M} P_{kij}^\star \mathbf{x}_{ki}][\sum_{i=1}^{N_k}\sum_{j=1}^{M} P_{kij}^\star]^{-1} - s_k \mathcal{R}_k [\sum_{i=1}^{N_k}\sum_{j=1}^{M} P_{kij}^\star \boldsymbol{\mu}_j][\sum_{i=1}^{N_k}\sum_{j=1}^{M} P_{kij}^\star]^{-1},$$

$$\qquad (3a)$$

$$\mathcal{C}_k = [\sum_{i=1}^{N_k}\sum_{j=1}^{M} P_{kij}^\star[(\mathbf{x}_{ki} - \mathbf{t}_k)\boldsymbol{\mu}_j^T]][\sum_{i=1}^{N_k}\sum_{j=1}^{M} P_{kij}^\star \boldsymbol{\mu}_j \boldsymbol{\mu}_j^T]^{-1}, \qquad (3b)$$

$$s_k = [Tr\{\sum_{i=1}^{N_k}\sum_{j=1}^{M} P_{kij}^\star \mathcal{R}_k^T (\mathbf{x}_{ki} - \mathbf{t}_k)\boldsymbol{\mu}_j^T\}][Tr\{\sum_{i=1}^{N_k}\sum_{j=1}^{M} P_{kij}^\star \boldsymbol{\mu}_j \boldsymbol{\mu}_j^T\}]^{-1}. \qquad (3c)$$

While the degrees of freedom ν_j are estimated numerically, expectations in the E-step and estimates for the remaining model parameters are derived analytically, similar to [3,8]. $\mathcal{C}_k$ represents a real covariance matrix from which the orthogonal rotation matrix $\mathcal{R}_k$ is computed by singular value decomposition similar to [2], $\mathbf{t}_k$ represents the translation, and s_k represents the scaling. $\{\mathcal{R}_k, s_k, \mathbf{t}_k\}$ together form the rigid transformation $\mathcal{T}_k$ mapping the current estimate of the mean model to the kth shape.

2.2   Multi-resolution Registration by Adaptive Sampling

A multi-resolution approach (mrTMM), wherein the density of the mean model is increased (and consequently, the model variance is decreased) at each successive resolution, was formulated to further improve the performance of the proposed method. We argue that such a framework reduces the influence of local minima which may be introduced during initialisation (by k-means clustering) and estimation of the mean model, and thereby improves registration accuracy and quality of SSMs trained. Multi-resolution schemes are often employed in image registration [9]. A probabilistic approach to multi-resolution registration of point sets, however, is novel to the best of our knowledge.

Increase in mean model density is achieved through adaptive sampling by imposing a multinomial distribution over the estimated mixture coefficients π_j and drawing N_s random samples from a subset of M TMM components, i.e. those with high responsibilities in explaining the observed data. The number of new model points s_j sampled from the jth mixture component is described by the multinomial distribution as $p(s_j|\pi_j, N_s) = \text{Mult}(s_1...s_M|\pi_j, N_s)$. New model points are generated by drawing random samples from a zero-centered multivariate Gaussian distribution and an inverse chi-squared distribution (with ν_j degrees of freedom), since t-distributed random variables can be expressed as $\mathbf{s}_j = \boldsymbol{\mu}_j + \mathcal{N}(0, \sigma^2)\sqrt{\nu_j/\chi^2(\nu_j)}$. The registration proceeds in a hierarchical coarse-to-fine fashion, with the mean model increasing in density at each successive level and the rigid transformations estimated at each level initialising the subsequent resolution.

3   Results

Two clinical data sets were used for validation: (1) a 2D set of 100 femur boundaries segmented automatically using a clinically employed software (Hologic Apex 3.2) from dual-energy X-ray absorptiometry images of healthy subjects; (2) a 3D set of 30 caudate nuclei, segmented automatically [10] from T1-weighted MR images[1] of healthy subjects. Point sets were generated from these segmentations using a marching cubes-based surface extraction algorithm. Alignments were then performed, and correspondences computed using the TMM and mrTMM approaches (results from the latter shown in Fig. 1(a–e)). Finally, SSMs were constructed (example presented in Fig. 1(f, g)) from the estimated correspondences using PCA. The process was repeated using the state-of-the-art sparse statistical shape model (SpSSM [2]) approach for comparison. SpSSM was chosen as in [2] the authors demonstrated its ability to generate SSMs of higher quality than a traditional GMM-based approach [3].

Comparisons were made on the basis of (1) rigid alignment accuracy of the estimated probabilistic correspondences across each group of shapes, and (2) quality of the corresponding SSMs. The former were quantified by Hausdorff

---

[1] Public database: http://www.brain-development.org (c) Copyright Imperial College of Science, Technology and Medicine 2007. All rights reserved.

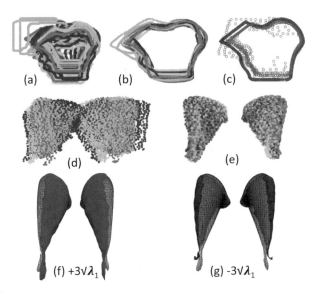

Fig. 1. Top row: (a) raw 2D femur point sets prior to alignment, (b) aligned probabilistic correspondences using mrTMM, (c) estimated mean shapes using mrTMM (blue) and SpSSM (red); Middle row: (d) raw 3D caudate point sets prior to alignment, (e) aligned probabilistic correspondences using mrTMM; Bottom row: first mode of variation of caudate SSM trained using mrTMM, overlaid on mean shape (transparent outline), (f) $+3\sqrt{\lambda_1}$ and (g) $-3\sqrt{\lambda_1}$. (Color figure online)

(HD) and quadratic surface distance (QSD), computed between the estimated mean shapes and all transformed samples in each corresponding group; the latter from the generality of the trained models in five-fold, leave-one-out, cross validation experiments. For each method tested, the optimal number of mixture components M_{opt} was identified by plotting their respective generalisation errors against the number of mixture components employed to align each clinical data set. M_{opt} values for both data sets and each registration method are summarised in Table 1. The corresponding average alignment accuracy of the estimated probabilistic correspondences are also presented in the table. SSMs trained using the identified M_{opt} values for both data sets were also assessed by evaluating their generality and specificity with respect to the number of modes of variation through full-fold cross-validation experiments.

The gain in computational efficiency, relative to [7], afforded by the proposed algorithm was assessed by aligning the caudate data set using 300 mixture components. A substantial improvement in speed was achieved using the proposed method: execution time: 317 s vs. 987 s. Furthermore, in [7], numerical estimation of the rigid transformation parameters required an additional user specified parameter (i.e. optimiser step size) which may need to be tuned to different data sets. This parameter is obviated in the proposed algorithm and consequently analysis is more automated and its application on large data sets is more robust.

Registration Errors. The registration errors quantified in Table 1 for the caudate data set indicate that the proposed single- and multi-resolution TMM-based methods outperform SpSSM in terms of registration accuracy, with mrTMM being the most accurate. The femur data set included many instances of oversegmented boundary masks, making it heavy with outliers (as depicted in Fig. 1(a)). In this case, the TMM-based methods conferred significantly higher accuracy and were able to estimate mean femur shapes in a manner robust to these outliers. This is depicted in Fig. 1(c), which shows the adverse effect outliers have on the estimated mean shape using SpSSM and the advantage mrTMM affords in this respect. In the experiments conducted, the TMM-based methods consistently outperform SpSSM and are more robust for group-wise rigid point set registration. Statistical significance of the computed registration errors for TMM and mrTMM with respect to SpSSM were assessed using a paired-sample t-test, considering a significance level of 1 %. Significant improvements on SpSSM are highlighted in bold in Table 1.

Table 1. Registration accuracy for clinical data sets evaluated using HD and QSD metrics at optimal mean model density M_{opt}

Registration method	3D Caudate Nuclei (K = 30)			2D Femur (K = 100)		
	M_{opt}	HD (mm)	QSD (mm)	M_{opt}	HD (mm)	QSD (mm)
SpSSM	1182	5.95 ± 1.36	1.05 ± 0.12	838	41.32 ± 3.54	2.90 ± 0.70
TMM	2560	**4.60 ± 2.38**	**0.95 ± 0.15**	640	**11.07 ± 5.17**	**2.15 ± 1.11**
mrTMM	2560	**3.76 ± 1.85**	**0.93 ± 0.14**	640	**11.49 ± 5.48**	**2.18 ± 0.96**

Additionally, by estimating valid mean shapes for the femur data set, the TMM-based methods were able to establish valid probabilistic correspondences (as shown in Fig. 1(b)). SpSSM on the other hand, was affected by the presence of outliers, resulting in the estimation of wrong mean shapes and correspondences, and consequently, incorrect modes of variation in the trained SSM.

SSM Quality. SSM generalisation errors evaluated with respect to number of mixture components are shown in Fig. 2(a, b). The proposed TMM and mrTMM approaches generated SSMs of both the caudate and femur that generalise better to unseen test shapes than does SpSSM. Generalisation errors with respect to number of modes of variation (for the first ten modes, using M_{opt} identified from the former experiments), evaluated by full-fold cross-validation, are depicted in Fig. 2(c, d). The first mode of variation achieved the lowest errors for the caudate, while two modes were optimal for the femur, using TMM and mrTMM.

As the caudate nuclei segmentations were of high quality, with no apparent outliers (from visual inspection), the performance of TMM and SpSSM were similar. In such cases, the constituent t-distribution components are little different

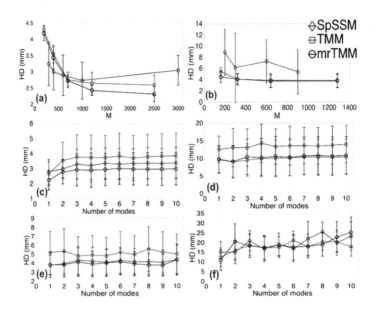

Fig. 2. SSM quality using SpSSM, TMM and mrTMM for caudate and femur data sets. Top row: generalisation errors (using HD) vs. number of mixture components M; middle row: generalisation errors vs. number of modes of variation N; bottom row: specificity errors vs. N. Left and right columns show results for caudate and femur data sets, respectively.

from Gaussian distributions. Nonetheless, for this set, mrTMM consistently outperformed both other methods in all generalisation experiments. The improvement afforded by mrTMM is also reflected in the specificity errors presented in Fig. 2(e).

For the femur data set, both TMM-based methods achieved significantly lower generalisation errors with respect to number of mixture components (Fig. 2(b)) and number of modes of variation (Fig. 2(d)); SpSSM estimated incorrect modes of variation in the femur shape, due to the wrong probabilistic correspondences established. This also resulted in higher specificity errors using SpSSM, as shown in Fig. 2(f).

4   Conclusion

Single- and multi-resolution TMM-based methods for group-wise rigid registration of unstructured point sets (such as derived from medical images) have been described and shown to be particularly advantageous over a state-of-the-art GMM-based method (SpSSM) for data containing outliers. For clinical data sets containing few or no outliers, the proposed methods showed some improvements over SpSSM, in terms of registration accuracy and quality of corresponding SSMs, though these were modest. Conversely, for clinical data with high levels of outliers, the proposed methods significantly outperformed SpSSM and showed excellent robustness. In most cases, the multi-resolution extension (mrTMM) afforded further improvement over the single-resolution (TMM) formulation. The presented approaches should be especially advantageous for applications involving large data sets, which correspondingly require automated processing techniques that are robust to outliers.

Acknowledgments. This study was funded by the European Unions Seventh Framework Programme (FP7/2007 2013) as part of the project VPH-DARE@IT (grant agreement no. 601055) and partly supported by the Marie Curie Individual Fellowship (625745, A. Gooya). The authors would like to thank Dr. Fabian Wenzel, Philips Research Laboratories, Hamburg, Germany, for providing access to their fully automated tool, to segment the caudate nuclei.

References

1. Evangelidis, G.D., Kounades-Bastian, D., Horaud, R., Psarakis, E.Z.: A generative model for the joint registration of multiple point sets. In: Fleet, D., Pajdla, T., Schiele, B., Tuytelaars, T. (eds.) ECCV 2014. LNCS, vol. 8695, pp. 109–122. Springer, Heidelberg (2014). doi:10.1007/978-3-319-10584-0_8
2. Gooya, A., Davatzikos, C., Frangi, A.F.: A bayesian approach to sparse model selection in statistical shape models. SIAM J. Imaging Sci. **8**(2), 858–887 (2015)
3. Hufnagel, H., Pennec, X., Ehrhardt, J., Ayache, N., Handels, H.: Generation of a statistical shape model with probabilistic point correspondences and the expectation maximization-iterative closest point algorithm. Int. J. Comput. Assist. Radiol. Surg. **2**(5), 265–273 (2008)
4. Chen, T., Vemuri, B.C., Rangarajan, A., Eisenschenk, S.J.: Group-wise point-set registration using a novel CDF-based Havrda-Charvát divergence. Int. J. Comput. Vis. **86**(1), 111–124 (2010)
5. Gerogiannis, D., Nikou, C., Likas, A.: The mixtures of Students t-distributions as a robust framework for rigid registration. Image Vis. Comput. **27**(9), 1285–1294 (2009)
6. Zhou, Z., Zheng, J., Dai, Y., Zhou, Z., Chen, S.: Robust non-rigid point set registration using Student's-t mixture model. plos one **9**(3), e91381 (2014)
7. Ravikumar, N., Gooya, A., Frangi, A.F., Taylor, Z.A.: Robust group-wise rigid registration of point sets using t-mixture model. In: SPIE Medical Imaging, pp. 97840S–97840S. International Society for Optics and Photonics (2016)
8. Peel, D., McLachlan, G.J.: Robust mixture modelling using the t distribution. Stat. Comput. **10**(4), 339–348 (2000)
9. Schnabel, J.A., et al.: A generic framework for non-rigid registration based on non-uniform multi-level free-form deformations. In: Niessen, W.J., Viergever, M.A. (eds.) MICCAI 2001. LNCS, vol. 2208, pp. 573–581. Springer, Heidelberg (2001). doi:10.1007/3-540-45468-3_69
10. Zagorchev, L., Meyer, C., Stehle, T., Wenzel, F., Young, S., Peters, J., Weese, J., et al.: Differences in regional brain volumes two months and one year after mild traumatic brain injury. J. Neurotrauma **33**(1), 29–34 (2016)

Quantifying Shape Deformations by Variation of Geometric Spectrum

Hajar Hamidian, Jiaxi Hu, Zichun Zhong, and Jing Hua$^{(\boxtimes)}$

Wayne State University, Detroit, MI 48202, USA
{nasim.hamidian,jinghua}@wayne.edu

Abstract. This paper presents a registration-free method based on geometry spectrum for mapping two shapes. Our method can quantify and visualize the surface deformation by the variation of Laplace-Beltrami spectrum of the object. In order to examine our method, we employ synthetic data that has non-isometric deformation. We have also applied our method to quantifying the shape variation between the left and right hippocampus in epileptic human brains. The results on both synthetic and real patient data demonstrate the effectiveness and accuracy of our method.

Keywords: Laplace-Beltrami spectrum · Registration-free mapping · Shape deformation

1 Introduction

Morphometric analysis is very important in many biomedical applications and clinical diagnoses. In general, there are two types of methods for mapping two shapes: spatial registration methods and spectral methods. Spatial registration methods usually require landmarks to map two shapes [1,2] which are often labor-intensive for users to define those large number of landmarks. It becomes even more challenging when the landmarks are difficult to define complicated shapes, such as hippocampus [3], heart, etc. Spectral methods, on the other hand, do not need any landmarks. Shape spectrum is a method inspired by Fourier transform in signal processing. From the computational geometry aspect, the shape geometry can be described with the differentiable manifold. Along this direction, Reuter et al. [4] and Levy [5] defined shape spectrum, using the shape spectrum approach, as the eigenvalues of the Laplace-Beltrami operator on a manifold and employed the eigenvalues and eigenfunctions as a global shape descriptor [6,7]. Konukoglu et al. [8] measured shape differences by using the weighted spectral distance. There are some great advantages for shape analysis using shape spectrum as it is invariant to isometric deformation [9], different triangulations and meshing [4]. It carries the intrinsic geometry of manifold. As the shape geometry changes, the shape spectrum will change as well. Therefore, the similarity and difference among shapes can be described using this method.

© Springer International Publishing AG 2016
S. Ourselin et al. (Eds.): MICCAI 2016, Part III, LNCS 9902, pp. 150–157, 2016.
DOI: 10.1007/978-3-319-46726-9_18

However, through the direct use of the decomposed eigenvalues and eigenfunctions [10], these spectral methods can only describe the global difference between shapes. They are neither able to localize the shape difference nor sensitive to small deformations. The variation of shape spectrum is less studied in the literature. A recent study shows that the shape spectrum can be controlled using a function on the Riemann metric [11] but shape difference defined by eigenvalue variations is never explored.

In this paper we focus on spectrum alignment of general shapes using the eigenvalue variation and present a spectral geometry method for localizing and quantifying non-isometric deformations between surface shapes. In our approach, shapes are automatically registered by calculating the metric scaling on both shapes. Our method allows to define the surface shape deformation by the variation of Laplace-Beltrami spectrum of the shapes. Compared to the traditional approaches, it can detect and localize small deformations in addition to global difference of the shapes. Our method is registration-free in nature. It does not need landmarks for mapping two manifolds and the spectrum only depends on the intrinsic geometry of the shape and invariant to spacial translation, rotation, scaling and isometric deformation. This method is computationally affordable and suitable to map surface shapes for non-isometric deformation analysis.

2   Method

In this paper, we use Laplace-Beltrami operator to compute the geometric spectrum of a manifold. Let $f \in C^2$ be a real function defined on a Riemannian manifold M. The Laplace-Beltrami operator $\triangle$ is defined as, $\triangle f = \nabla \cdot (\nabla f)$, where ∇f is te gradient of f and $\nabla \cdot$ is the divergence on the Manifold M. In this paper, we compute the eigenvalue of the Laplacian equation defined as $\triangle f = -\lambda f$ using discrete differential operator. In this equation, the family solution $\{\lambda_i\}$ is a real nonnegative scalar and will result in the corresponding real family functions of $\{f_i\}$ for $i = 0, 1, 2, \dots$. In this framework, a 2D manifold data is discretized to triangle meshes. Assuming the neighborhood of a vertex is approximated with the area of its Voronoi region, a discrete Laplace-Beltrami operator can be defined with the average value over the area of the Voronoi region as following:

$$L_{ij} = \begin{cases} -\frac{\cot \alpha_{ij} + \cot \beta_{ij}}{2A_i} & \text{if } i, j \text{ are adjacent,} \\ \sum_k \frac{\cot \alpha_{ik} + \cot \beta_{ik}}{2A_i} & \text{if } i = j, \\ 0 & \text{otherwise,} \end{cases} \tag{1}$$

where α_{ij} and β_{ij} are the two angles opposite to the sharing edge ij of two triangles, and A_i is the area of Voronoi region at vertex i. k is the index of triangles within 1-ring neighborhood of the vertex i. This equation is solved numerically by constructing a sparse matrix $\mathbf{W}$ and a diagonal matrix $\mathbf{S}$ in which $S_{ii} = A_i$ and $W_{i,j} = L_{i,j} \times S_{ii}$. Therefore, the generalized eigenvalue problem can be presented as $\mathbf{W}\mathbf{v} = \lambda \mathbf{S}\mathbf{v}$ where $\mathbf{v}$ is the eigenvector and λ is the eigenvalue of the matrix $\mathbf{L}$. When the deformations are mostly non-isometric, the eigenvalue and eigenfunction of the shape dramatically change. On a compact closed manifold M with Riemannian metric g (such as organ dilation and shrink with scaling information), we define deformation as a time variant positive scale function $\omega(t) : M \rightarrow R^+$ such that $g_{ij}^\omega = \omega g_{ij}$ and $d\sigma^\omega = \omega d\sigma$, where $\omega(t)$ is nonnegative and continuously differentiable. By definition, the weighted Laplace-Beltrami operator becomes $\Delta^{g^\omega} = \frac{1}{\omega}\Delta^g$. Consider the ith solution of the weighted eigen problem, this equation can be rewritten as $\Delta^g f_i = -\lambda_i \omega f_i$. Using these equations we have proved the theorem as follows.

Theorem 1. λ_i *is piecewise analytic and, at any regular point, the t-derivative of λ_i is given by:*

$$\dot{\lambda}_i = -\lambda_i \mathbf{v}_i^T \dot{\mathbf{\Omega}} \mathbf{S} \mathbf{v}_i, \qquad (2)$$

in which $\mathbf{\Omega}$ is a nonnegative, continuously differentiable, and diagonal matrix.

Our theorem shows that the spectrum is smooth and analytical to non-isometric local scale deformation. It supports the variation of eigenvalues for the alignment of non-isometrically deformed shapes, hence a registration free method for deformation analysis. In this paper, for aligning two shapes we use first k eigenvalues. The number of k may be different depending on the total number of the manifold nodes. Also by increasing k, some high frequency deformation may be detected. Consider two closed manifolds, M and N, represented with discrete triangle meshes. In order to align the first k eigenvalues of N to those of M, a scale diagonal matrix $\mathbf{\Omega}(t)$ is applied on N. $\mathbf{\Omega}$ is an n by n matrix, where n is number of vertices on N. The element Ω_{ii} at the diagonal is a scale factor defined on each vertex on N. According to Theorem 1, the derivative of each eigenvalue is expressed by those of Ω_{ii} analytically. Thus, the scale matrix $\mathbf{\Omega}$ will introduce an alignment from N to M on eigenvalues. The following will explain the details how to calculate the diagonal matrix $\mathbf{\Omega}$ numerically.

We assume that the eigenvalues of N vary linearly towards those of M. This linear interpolation is represented as:

$$\lambda_i(t) = (1-t)\lambda_{N_i} + t\lambda_{M_i}, t \in [0,1] \Rightarrow \dot{\lambda}_i(t) = \lambda_{M_i} - \lambda_{N_i}, t \in [0,1]. \qquad (3)$$

At the beginning, $t = 0$, and $\lambda_i(0)$ starts as λ_{N_i}, while t reaches 1, $\lambda_i(1)$ aligned to λ_{M_i}. Combining Eqs. 3 and 2, the derivative of each $\lambda_i(t)$ leads to an equation of $\mathbf{\Omega}$ as $-\lambda_i(t)\mathbf{v}_i(t)^T \dot{\mathbf{\Omega}} \mathbf{S} \mathbf{v}_i(t) = \lambda_{M_i} - \lambda_{N_i}, t \in [0,1]$. Each diagonal element Ω_{ii} represents a scale factor at vertex i on manifold N. Although the time derivative of $\mathbf{\Omega}$ can be calculated in Eq. 3 but solving this equation is not straightforward. We need to transform the individual integration equation into a linear system. We achieve this by extracting the diagonals as vectors $\mathbf{v_\Omega}$ and $\mathbf{v_S}$ and then employing Hadamard production [12]. Finally, by combining the Eqs. 2 and 3, and using Hadamard production theory, we can obtain a linear form as:

$$(\mathbf{v_S} \circ \mathbf{v}_i \circ \mathbf{v}_i)^T \cdot \mathbf{v_{\dot{\Omega}}} = \frac{\lambda_{N_i} - \lambda_{M_i}}{\lambda_i(t)}, t \in [0,1]. \qquad (4)$$

Considering that practically k is much less than the number of nodes in the mesh, the system is undetermined and has no unique solution. Thus, more constrains are necessary to provide an optimized solution for the linear system.

In our paper, we focus on the global smoothness of scale factors distributed on N. Consider a scalar function $f \in C^2$ is define on the continuous manifold $< N_c, g >$. The gradient of f describes the local change of f. For example, if f is a constant function, which is considered as the smoothest distribution, the gradient ∇f is zero everywhere. A smoothness energy of f is defined with total square magnitude of the gradient ∇f on N_c as $E = \int_{N_c} \|\nabla f\|^2 d\sigma$. On the discrete triangle mesh N, the scale function is a vector $\mathbf{v}_\Omega$, which is the diagonal of matrix Ω. The integral is a matrix product which can be determined as:

$$E = <\mathbf{v}_\Omega + \mathbf{v}_{\dot\Omega}, L \cdot (\mathbf{v}_\Omega + \mathbf{v}_{\dot\Omega}) >_s \Rightarrow E_q = \mathbf{v}_{\dot\Omega}^T \cdot \mathbf{W} \cdot \mathbf{v}_{\dot\Omega} + 2\mathbf{c}^T \cdot \mathbf{v}_{\dot\Omega}, \quad (5)$$

where $\mathbf{c} = \mathbf{W} \cdot \mathbf{v}_\Omega$. Assume that $\mathbf{v}_\Omega$ is known at each time t and $\mathbf{v}_{\dot\Omega}$ is to be solved in Eq. 4. $\mathbf{v}_{\dot\Omega}$ is going to minimize the quadratic smooth energy E_q at any time. In order to preserve the physical availability, $\mathbf{v}_\Omega$ must be bounded. The scale factor cannot be zero or negative. Furthermore, any point cannot be infinity either. We denote a lower bound and an upper bound with $\mathbf{h}_l, \mathbf{h}_u > 0$, where $\mathbf{h}_l$ and $\mathbf{h}_u$ are n dimensional constant vector. $\mathbf{v}_{\dot\Omega}$ must satisfy:

$$\mathbf{h}_l \leq \mathbf{v}_\Omega + \mathbf{v}_{\dot\Omega} \leq \mathbf{h}_u. \quad (6)$$

The linear system (Eq. 4), smoothness constraint (Eq. 5) and constant bound (Eq. 6) introduce a quadratic programming problem at each time t. This integration is discretely approximated with an iteration. We divide the time interval $[0, 1]$ into K steps which we index them as j. Assume the eigenvalues and eigenvectors are known at each time j, the derivative of the scale matrix $\dot\Omega$ is the solution of such quadratic programming. The result $\dot\Omega(j)$ can be used to calculate $\Omega(j + 1)$ using $\Omega(j + 1) = \Omega(j) + \dfrac{1}{K - j}\dot\Omega(j)$. After K steps, the desire $\Omega(K)$ is achieved and manifold M will be aligned to manifold N.

3   Experiments and Results

The proposed algorithm is implemented using Python and C++ on a 64-bit Linux platform. The experiments are conducted on a computer with an Intel Core i7-3770 3.4 GHz CPU and 8 GB RAM. We apply our algorithm on 2D manifold, represented with triangle meshes. In the experiments, we use hippocampi extracted from brain MR images and the surface mesh has around 5000 vertices. Besides the vertex number, there are two constants, K iteration and the first k nonzero eigenvalues to be aligned. According to the algorithm described in Sect. 2, each iteration is an independent quadratic programming problem. Thus the complexity is linear to the step number K. k determines how many eigenvalues to be re-initialized at the beginning of each step. The algorithm calculates the eigenvalues by iterations with the complexity of $O(n^2)$ to the number of vertices and linear to k. The average computing time for around 5000 nodes, $k = 100$ and $K = 10$ is around 17 s. Note that, the larger the K is, the more accurate the approximation is, in terms of the linear interpolation.

In practice, we found $K = 10$ is sufficient to get the accurate result with a reasonable computational time. Ideally, including more eigenvalues for alignment can be more accurate as well. However, the numeric eigenvalue calculation is not reliable on higher indexed eigenvalues, which will bring more unsuitability. It is noted that the unstable eigenfunctions are introduced by the symmetry. This is avoided by applying some preprocessing with existing symmetry analysis algorithms. Our experiments show that the first 100 eigenfunctions carry sufficient geometry information and are also quite reliable. The middle range frequencies provide sufficient geometry information for the fine deformation. So we usually choose $k = 100$ in our experiments.

3.1   Synthetic Data

In order to evaluate the efficacy of our method, we synthetically generate some non-isometric deformations based on an initial shape. In this experiment, we use a hippocampus segmented from 3D brain images. The surface is then deformed using Blender to make non-isometric deformations. Our spectrum alignment is applied on the first 100 nonzero eigenvalues. Note that, no correspondence information is used in the experiments.

First, we generate a bump on the surface. Then we align the original object to the bumped one to obtain the scale function. Figure 1a and b show original and deformed objects, respectively. Figure 1c shows the result of mapping the original shape to the deformed one. The spectrum variation can detect non-isometric deformation clearly. The red color indicates the dilating area in order to map the original manifold to the deformed one. Second, we shrink one part of the original manifold using Blender. Then, we align the original shape to the shrunk one. Figure 1a and d shows the original and deformed shapes. Figure 1e shows the results of mapping. The field of Ω is the intrinsic component of the full deformation, which is normalized in Fig. 1c and e. It is much more than the isometric one. Although itself does not fully recover the deformation, it is sufficient to represent the desired local deformations with the original spatial meshes. As can be seen, the local deformation of shrunk region is detected using our method. The blue color shows the contraction of the area. Finally, we scale the manifold by a factor of 0.5 using blender and then align the original shape to the scaled one. Figure 1f shows the comparison of the original and scaled objects. Figure 1g shows the result of mapping the original shape to the scaled one. As can be seen the whole surface is blue, which means it is globally shrunk. These experiments clearly demonstrate that our method is able to detect and quantify local deformations as well as global deformations.

We compare our method with non-rigid Iterative Closest Point (ICP) algorithm [13] on the synthetic data and experiments demonstrate that our method outperforms the non-rigid ICP method in these shapes with few landmarks and features, as follows: average accuracy: 92 % (our method), 81 % (non-rigid ICP); computational time: <20 s (our method), >60 s (non-rigid ICP). Furthermore, our method is invariant to different triangulation methods, such as uniform and non-uniform triangulations, by testing on the synthetic data.

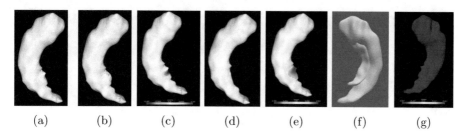

(a)   (b)   (c)   (d)   (e)   (f)   (g)

Fig. 1. The results of mapping the original shape to the synthetically deformed ones. (a) shows the original object. (b) is obtained by generating a bump on the original shape. (c) shows the result of mapping the shape in (a) to the one in (b) where the expansion is determined and located. (d) shows the synthetic data generated by shrinking one part of the original shape. (e) shows the result of mapping the original shape in (a) to the shrunk shape in (c) where shrinkage is localized. (f) shows the synthetically scaled shape with the scale factor of 0.5. (f) shows the result of mapping the original shape to the scaled one. The red color illustrates the expansion area and the blue color shows the shrinkage area. (Color figure online)

3.2 Epilepsy Imaging Study

We also apply our method to mesial temporal lobe (mTLE) epilepsy study. mTLE is one of the most common types of focal epilepsy. Among mTLE structural abnormalities, hippocampus is one of the most frequent structures that can be affected. As indicated in [14], epilepsy may cause shrinkage of the affected hippocampus in comparison to the non-affected one. In this experiment, we have applied our method on twenty TLE patients to quantify the shape variation between left and right hippocampus. Half number of the patients are reported to have left defected hippocampus and the other half have abnormality in the right hippocampus. For generating the 3D hippocampus surfaces, right and left hippocampi are segmented from 3D T1 images. Right hippocampi are then mirrored in order to have the same direction as the left ones. In Fig. 2a and b, column 1 and 2 show samples of left and right hippocampi. Column 3 shows the computed scale function distributions on the left hippocampus surface when mapping from the left one to the right. The colors denote the values of scale function in each vertices of original surface. Red means dilating, blue means contraction, and white means no distortion. According to the clinical record, Fig. 2a is for a patient case that has left abnormal hippocampus, therefore, mapping from the left hippocampus to the right displays more expansion (indicated in red), i.e., the left hippocampus is shrunk (i.e., diseased) compared to the right, normal one. Figure 2b depicts another patient case that has the right defected hippocampus. When mapping from the left hippocampus to the right, the scale distribution displayed on the left hippocampus surface mainly shows the shrinkage (indicated in blue) which indicates the right hippocampus is shrunk (diseased) in comparison to the left hippocampus.

To see how eigenfunctions vary after changing eigenvalues, we select the 12th eigenvalue and show the eigenfunctions corresponding to this eigenvalue on the

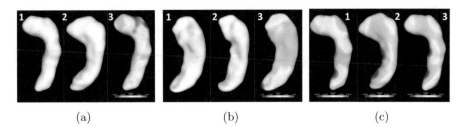

(a)   (b)   (c)

Fig. 2. (a) and (b) show the results of mapping the left hippocampus to the right one for two patient cases. (c) shows the 12th eigenfunction of the left hippocampus (column 1), right hippocampus (column 2), and the left hippocampus after being mapped (column 3). The pattern of the eigenfunction for the left hippocampus shape has been changed in order to map the right one. (Color figure online)

Table 1. The result of aligning eigenvalues of the left hippocampus to the right one using the same case as in Fig. 2a.

Manifold	$\lambda_i/\lambda_1, i \in [2,8]$
Left hippocampus	3.87, 7.76, 11.93, 14.22, 15.88, 18.49, 20.62
Right hippocampus	4.36, 7.75, 11.20, 12.62, 16.60, 18.35, 21.73
Left hippocampus (after being aligned to the Right)	4.36, 7.75, 11.19, 12.62, 16.59, 18.34, 21.73

source manifold before and after mapping to the target manifold. Figure 2c shows the 12th eigenfunction of left hippocampus (first column), right hippocampus (second column), and the mapped hippocampus (third column). The eigenfunctions are normalized between -1 and 1. The values of eigenfunction at each vertex are expressed with color map, where red means larger value, blue means smaller ones, and white means zero. Comparing the eigenfunction patterns before and after alignment, great improvement is obtained and the pattern of the eigenfunction in source manifold has changed to well map into the target manifold.

In order to show the variation of eigenvalues of manifolds before and after mapping, we list the 2nd to 8th eigenvalues of left hippocampus (before and after mapping) and the right hippocampus in Table 1. The eigenvalues are normalized by the first nonzero one to remove the scale factor. It can be seen that after applying the spectrum alignment algorithm, the eigenvalues of the source manifold have been changed in order to well align with the target ones.

4   Conclusion

In this paper, we present a registration-free method to quantify the deformation between shapes. The result of spectral alignment of shape spectrum can provide the scale function which defines the deformation of each vertex. This method can be used for diagnosing the local deformation of hippocampus that is affected by epilepsy. It can be applied to other morphometry analyses as well. The proposed method can handle complicated meshes with more than 5000 or 10,000 vertices on regular desktops and laptops. The algorithm relies on the linear system, which will be highly scalable on GPU or cloud computing. Furthermore, we will apply our method on the brain and other surfaces in the future.

Acknowledgements. We would like to thank Dr. Hamid Soltanian-Zadeh from Department of Radiology at Henry Ford Health System to provide the data for mTLE study. The research is supported in part by grants NSF IIS-0915933, IIS-0937586 and LZ16F020002.

References

1. Tsuzukia, D., Watanabec, H., Danb, I., Taga, G.: Minr 10/20 system: quantitative and reproducible cranial landmark setting method for mri based on minimum initial reference points. Neurosci. Methods **264**, 86–93 (2016)
2. Zou, G., Hua, J., Lai, Z., Gu, X., Dong, M.: Intrinsic geometric scale space by shape diffusion. IEEE Trans. Vis. Comput. Graph. **15**, 1193–1200 (2009)
3. Jenkinson, M., Bannister, P., Brady, J., Smith, S.: Improved optimisation for the robust and accurate linear registration and motion correction of brain images. NeuroImage **17**, 825–841 (2002)
4. Reuter, M., Wolter, F., Peinecke, N.: Laplace-beltrami spectra as "shape-DNA" of surfaces and solids. Comput. Aided Des. **38**, 342–366 (2006)
5. Levy, B.: Laplace-beltrami eigenfunctions: towards an algorithm that understands geometry. In: IEEE International Conference on Shape Modeling and Applications, invited talk (2006)
6. Reuter, M., Wolter, F., Shenton, M., Niethammer, M.: Laplace beltrami eigenvalues and topological features of eigenfunctions for statistical shape analysis. Comput. Aided Des. **35**, 2284–2297 (2009)
7. Reuter, M.: Hierarchical shape segmentation and registration via topological features of laplace-beltrami eigenfunctions. Inter. J. Comput. Vis. **89**, 287–308 (2010)
8. Konukoglu, E., Glocker, B., Criminisi, A., Pohl, K.M.: WESD-weighted spectral distance for measuring shape dissimilarity. IEEE Trans. Pattern. Anal. Mach. Intell. **89**, 287–308 (2013)
9. Ruggeri, M.R., Patanè, G., Spagnuolo, M., Saupe, D.: Spectral-driven isometry-invariant matching of 3D shapes. Inter. J. Comput. Vis. **89**, 248–265 (2010)
10. Shi, Y., Lai, R., Kern, K., Sicotte, N., Dinov, I., Toga, A.W.: Harmonic surface mapping with Laplace-Beltrami eigenmaps. In: Metaxas, D., Axel, L., Fichtinger, G., Székely, G. (eds.) MICCAI 2008. LNCS, vol. 5242, pp. 147–154. Springer, Heidelberg (2008). doi:10.1007/978-3-540-85990-1_18
11. Shi, Y., Lai, R., Gill, R., Pelletier, D., Mohr, D., Sicotte, N., Toga, A.W.: Conformal metric optimization on surface (CMOS) for deformation and mapping in Laplace-Beltrami embedding space. In: Fichtinger, G., Martel, A., Peters, T. (eds.) MICCAI 2011. LNCS, vol. 6892, pp. 327–334. Springer, Heidelberg (2011). doi:10.1007/978-3-642-23629-7_40
12. Grinfeld, P.: Hadamard's formula inside and out. J. Optim. Theory Appl. **146**, 654–690 (2010)
13. Besl, P., McKay, N.: A method for registration of 3-D shapes. IEEE Trans. Pattern. Anal. Mach. Intell. **14**, 239–256 (1992)
14. Jafari-Khouzania, K., Elisevichb, K., Patela, S., Smithc, B., Soltanian-Zadeh, H.: Flair signal and texture analysis for lateralizing mesial temporal lobe epilepsy. NeuroImage **49**, 1159–1571 (2010)

Myocardial Segmentation of Contrast Echocardiograms Using Random Forests Guided by Shape Model

Yuanwei Li[1], Chin Pang Ho[2], Navtej Chahal[3], Roxy Senior[3],
and Meng-Xing Tang[1(✉)]

[1] Department of Bioengineering, Imperial College London, London, UK
mengxing.tang@imperial.ac.uk
[2] Department of Computing, Imperial College London, London, UK
[3] Department of Echocardiography, Royal Brompton Hospital, London, UK

Abstract. Myocardial Contrast Echocardiography (MCE) with micro-bubble contrast agent enables myocardial perfusion quantification which is invaluable for the early detection of coronary artery diseases. In this paper, we proposed a new segmentation method called Shape Model guided Random Forests (SMRF) for the analysis of MCE data. The proposed method utilizes a statistical shape model of the myocardium to guide the Random Forest (RF) segmentation in two ways. First, we introduce a novel Shape Model (SM) feature which captures the global structure and shape of the myocardium to produce a more accurate RF probability map. Second, the shape model is fitted to the RF probability map to further refine and constrain the final segmentation to plausible myocardial shapes. Evaluated on clinical MCE images from 15 patients, our method obtained promising results (Dice = 0.81, Jaccard = 0.70, MAD = 1.68 mm, HD = 6.53 mm) and showed a notable improvement in segmentation accuracy over the classic RF and its variants.

1 Introduction

Myocardial Contrast Echocardiography (MCE) is a cardiac ultrasound imaging technique that utilizes vessel-bound microbubbles as contrast agents. In contrast to conventional B-mode echocardiography which only captures the structure and motion of the heart, MCE also allows for the assessment of myocardial perfusion through the controlled destruction and replenishment of microbubbles [13]. The additional perfusion information gives it great potential for the detection of coronary artery diseases. However, current perfusion analysis of MCE data mainly relies on human visual assessment which is time consuming and not reproducible [9]. There is generally a lack of automatic computerized algorithms and methods to help clinician perform accurate perfusion quantification [9]. One major challenge is the automatic segmentation of the myocardium before subsequent perfusion analysis can be carried out.

In this paper, we extend the Random Forests (RF) framework [1] to segment the myocardium in our MCE data. RF is a machine learning technique that has

© Springer International Publishing AG 2016
S. Ourselin et al. (Eds.): MICCAI 2016, Part III, LNCS 9902, pp. 158–165, 2016.
DOI: 10.1007/978-3-319-46726-9_19

gained increasing use in the medical imaging field for tasks such as segmentation [7] and organ localization [3]. RF has been successful due to its accuracy and computational efficiency. Promising results of myocardial delineation on 3D B-mode echo has also been demonstrated in [7]. However, classic RF has two limitations. First, our MCE data exhibit large sources of intensity variations [11] due to factors such as speckle noise, low signal-to-noise ratio, attenuation artefacts, unclear and missing myocardial borders, presence of structures (papillary muscle) with similar appearance to the myocardium. These intensity variations reduce the discriminative power of the classic RF that utilizes only local intensity features. Second, RF segmentation operates on a pixel basis where the RF classifier predicts a class label for each pixel independently. Structural relationships and contextual dependencies between pixel labels are ignored [6,10] which results in segmentation with inconsistent pixel labelling leading to unsmooth boundaries, false detections in the background and holes in the region of interest. To overcome the above two problems, we need to incorporate prior knowledge of the shape of the structure and use additional contextual and structural information to guide the RF segmentation.

There are several works which have incorporated local contextual information into the RF framework. Lempitsky et al. [7] use the pixel coordinates as position features for the RF so that the RF learns the myocardial shape implicitly. Tu and Bai [12] introduce the concept of auto-context which can be applied to RF by using the probability map predicted by one RF as features for training a new RF. Montillo et al. [10] extend the auto-context RF by introducing entanglement features that use intermediate probabilities derived from higher levels of a tree to train its deeper levels. Kontschieder et al. [6] introduce the structured RF that builds in structural information by using RF that predicts structured class labels for a patch rather than the class label of an individual pixel. Lombaert et al. [8] use spectral representations of shapes to classify surface data.

The above works use local contextual information that describes the shape of a structure implicitly. The imposed structural constraint are not strong enough to guide the RF segmentation in noisy regions of MCE data. In this paper, we proposed the Shape Model guided Random Forests (SMRF) which provides a new way to incorporate global contextual information into the RF framework by using a statistical shape model that captures the explicit shape of the entire myocardium. This imposes stronger, more meaningful structural constraints that guide the RF segmentation more accurately. The shape model is learned from a set of training shapes using Principal Component Analysis (PCA) and is originally employed in Active Shape Model (ASM) where the model is constrained so that it can only deform to fit the data in ways similar to the training shapes [2]. However, ASM requires a manual initialization and the final result is sensitive to the position of this initialization. Our SMRF is fully automatic and enjoys both the local discriminative power of the RF and the prior knowledge of global structural information contained in the statistical shape model. The SMRF uses the shape model to guide the RF segmentation in two ways. First, it directly incorporates the shape model into the RF framework by introducing a novel Shape

Model (SM) feature which has outperformed the other contextual features and produced a more accurate RF probability map. Second, the shape model is fitted to the probability map to generate a smooth and plausible myocardial boundary that can be used directly for subsequent perfusion analysis.

2   Method

In this section, we first review some basic background on statistical shape model and RF. We then introduce the two key aspects of our SMRF—the novel SM feature and the fitting of the shape model.

Statistical Shape Model: A statistical shape model of the myocardium is built from 89 manual annotations using PCA [2]. Each annotation has $N = 76$ landmarks comprising 4 key landmarks with 18 landmarks spaced equally in between along the boundary of manual tracing (Fig. 1a left). The shape model is represented as:

$$x = \bar{x} + Pb \tag{1}$$

where x is a $2N$-D vector containing the 2D coordinates of the N landmark points, $\bar{x}$ is the mean coordinates of all training shapes, b is a set of K shape parameters and P contains K eigenvectors with their associated eigenvalues λ_i. K is the number of modes and set to 10 to explain 98 % of total variance so that fine shape variations are modeled while noise is removed. Values of b_i are bounded between $\pm s\sqrt{\lambda_i}$ so that only plausible shape similar to the training set is generated (Fig. 1a right). Refer to [2] for details on statistical shape model.

Random Forests: Myocardial segmentation can be formulated as a problem of binary classification of image pixels. An RF classifier [1] is developed that predicts the class label (myocardium or background) of a pixel using a set of features. The RF is an ensemble of decision trees. During training, each branch node of a tree learns a pair of feature and threshold that results in the best split of the training pixels into its child nodes. The splitting continues recursively until the maximum tree depth is reached or the number of training pixels in the node falls below a minimum. At this time, a leaf node is created and the class distribution of the training pixels reaching the leaf node is used to predict the class label of unseen test pixels. The average of the predictions from all the trees gives a segmentation probability map. Refer to [1,7] for details on RF.

Shape Model Feature: The classic RF uses local appearance features which are based on surrounding image intensities of the reference pixel [3]. We introduced an additional novel SM feature that is derived from the shape model. The SM feature randomly selects some values for the shape model parameters b and generates a set of landmarks x using (1) (Fig. 1b left). The landmarks can be joined to form a myocardial boundary. Let $B(\bar{x} + Pb)$ be the myocardial boundary formed by joining the landmarks generated using some values of b. The SM feature value is then given by the signed shortest distance d from the reference pixel p to the boundary B (Fig. 1b right). The distance is positive

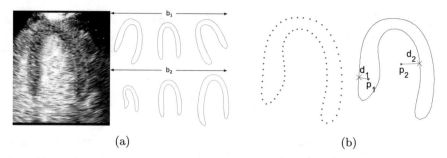

(a)   (b)

Fig. 1. (a) Left: A manual annotation from training set showing key landmarks (*red*) and other landmarks in between (*green*). Right: First two modes of variations of the shape model. (b) Left: Landmarks x (*blue dots*) generated randomly by the shape model in (1). Right: $d_1(d_2)$ is the SM feature value measuring the signed shortest distance from pixel $p_1(p_2)$ to the myocardial boundary $B(x)$ (*blue contour*). d_1 is positive and d_2 is negative. (Color figure online)

if p lies inside the boundary and negative if it lies outside. The SM feature is essentially the signed distance transform of a myocardial boundary generated by the shape model. Each SM feature is defined by the shape parameters b. During training, an SM feature is created by random uniform sampling of each b_i in the range of $\pm s_{feature}\sqrt{\lambda_i}$ where $s_{feature}$ is set to 1 in all our experiments. The binary SM feature test, parameterized by b and a threshold τ, is written as:

$$t_{\text{SM}}^{b,\tau}(p) = \begin{cases} 1, & \text{if} \quad D(p, B(\bar{x} + Pb)) > \tau \\ 0, & \text{otherwise.} \end{cases} \tag{2}$$

where $D(.)$ is the function that computes d. Depending on the binary test outcome, pixel p will go to the left (1) or right (0) child node of the current split node. During training, the RF learns the values of b and τ that best split the training pixels at a node. The SM features explicitly impose a global shape constraint in the RF framework. The random sampling of b also allows the RF to learn plausible shape variations of the myocardium.

Shape Model Fitting: The RF output is a probability map which cannot be used directly in subsequent analysis and application. Simple post-processing on the probability map such as thresholding and edge detection can produce segmentations with inaccurate and incoherent boundaries due to the nature of the pixel-based RF classifier. Our SMRF fits the shape model to the RF probability map to extract a final myocardial boundary that is smooth and which preserves the integrity of the myocardial shape. The segmentation accuracy is also improved as the shape constraint imposed by the shape model can correct some of the misclassifications made by the RF.

Let T_θ be a pose transformation defined by the pose parameter θ which includes translation, rotation and scaling. The shape model fitting is then an optimization problem where we want to find the optimal values of (b, θ) such that the model best matches the RF probability map under some shape constraints. We minimize the following objective function:

$$\min_{b,\theta} \quad \|\boldsymbol{I}_{\mathrm{RF}} - \boldsymbol{I}_{\mathrm{M}}(T_{\theta}(\bar{\boldsymbol{x}} + \boldsymbol{P}\boldsymbol{b}))\|^2 + \alpha \frac{1}{K} \sum_{i=1}^{K} \frac{|b_i|}{\sqrt{\lambda_i}} \tag{3}$$

$$\text{subject to} \quad -s_{fit}\sqrt{\lambda_i} < b_i < s_{fit}\sqrt{\lambda_i}, \; i = 1, \ldots, K.$$

The first term of the objective function compares how well the match is between the model and the RF probability map $\boldsymbol{I}_{\mathrm{RF}}$. $\boldsymbol{I}_{\mathrm{M}}(.)$ is a function that converts the landmarks generated by the shape model into a binary mask of the myocardial shape. This allows us to evaluate a dissimilarity measure between the RF segmentation and the model by computing the sum of squared difference between the RF probability map and the model binary mask. The second term of the objective function is a regularizer which imposes a shape constraint. It is related to the probability of a given shape [4] and ensures that it does not deviate too much away from its mean shape. α is the weighting given to the regularization term and its value is determined empirically. Finally, an additional shape constraint is imposed on the objective function by limiting the upper and lower bounds of b_i to allow for only plausible shapes. s_{fit} is set to 2 in all our experiments. The optimization is carried out using direct search which is a derivative-free solver from the MATLAB global optimization toolbox. At the start of the optimization, each b_i is initialized to zero. Pose parameters are initialized such that the model shape is positioned in the image center with no rotation and scaling.

3   Experiments

Datasets: 2D+t MCE sequences were acquired from 15 individuals using a Philips iE33 ultrasound machine and SonoVue as the contrast agent. Each sequence is taken in the apical 4-chamber view under the triggered mode which shows the left ventricle at end-systole. One 2D image was chosen from each sequence and the myocardium manually segmented by two experts to give inter-observer variability. This forms a dataset of 15 2D MCE images for evaluation. Since the appearance features of the RF are not intensity invariant, all the images are pre-processed with histogram equalization to reduce intensity variations between different images. The image size is approximately 351×303 pixels.

Validation Methodology: We compared our SMRF segmentation results to the classic RF that uses appearance features [3], as well as RFs that use other contextual features such as entanglement [10] and position features [7]. We also compared our results to repeated manual segmentations and the Active Shape Model (ASM) method [5]. Segmentation accuracy is assessed quantitatively using pixel classification accuracy, Dice and Jaccard indices, Mean Absolute Distance (MAD) and Hausdorff Distance (HD). To compute the distance error metrics (MAD and HD), a myocardial boundary is extracted from the RF probability

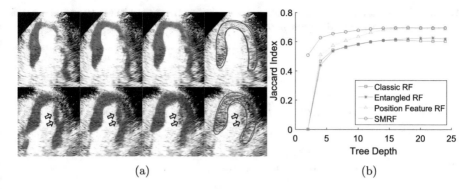

Fig. 2. (a) Visual segmentation results with one MCE example on each row. First three columns: Probability maps from classic RF, position feature RF and SMRF respectively. Last column: Ground truth boundary (*red*) and the SMRF boundary (*blue*) obtained from fitting the shape model to the SMRF probability map in the third column. *Black arrows* indicate papillary muscle. (b) Segmentation accuracy of different RF classifiers at different tree depths. (Color figure online)

map using the Canny edge detector. This is not required for the SMRF in which the shape model fitting step directly outputs a myocardial boundary.

We performed leave-one-out cross-validation on our dataset of 15 images. The RF parameters are determined experimentally and then fixed for all experiments. 20 trees are trained with maximum tree depth of 24. 10 % of the pixels from the training images are randomly selected for training. The RF and the shape model fitting were implemented in C# and MATLAB respectively. Given an unseen test image, RF segmentation took 1.5 min with 20 trees and shape model fitting took 8 s on a machine with 4 cores and 32 GB RAM. RF training took 38 min.

4   Results

Figure 2a qualitatively shows that our SMRF probability map (column 3) has smoother boundary and more coherent shape than the classic RF (column 1) and position feature RF (column 2). Fitting the shape model to the SMRF probability map produces the myocardial boundary (*blue*) in column 4. The fitting guides the RF segmentation especially in areas where the probability map has a low confidence prediction. In the example on the second row, our SMRF predicts a boundary that correctly excludes the papillary muscle (*black arrows*). This is often incorrectly included by the other RFs due to its similar appearance to the myocardium.

Table 1 compares the quantitative segmentation results of our SMRF to other methods. Both SM features and position features encode useful structural information that produces more accurate RF probability maps than the classic RF and entangled RF. This is reflected by the higher Dice and Jaccard indices. For MAD and HD metrics, SMRF outperforms all other RF methods because the

Table 1. Quantitative comparison of segmentation results between the proposed SMRF and other methods. Results presented as (Mean ± Standard Deviation).

	Accuracy	Dice	Jaccard	MAD (mm)	HD (mm)
Intra-observer	0.96±0.01	0.89±0.02	0.80±0.03	1.02±0.26	3.75±0.93
Inter-observer	0.94±0.02	0.84±0.05	0.72±0.07	1.59±0.57	6.90±3.24
ASM [5]	0.92±0.03	0.77±0.08	0.64±0.11	2.23±0.81	11.44±5.23
Classic RF	0.91±0.04	0.74±0.12	0.60±0.14	2.46±1.36	15.69±7.34
Entangled RF [10]	0.91±0.05	0.75±0.13	0.62±0.15	2.43±1.62	15.06±7.92
Position Feature RF [7]	**0.93±0.03**	**0.81±0.10**	0.69±0.13	1.81±0.84	9.51±3.80
SMRF	**0.93±0.03**	**0.81±0.10**	**0.70±0.12**	**1.68±0.72**	**6.53±2.61**

shape model fitting step in SMRF produces more accurate myocardial boundaries than those extracted using the Canny edge detector. In addition, SMRF also outperforms ASM [5] and comes close to the inter-observer variations.

Figure 2b compares the segmentation accuracy of the probability maps of different RF classifiers. Our SMRF obtained higher Jaccard indices than the classic and entangled RFs at all tree depths. At lower tree depths, SMRF shows notable improvement over the position feature RF. The SM features have more discriminative power than the position features as it captures the explicit geometry of the myocardium using the shape model. The SM feature binary test partitions the image space using more complex and meaningful myocardial shapes as opposed to position feature which simply partitions the image space using straight lines. This provides a stronger global shape constraint than the position feature and allows a decision tree to converge faster to the correct segmentation at lower tree depths. This gives the advantage of using trees with smaller depths which speeds up both training and testing.

5   Conclusion

We presented a new method SMRF for myocardial segmentation in MCE images. We showed how our SMRF utilizes a statistical shape model to guide the RF segmentation. This is particular useful for MCE data whose image intensities are affected by many variables and therefore prior knowledge of myocardial shape becomes important in guiding the segmentation. Our SMRF introduces a new SM feature which captures the global myocardial structure. This feature outperforms other contextual features to allow the RF to produce a more accurate probability map. Our SMRF then fits the shape model to the RF probability map to produce a smooth and coherent final myocardial boundary that can be used in subsequent perfusion analysis. In future work, we plan to validate our SMRF on a larger, more challenging dataset which includes different cardiac phases and chamber views.

Acknowledgments. The authors would like to thank Prof. Daniel Rueckert, Liang Chen and other members from the BioMedIA group for their help and advice. This work was supported by the Imperial College PhD Scholarship.

References

1. Breiman, L.: Random forests. Mach. Learn. **45**(1), 5–32 (2001)
2. Cootes, T.F., Taylor, C.J., Cooper, D.H., Graham, J.: Active shape models-their training and application. Comput. Vis. Image Underst. **61**(1), 38–59 (1995)
3. Criminisi, A., Robertson, D.P., Konukoglu, E., Shotton, J., Pathak, S., White, S., Siddiqui, K.: Regression forests for efficient anatomy detection and localization in computed tomography scans. Med. Image Anal. **17**(8), 1293–1303 (2013)
4. Cristinacce, D., Cootes, T.F.: Automatic feature localisation with constrained local models. Pattern Recogn. **41**(10), 3054–3067 (2008)
5. van Ginneken, B., Frangi, A.F., Staal, J., ter Haar Romeny, B.M., Viergever, M.A.: Active shape model segmentation with optimal features. IEEE Trans. Med. Imaging **21**(8), 924–933 (2002)
6. Kontschieder, P., Bulò, S.R., Bischof, H., Pelillo, M.: Structured class-labels in random forests for semantic image labelling. In: Metaxas, D.N., Quan, L., Sanfeliu, A., Gool, L.J.V. (eds.) ICCV 2011, pp. 2190–2197. IEEE, Washington, DC (2011)
7. Lempitsky, V., Verhoek, M., Noble, J.A., Blake, A.: Random forest classification for automatic delineation of myocardium in real-time 3D echocardiography. In: Ayache, N., Delingette, H., Sermesant, M. (eds.) FIMH 2009. LNCS, vol. 5528, pp. 447–456. Springer, Heidelberg (2009)
8. Lombaert, H., Criminisi, A., Ayache, N.: Spectral forests: learning of surface data, application to cortical parcellation. In: Navab, N., Hornegger, J., Wells, W.M., Frangi, A.F. (eds.) MICCAI 2015. LNCS, vol. 9349, pp. 547–555. Springer, Heidelberg (2015). doi:10.1007/978-3-319-24553-9_67
9. Ma, M., van Stralen, M., Reiber, J.H.C., Bosch, J.G., Lelieveldt, B.P.F.: Left ventricle segmentation from contrast enhanced fast rotating ultrasound images using three dimensional active shape models. In: Ayache, N., Delingette, H., Sermesant, M. (eds.) FIMH 2009. LNCS, vol. 5528, pp. 295–302. Springer, Heidelberg (2009)
10. Montillo, A., Shotton, J., Winn, J., Iglesias, J.E., Metaxas, D., Criminisi, A.: Entangled decision forests and their application for semantic segmentation of CT images. In: Székely, G., Hahn, H.K. (eds.) IPMI 2011. LNCS, vol. 6801, pp. 184–196. Springer, Heidelberg (2011)
11. Tang, M.X., Mulvana, H., Gauthier, T., Lim, A.K.P., Cosgrove, D.O., Eckersley, R.J., Stride, E.: Quantitative contrast-enhanced ultrasound imaging: a review of sources of variability. Interface Focus **1**(4), 520–539 (2011)
12. Tu, Z., Bai, X.: Auto-context and its application to high-level vision tasks and 3D brain image segmentation. IEEE Trans. Pattern Anal. Mach. Intell. **32**(10), 1744–1757 (2010)
13. Wei, K., Jayaweera, A.R., Firoozan, S., Linka, A., Skyba, D.M., Kaul, S.: Quantification of myocardial blood flow with ultrasound-induced destruction of microbubbles administered as a constant venous infusion. Circulation **97**(5), 473–483 (1998)

Low-Dimensional Statistics of Anatomical Variability via Compact Representation of Image Deformations

Miaomiao Zhang[1]([⊠]), William M. Wells III[1,2], and Polina Golland[1]

[1] Computer Science and Artificial Intelligence Laboratory, MIT, Cambridge, USA
miao86@mit.edu
[2] Brigham and Women's Hospital, Harvard Medical School, Boston, USA

Abstract. Using image-based descriptors to investigate clinical hypotheses and therapeutic implications is challenging due to the notorious "curse of dimensionality" coupled with a small sample size. In this paper, we present a low-dimensional analysis of anatomical shape variability in the space of diffeomorphisms and demonstrate its benefits for clinical studies. To combat the high dimensionality of the deformation descriptors, we develop a probabilistic model of principal geodesic analysis in a bandlimited low-dimensional space that still captures the underlying variability of image data. We demonstrate the performance of our model on a set of 3D brain MRI scans from the Alzheimer's Disease Neuroimaging Initiative (ADNI) database. Our model yields a more compact representation of group variation at substantially lower computational cost than models based on the high-dimensional state-of-the-art approaches such as tangent space PCA (TPCA) and probabilistic principal geodesic analysis (PPGA).

1 Introduction

Shape analysis is critical for image-based studies of disease as it offers characterizations of anatomical variability between different groups, or in the course of a disease. Analysis of shape changes can provide new insights into the nature of the disease and support treatment. For example, brain atrophy has been identified in patients affected by neuro-degenerative diseases such as Parkinson's, Huntington's, and Alzheimer's [5,10]. When combined with other clinical information, characterization of shape differences between clinical cohorts and a healthy population can be useful in predicting disease progression. Landmarks [3], distance transforms [6,9], and medial cores [11] are examples of image-based shape descriptors often used in medical image analysis. Most of these descriptors require informative feature points or a segmented binary image as input to the shape extraction procedure. In this paper, we focus on diffeomorphic transformations estimated from full images as a way to represent shape in a group of images [12,14].

The high-dimensional nature of the data (e.g., a 128^3 displacement grid as a shape descriptor for a 3D brain MRI) presents significant challenges for the

S. Ourselin et al. (Eds.): MICCAI 2016, Part III, LNCS 9902, pp. 166–173, 2016.
DOI: 10.1007/978-3-319-46726-9_20

statistical methods when extracting relevant latent structure from image transformations. The barriers for effective statistical analysis include (i) requiring greater computational resources and special programming techniques for statistical inference and (ii) numerous local minima. Two main ways of overcoming this problem via data dimensionality reduction have been recently proposed in the diffeomorphic setting. One is to perform statistical modeling of the transformations as a step that follows the estimation of deformations, for instance, by carrying out principal component analysis (PCA) in the tangent space of diffeomorphisms (TPCA) [14]. An empirical shape distribution can be constructed by using TPCA to estimate the intrinsic dimensionality of the diffeomorphic surface variation [12]. Later, a Bayesian model of shape variability was demonstrated to extract the principal modes after estimating a covariance matrix of transformations [7]. Alternatively, one could infer the principal modes of variation and transformations simultaneously. Principal geodesic analysis (PGA) generalized PCA to finite-dimensional manifolds and estimated the geodesic subspaces by minimizing the sum-of-squared geodesic distances to the data [4]. This enabled factor analysis of diffeomorphisms that treats data variability as a joint inference problem in a probabilistic principal geodesic analysis (PPGA) [17]. While these models were designed to find a concise low-dimensional space to represent the data, the estimation must be performed numerically on dense image grids in a high-dimensional space.

In contrast, we use the finite-dimensional representation of the tangent space of diffeomorphisms [18] to investigate shape variability using bandlimited velocity fields as a representation. We call this approach *low-dimensional probabilistic principal geodesic analysis* (LPPGA). We define a low-dimensional probabilistic framework for factor analysis in the context of diffeomorphic atlas building. Our model dramatically reduces the computational cost by employing a low-dimensional parametrization in the Fourier space. Furthermore, we enforce the orthogonality constraints on the principal modes, which is computationally intractable in high-dimensional models like PPGA [17]. We report estimated principal modes in the ADNI brain MRI dataset [8] and compare them with the results of TPCA and PPGA of diffeomorphisms in the full dimensional space. The experimental results show that the low-dimensional statistics encode the features of interest in the data, better capture the group variation and improve data interpretability. Moreover, our model requires much less computational resources.

2   Diffeomorphic Atlas Building with Geodesic Shooting

We first briefly review the mathematical background of diffeomorphic atlas building in the setting of large deformation diffeomorphic metric mapping (LDDMM) [1] with geodesic shooting [15,16].

We let $J_1, \cdots, J_N$ be the N input images that are assumed to be square integrable functions defined on d-dimensional torus domain $\Omega = \mathbb{R}^d/\mathbb{Z}^d$ ($J_n \in L^2(\Omega, \mathbb{R}), n \in \{1, \cdots, N\}$). We use I to denote the atlas template and ϕ_n to denote the deformation from template I to image J_n. The time-varying deformation $\phi_n(t, x) : t \in [0, 1], x \in \Omega$ is defined as the integral flow of time-varying velocity field $v_n(t, x)$ in a reproducing kernel Hilbert space V:

$$d/dt\,\phi_n(t, x) = v_n(t, \phi_n(t, x)).$$

The geodesic path of the deformation is uniquely determined by integrating the Euler-Poincaré differential equation (EPDiff) [18] with an initial condition of $v_n(t, x)$ at $t = 0$:

$$\frac{\partial v_n}{\partial t} = -\mathcal{K}\left[(Dv_n)^T m_n + Dm_n\, v_n + m_n \operatorname{div}(v_n)\right], \tag{1}$$

where D is the Jacobian matrix and $\div$ is the divergence operator. The operator $\mathcal{K}$ is the inverse of a symmetric, positive-definite differential operator $\mathcal{L} : V \to V^*$ that maps a velocity field $v_n \in V$ to a momentum vector $m_n \in V^*$ such that $m_n = \mathcal{L}v_n$ and $v_n = \mathcal{K}m_n$. This process is known as *geodesic shooting* [15, 16].

With a slight abuse of notation, we define $\phi_n = \phi_n(1, \cdot)$, $v_n = v_n(0, \cdot)$, allowing us to drop the time index in the subsequent derivations. Geodesic shooting (1) enables differentiation of the image differences with respect to the initial velocity field, leading to a gradient decent minimization of the energy function

$$E(v_n, I) = \sum_{n=1}^{N} \frac{1}{2\sigma^2} \left\| J_n - I \circ \phi_n^{-1} \right\|_{L^2}^2 + (\mathcal{L}v_n, v_n), \tag{2}$$

where σ^2 is the image noise variance. In this paper, we use $\mathcal{L} = (-\alpha\Delta + e)^c$, where Δ is the discrete Laplacian operator, e is the identity matrix, c is a positive scalar controlling smoothness, and α is a positive regularity parameter. The notation $(\cdot, \cdot)$ denotes the pairing of a momentum vector with a tangent vector, similar to an inner product.

It has been recently demonstrated that the initial velocity v_n can be efficiently captured via a discrete low-dimensional bandlimited representation in the Fourier space [18]. We adopt this low-dimensional representation for statistical shape analysis.

3   Generative Model

We build our generative model in the discrete finite-dimensional space $\tilde{V}$ that represents bandlimited velocity fields. Elements of this space $\tilde{v} \in \tilde{V}$ are complex-valued vector fields in the Fourier domain that represent conjugate frequencies: $v = \mathcal{F}\tilde{v}$, where $\mathcal{F}$ is the Fourier basis that maps from the frequency domain to the image domain.

Let $\tilde{W} \in \mathbb{C}^{p \times q}$ be a matrix in the Fourier space whose q columns ($q < N$) are orthonormal principal initial velocities in a low p-dimensional space ($p \ll d$), $\Lambda \in \mathbb{R}^{q \times q}$ be a diagonal matrix of scale factors for the columns of $\tilde{W}$, and $s \in \mathbb{R}^q$ be a vector that parameterizes the space of transformations. The initial velocity is therefore represented as $\tilde{v} = \tilde{W}\Lambda s$ in the low-dimensional space. Assuming i.i.d. Gaussian noise on image intensities, we obtain

$$p(J_n \mid s_n; \tilde{W}, \Lambda, I, \sigma) = \mathcal{N}(J_n ; I \circ \phi_n^{-1}, \sigma^2), \tag{3}$$

where ϕ_n is a deformation that corresponds to the initial velocity $v_n = \mathcal{F}\tilde{W}\Lambda s_n$ in the image space, that is, $d/dt\,\phi_n = \mathcal{F}\tilde{W}\Lambda s_n$, and $\mathcal{N}(\cdot ; \mu, \sigma^2)$ is a Gaussian distribution with mean μ and variance σ^2.

The prior on the loading coefficients s_n is the combination of a Gaussian distribution $\mathcal{N}(0, e)$ (e is the identity matrix) with a complex multivariate Gaussian distribution $\mathcal{N}(0, (\tilde{\mathcal{L}}\tilde{W}^T\Lambda^2\tilde{W})^{-1})$ that ensures the smoothness of the geodesic path. Similar to the $\mathcal{L}$ operator, $\tilde{\mathcal{L}} : \tilde{V} \to \tilde{V}^*$ is also a symmetric, positive definite operator that maps a complex tangent vector $\tilde{v} \in \tilde{V}$ in the Fourier domain to its dual momentum vector $\tilde{m} \in \tilde{V}^*$. For a $D_1 \times D_2 \times D_3$ grid, the operator value $\tilde{L}_{d_1 d_2 d_3}$ at location (d_1, d_2, d_3) is given by

$$\tilde{L}_{d_1 d_2 d_3} = \left[-2\alpha \left(\cos \frac{2\pi d_1}{D_1} + \cos \frac{2\pi d_2}{D_2} + \cos \frac{2\pi d_3}{D_3} - 3 \right) + 1 \right]^c,$$

and its inverse is $\tilde{L}_{d_1 d_2 d_3}^{-1} = \tilde{K}_{d_1 d_2 d_3}$. Finally, we formulate the prior as

$$p(s_n \mid \tilde{W}, \Lambda) = \mathcal{N}(s_n ; 0, (\tilde{\mathcal{L}}\tilde{W}^T\Lambda^2\tilde{W})^{-1} + e). \tag{4}$$

We now arrive at the posterior distribution of $s_1, \cdots, s_N$

$$\begin{aligned}
Q &\triangleq \log p(s_1, \cdots, s_N \mid J_1, \cdots, J_N; \tilde{W}, \Lambda, I, \sigma^2) \\
&= \sum_{n=1}^{N} \log p(J_n \mid s_n; \tilde{W}, \Lambda, I, \sigma) + \log p(s_n \mid \tilde{W}, \Lambda) + \text{const.} \\
&= \sum_{n=1}^{N} -\frac{\|J_n - I \circ \phi_n^{-1}\|_{L^2}^2}{2\sigma^2} - \frac{s_n^T(\tilde{\mathcal{L}}\tilde{W}^T\Lambda^2\tilde{W} + e)s_n}{2} - \frac{dN}{2}\log\sigma + \text{const.} \tag{5}
\end{aligned}$$

4   Inference

We use alternating gradient accent to maximize the posterior probability (5) with respect to the model parameters $\theta = \{\tilde{W}, \Lambda, I, \sigma^2\}$ and latent variables $\{s_1, \cdots, s_N\}$.

By setting the derivative of Q with respect to I and σ to zero, we obtain closed-form updates for the atlas template I and noise variance σ^2:

$$I = \frac{\sum_{n=1}^{N} J_n \circ \phi_n |D\phi_n|}{\sum_{n=1}^{N} |D\phi_n|}, \qquad \sigma^2 = \frac{1}{dN}\sum_{n=1}^{N} \|J_n - I \circ \phi_n^{-1}\|_{L^2}^2.$$

To estimate the principal initial velocity basis $\tilde{W}$, the scaling factor Λ, and the loading coefficients $\{s_n\}$, we follow the derivations in [18] and first obtain the gradient of Q w.r.t. the initial velocity $\tilde{v}_n$ as follows:

(i) Forward integrate the geodesic evolution equation (1) to generate time-dependent diffeomorphic deformation $\phi_n(t, x)$.
(ii) Compute the gradient $\nabla_{\tilde{v}_n} Q$ at time point $t = 1$ as

$$[\nabla_{\tilde{v}_n} Q]_{t=1} = -\tilde{K} \left[\frac{1}{\sigma^2} (J_n - I \circ \phi_n^{-1}) \cdot \nabla(I \circ \phi_n^{-1}) + \tilde{L}\tilde{v}_n \right]. \tag{6}$$

(iii) Backward integrate the gradient (6) to $t = 0$ to obtain $[\nabla_{\tilde{v}_n} Q]_{t=0}$.

After applying the chain rule, we have the gradient of Q for updating the loading factor s_n:

$$\nabla_{s_n} Q = -\Lambda \tilde{W}^T [\nabla_{\tilde{v}_n} Q]_{t=0} - s_n.$$

The gradients of Q w.r.t. $\tilde{W}, \Lambda$ are given as follows:

$$\nabla_{\tilde{W}} Q = -\sum_{n=1}^{N} [\nabla_{\tilde{v}_n} Q]_{t=0} s_n^T \Lambda, \qquad \nabla_{\Lambda} Q = -\sum_{n=1}^{N} \tilde{W} s_n^T [\nabla_{\tilde{v}_n} Q]_{t=0}.$$

Unlike the PPGA model [17], we can readily enforce the mutual orthogonality constraint on the columns of $\tilde{W}$. Here, we choose to employ Gram-Schmidt orthogonalization [2] on the column vectors of $\tilde{W}$ in a complex inner product space.

5 Results

Data. To evaluate the effectiveness of the proposed *low-dimensional principal geodesic analysis* (LPPGA), we applied the algorithm to brain MRI scans of 90 subjects from the ADNI [8] study, aged 60 to 90. Fifty subjects have Alzheimer's disease and the remaining 40 subjects are healthy controls. All MRIs have the same resolution $128 \times 128 \times 128$ with the voxel size of $1.25 \times 1.25 \times 1.25 \text{ mm}^3$. All images underwent skull-stripping, downsampling, intensity normalization, bias field correction, and co-registration with affine transformations.

Experiments. We first estimate a full collection of principal modes $q = 89$ for our model, using $\alpha = 3.0, c = 3.0$ for the operator $\tilde{\mathcal{L}}$ with $p = 16^3$ dimensions of initial velocity $\tilde{v}$, similar to the settings used in pairwise diffeomorphic image registration [18]. The number of time steps for integration in geodesic shooting is set to 10. We initialize the atlas I to be the average of image intensities, Λ to be the identity matrix, s_n to be the all-ones vector, and the initial velocity matrix $\tilde{W}$ to be the principal components estimated by TPCA [14]. We then compare the results with PPGA [17] and TPCA on the same dataset. In order to conduct a fair comparison, we keep all the parameters including regularization and time steps for numerical integration fixed across the three algorithms. To evaluate the model stability, we randomly select 50 images out of 90 and rerun the entire experiment 50 times.

To investigate the ability of our model to capture anatomical variability, we use the loading coefficients $s = \{s_1, \cdots, s_N\}$ as a shape descriptor in a

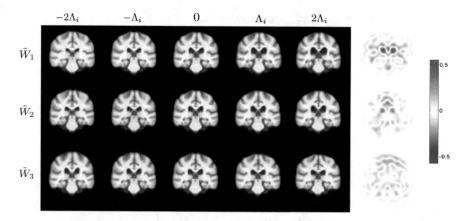

Fig. 1. Top to bottom: first, second and third principal modes of brain shape variation evaluated for varying amounts of the corresponding principal mode, and log determinant of Jacobians at $2\Lambda_i$. Coronal views are shown.

statistical study. The idea is to test the hypothesis that the principal modes estimated by our method are correlated significantly with clinical information such as mini-mental state examination (MMSE), Alzheimer's Disease Assessment Scale (ADAS), and Clinical Dementia Rating (CDR). We focus on MMSE and fit it to a linear regression model using the loadings for all 90 subjects in the training dataset as predictors. Similar analysis is performed on the results of PPGA and TPCA.

Experimental Results. Figure 1 visualizes the first three modes of variation in this cohort by shooting the estimated atlas I along the initial velocities $\tilde{v} = a_i \tilde{W}_i \Lambda_i$ ($a_i = \{-2, -1, 0, 1, 2\}, i = 1, 2, 3$). We also show the log determinant of Jacobians at $a_i = 2$ (regions of expansion in red and contraction in blue). The first mode of variation clearly shows that changes in ventricle size is the dominant source of variability in the brain shape. The algorithm estimates standard deviation of the image noise to be $\sigma = 0.02$.

Figure 2 reports the cumulative variance explained by the model as a function of the model size. Our approach achieves higher representation accuracy than the two state-of-the-art baseline algorithms across the entire range of model sizes.

Table 1 compares the regression results of our model and the two baseline algorithms using the first principal mode. The higher F and R^2 statistics indicate that our approach captures more variation of the MMSE score than the other models. Table 1 also reports run time and memory consumption for building the full model of anatomical variability. It demonstrates that our approach offers an order of magnitude improvement in both the run time and memory requirements while providing a more powerful model of variability.

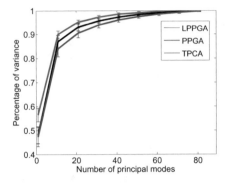

Model	90%	95%
LPPGA	11	20
PPGA	15	27
TPCA	19	35

Fig. 2. Left: cumulative variance explained by principal modes estimated through our method (LPPGA) and baseline algorithms (PPGA and TPCA). Right: number of principal modes that explain 90 % and 95 % of total variance respectively.

Table 1. Left: Comparison of linear regression models on the first principal mode for our model (LPPGA) and the baseline algorithms (PPGA and TPCA) on 90 brain MRIs from ADNI. Right: Comparison of run time and memory consumption. The implementation employed a message passing interface (MPI) parallel programming for all methods and distributed 90 subjects to 10 processors.

Model	Residual	R^2	F	p-value	Time (Hours)	Memory (MB)
LPPGA	**4.45**	**0.18**	**19.47**	**$2.18e^{-5}$**	**1.2**	**168.4**
PPGA	4.49	0.16	17.96	$5.54e^{-5}$	17.8	1708.1
TPCA	4.53	0.14	16.34	$1.10e^{-4}$	16.7	1708.1

6 Conclusion

We presented a low-dimensional probabilistic framework for factor analysis in the space of diffeomorphisms. Our model reduces the computational cost and amplifies the statistical power of shape analysis by using a low-dimensional parametrization. This work represents the first step towards *efficient* probabilistic models of shape variability based on high-dimensional diffeomorphisms. Future work will explore Bayesian variants of shape analysis. A multiscale strategy like [13] can be added to our model to make the inference even faster.

Acknowledgments. This work was supported by NIH NIBIB NAC P41EB015902, NIH NINDS R01NS086905, NIH NICHD U01HD087211, and Wistron Corporation.

References

1. Beg, M., Miller, M., Trouvé, A., Younes, L.: Computing large deformation metric mappings via geodesic flows of diffeomorphisms. Int. J. Comput. Vis. **61**(2), 139–157 (2005)

2. Cheney, W., Kincaid, D.: Linear Algebra: Theory and Applications, vol. 110. The Australian Mathematical Society, Canberra (2009)
3. Cootes, T.F., Taylor, C.J., Cooper, D.H., Graham, J.: Active shape models-their training and application. Comput. Vis. Image Underst. **61**(1), 38–59 (1995)
4. Fletcher, P.T., Lu, C., Joshi, S.: Statistics of shape via principal geodesic analysis on Lie groups. Comput. Vis. Pattern Recogn. **1**, 1–95 (2003). IEEE
5. Gerig, G., Styner, M., Shenton, M.E., Lieberman, J.A.: Shape versus size: improved understanding of the morphology of brain structures. In: Niessen, W.J., Viergever, M.A. (eds.) MICCAI 2001. LNCS, vol. 2208, pp. 24–32. Springer, Heidelberg (2001). doi:10.1007/3-540-45468-3_4
6. Golland, P., Grimson, W.E.L., Shenton, M.E., Kikinis, R.: Small sample size learning for shape analysis of anatomical structures. In: Delp, S.L., DiGoia, A.M., Jaramaz, B. (eds.) MICCAI 2000. LNCS, vol. 1935, pp. 72–82. Springer, Heidelberg (2000). doi:10.1007/978-3-540-40899-4_8
7. Gori, P., Colliot, O., Worbe, Y., Marrakchi-Kacem, L., Lecomte, S., Poupon, C., Hartmann, A., Ayache, N., Durrleman, S.: Bayesian atlas estimation for the variability analysis of shape complexes. In: Mori, K., Sakuma, I., Sato, Y., Barillot, C., Navab, N. (eds.) MICCAI 2013, Part I. LNCS, vol. 8149, pp. 267–274. Springer, Heidelberg (2013)
8. Jack, C.R., Bernstein, M.A., Fox, N.C., Thompson, P., Alexander, G., Harvey, D., Borowski, B., Britson, P.J., Whitwell, J.L., Ward, C., et al.: The alzheimer's disease neuroimaging initiative (ADNI): MRI methods. J. Magn. Reson. Imaging **27**(4), 685–691 (2008)
9. Leventon, M.E., Grimson, W.E.L., Faugeras, O.: Statistical shape influence in geodesic active contours. In: Proceedings of IEEE Conference on Computer Vision and Pattern Recognition, vol. 1, pp. 316–323. IEEE (2000)
10. Nemmi, F., Sabatini, U., Rascol, O., Péran, P.: Parkinson's disease and local atrophy in subcortical nuclei: insight from shape analysis. Neurobiol. Aging **36**(1), 424–433 (2015)
11. Pizer, S.M., Fritsch, D.S., Yushkevich, P.A., Johnson, V.E., Chaney, E.L.: Segmentation, registration, and measurement of shape variation via image object shape. IEEE Trans. Med. Imaging **18**(10), 851–865 (1999)
12. Qiu, A., Younes, L., Miller, M.I.: Principal component based diffeomorphic surface mapping. IEEE Trans. Med. Imaging **31**(2), 302–311 (2012)
13. Sommer, S., Lauze, F., Nielsen, M., Pennec, X.: Sparse multi-scale diffeomorphic registration: the kernel bundle framework. J. Math. Imaging Vis. **46**(3), 292–308 (2013)
14. Vaillant, M., Miller, M.I., Younes, L., Trouvé, A.: Statistics on diffeomorphisms via tangent space representations. NeuroImage **23**, S161–S169 (2004)
15. Vialard, F.X., Risser, L., Rueckert, D., Cotter, C.J.: Diffeomorphic 3D image registration via geodesic shooting using an efficient adjoint calculation. Int. J. Comput. Vis. **97**(2), 229–241 (2012)
16. Younes, L., Arrate, F., Miller, M.: Evolutions equations in computational anatomy. NeuroImage **45**(1), S40–S50 (2009)
17. Zhang, M., Fletcher, P.T.: Bayesian principal geodesic analysis in diffeomorphic image registration. In: Golland, P., Hata, N., Barillot, C., Hornegger, J., Howe, R. (eds.) MICCAI 2014. LNCS, vol. 8675, pp. 121–128. Springer, Heidelberg (2014). doi:10.1007/978-3-319-10443-0_16
18. Zhang, M., Fletcher, P.T.: Finite-dimensional Lie algebras for fast diffeomorphic image registration. In: Ourselin, S., Alexander, D.C., Westin, C.-F., Cardoso, M.J. (eds.) IPMI 2015. LNCS, vol. 9123, pp. 249–260. Springer, Heidelberg (2015)

A Multiscale Cardiac Model for Fast Personalisation and Exploitation

Roch Mollero$^{(\boxtimes)}$, Xavier Pennec, Hervé Delingette, Nicholas Ayache, and Maxime Sermesant

Inria - Asclepios Research Project, Sophia Antipolis, France
roch-philippe.mollero@inria.fr

Abstract. Computer models of the heart are of increasing interest for clinical applications due to their discriminative and predictive abilities. However a single 3D simulation can be computationally expensive and long, which can make some practical applications such as the personalisation phase, or a sensitivity analysis of mechanical parameters over the simulated behaviour quite slow. In this manuscript we present a multiscale 0D/3D model which allows us to have a reliable (and extremely fast) approximation of the behaviour of the 3D model under a few simplifying assumptions. We first detail the two different models, then explain the coupling of the two models to get fast 0D approximation of 3D simulations. Finally we demonstrated how the multiscale model can speed-up an efficient optimization algorithm, which enables a fast personalisation of the 3D simulations by leveraging on the advantages of each scale.

1 Introduction

Three-D personalised cardiac models simulate the physical behaviour of a patient heart, in order to perform advanced analysis of the cardiac function. The movement of the myocardium is calculated under the influence of simulated electromechanics and haemodynamic condition, which requires complex and expensive calculations, particularly as the spatial and temporal resolution of the model increases (1 h per heart beat, even several days for some models).

This computational burden particularly impacts applications of the models where many simulations are required. The model personalisation phase (fitting the available clinical data) is particularly impacted, slowing the study of clinical applications such as disease caracterisation and prediction of case evolution

To tackle this computational burden, surrogate models of the cardiac function have been developed, for example for uncertainty quantification [1] or probability estimation [2] over the cardiac parameters. Those models usually rely on regression models which require many pre-computations to approximate nonlinear behaviours, thus scaling badly as the number of varying parameters increases.

Here we built a multiscale cardiac model by developing an novel coupling method between an original 3D cardiac model and a reduced lumped "0D" version of the same model. While the coupling of different scales has been used to improve boundary conditions in cardiac modelling and computational fluid

© Springer International Publishing AG 2016
S. Ourselin et al. (Eds.): MICCAI 2016, Part III, LNCS 9902, pp. 174–182, 2016.
DOI: 10.1007/978-3-319-46726-9_21

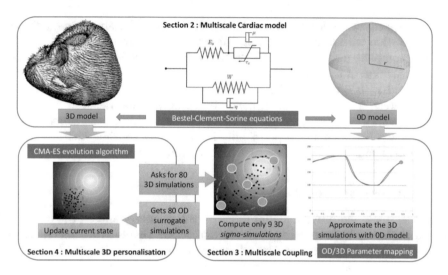

Fig. 1. Multiscale model and personalisation pipeline

dynamics [3], we propose here the simultaneous simulation of the same model at different scales, which enables extremely fast approximations of the behaviour of the 3D model with 0D simulations. It provides a natural approximation of all the desired cardiac values. Furthermore, we demonstrate the efficiency of the multiscale 0D/3D model when plugged into a personalisation process driven by the genetic algorithm CMA-ES. This creates a very fast and computationally efficient personalisation agent, successfully tested on the personalisation of 34 hearts with different geometries (Fig. 1).

2 Multiscale Cardiac Model

In order to build a computer model of the myocardium, one needs different components to represent the passive stiffness, the active contraction and the boundary conditions (hemodynamics). We use here the Bestel-Clement-Sorine model (BCS) of the sarcomere contraction, in conjonction with the Mooney-Rivlin model for passive elasticity as described in [4]. Hemodynamics are represented through global values of pressures and flows in the cardiac chambers.

2.1 Three-D Cardiac Model

Here we first use 3D biventricular mesh geometry extracted from MRI images, with synthetic myocardial fibres. The active sarcomere force and the passive force are computed at each point of the mesh with the Bestel-Clement-Sorine (BCS) model under the influence of the pre-computed electrophysiology. The boundary condition is a circulation model with the 4 phases of the cardiac cycle based using a 3-parameters Windkessel model of blood pressure as after-load.

We also specify a *resting mesh* in addition of the initial mesh geometry to start the simulation with a geometry which already includes residual stress.

The complete details of the 3D electromechanical model as well as the C++ implementation of the finite element solver are discussed in [5]. With meshes of 10 000 and 15 000 points and a time step of 5 ms, a single beat (around 0.9 s) takes between 25 min and 1 h to compute. Finally, since we want to consider cardiac beats which are not affected by the initialization of the simulation, we compute 3 subsequent beats per simulation and only consider the last one, so the full 3D simulation takes between 75 min and 3 h to be computed.

2.2 0D Cardiac Model

If we then make simplifying assumptions on the geometry and on the properties of the material, by approximating the ventricular shape as a sphere, we can derive the equations of a fast *lumped model of the heart* as detailed in [6].

The myocardial motion is then only described by the inner radius **r** of the ventricle (the "Resting Mesh" in 3D becomes simply a "Resting Radius" **r0**), the material is considered incompressible and has idealised tangential fibres. The electrophysiological activation is supposed synchronous and homogeneous over the sphere as well as the resulting active sarcomere force. Finally we use the same circulation model and Mooney Rivlin equations than in the 3D model.

We implemented the 0D model within the CellML framework, then converted into C code with OpenCOR [7]. With a temporal discretisation of 0.1 ms, we can simulate 10 to 20 heart beats per seconds.

3   Multiscale Coupling

Although with different mechanical assumptions, both models follow the same trends in behaviour when we change the global parameters. The idea of the coupling is to have those trends match within a specific domain of 3D parameters, in order to predict the behaviour of many 3D simulations by only computing 0D simulations. This is done by first matching several 3D simulations of the domain (called the *sigma-simulations*) with the 0D model, then learning a mapping between the 3D parameters and the 0D parameters.

3.1   Personalisation of the 0D Model to a 3D Simulation

The first step of the coupling is to make the two models match on a single simulated beat. Given one 3D simulated heartbeat, we want to accurately reproduce the pump behaviour of the heart with the 0D model (under the same boundary conditions). In particular we focus on reproducing 6 features of the volume curve by setting 5 main electromechanical parameters in the 0D model, both listed in Table 1.

We estimate the parameters by performing a derivative-free optimisation with the genetic algorithm CMA-ES [8]. This powerful algorithm combines Bayesian

Table 1. Features and parameters in the 0D model personalisation over a 3D simulation

Features	0D parameters
Maximal Volume **Vmax**	*Maximal Contraction* σ
Minimal Volume **Vmin**	*Stiffness* **c1**
Percentage of filling when the atrium contracts **FVat**	*Resting radius* **r0**
Flow when the atrium contracts **Qat**	*damping* **eta**
Time where the volume is minimum **tVmin**	*Atrio-Ventricular Delay* **AV.**
Time when ejection starts **teject**	

principles of Maximum Likelihood with a local gradient descent on the members of each generation, by updating at each iteration both an internal covariance **Ic** and mean **Im** of the parameters to explore at the next iteration. We define the fitness (score) of each simulation by:

$$fitness(x) = \|(Values(x) - TargetValues)/Normalization\|$$

which is the L_2 distance between the simulated and the objective values, normalized to be able to compare *volumes* (unit_volume = 10 ml) with *times* (unit_time = 20 ms), *percentages* (unit_percent = 5 %) and *flow* (unit_flow = 10 ml/s).

We use a population of 20 simulations per generation, and optimize over 100 generations. This takes less than 10 min on a multi-core computer with parallel computation of the simulations within each generation. Figure 2 shows the matching behaviours of a 3D simulation and its 0D counterpart.

3.2   Prediction of 3D Behaviour from 0D Simulations

We want to be able to get reliable approximations of other 3D simulations within a domain Ω_{3D} of 3D parameters by doing 0D simulations, so we need to be able to convert a vector $X \in \Omega_{3D}$ into a relevant vector Y of 0D parameters which best approximates the 3D simulations. Here we focus in the mapping of $N_1=4$ 3D parameters toward $N_2=5$ 0D parameters listed in Table 2.

The parameters do not behave necessarily the same for both models (and not in the same range of values). For example the 3D and 0D dampings are not calculated in the same way, and the "resting position" variable is a unitless value from 0 to 10 in the 3D case, whereas it is the "inner radius" (in cm) in the 0D mdoel. Also even for parameters coming from the same equations in both models (such as σ and **c1**) the values might be different for two matching 0D and 3D simulations. For example we can get the same volume curve with contractility and stiffness values which are 10 times smaller in the 0D implementation than in the 3D setting). The mapping is thus not trivial and is done through the following steps:

1. We first perform $2N_1+1$ 3D simulations at 2 points of each of the N_1 principal directions of the domain of interest Ω_{3D} and its center (called the *sigma-simulations* with parameters S_i).

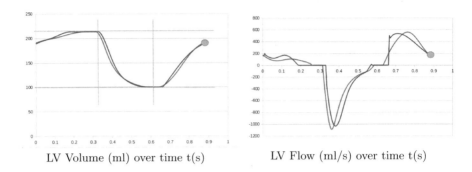

LV Volume (ml) over time t(s)   LV Flow (ml/s) over time t(s)

Fig. 2. Comparison between a volume curve simulated with the 3D model (blue) and the matched 0D simulation (red). Orange lines and points outline the 6 fitted values (Color figure online)

2. We then fit the 0D model on each of those $2N_1+1$ simulations with the method explained in the previous subsection, which gives the $2N_1 + 1$ corresponding vectors of 0D parameters V_i.
3. Then we compute a least square linear regression ϕ between the parameters of S_i and the parameters V_i.
4. Finally for each vector X of Ω_{3D}, we get the relevant vector $Y = \phi(X)$ of 0D parameters by using this linear regression.

3.3   Results of the Parameter Mapping

Here we evaluate the approximation of 80 other 3D simulations with parameters $X_j \in \Omega_{3D}$ by their corresponding 0D simulations with parameters $Y_j = \phi(X_j)$. We focus on the error made on 7 features, which we compare with the error made by a direct linear regression between the parameters of the *sigma-simulations* and the 7 features (which is the best regression model we can run with this small number of points). Results are shown in Table 3.

Both methods provide good approximations of the features. However if we exclude **tVmin** (which is harder to approximate because of the temporal discretisation of the models), the simulations with the 0D model provide overall better approximations of the values, particularly of those with the most nonlinear behaviour such as the percentage of filling (**FVat**) and the flow (**Qat**) when the atrium opens (resp by 43 % and 40 %). This is because the 0D model naturally captures the nonlinear behaviour of those features which would require many simulations to be well approximated by a nonlinear regression model.

4   Efficient Personalisation of the Multiscale Model

Personalisation is the first step for the application of 3D cardiac modelling to patient-specific data. After extracting a patient-specific mesh geometry from the

Table 2. Three-D and 0D parameters of the mapping

Three-D parameters	0D parameters
Maximal Contractionσ	*Maximal Contraction* σ
Stiffness **c1**	*Stiffness* **c1**
Resting Mesh **RM**	*Resting radius* **r0**
3D damping μ	*0D damping* **eta**
	Atrio-Ventricular Delay **AV**

Table 3. Feature approximation by the mapping: range of values of each feature, mean absolute error with the mapping (MAE_m) and mean absolute error with the direct regression (MAE_r)

Feature	tVmin (ms)	Vmax (ml)	Vmin (ml)	EF (%)	SV (ml)	FVat (%)	Qat (ml/s)
Range	30.3	9.97	34.6	27.7	29.7	11.1	93.9
MAE_m	6.35	**2.03**	1.06	0.17	**0.98**	**0.78**	**3.62**
MAE_r	**3.86**	2.09	**0.89**	**0.15**	1.21	1.38	5.99

images, we want the 3D simulation to match specific clinical data. This can be done as in Sect. 3.1, by optimizing some parameters of the 3D cardiac model with CMA-ES to minimize a score related to the distance between the simulation and the target clinical data.

Since the convergence speed of CMA-ES increases with the size of the population evaluated at each iteration, we want to set this size as high as possible, but the computational cost of each 3D simulation is the limiting factor. However with the coupled model, we show that we can evaluate the scores of the members of a large population with a limited number of 3D simulations, which allows to benefit from the increased speed of convergence while keeping a reasonable computational burden.

4.1 Full Personalisation Pipeline

In the personalisation process of the 3D model, we want to reproduce 5 features of the volume curve (listed in Table 4) by optimizing the 4 parameters described in Sect. 3.2. We initialize a CMA-ES optimization process with a high population size m = 80, and derive the **Coupled-CMA** optimization method by adapting the original CMA-ES as follows:

At each iteration, the CMA-ES algorithm asks for the scores of m 3D simulations X_j whose parameters are drawn from a multivariate distribution, ruled by its own internal mean **Im** and covariance **Ic**.

Instead of performing these m 3D simulations, we calculate a mapping ϕ and m surrogate 0D simulations with parameters $Y_j = \phi(X_j)$, as explained in

Table 4. Features and parameters in the 3D model personalisation to a real volume curve

Features	3D parameters
Maximal Volume **Vmax**	*Maximal Contraction* σ
Stroke Volume **SV**	*Stiffness* **c1**
Percentage of filling when the atrium contracts **FVat**	*Resting Mesh* **RM**
Flow when the atrium contracts **Qat**	*3D damping* μ
Time where the volume is minimum **tVmin**	

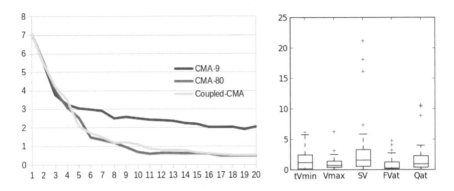

Fig. 3. Left: Score per iteration for the 3D methods. **Right:** Fitting error of each feature for the 34 patients (in percentage of the mean observed value of each feature)

Sect. 3.2. Only the $2N_1 + 1 = 9$ 3D *sigma-simulations* are required, which are drawn at the center and within the principal axis of the multivariate distribution (two simulations per axis at $\pm$ *standard deviation of the axis* from the mean).

Then we calculate the scores of these m surrogate simulations $Y_j = \phi(X_j)$ and provide the scores to the CMA-ES algorithm "as if" they were the scores of the m 3D simulations.

4.2   Results

In order to compare the efficiency of the **Coupled-CMA** optimization, we compare it with the full CMA optimization with a population size of 80 (**CMA-80**), as well as with a direct CMA optimization with a population size of 9 (**CMA-9**) which has the same computational burden than the Coupled-CMA.

This is done by comparing the scores of the 3D simulations made with the algorithm's internal mean **Im** at each iteration, which is the algorithm's current best estimate of the minimal parameters (In the case of Coupled-CMA, it is the score of the central *sigma-simulation*). Results are shown in Fig. 3 (left).

The CMA-80 expectedly converges a lot faster than the CMA-9, but the main result is that the Coupled-CMA optimization converges at the same speed than the CMA-80. From a computing viewpoint, the Coupled-CMA lowers the number of 3D simulations from 80 to 9 at each iteration while keeping the accuracy, thus saving between 50 and 150 h of CPU time at each iteration.

This similarity of convergence between CMA-80 and Coupled-CMA was confirmed on other geometries and values to fit, and overall we applied this method to the personalisation of 34 patient hearts, sucessfully matching the features to their target clinical values, within 6 % of the mean value of each feature in the population, for at least 90 % of the cases, as show on Fig. 3 (right).

5   Conclusion

In this manuscript we detailed how a fast reduced "0D" model relying on the same equations but simplifying assumptions can be coupled to the original 3D model to approximate computationally-costly 3D simulations with fast 0D simulations within a domain of 3D parameters. For this we developed a novel method to learn a mapping between the parameters of 3D *sigma-simulations* within the domain, and the parameters of corresponding 0D simulations with the same mechanical behaviour. In learning how to go from 3D parameters to 0D parameters, we learned the difference between the 0D (lumped) hypothesis and the 3D hypothesis. We then used the coupled model to build a fast personalisation agent, by substituting many 3D simulations in the optimization process by their 0D counterparts. This enabled us to benefit from the higher speed of convergence while considerably reducing the computational burden.

Several aspects of this method can be directly extended to more (nonlinear) features and parameters, such as the pressure, heart rate and the boundary conditions. We could also improve the computational gain by reusing the mapping from one iteration of the CMA-ES to the next one when the domains are similar enough instead of recomputing it. Finally, we expect the personalisation method to scale well to more complex optimization problems with a larger parameter space, since CMA-ES is well suited for those problems.

Ackowledgements. This work has been partially funded by the EU FP7-funded project MD-Paedigree (Grant Agreement 600932) and contributes to the objectives of the ERC advanced grant MedYMA (2011-291080).

References

1. Neumann, D., et al.: Robust image-based estimation of cardiac tissue parameters and their uncertainty from noisy data. In: Golland, P., Hata, N., Barillot, C., Hornegger, J., Howe, R. (eds.) MICCAI 2014, Part II. LNCS, vol. 8674, pp. 9–16. Springer, Heidelberg (2014)
2. Konukoglu, E., Relan, J., Cilingir, U., Menze, B.H., Chinchapatnam, P., Jadidi, A., Cochet, H., Hocini, M., Delingette, H., Jaïs, P., et al.: Efficient probabilistic model personalization integrating uncertainty on data and parameters: application to eikonal-diffusion models in cardiac electrophysiology. Prog. Biophys. Mol. Biol. **107**(1), 134–146 (2011)

3. Moghadam, M.E., Vignon-Clementel, I.E., Figliola, R., Marsden, A.L.: A modular numerical method for implicit 0d/3d coupling in cardiovascular finite element simulations. J. Comput. Phys. **244**, 63–79 (2013)
4. Chapelle, D., Le Tallec, P., Moireau, P., Sorine, M.: Energy-preserving muscle tissue model: formulation and compatible discretizations. Int. J. Multiscale Comput. Eng. **10**(2), 189–211 (2012)
5. Marchesseau, S., Delingette, H., Sermesant, M., Ayache, N.: Fast parameter calibration of a cardiac electromechanical model from medical images based on the unscented transform. Biomech. Model. Mechanobiol. **12**(4), 815–831 (2013)
6. Caruel, M., Chabiniok, R., Moireau, P., Lecarpentier, Y., Chapelle, D.: Dimensional reductions of a cardiac model for effective validation and calibration. Biomech. Model. Mechanobiol. **13**(4), 897–914 (2014)
7. Garny, A., Hunter, P.J.: Opencor: a modular and interoperable approach to computational biology. Front. Physiol. **6**, 26 (2015)
8. Hansen, N.: The CMA evolution strategy: a comparing review. In: Lozano, J.A., Larrañaga, P., Inza, I., Bengoetxea, E. (eds.) Towards a New Evolutionary Computation. Advances in the Estimation of Distribution Algorithms. Studies in Fuzziness and Soft Computing, vol. 192, pp. 75–102. Springer, Berlin, Heidelberg (2006)

Transfer Shape Modeling Towards High-Throughput Microscopy Image Segmentation

Fuyong Xing[1,2], Xiaoshuang Shi[2], Zizhao Zhang[3], JinZheng Cai[2],
Yuanpu Xie[2], and Lin Yang[1,2,3(✉)]

[1] Department of Electrical and Computer Engineering,
University of Florida, Gainesville, FL 32611, USA
[2] J. Crayton Pruitt Family Department of Biomedical Engineering,
University of Florida, Gainesville, FL 32611, USA
lin.yang@bme.ufl.edu
[3] Department of Computer and Information Science and Engineering,
University of Florida, Gainesville, FL 32611, USA

Abstract. In order to deal with ambiguous image appearances in cell segmentation, high-level shape modeling has been introduced to delineate cell boundaries. However, shape modeling usually requires sufficient annotated training shapes, which are often labor intensive or unavailable. Meanwhile, when applying the model to different datasets, it is necessary to repeat the tedious annotation process to generate enough training data, and this will significantly limit the applicability of the model. In this paper, we propose to transfer shape modeling learned from an existing but different dataset (e.g. lung cancer) to assist cell segmentation in a new target dataset (e.g. skeletal muscle) without expensive manual annotations. Considering the intrinsic geometry structure of cell shapes, we incorporate the shape transfer model into a sparse representation framework with a manifold embedding constraint, and provide an efficient algorithm to solve the optimization problem. The proposed algorithm is tested on multiple microscopy image datasets with different tissue and staining preparations, and the experiments demonstrate its effectiveness.

1 Introduction

Automatic cell segmentation is a critical step in microscopy image analysis, and serves as a basis of many subsequent quantitative analyses [4], such as cellular morphology calculation and individual cell classification. It is challenging to achieve robust cell segmentation due to ambiguous image appearance, such as weak cell boundaries, inhomogeneous intracellular intensity, and partial occlusion of cells, etc. Therefore, instead of purely relying on low-level image appearances, high-level shape modeling has been introduced to improve object boundary delineation [2,15,18,19].

© Springer International Publishing AG 2016
S. Ourselin et al. (Eds.): MICCAI 2016, Part III, LNCS 9902, pp. 183–190, 2016.
DOI: 10.1007/978-3-319-46726-9_22

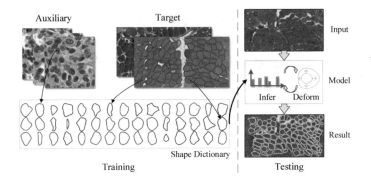

Fig. 1. The overview of the proposed shape transfer model. It aims at learning a cell shape dictionary, which can produce data representations applicable to the target set.

Effective shape modeling usually requires a sufficient number of annotated training data, which might be labor intensive or even unavailable in some applications. Meanwhile, it is necessary to repeat the tedious annotation process to generate training shapes for different microscopy image datasets, thereby significantly limiting the generality of shape modeling. In this paper, we propose to transfer shape modeling from an auxiliary dataset with sufficient training cell shapes to a target dataset with a limited number of training samples for automatic cell segmentation. In order to respect the intrinsic geometry structure of cell shapes [16], we incorporate the shape transfer model into a sparse representation framework with a manifold embedding constraint. Cell shape transfer is modeled as learning a compact dictionary that can construct robust representations for cells from different datasets, and model optimization is achieved by using an efficient sparse encoding algorithm. In this scenario, we can significantly reduce the manual annotation efforts and improve the generality of the shape modeling across multiple datasets so as to produce high-throughput cell segmentation in microscopy image analysis.

2   Methodology

An overview of the proposed shape transfer modeling for cell segmentation is shown in Fig. 1. In the training stage, the shape dictionary is learned by regularizing the distribution differences of cell training shapes between the auxiliary and target datasets, and thus the dictionary can serve as a reference repository to generate robust data representations across both datasets. Convolutional neural networks (CNNs) [5,15] are learned to conduct pixel-wise classification for generating initial cell contours/shapes. In the testing stage, the framework moves the contours towards cell boundaries until convergence in an alternate manner [18]: deform shapes with an efficient active contour model [20] and infer shapes with the transferred shape priors based on the learned dictionary. Due to page limits, this paper only focuses on shape transfer modeling.

2.1   Shape Transfer Modeling

Problem Definition: Denote auxiliary data by $\mathcal{D}_a = \{x_1, x_2, ..., x_{N_a}\}$ with N_a training cell shapes and target data by $\mathcal{D}_t = \{x_{N_a+1}, x_{N_a+2}, ..., x_{N_a+N_t}\}$ with N_t training shapes, where each shape is described by the concatenated 2D coordinates of p evenly-sampled control points and aligned by removing global transformation. Based on $\mathcal{D}_a$ and $\mathcal{D}_t$, our goal is to learn a compact shape dictionary $B = [b_1, ..., b_K] \in \mathbb{R}^{2p \times K}$ such that for any cell shape $x \in \mathbb{R}^{2p \times 1}$, a solution to $x = B\alpha$, with sparse constraints on the coefficient α, is robust and effective across both datasets. In this way, the cell shape information from the auxiliary dataset would be transferred and thus assist the data representation generation for cell segmentation in the target dataset.

Shape Transfer Model: Let $X = [x_1, x_2, ..., x_N] \in \mathbb{R}^{2p \times N}$ with $N = N_a + N_t$ be the input data matrix consisting of $\mathcal{D}_a$ and $\mathcal{D}_t$, sparse shape modeling aims to learn a dictionary by minimizing the reconstruction error with specific constraints on the coefficients [18,19]. In this paper, we model dictionary learning as a subsect selection problem which seeks a small set of representatives to summarize and describe the whole dataset X, thereby removing outliers that are not true representatives and improving the runtime computational efficiency. A straightforward way to conduct sparse subsect selection is to regularize the coefficient matrix with an $\ell_{2,1}$ or $\ell_{\infty,1}$ norm [6]. Meanwhile, since the number of constraints for shape control is limited, cell shapes actually lie on a low-dimensional manifold [16]. Therefore, we can formulate the subset selection as a graph and row-sparsity regularized optimization problem

$$\min_A ||X - XA||_F^2 + \gamma \mathrm{Tr}(ALA^T) + \lambda ||A||_{2,1}, \text{ s.t. } \mathbf{1}_N^T A = \mathbf{1}_N, \quad (1)$$

where $A \in \mathbb{R}^{N \times N}$ is the sparse coefficient matrix. $L = D - W$ is the graph Laplacian, where W is a n-nearest neighbor graph ($n = 5$) with nodes representing the training shapes: $W_{ij} = 1$ if x_i is among the n-nearest neighbors of x_j, otherwise 0; D is a diagonal matrix with $D_{ii} = \sum_{j=1}^{N} W_{ij}$. $\mathrm{Tr}(\cdot)$ denotes the trace operation, and it encourages those adjacent shapes in the intrinsic geometry to be represented with similar codes. $||A||_{2,1} = \sum_{i=1}^{N} ||\alpha^i||_2$ (α^i representing the i-th row of A) is the sum of the ℓ_2 norms of the rows and is a convex relaxation for counting the number of nonzero rows of A. The affine constraint ensures shift invariance, and $\mathbf{1}_N \in \mathbb{R}^{N \times 1}$ is a vector with all elements equal to one. Since each row α^i corresponds to one input cell shape x_i, after solving (1) we can simply form the dictionary $B = [x_{b_1}, ..., x_{b_K}]$ by selecting the representatives corresponding to the nonzero rows of A and apply it to cell shape encoding based on sparse reconstruction in the testing stage.

In order to transfer the shape prior knowledge from the auxiliary to target dataset, the sparse encoding needs to be robust across both datasets. An intuitive strategy is to enable the selected representatives or the dictionary to capture the common composition of the two datasets instead of only the individual characteristics of the auxiliary shapes, and this can be realized by reducing the distribution differences of the representations between two datasets. Inspired by [8,11], we propose to penalize the distance in Maximum Mean Discrepancy (MMD), which is a nonparametric criterion to measure the distribution difference between the means of samples from two datasets in a transformed representation space. In our model, cell shapes are mapped into a representation space via the learned dictionary, and thus we need to penalize the distance between the auxiliary and target datasets in the sparse coefficients

$$\left\| \frac{1}{N_a} \sum_{i=1}^{N_a} \boldsymbol{\alpha}_i - \frac{1}{N_t} \sum_{j=N_a+1}^{N_a+N_t} \boldsymbol{\alpha}_j \right\|^2 = \sum_{i,j=1}^{N_a+N_t} \boldsymbol{\alpha}_i^T \boldsymbol{\alpha}_j M_{ij} = \mathrm{Tr}(\boldsymbol{AMA}^T), \qquad (2)$$

where $\boldsymbol{\alpha}_i \in \mathbb{R}^{N \times 1}$ is the i-th column of $\boldsymbol{A}$, and $\boldsymbol{M} \in \mathbb{R}^{N \times N}$ is the MMD matrix with the ij-th element computed as $M_{ij} = \frac{1}{N_a^2}$ when $\boldsymbol{x}_i, \boldsymbol{x}_j \in \mathcal{D}_a$; $M_{ij} = \frac{1}{N_t^2}$ when $\boldsymbol{x}_i, \boldsymbol{x}_j \in \mathcal{D}_t$ and $M_{ij} = \frac{-1}{N_a N_t}$ otherwise.

One of significant benefits for choosing the MMD criterion is that it does not require an intermediate density estimate, which is usually a non-trivial task. By incorporating (2) into (1), we obtain the proposed objective function for cell shape knowledge transfer

$$\min_{\boldsymbol{A}} ||\boldsymbol{X} - \boldsymbol{XA}||_F^2 + \gamma \mathrm{Tr}(\boldsymbol{ALA}^T) + \mu \mathrm{Tr}(\boldsymbol{AMA}^T) + \lambda ||\boldsymbol{A}||_{2,1}, \text{ s.t. } \mathbf{1}_N^T \boldsymbol{A} = \mathbf{1}_N, \quad (3)$$

where $\mu > 0$ is a weight parameter controlling the MMD regularization. MMD asymptotically approaches to zero if the auxiliary and target datasets exhibit the same distribution [8]. By mapping cell shapes into a common representation space, solving (3) can refine the subset selection of representatives and transfer the shape knowledge of the auxiliary dataset, thereby producing representations that are applicable to the target dataset.

2.2   Efficient Local Encoding

The model in (3) can be solved by the Alternating Direction Method of Multipliers (ADMM) framework [3]. However, ADMM might introduce additional parameters in the optimization procedure. Note that the graph regularization in (3) respects the intrinsic Riemannian structure of cell shapes by obeying the manifold assumption: if $\boldsymbol{x}_i$ and $\boldsymbol{x}_j$ are adjacent in the manifold, then their representations, $\boldsymbol{\alpha}_i$ and $\boldsymbol{\alpha}_j$, with respect to the learned dictionary should be close to each other. Actually this can be approximated in a more efficient way: using a globally linear function with respect to a set of learned local coordinates [17] and solving a much smaller linear system. Therefore, instead of directly penalizing the differences of the representations between neighboring shapes, during the sparse coding we can weight the codes with the similarity between the shapes and the dictionary bases. More importantly, the time complexity can be significantly reduced. Therefore, we can revise the model in (3) by replacing the graph regularization with a locality-constrained term and explicitly modeling the dictionary $\boldsymbol{B}$

$$\min_{\boldsymbol{B}, \tilde{\boldsymbol{A}}} J = ||\boldsymbol{X} - \boldsymbol{B}\tilde{\boldsymbol{A}}||_F^2 + \gamma \sum_{i=1}^{N} \tilde{\boldsymbol{\alpha}}_i^T \boldsymbol{Q}^i \tilde{\boldsymbol{\alpha}}_i + \mu \mathrm{Tr}(\tilde{\boldsymbol{A}} \boldsymbol{M} \tilde{\boldsymbol{A}}^T), \text{ s.t. } \mathbf{1}_K^T \tilde{\boldsymbol{A}} = \mathbf{1}_K, \quad (4)$$

where $Q^i \in \mathbb{R}^{K \times K}$ is a diagonal matrix with $Q^i_{kk} = ||x_i - b_k||^2$ representing the distance between shape x_i and dictionary basis b_k. The introduced locality constraint encourages each shape to be represented with its neighbors in B. $\tilde{A} \in \mathbb{R}^{K \times N}$ is the coefficient matrix. We remove the sparsity regularization in (4) since locality guarantees sparsity but not necessary vice versa [14,17].

It is difficult to simultaneously compute the two unknown variables in (4), and thus we solve it in an alternate way: calculate coefficients $\tilde{A}$ with dictionary B fixed and learn dictionary B with coefficients $\tilde{A}$ fixed. We can derive the i-th coefficient analytically with a fixed dictionary as

$$\tilde{\alpha}_i = (Y + \mu(M_{ii}I_K + 1_K r_i^T + r_i 1_K^T) + \gamma Q^i)^{-1} 1_K, \tag{5}$$

where $Y = (1_K x_i^T - B^T)(x_i 1_K^T - B)$ and $r_i = \sum_{j \neq i} M_{ij} \tilde{\alpha}_j$. In order to preserve the affine constraint, we further normalize $\tilde{\alpha}_i$ such that $1_K^T \tilde{\alpha}_i = 1$. In our implementation, we anchor each shape in its local coordinate system for fast encoding.

With coefficients $\tilde{A}$ fixed, dictionary B is updated by gradient decent [10]. The derivative of the objective function with respect to the k-th basis b_k is derived in (6). To ensure that the dictionary bases coincide with a subset of actual cell shapes, in each iteration we update the basis b_k by selecting the shape x_l that exhibits the largest correlation between the displacement and the negative gradient in (7)

$$\nabla J_{b_k} = -2 \sum_{i=1}^{N} (x_i - B\tilde{\alpha}_i)\tilde{\alpha}_{ik} + (x_i - b_k)\tilde{\alpha}_{ik}^2, \tag{6}$$

$$b_k = \arg \max_{x_l \in X} \frac{(x_l - b_k)^T(-\nabla J)}{||x_l - b_k||_2|| - \nabla J||_2}. \tag{7}$$

The dictionary basis update and the coefficient computation are alternately conducted until convergence. In the testing stage, a new cell shape x from the target dataset can be encoded by solving (4) with a fixed B and without the MMD term.

3   Experiments

Datasets and Experimental Setup: The proposed shape transfer model is extensively tested on multiple microscopy image datasets: lung cancer, pancreatic neuroendocrine tumor (NET), and skeletal muscle. The gold standards of cell boundaries are manually annotated. Lung cancer has over 20000 annotated cell shapes, and thus it is used as the auxiliary dataset with randomly selected about one-tenth for training. The target datasets include 45 NET images with half for training (the left for testing) and 41 skeletal muscle images with about three-fourths for training. The parameters in (4) are chosen as $\gamma = 0.001$ and $\mu = 10$. The dictionary size is chosen as one-tenth of the training data. Many metrics [9,13] can be applied to quantitative analysis, and we choose three generic segmentation-based criteria [15]: Dice similarly coefficient (DSC), Hausdorff distance (HD), and mean absolute distance (MAD).

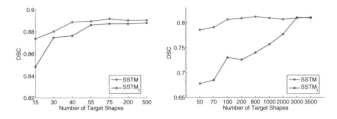

Fig. 2. Comparative segmentation accuracy (DSC) between the shape transfer model, SSTM, and the model trained with only target shapes, $SSTM_t$, on the NET (left) and muscle (right) datasets.

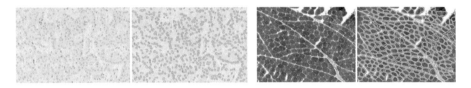

Fig. 3. Cell segmentation results on two sample images from the NET (left two) and muscle (right two) datasets. Cells touching image boundaries are ignored.

We train the CNN models by following [15] on the NET and [5] on the skeletal muscle images. For the former, the CNN model is trained with over 6×10^5 positive and 9×10^5 negative image patches. The parameters are with: total iterations of 2.5×10^5, learning rate of 0.001, momentum of 0.8, and batch size of 128. For the latter, the model is trained with one million patches with half positives and half negatives. The parameters are with: total iterations of 2×10^5, learning rate of 0.01, momentum of 0.9, weight decay of 0.1 (every 50000 iterations), and batch size of 256. CNN models provide coarse segmentation for subsequent contour deformation and refinement.

Shape Transfer Model Evaluation: Figure 2 shows the segmentation accuracy of the proposed model, SSTM, with respect to the number of target cell shapes and two hundred auxiliary data samples. The model learned using only target cell shapes (denoted by $SSTM_t$) is also provided for comparison. It is clear that when there exist limited target training samples, shape transfer modeling improves the segmentation accuracy and outperforms $SSTM_t$. When sufficient target shapes are applied to training, there exist no significant performance improvement using transfer shapes. Since muscle cells exhibit more significant shape variations than NET cells, $SSTM_t$ requires much more target shapes to produce competitive performance to SSTM. We can see that when fixing a desired segmentation accuracy, transfer models require less target data. Figure 3 shows qualitative segmentation results on the two datasets, where many cells with weak boundaries are segmented.

Comparison with State of the Arts: We compare SSTM with four state of the arts: isoperimetric graph partition (IGP) [7], superpixel-based segmentation (SUP) [12], graph cut and coloring (GCC) [1], and repulsive level set (RLS) [13].

Table 1. Comparative pixel-wise segmentation accuracy on NET and muscle datasets. For each metric (DSC, HD, and MAD), the mean and standard deviation are listed.

	NET			Muscle		
	DSC	HD	MAD	DSC	HD	MAD
IGP [7]	0.49 ± 0.21	10.58 ± 14.07	8.16 ± 7.15	0.63 ± 0.24	12.81 ± 11.22	7.73 ± 5.62
SUP [12]	0.74 ± 0.18	7.30 ± 7.69	4.08 ± 3.76	0.63 ± 0.16	16.71 ± 9.52	8.86 ± 4.99
GCC [1]	0.60 ± 0.22	6.57 ± 4.38	5.18 ± 2.85	0.70 ± 0.22	12.47 ± 16.11	7.48 ± 9.13
RLS [13]	0.84 ± 0.09	4.25 ± 3.48	2.35 ± 2.11	0.84 ± 0.12	8.64 ± 10.53	4.97 ± 6.72
SSTM	0.89 ± 0.12	2.98 ± 3.14	2.01 ± 2.11	0.85 ± 0.13	4.88 ± 4.80	3.11 ± 2.63

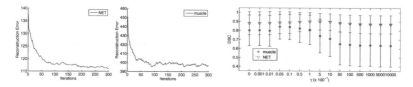

Fig. 4. Convergence study (left and middle) and parameter sensitivity analysis (right).

Table 1 lists the comparative performance on the two target datasets. As we can see, SSTM outperforms the others in terms of three segmentation criteria, especially in HD that measures the largest error for each segmentation. In addition, the lowest standard deviations in the metrics (for almost all cases) indicate the strong stability of the proposed approaches.

Convergence and Parameter Sensitivity Analysis: The reconstruction errors for model training with respect to the number of iterations are shown in Fig. 4, which indicates that the algorithm can converge in a limited number of iterations. We set $\mu = \{10, 100, 1000\}$ and find that there exist no statistically significant variations on the accuracy. The effects of parameter γ on the performance is provided in the right panel of Fig. 4, which shows our algorithm can achieve stable performance within a wide range of values.

4   Conclusion

In this paper, we propose a shape transfer model for cell segmentation in microscopy images. By learning a compact shape dictionary using an auxiliary dataset, it can generate shape representations that are applicable to the target dataset. In this scenario, it can significantly reduce expensive manual annotations of target training data. Extensive experiments on multiple microscopy image datasets demonstrate the effectiveness of the proposed method.

References

1. Al-Kofahi, Y., Lassoued, W., Lee, W., Roysam, B.: Improved automatic detection and segmentation of cell nuclei in histopathology images. TBME **57**(4), 841–852 (2010)

2. Ali, S., Madabhushi, A.: An integrated region-, boundary-, shape-based active contour for multiple object overlap resolution in histological imagery. TMI **31**(7), 1448–1460 (2012)
3. Boyd, S., Parikh, N., Chu, E., Peleato, B., Eckstein, J.: Distributed optimization and statistical learning via the alternating direction method of multipliers. Found. Trends Mach. Learn. **3**(1), 1–122 (2011)
4. Chang, H., Han, J., Borowsky, A., Loss, L., Gray, J., Spellman, P., Parvin, B.: Invariant delineation of nuclear architecture in glioblastoma multiforme for clinical and molecular association. TMI **32**(4), 670–682 (2013)
5. Cireşan, D., Giusti, A., Gambardella, L.M., Schmidhuber, J.: Deep neural networks segment neuronal membranes in electron microscopy images. In: NIPS, pp. 2843–2851 (2012)
6. Elhamifar, E., Sapiro, G., Sastry, S.: Dissimilarity-based sparse subset selection. TPAMI **PP**(99), 1 (2016)
7. Grady, L., Schwartz, E.L.: Isoperimetric graph partitioning for image segmetentation. TPAMI **28**(1), 469–475 (2006)
8. Gretton, A., Borgwardt, K.M., Rasch, M., Schölkopf, B., Smola, A.J.: A kernel method for the two-sample-problem. In: NIPS, pp. 513–520 (2007)
9. Konukoglu, E., Glocker, B., Criminisi, A., Pohl, K.M.: Wesd-weighted spectral distance for measuring shape dissimilarity. TPAMI **35**(9), 2284–2297 (2013)
10. Liu, B., Huang, J., Kulikowski, C., Yang, L.: Robust visual tracking using local sparse appearance model and k-selection. TPAMI **35**(12), 2968–2981 (2013)
11. Long, M., Ding, G., Wang, J., Sun, J., Guo, Y., Yu, P.S.: Transfer sparse coding for robust image representation. In: CVPR, pp. 407–414 (2013)
12. Mori, G.: Guiding model search using segmentation. In: ICCV, vol. 2, pp. 1417–1423 (2005)
13. Qi, X., Xing, F., Foran, D.J., Yang, L.: Robust segmentation of overlapping cells in histopathology specimens using parallel seed detection and repulsive level set. TBME **59**(3), 754–765 (2012)
14. Wang, J., Yang, J., Yu, K., Lv, F., Huang, T., Gong, Y.: Locality-constrained linear coding for image classification. In: CVPR, pp. 3360–3367 (2010)
15. Xing, F., Xie, Y., Yang, L.: An automatic learning-based framework for robust nucleus segmentation. TMI **35**(2), 550–566 (2016)
16. Xing, F., Yang, L.: Fast cell segmentation using scalable sparse manifold learning and affine transform-approximated active contour. In: Navab, N., Hornegger, J., Wells, W.M., Frangi, A.F. (eds.) MICCAI 2015. LNCS, vol. 9351, pp. 332–339. Springer, Heidelberg (2015). doi:10.1007/978-3-319-24574-4_40
17. Yu, K., Zhang, T., Gong, Y.: Nonlinear learning using local coordinate coding. In: NIPS, pp. 1–9 (2009)
18. Zhang, S., Zhan, Y., Metaxas, D.N.: Deformable segmentation via sparse representation and dictionary learning. MedIA **16**(7), 1385–1396 (2012)
19. Zhang, S., Zhan, Y., Dewan, M., Huang, J., Metaxas, D.N., Zhou, X.S.: Deformable segmentation via sparse shape representation. In: Fichtinger, G., Martel, A., Peters, T. (eds.) MICCAI 2011. LNCS, vol. 6892, pp. 451–458. Springer, Heidelberg (2011). doi:10.1007/978-3-642-23629-7_55
20. Zimmer, C., Olivo-Marin, J.C.: Coupled parametric active contours. TPAMI **27**(11), 1838–1842 (2005)

Hierarchical Generative Modeling and Monte-Carlo EM in Riemannian Shape Space for Hypothesis Testing

Saurabh J. Shigwan$^{(\boxtimes)}$ and Suyash P. Awate

Computer Science and Engineering Department,
Indian Institute of Technology (IIT) Bombay, Mumbai, India
saurabh.shigwan@cse.iitb.ac.in

Abstract. Statistical shape analysis has relied on various models, each with its strengths and limitations. For multigroup analyses, while typical methods pool data to fit a single statistical model, partial pooling through hierarchical modeling can be superior. For *pointset shape* representations, we propose a novel *hierarchical model* in *Riemannian shape space*. The inference treats individual shapes and group-mean shapes as latent variables, and uses expectation maximization that relies on sampling shapes. Our generative model, including shape-smoothness priors, can be robust to segmentation errors, producing more compact per-group models and realistic shape samples. We propose a method for efficient sampling in Riemannian shape space. The results show the benefits of our hierarchical Riemannian generative model for hypothesis testing, over the state of the art.

Keywords: Kendall shape space · Hierarchical model · MCEM · Shape sampling

1 Introduction and Related Work

Statistical shape analysis typically relies on boundary point distribution models [4,12], implicit models [5], medial models [17], or nonlinear dense diffeomorphic warps [2,6,10,19]. Unlike some models based on pointsets [3,4,8,21] or distance transforms [5], medial [7] and warp-based models [6] represent shape as an equivalence class of object boundaries and lead to statistical analyses in the associated Riemannian shape space. While medial representations are limited to non-branching objects, methods based on diffeomorphisms involve very large dimensional Riemannian spaces where the analysis can be expensive and challenged by noise and limited sample sizes of training data [16]. All these approaches are active areas of research in their own right.

S.P. Awate—The authors thank funding via IIT Bombay Seed Grant 14IRCCSG010.

S. Ourselin et al. (Eds.): MICCAI 2016, Part III, LNCS 9902, pp. 191–200, 2016.
DOI: 10.1007/978-3-319-46726-9_23

Typical cross-sectional studies, e.g., hypothesis testing [3,18], pool the data from multiple groups to fit a single model. However, when data has is naturally organized in groups, partial pooling through hierarchical modeling [9] offers several benefits, including more compact models per group and reduced risk of overfitting (e.g., for low sample size or in presence of outliers) through shrinkage. We propose a *hierarchical model* for pointset shape representations in Kendall shape space. While [21] also uses a hierarchical generative model that estimates all shape covariances in Euclidean space, our method models shape variability in *Riemannian shape space*, at the group and population levels. While [1,2] model nonlinear warps as latent variables and treats the segmentations as error free, we model individual shapes as latent variables (treating data-shape similarity transforms as parameters) and allow for errors in segmentations. Nevertheless, [1,2] do *not* use a hierarchical model for multigroup data.

We fit our model to the data using Monte-Carlo (MC) expectation maximization (EM). For EM, we propose a Markov chain Monte Carlo (MCMC) method for sampling in Riemannian space, by extending Skilling's leapfrog [13] to Riemannian space, and then adapting it to shape space. This sampler is virtually parameter free, unlike the one in [21] that is sensitive to internal parameter values.

In this paper, we propose a hierarchical generative model using pointset-based shape representations for multigroup shape analysis, incorporating statistical analysis in the associated Riemannian (Kendall) shape space. We treat individual and group-mean shapes as latent variables within an EM inference framework. The generative model incorporating shape-smoothness priors to regularize model learning, helps counter errors in imaging and segmentation, producing more compact per-group models and realistic shape samples. We also propose a MCMC sampling algorithm in Riemannian space and adapt it to shape space. We use the model for hypothesis testing on simulated and medical images showing its benefits over the state of the art.

2   Methods

We describe algorithms for modeling, inference, sampling, and hypothesis testing.

2.1   Hierarchical Generative Statistical Model for Multiple Groups of Shapes

We model each shape as an equivalence class of pointsets, where equivalence is defined through the similarity transform comprising translation, rotation, and isotropic scaling [12]. We model all shape-representing pointsets to be of equal cardinality to use the Procrustes distance [11] between shapes. Model fitting fixes point correspondences across all shapes and optimizes point locations based on the data. The fixed correspondences lead to a pointset representation as an ordered set of points or as a vector.

Notation. Consider a population comprising M groups, where group m has N_m individuals. Let *data* x_{mi} represent the set of pixel locations on the boundary of the segmented anatomical object in individual i in group m. Let y_{mi} be the (unknown) pointset representing object shape for individual i in group m. Let z_m be the (unknown) pointset representing the mean object shape for group m. Let C_m model the covariance of shapes in group m. Let μ be the (unknown) pointset representing the population-level mean object shape and let (unknown) C model the associated covariance; μ and C capture the variability of the group-mean shapes z_m.

Each shape-representing pointset (or *shape pointset*) has J points in 3D; so $y_{mi} \in \mathbb{R}^{3J}$, $z_m \in \mathbb{R}^{3J}$. Each data-representing pointset (or *data pointset*) x_{mi} has arbitrary cardinality. We model the population mean μ and covariance C and the group covariances $\{C_m\}_{m=1}^M$ as *parameters*. We model the shape pointsets Y_{mi} and Z_m as *latent variables*. Each shape pointset also lies in preshape space [11, 12], with centroid at the origin and unit L^2 norm. For shape pointsets a and b, the Procrustes distance is $d_{\text{Pro}}(a,b) := \min_{\mathcal{R}} d_g(a, \mathcal{R}b)$, where operator $\mathcal{R}$ applies a rotation to each point in the pointset and $d_g(\cdot, \cdot)$ is the geodesic distance on the unit hypersphere in preshape space.

Prior Models. We model a probability density function (PDF) to capture the covariance structures of (i) group-mean variation and (ii) individual shape variation, by extending the approximate Normal law on Riemannian manifolds [15] to shape space, as motivated in [8]. For a and b on the unit hypersphere, let $\text{Log}_a(b)$ be the logarithmic map of b with respect to a. Considering the tangent space of *shape* space at μ to relate to preshapes that are rotationally aligned to μ, the logarithmic map of shape a to the tangent space of the shape space at μ is $\text{Log}_\mu^S(a) := \text{Log}_\mu(\mathcal{R}^* a)$, where $\mathcal{R}^* := \arg\min_{\mathcal{R}} d_g(\mathcal{R}a, \mu)$. Extending the Procrustes distance, the squared Mahalanobis distance of shape a with respect to μ and C is $d_{\text{Mah}}^2(a; \mu, C) := \text{Log}_\mu^S(a)^\top C^{-1} \text{Log}_\mu^S(a)$. To model a PDF that gives larger probabilities to smoother shapes a, we use a prior that penalizes distances between each point a_j and its neighbors. Let the neighborhood system $\mathcal{N} := \{\mathcal{N}_j\}_{j=1}^J$, where set $\mathcal{N}_j$ has the neighbor indices of j-th point. In practice, we get $\mathcal{N}$ by fitting a triangular mesh to the segmented object boundary. Thus, the probability for shape a is

$$P(a|\mu, C, \beta) := \frac{1}{\eta(\mu, C, \beta)} \exp\left(-\frac{d_{\text{Mah}}^2(a; \mu, C)}{2} - \frac{\beta}{2} \sum_j \sum_{k \in \mathcal{N}_j} \|a_j - a_k\|_2^2\right), \quad (1)$$

where $\beta \geq 0$ controls the prior strength and $\eta(\mu, C, \beta)$ is the normalization constant. We use this design to model (i) the conditional PDF $P(z_m|\mu, C, \beta)$ of group mean shapes z_m and (ii) the conditional PDF $P(y_{mi}|z_m, C_m, \beta_m)$ of individual shapes y_{mi}. The second term in the exponent equals $0.5a^\top \Omega a$, where Ω is a sparse precision matrix with diagonal elements 2β and the only non-zero off diagonal elements equal $(-\beta)$ when the corresponding points are neighbors in $\mathcal{N}$.

Likelihood Model. To measure dissimilarity between data pointset x_{mi} and individual shape pointset y_{mi}, of differing cardinality, we use a measure $\Delta(x_{mi}, y_{mi}) :=$ $\min_{\mathcal{S}_{mi}} \left(\sum_{j=1}^{J} \min_l \|\mathcal{S}_{mi} x_{mil} - y_{mij}\|_2^2 + \sum_{l=1}^{L} \min_j \|\mathcal{S}_{mi} x_{mil} - y_{mij}\|_2^2 \right)$, where the operator $\mathcal{S}_{mi}$ applies a similarity transform to point x_{mil} in the pointset x to factor out similarity transforms on data. Unlike methods [6,21] that use current distance [19] having quadratic complexity in either pointset's cardinality, $\Delta(x, z)$ can be well approximated efficiently using algorithms of complexity close to $O((J + L)(\log J + \log L))$, described later. We model $P(x_{mi}|y_{mi}) \propto \exp(-\Delta(x_{mi}, y_{mi}))$.

2.2   Model Fitting Using Monte-Carlo Expectation Maximization

We use EM to fit the hierarchical model to the data pointsets $x :=$ $\{\{x_{mi}\}_{i=1}^{N_m}\}_{m=1}^{M}$. In this paper, $\beta_m := \beta, \forall m$ and β is user defined. Let the parameter set be $\theta := \{\mu, C, \{C_m\}_{m=1}^{M}\}$. At iteration t, given parameter estimates $\theta^t := \{\mu^t, C^t, \{C_m^t\}_{m=1}^{M}\}$, the *E step* defines $Q(\theta; \theta^t) :=$ $E_{P(Y,Z|x,\theta^t)}[\log P(x, Y, Z|\theta)]$ where the complete data likelihood $P(x, y, z|\theta) =$ $\prod_m \prod_i P(x_{mi}|y_{mi})P(y_{mi}|z_m, C_m, \beta_m)P(z_m|\mu, C, \beta)$. Because the expectation is analytically intractable, we use a Monte-Carlo approximation

$$Q(\theta; \theta^t) \approx \frac{1}{S} \sum_{s=1}^{S} \log P(x, y^s, z^s|\theta) \text{ where the pair } (y^s, z^s) \sim P(Y, Z|x, \theta^t). \quad (2)$$

The *M step* obtains parameter updates $\theta^{t+1} := \arg\max_\theta \widehat{Q}(\theta; \theta^t)$. Given data x and the sampled shape pairs $\{(y^s, z^s)\}_{s=1}^{S}$, we alternately optimize the shape-distribution parameters θ and the internal parameters $\mathcal{S}_{mi}$, until convergence to a local optimum.

Update Similarity Transforms $\mathcal{S}_{mi}$. The optimal similarity transform $\mathcal{S}_{mi}$ is

$$\arg\min_{\mathcal{S}_{mi}} \sum_{s=1}^{S} \left(\sum_{j=1}^{J} \min_l \|\mathcal{S}_{mi} x_{mil} - y_{mij}^s\|_2^2 + \sum_{l=1}^{L} \min_j \|\mathcal{S}_{mi} x_{mil} - y_{mij}^s\|_2^2 \right), \quad (3)$$

which aligns the data pointset x_{mi} to the set of sampled shape pointsets $\{y_{mi}^s\}_{s=1}^{S}$. We optimize the parameter for translation, scaling, and rotation, $\mathcal{S}_{mi}$ using gradient descent that approximates the objective function efficiently. The objective function value depends on the nearest point in one pointset to each point in the other pointset. For shapes x_{mi} (cardinality L) and y_{mi} (cardinality J), we can find the required pairs of nearest neighbors in $O((J+L)(\log J + \log L))$ time by building k-d trees $(O(J \log J) + O(L \log L))$ followed by nearest neighbor searches $(O(J \log L) + O(L \log J))$. Assuming the parameter updates to be sufficiently small, (i) for most data points x_{mil}, the nearest shape point $y_{mi\phi(l)}^s$ is the same before and after the update and (ii) for most shape points y_{mij}^s, the displacement vector to the nearest data point $x_{mi\psi(j)}$ is the same before and after the update. Thus, constraining parameter updates to be small, we approximate the gradients of the desired objective function by first finding the pairs of nearest points $(l, \phi(l))$ and $(j, \phi(j))$ and then taking the gradients of

$$\sum_{s=1}^{S} \left(\sum_{j=1}^{J} \|\mathcal{S}_{mi} x_{mi\phi(j)} - y_{mij}^s\|_2^2 + \sum_{l=1}^{L} \|\mathcal{S}_{mi} x_{mil} - y_{mi\phi(l)}^s\|_2^2 \right). \tag{4}$$

Updates for translation and scale are in closed form. We optimize rotation using gradient descent on the manifold of orthogonal matrices with determinant 1.

Update Mean μ. The optimal $\widehat{\mu}$ comes from the constrained nonlinear optimization

$$\arg\min_{\mu} \sum_{s=1}^{S} \sum_{m=1}^{M} \mathrm{Log}_{\mu}(z_m^s)^{\top} C^{-1} \mathrm{Log}_{\mu}(z_m^s) \text{ such that } \|\mu\| = 1, \tag{5}$$

Differentiating the Log function, we optimize μ using projected gradient descent.

Update Covariances C_m. The optimal covariance C_m minimizes

$$\sum_{i=1}^{N_m} \sum_{s=1}^{S} \mathrm{Log}_{z_m^s}^{S}(y_{mi}^s)^{\top} C_m^{-1} \mathrm{Log}_{z_m^s}^{S}(y_{mi}^s) + (y_{mi}^s)^{\top} \Omega y_{mi}^s + 2 \log \eta(z_m^s, C_m, \beta_m). \tag{6}$$

Although the normalization term $\eta(z_m^s, C_m, \beta_m)$ is difficult to evaluate analytically, it can be approximated well enough in practice. Assuming that the shape distribution $P(y_{mi}^s | z_m^s, C_m)$ has sufficiently low variance, the tangent vector $\mathrm{Log}_{z_m^s}^{S}(y_{mi}^s)$ is close to the difference vector $y_{mi}^s - z_m^s$, in which case $P(y_{mi}^s | z_m^s, C_m)$ appears as a product of a multivariate Gaussian $G(y_{mi}^s; z_m^s, C_m)$ with another multivariate Gaussian $G(y_{mi}^s; \mathbf{0}, \Omega)$. The product distribution equals $G(y_{mi}^s; z_m^s, C_m^{\mathrm{reg}})$ where the regularized covariance $C_m^{\mathrm{reg}} := (C_m^{-1} + \Omega)^{-1}$ restricts all variability to the tangent space at the mean z_m and the normalization term $\eta(z_m^s, C_m, \beta_m) \approx (2\pi)^{D/2} |C^{\mathrm{reg}}|^{0.5}$. Then, the optimal covariance $\widehat{C}_m^{\mathrm{reg}}$ is the sample covariance of tangent vectors $\mathrm{Log}_{z_m^s}^{S}(y_{mi}^s)$ in the tangent spaces at z_m^s. Thus, the optimal covariance $\widehat{C}_m$ is obtained in closed form.

Update Covariance C. The strategy for optimizing C is analogous to the one just described for estimating C^m. We first compute $\widehat{C}^{\mathrm{reg}}$ as the sample covariance of tangent vectors $\mathrm{Log}_{\mu}^{S}(z_m^s)$ in the tangent space at μ. Then, the optimal $\widehat{C} = ((\widehat{C}^{\mathrm{reg}})^{-1} - \Omega)^{-1}$.

2.3   Robust Efficient MCMC Sampling on Riemannian Manifolds

EM entails sampling shape-pointset pairs (y^s, z^s) from their posterior PDF $P(Y, Z | x, \theta^t)$ in shape space. We propose a generic scheme for efficient sampling in high-dimensional spaces on a Riemannian manifold and adapt it for sampling in shape space. Standard Metropolis-Hastings or Gibbs MCMC samplers are inefficient in high-dimensional spaces [13] where the data typically shows strong correlations between dimensions. We propose to adapt Skilling's multi-state leapfrog method [13], an efficient MCMC sampler, to Riemannian spaces.

Alternate efficient MCMC methods, e.g., Hamiltonian Monte Carlo used in [21], are sensitive to tuning of the underlying parameters [20]. We propose a sampler that is robust in practice, requiring little parameter tuning.

Consider a multivariate random variable F taking values f on a Riemannian manifold $\mathbb{F}$ with associated PDF $P(F)$. We initialize the MCMC sampler with a set of states $\{f^q \in \mathbb{F}\}_{q=1}^{Q}$. We propose to leapfrog a randomly-chosen current state f^{q_1} over a randomly-chosen state f^{q_2} to give a proposal state $f^{q_3} := \mathrm{Exp}_{f^{q_2}}^{\mathbb{F}}(-\mathrm{Log}_{f^{q_2}}^{\mathbb{F}}(f^{q_1}))$, where the logarithmic and exponential maps are with respect to the manifold $\mathbb{F}$. The proposal state f^{q_3} is accepted, according to the Metropolis method, with probability equal to the ratio $P(f^{q_3})/P(f^{q_1})$. The sampler only needs to evaluate probabilities, without needing the gradients of $P(F)$. Such leapfrog jumps are repeated and after sufficient burn in, the set of Q states are considered to be a sample from $P(F)$.

We adapt the proposed leapfrog sampling scheme to shape space for sampling from the Normal law $P(z|\mu, C, \beta)$ that defines a Gaussian distribution in the tangent space of shape space at μ, where the tangent space comprises all shapes aligned to μ. We initialize the set of states to the pointsets $\{z^q\}_{q=1}^{Q}$ in preshape space and rotationally aligned to the mean μ. In shape space, we propose the leapfrog step $z^{q_3} := \arg\min_{c:=\mathcal{R}b} d_g(c, \mu)$, where $b := \mathrm{Exp}_{z^{q_2}}(-\mathrm{Log}_{z^{q_2}}(z^{q_1}))$, which approximates the geodesic from z^{q_1} to z^{q_2} and uses that to "leap" to z^{q_3} in shape space.

2.4 Hypothesis Testing on Riemannian Manifolds

Unlike parametric hypothesis, permutation tests are nonparametric, rely on the generic assumption of exchangeability, lead to stronger control over Type-1 error, and are more robust to random errors in the measurements/post-processing of image data. We use permutation testing to test the null hypothesis of the equality of two group distributions in shape space. After estimating the group means and covariances $\{\mu^m, C^m\}_{m=1}^{M}$, we propose a test statistic to measure the differences between the shape distributions arising from two cohorts, say, A and B, by adding the squared Mahalanobis geodesic distance between the group means with respect to each group covariance, i.e., $T := d_{\mathrm{Mah}}^2(\mu^A; \mu^B, C^B) + d_{\mathrm{Mah}}^2(\mu^B; \mu^A, C^A)$. The test-statistic distribution is unknown analytically and we infer it using bootstrap sampling (150 repeats).

3   Results and Conclusion

We compare our method with ShapeWorks [3] that does *not* employ a hierarchical model, restricts point locations within shapes to the object-boundary, and does *not* enforce shape smoothness. We also compare our method with an improved version of the hierarchical non-Riemannian method in [21] by adding the shape smoothness prior and replacing the current distance with the cost-effective one in [8]. After EM gives the optimal parameters θ^*, we get optimal individual shapes y_{mi}^* and group-mean shapes z_m^* as the maximum-a-posteriori (MAP) estimates $\arg\max_{z_m, y_{mi}} P(z_m, y_{mi}|x, \theta^*, \beta)$.

Validation on Simulated Data. We generate 2 groups, with subtle differences, of 40 ellipsoids each. Each group has 1 major mode of variation, where we fix 2 of the ellipsoid axes lengths to 10 mm and vary the third. The third axis lengths for group I are Gaussian distributed with mean 7.25 mm and standard deviation (SD) 0.4 mm and for group II are Gaussian distributed with mean 8.5 mm and SD 0.5 mm. To mimic realistic segmentations in typical applications, we *corrupt* the segmentations with random coarse-scale and fine-scale (noise) perturbations to each object boundary (Fig. 1(a)).

Figures 1(b)–(c) show example sampled shapes, which are well regularized because of the smoothness prior controlled by β. The population mean estimate (Figs. 1(d)) expectedly lies "between" the MAP estimates for the group means (Figs. 1(e)–(f)). The proposed hierarchical Riemannian approach leads to a more compact model (Fig. 2(d)–(f)), i.e., larger fraction of variability captured in fewer modes, compared to the hierarchical non-Riemannian approach and non-hierarchical non-Riemannian ShapeWorks. ShapeWorks's eigenspectra decay slowly because (i) it does *not* use partial pooling and (ii) assumes

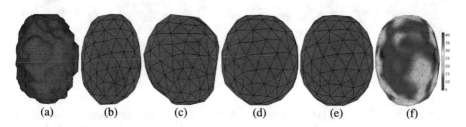

Fig. 1. Simulated Data, Proposed Method. (a) Example noisy ellipsoid segmentation, whose boundary gives data x_{mi}. **(b)**, **(c)** Example sampled shapes y_{mi}^s. **(d)**, **(e)** Group mean MAP estimates z_1^*, z_2^*, obtained after EM optimization for parameters θ^*. **(f)** Population mean estimate μ^* with Cohen's effect sizes at each vertex j computed via means z_{1j}^*, z_{2j}^* and variances C_{1jj}, C_{2jj}.

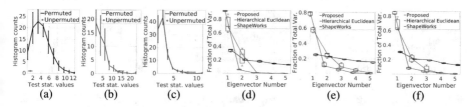

Fig. 2. Simulated Data, Comparison with Other Methods. Permutation-test histograms of test statistics, along with their variability estimated through bootstrap sampling of cohorts, for **(a)** ShapeWorks, **(b)** a hierarchical model with Euclidean analysis, **(c)** the **proposed** hierarchical model with Riemannian analysis. Eigenvalue spectra of estimated **(d)** population covariance C, **(e)** group covariance C_1, **(f)** group covariance C_2, for each of the 3 aforementioned methods.

the segmentation to be devoid of errors that can lead to fine-scale or coarse-scale perturbations, resulting from noise or artifacts (e.g., inhomogeneity) or human errors. Repeated permutation testing through bootstrap sampling of cohorts (Fig. 2(a)–(c)) gives the smallest p values (significantly) for the proposed hierarchical Riemannian approach, correctly favoring the rejection of the null hypothesis.

Evaluation on Medical Data. We test for gender differences in 4 wrist bone shapes; 15 subjects per bone per group [14]. For the capitate bone (Fig. 3), the proposed method gives smaller permutation-test p values (Fig. 4(a)–(c)), compared to ShapeWorks and the hierarchical non-Riemannian approach, stemming from a more compact model (Fig. 4(d)–(f)). Bootstrap sampling of the cohort yielded variability of the p values, which we summarize through the mean (and SD in parentheses): (i) proposed approach: 0.04(0.04), (ii) Shape-Works: 0.60(0.13), (iii) hierarchical non-Riemannian 0.36(0.11). For both trapezoid and trapezium bones, the p values were: (i) proposed approach: 0.04(0.02) and (ii) ShapeWorks: 0.13(0.04). For the pisiform bone, the p values were (i) proposed approach: 0.08(0.03) and (ii) ShapeWorks: 0.10(0.04).

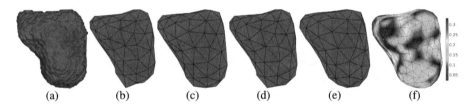

(a)   (b)   (c)   (d)   (e)   (f)

Fig. 3. Bone Imaging Data, Proposed Method. (a) Example segmentation for the capitate wrist bone, whose boundary gives data x_{mi}. (b), (c) Example sampled shapes y_{mi}^s. (d), (e) Group mean MAP estimates z_1^*, z_2^*, obtained after EM optimization for parameters θ^*. (f) Population mean estimate μ^* with Cohen's effect sizes at each vertex; computed as in Fig. 1(f).

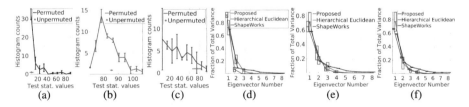

(a)   (b)   (c)   (d)   (e)   (f)

Fig. 4. Bone Imaging Data, Comparison with Other Methods. Permutation-test histograms of test statistics, along with their variability estimated through bootstrap sampling of cohorts, for (a) ShapeWorks, (b) a hierarchical model with Euclidean analysis, (c) the **proposed** hierarchical model with Riemannian analysis. Eigenvalue spectra of estimated (d) population covariance C, (e) group covariance C_1, (f) group covariance C_2, for each of the 3 aforementioned methods.

We evaluate the quality of the shape fit y^*_{mi} by measuring the distances between each point in shape y^*_{mi} to the nearest point in data x_{mi}. These distances, as a percentage of the distance between the two farthest points of the population mean μ^* (that has norm 1) were small for the bone populations: mean 0.98 %, median 0.88 %, SD 0.5 %.

Conclusion. We propose a hierarchical model in Riemannian shape space. The generative model counter errors in the data and the shape-smoothness prior acts as regularization. We propose novel methods for robust efficient sampling and hypothesis testing in Riemannian shape space. Our method detects subtle differences between small cohorts, simulated and medical, more accurately than the state of the art.

References

1. Allassonniere, S., Amit, Y., Trouve, A.: Toward a coherent statistical framework for dense deformable template estimation. J. R. Stat. Soc. Ser. B **69**(1), 3–29 (2007)
2. Allassonniere, S., Kuhn, E., Trouve, A.: Construction of bayesian deformable models via a stochastic approximation algorithm: a convergence study. Bernoulli **16**(3), 641–678 (2010)
3. Cates, J., Fletcher, T., Styner, M., Shenton, M., Whitaker, R.: Shape modeling and analysis with entropy-based particle systems. Proc. Inf. Process. Med. Imaging **20**, 333–45 (2007)
4. Cootes, T., Taylor, C., Cooper, D., Graham, J.: Active shape models - their training and application. Comput. Vis. Image Underst. **61**(1), 38–59 (1995)
5. Dambreville, S., Rathi, Y., Tannenbaum, A.: A framework for image segmentation using shape models kernel space shape priors. IEEE Trans. Pattern Anal. Mach. Intell. **30**(8), 1385–1399 (2008)
6. Durrleman, S., Pennec, X., Trouve, A., Ayache, N.: Statistical models of sets of curves and surfaces based on currents. Med. Imaging Anal. **13**(5), 793–808 (2009)
7. Fletcher, T., Lu, C., Pizer, S., Joshi, S.: Principal geodesic analysis for the study of nonlinear statistics of shape. IEEE Trans. Med. Imaging **23**(8), 995–1005 (2004)
8. Gaikwad, A.V., Shigwan, S.J., Awate, S.P.: A statistical model for smooth shapes in kendall shape space. In: Navab, N., Hornegger, J., Wells, W.M., Frangi, A.F. (eds.) MICCAI 2015. LNCS, vol. 9351, pp. 628–635. Springer, Heidelberg (2015). doi:10.1007/978-3-319-24574-4_75
9. Gelman, A.: Multilevel (hierarchical) modeling: what it can and cannot do. Am. Stat. Assoc. **48**(3), 432–435 (2006)
10. Glasbey, C.A., Mardia, K.V.: A penalized likelihood approach to image warping. J R. Stat. Soc. Ser. B **63**(3), 465–514 (2001)
11. Goodall, C.: Procrustes methods in statistical analysis of shape. J. R. Stat. Soc. **53**(2), 285–339 (1991)
12. Kendall, D.: A survey of the statistical theory of shape. Stat. Sci. **4**(2), 87–99 (1989)
13. MacKay, D.: Information Theory, Inference, Learning Algorithms. Cambridge University Press, Cambridge (2012)
14. Moore, D., Crisco, J., Trafton, T., Leventhal, E.: A digital database of wrist bone anatomy and carpal kinematics. J. Biomech. **40**(11), 2537–2542 (2007)

15. Pennec, X.: Intrinsic statistics on Riemannian manifolds: basic tools for geometric measurements. J. Math. Imaging Vis. **25**(1), 127–154 (2006)
16. Pizer, S., Jung, S., Goswami, D., Vicory, J., Zhao, X., Chaudhuri, R., Damon, J., Huckemann, S., Marron, J.: Nested sphere statistics of skeletal models. Innov. Shape Anal. 93 (2012)
17. Siddiqi, K., Pizer, S.: Medial Representations: Mathematics, Algorithms and Applications. Springer, Netherlands (2008)
18. Terriberry, T.B., Joshi, S.C., Gerig, G.: Hypothesis testing with nonlinear shape models. In: Christensen, G.E., Sonka, M. (eds.) IPMI 2005. LNCS, vol. 3565, pp. 15–26. Springer, Heidelberg (2005). doi:10.1007/11505730_2
19. Vaillant, M., Glaunès, J.: Surface matching via currents. In: Christensen, G.E., Sonka, M. (eds.) IPMI 2005. LNCS, vol. 3565, pp. 381–392. Springer, Heidelberg (2005)
20. Wang, Z., Mohamed, S., Freitas, N.: Adaptive Hamiltonian and Riemann manifold monte carlo samplers. Proc. Int. Conf. Mach. Learn. **3**, 1462–1470 (2013)
21. Yu, Y.-Y., Fletcher, P.T., Awate, S.P.: Hierarchical bayesian modeling, estimation, and sampling for multigroup shape analysis. In: Golland, P., Hata, N., Barillot, C., Hornegger, J., Howe, R. (eds.) MICCAI 2014. LNCS, vol. 8675, pp. 9–16. Springer, Heidelberg (2014). doi:10.1007/978-3-319-10443-0_2

Direct Estimation of Wall Shear Stress from Aneurysmal Morphology: A Statistical Approach

Ali Sarrami-Foroushani, Toni Lassila, Jose M. Pozo, Ali Gooya,
and Alejandro F. Frangi$^{(\boxtimes)}$

Department of Electronic and Electrical Engineering,
Centre for Computational Imaging and Simulation Technologies in Biomedicine,
The University of Sheffield, Sheffield, UK
a.frangi@sheffield.ac.uk

Abstract. Computational fluid dynamics (CFD) is a valuable tool for studying vascular diseases, but requires long computational time. To alleviate this issue, we propose a statistical framework to predict the aneurysmal wall shear stress patterns directly from the aneurysm shape. A database of 38 complex intracranial aneurysm shapes is used to generate aneurysm morphologies and CFD simulations. The shapes and wall shear stresses are then converted to clouds of hybrid points containing both types of information. These are subsequently used to train a joint statistical model implementing a mixture of principal component analyzers. Given a new aneurysmal shape, the trained joint model is firstly collapsed to a shape only model and used to initialize the missing shear stress values. The estimated hybrid point set is further refined by projection to the joint model space. We demonstrate that our predicted patterns can achieve significant similarities to the CFD-based results.

1 Introduction

We address the problem of estimating wall shear stress (WSS) on the surface of patient-specific image-based models of vascular aneurysms. Such estimates are clinically relevant as the endothelial cell response to WSS variations is one of the driving factors in the inflammatory process that leads to aneurysm growth and rupture. Boussel et al. [1], for example, have reported a correlation between aneurysm growth and areas of low time-averaged WSS. However, WSS in small vessels is difficult to be estimated accurately from flow imaging, so that it is often evaluated indirectly through computational fluid dynamics (CFD) simulations.

CFD simulations can be very time-consuming, especially in the context of rapid clinical decision making. Thus there is a need to develop methods that predict WSS directly from image-based models of aneurysms, preferably without relying on costly CFD simulations. One way to do this is by applying machine learning algorithms to build statistical models. This has been previously proposed e.g. by Schiavazzi et al. [5] to learn the relation between inlet/outlet flow

© Springer International Publishing AG 2016
S. Ourselin et al. (Eds.): MICCAI 2016, Part III, LNCS 9902, pp. 201–209, 2016.
DOI: 10.1007/978-3-319-46726-9_24

and pressure in vascular flows. In contrast, statistical models for aneurysms are not found in the literature, possibly due to the heterogeneity of shapes and the consequent problems in establishing point correspondences.

To successfully predict WSS based only on the morphology of the aneurysm, we hypothesize that we deal with *geometry-driven flow*. This means that the time-averaged flow (and consequently the time-averaged WSS) is determined mainly by the morphology of the vasculature, and that other factors such as the mean input flow and the blood viscosity only contribute negligible fluctuation terms. Cebral *et al.* [2] performed a sensitivity analysis of various hemodynamic parameters in intracranial aneurysms (IAs), and showed that the greatest impact on the computed flow fields was indeed due to the morphology.

We propose a framework to predict the time-averaged WSS (TAWSS) on the surface of patient-specific saccular IAs. A joint statistical model (JSM) is trained by a hybrid dataset of IA shapes and CFD-predicted aneurysmal TAWSS. We apply the method of Gooya *et al.* [4] for joint clustering and principal component analysis for building statistical models. However, the published method does not provide a mechanism to predict missing values from partially observed data. We further extend it by collapsing the JSM to a shape only model, obtaining initial TAWSS values, and further refining the result by projecting it to the JSM space.

The JSM is trained using a database of 38 patient-specific IA morphologies plus 114 TAWSS patterns (three different flow scenarios for each IA morphology). The optimal model is first selected by maximizing the model evidence, and used to predict the TAWSS pattern given the IA morphology of the test aneurysm. To the best of our knowledge, this represents the first development of a statistical model for complex IA shapes that also provides predictions of WSS. While the focus here is on the TAWSS, the method is general and can also predict flow quantities in other cases where the geometry-driven flow assumption holds.

2   Methods

2.1   Vascular Modeling and Pre-processing of Shapes

A cohort of 38 IA cases are selected from the @neurIST database. Surface models of the parent vessels, the neck surface, and the aneurysm sac have been previously reconstructed using the @neurIST processing toolchain as described by Villa-Uriol *et al.* in [7]. In all these cases, the IA is located at the sylvian bifurcation of the middle cerebral artery (MbifA-type), which is the most prevalent location for IAs. For each vascular model, the inlet branches are truncated at the beginning of the internal carotid artery (ICA) cavernous segment and extruded by an entry length of 5× the inlet diameter to allow for fully developed flow. Outlet branches are automatically clipped 20 mm after their proximal bifurcation. Branches shorter than 20 mm are extruded before truncation. The processed vascular surface models are then used for CFD simulation of blood flow as described in the next section.

2.2 Flow Simulation and Post-processing of TAWSS

For each surface model, a volumetric mesh of unstructured tetrahedrons with a maximum side length of 0.2 mm is generated in ANSYS ICEM v16.2 (Ansys Inc., Canonsburg, PA, USA). Three boundary layers of prismatic elements with edge size of 0.1 mm are used to provide convergence of WSS-related quantities. Blood is considered incompressible and Newtonian with density of 1066 kg/m^3 and dynamic viscosity of 0.0035 Pa·s. Arterial distensibility is not considered.

Time-varying inlet boundary conditions are prescribed at the ICA. To account for intra-subject flow variability on the aneurysmal TAWSS, we perform multiple flow simulations with different inflow boundary conditions for each case. A Gaussian process -model (GPM) is used to generate multiple inflow waveforms over the physiological range of variability at the ICA. This GPM is trained on subject-specific data from the study of Ford et al. [3], describing the statistical variance of 14 fiducial landmarks on the waveform. To simulate the high, moderate, and low flow conditions, we select three representative waveforms from the GPM generated samples and use them as inlet boundary conditions for flow simulations. A Poiseuille profile is imposed at all times of the inlet, and zero pressure at the outlets.

The unsteady Navier-Stokes equations are solved in ANSYS CFX v16.2 (Ansys Inc., Canonsburg, PA, USA) using a finite-volume method. Mesh convergence tests are performed on WSS, pressure, and flow velocity at several points in the computational domain. Unsteady simulations are run for 3 heartbeats until a periodic solution with stationary mean pressure is achieved. A total of $38 \times 3 = 114$ flow simulations are performed. Thereafter, the WSS vector field $\boldsymbol{\tau}_w(x, t)$ on the surface is reconstructed and TAWSS is computed as:

$$\text{TAWSS}(x) = \frac{1}{T_{\text{period}}} \int_{T_0}^{T_0 + T_{\text{period}}} |\boldsymbol{\tau}_w(x, t)| \, dt. \tag{1}$$

The area of interest for building the statistical model contains only the IA aneurysm sac. This choice was made to reduce the shape complexity due to variations of the branch vessels. For each of the 114 simulated cases, aneurysm sacs along with the TAWSS data are extracted from the complete vascular model and semi-automatically aligned by Procrustes registration according to their neck surfaces. Joint aneurysm sac and TAWSS field data sets are then decimated to point sets of around 600 points, so that the statistical model could be trained in a reasonable amount of time (< 30 mins).

2.3 Construction of Hybrid Point Sets

Our combined 4-D data vectors mix both spatial (coordinates (x, y, z) of the points) ans flow components (TAWSS in units of Pa). The relative magnitudes of the different components thus need to be carefully selected to avoid biasing the joint model towards either pure shape or pure TAWSS approximations. As initial scaling, the Euclidean distance (d) of each point in the point sets from the global centroid of point sets is computed and the maximum, $d_{\max}$, is used to scale the spatial coordinates as $(\widetilde{x}, \widetilde{y}, \widetilde{z}) = (x, y, z)/d_{\max}$. TAWSS values are scaled to fall between [0,1] by dividing them with the peak TAWSS value computed across all the vectors in the training set. To open up a possibility to investigate the effect of relative weight of shape and TAWSS in the JSM, we introduce a weighting factor (α). Thus, for each case $(k = 1, \ldots, 114)$ the 4D point set is, $\mathcal{X}_k(\alpha) = [\widetilde{\mathcal{Y}}_k, \alpha\widetilde{\mathcal{F}}_k]$, where $\widetilde{\mathcal{Y}}_k$ is the shape vector and $\widetilde{\mathcal{F}}_k$ is the TAWSS vector. Note that as there is no point-to-point correspondence between different shapes.

2.4   Joint Statistical Flow-and-Shape Model Construction

[1]Let $\mathcal{X}_k = \{\mathbf{x}_{kn}\}_{n=1, k=1}^{N_k, K}$ denote the kth point set, where $\mathbf{x}_{kn}$ is a $D = 4$ dimensional vector containing spatial and TAWSS coordinates of the nth landmark. Our statistical model can be explained by considering a hierarchy of two interacting mixture models. In D dimensions, points in $\mathcal{X}_k$ are assumed to be samples from a Gaussian Mixture Model (GMM) having M components. Furthermore, by consistently concatenating the coordinates of those components, $\mathcal{X}_k$ can be represented as an MD dimensional vector. These are assumed to be samples from a mixture of J probabilistic principal component analyzers (PPCA) [6]. Clustering and linear component analysis for $\mathcal{X}_k$ takes place in this high-dimensional space. The jth PPCA is an MD dimensional Gaussian specified by the mean vector $\bar{\boldsymbol{\mu}}_j$, and the covariance matrix given by $\mathbf{W}_j\mathbf{W}_j^T + \beta^{-1}\mathbf{I}$. Here, $\mathbf{W}_j$ is an $MD \times L$ dimensional matrix, whose columns encode the variation modes in the cluster j. Let $\mathbf{v}_k$ be an L dimensional vector and define $\boldsymbol{\mu}_{jk} = \mathbf{W}_j\mathbf{v}_k + \bar{\boldsymbol{\mu}}_j$, a *re-sampled* representation of $\mathcal{X}_k$ in the space spanned by principal components of the jth cluster. Meanwhile, if we partition $\boldsymbol{\mu}_{jk}$ into a series of M subsequent vectors and denote each as $\boldsymbol{\mu}_{jk}^{(m)}$, we obtain the means of the corresponding GMM.

To specify point correspondences, let $\mathcal{Z}_k = \{\mathbf{z}_{kn}\}_{n=1}^{N_k}$, and $\mathbf{z}_{kn} \in \{0,1\}^M$. The latter is a vector of zeros except for its arbitrary mth component, where $z_{knm} = 1$, indicating that $\mathbf{x}_{kn}$ is a sample from the D-dimensional Gaussian m. Moreover, let $\mathbf{t}_k \in \{0,1\}^J$, whose component j being one, $(t_{kj} = 1)$, indicates that $\mathcal{X}_k$ belongs to cluster j. We define

$$p(\mathbf{x}_{kn}|\mathbf{z}_{kn}, \mathbf{t}_k, \beta, \mathbb{W}, \mathbf{v}_k) = \prod_{j,m} \mathcal{N}(\mathbf{x}_{kn}|\boldsymbol{\mu}_{jk}^{(m)}, \beta^{-1}\mathbf{I}_D)^{z_{knm}t_{kj}}. \tag{2}$$

Finally, we impose prior multinomial distributions on $\mathbb{Z} = \{\mathcal{Z}_k\}$ and $\mathbb{T} = \{\mathbf{t}_k\}$ variables, normal distributions on $\mathbb{W} = \{\mathbf{W}_j\}$ and $\mathbb{V} = \{\mathbf{v}_k\}$ variables, and assume conditional independence (see [4] for further details).

To train the joint flow-shape model, we consider estimating the posterior probability of $p(\boldsymbol{\theta}|\mathbb{X}, M, L, J)$, where $\mathbb{X} = \{\mathcal{X}_k\}$ and $\boldsymbol{\theta} = \{\mathbb{Z}, \mathbb{T}, \mathbb{W}, \mathbb{V}\}$. Since this is not analytically tractable, an approximate posterior is sought by maximizing a lower bound (LB) on the $p(\mathbb{X}|M, L, J)$ (also known as *model evidence*). This is

---

[1] The details of statistical model has been given in [4]. A brief overview is provided here for the sake of completeness.

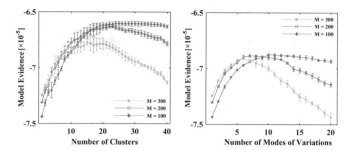

Fig. 1. Lower bound of model evidence used for optimising the number of clusters J when $L = 1$ (left), and the number of modes of variation per cluster L when $J = 1$ (right). Results shown for different M, the number of sampling points in each cluster.

achieved by assuming a factorized form of posteriors, following the Variational Bayesian (VB) principal. On the convergence, the approximated posteriors are computed, hence expectations (denoted by $\langle \cdot \rangle$) of latent variables with regard to these variational posteriors become available. For a new test point set $\mathcal{X}_r$, we can then compute the model projected point set using the definition of the expectation: $\langle \hat{\mathbf{x}}_{rn} \rangle = \int \hat{\mathbf{x}}_{rn} p(\hat{\mathbf{x}}_{rn} | \mathcal{X}_r, \mathbb{X}) d\hat{\mathbf{x}}_{rn}$. The latter can be shown to lead into the following result.

$$\langle \hat{\mathbf{x}}_{rn} \rangle = \sum_{j,m} \langle t_{jr} \rangle \langle z_{rnm} \rangle \langle \boldsymbol{\mu}_{jr} \rangle^{(m)} \tag{3}$$

To predict TAWSS values from a shape, we first collapse the trained joint model to a shape-only model, by discarding flow related rows from the $\mathbf{W}_j$ matrices and $\bar{\boldsymbol{\mu}}_j$ vectors. Using this collapsed model, we then perform VB iterations and obtain the initial posteriors for the corresponding $\mathbf{t}_r$, $\mathcal{Z}_r$ and $\mathbf{v}_r$ variables. Following this, we retrieve $\langle \mathbf{W}_j \rangle$ and $\bar{\boldsymbol{\mu}}_j$ from the joint model and set: $\langle \boldsymbol{\mu}_{jr} \rangle = \langle \mathbf{W}_j \rangle \langle \mathbf{v}_r \rangle + \bar{\boldsymbol{\mu}}_j$. Subsequently, we use (3) to estimate initial TAWSS values. These estimates are then further refined by performing VB iterations (using the joint model), updating $\mathbf{t}_r$, $\mathcal{Z}_r$ and $\mathbf{v}_r$, and interlacing imputations from (3). We observed that a convergence is achieved within 10 iterations (< 5 mins).

3 Results

3.1 Model Selection and Validation

The lower bound of the model evidence, $p(\mathbb{X} \mid M, L, J)$, was used as a criterion to select optimal numbers of: 4-dimensional Gaussians (M), PPCA clusters (J), and modes of variations (L) in each cluster. A nine-fold cross validation was then performed using 36 IA shapes and flows to assess the generality and specificity of the model. The scaling parameter α, representing the relative weight of shape and TAWSS information in each point set, was then chosen to minimize the generalization and specificity errors. It was observed that the specificity and

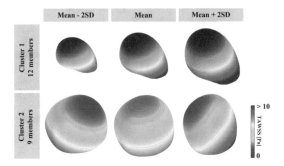

Fig. 2. Mean and first mode of variation for the two most populated clusters. The mode of the first cluster (top row) represents mainly the IA size, while the mode of the second cluster (bottom row) represents mainly changes in TAWSS patterns.

generalization errors was minimized for the default choice of scaling, i.e. $\alpha = 1$. These parameters were used for the flow prediction test.

Figure 1 shows the variation of model evidence with respect to the model parameters (J, L, and M). For each $1 \leq J \leq 40$ and $1 \leq L \leq 20$, we repeated the training for 10 rounds of initializations. The mean and standard deviation of the model evidences obtained are reported. As shown in Fig. 1, maximal model evidence was observed for $J = 23$, $L = 1$, and $M = 100$.

Figure 2 shows the mean shape and the first (and only) mode of variation for the two most populated clusters (the largest cluster having 12 point sets, and the second largest cluster containing 9 point sets). It can be seen that the IA size is the leading mode of the first cluster. However, in the second cluster, the leading mode of variation acts mainly to reorient the TAWSS pattern while the aneurysm shape remains similar. This demonstrates that the modes identified in the model training capture both flow and shape variabilities.

3.2   TAWSS Prediction from Shape

To evaluate the ability of the JSM to predict TAWSS for a given test shape, we performed leave-one-out cross-validations. Since CFD model inputs have been shown to only affect the TAWSS magnitude and not the distribution of TAWSS on the aneurysm sac [8], Pearson correlation test was used to perform a statistical point-by-point comparison between the model predicted TAWSS and that obtained from the full CFD simulation. Among a total of 38, the following correlation coefficients were found: $\rho \geq 0.6$ for 18 cases, $0.4 \leq \rho \leq 0.6$ for 13 cases, and $\rho \leq 0.4$ for the rest. It was observed that IAs with worst correlation coefficients fell into clusters with only one aneurysm shape in them. This revealed that the unsuccessful WSS prediction cases were associated with what appeared to be outlier shapes from the training data set; mainly complex multi-bleb aneurysm shapes. Figure 3 shows the model predicted TAWSS compared with the ground truth CFD solutions for the four best and worst cases. For each aneurysm, we report correlation coefficient ρ and the most probable cluster size (MPCS). The

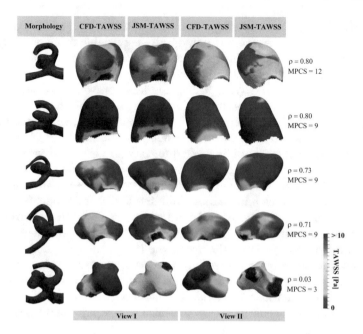

Fig. 3. Leave-one-out cross validation test for TAWSS estimation. Shown are the four best cases and the worst case (in terms of Pearson's ρ). The JSM accurately predicts flow impingement regions (case 1) and absence of flow (case 2). Case 5 is a complex outlier shape that does not resemble any of the other IA shapes used for training. All correlations significant to $p < 0.001$ except case 5, $p = 0.05$.

latter refers to the size of the cluster that appeared most similar to the test case. It can be seen that the IA with the worst ρ value (bottom row) fell into a cluster with size of three. While others with stronger predictions fell into more populated clusters containing at least 9 point sets in the training data.

4   Discussion

We have presented the first statistical model for complex saccular IAs that also predicts TAWSS patterns. The JSM was trained using a database of 38 patient-specific IA geometries and corresponding TAWSS values obtained from CFD simulations. A mixture PPCA model with 23 clusters and one mode of variation in each provided the best fit in terms of model evidence. Only the morphology and TAWSS on the aneurysmal sac were used for training, yet the TAWSS included implicitly information about the configuration of the host vessels. This enabled estimations of TAWSS on the IA wall based on the IA shape alone. Observation of the modes of variation of the largest clusters confirmed that the modes contained information on the variability of both TAWSS and shape.

The large inter-subject variability of IA shapes and their parent vessel configurations means that a sufficiently representative set of training data needs to be acquired. Even when choosing the most populous type of IA (MbifA-type) from the most comprehensive imaging database available to us, we only had 38 patient cases for training. To further study the prediction power of the proposed method, a larger cohort of synthetic aneurysms could however be generated and analyzed as a future work. As a result, the leave-one-out flow prediction test revealed that some IA shapes in the dataset were outlier shapes in which the TAWSS could not be well approximated. These outlier shapes included IAs with multiple daughter aneurysms and/or unusual positioning of the IA with respect to the vasculature. They could be flagged for further CFD analysis based on the size of the cluster in the training data that they were most likely to be part of.

We used IAs as an example of heterogeneous datasets with large variability in both flow patterns and shapes. Building the shape model is challenging since there is no straightforward method for establishing point correspondences between heterogeneous shapes. In the proposed method point correspondences are not required. Furthermore, the use of the PPCA mixture model allows outliers to be automatically separated into their own clusters. This is an improvement to single cluster PPCA models, which are known to be sensitive to outliers. The method presented here is therefore general and applicable to a number of other flow prediction scenarios in the presence of complex shape variations.

Acknowledgements. This project was partly supported by the Marie Curie Individual Fellowship (625745, A. Gooya). The aneurysm dataset has been provided by the European integrated project @neurIST (IST-027703).

References

1. Boussel, L., Rayz, V., McCulloch, C., Martin, A., Acevedo-Bolton, G., Lawton, M., Higashida, R., Smith, W.S., Young, W.L., Saloner, D.: Aneurysm growth occurs at region of low wall shear stress patient-specific correlation of hemodynamics and growth in a longitudinal study. Stroke **39**(11), 2997–3002 (2008)
2. Cebral, J.R., Castro, M.A., Appanaboyina, S., Putman, C.M., Millan, D., Frangi, A.F.: Efficient pipeline for image-based patient-specific analysis of cerebral aneurysm hemodynamics: technique and sensitivity. IEEE Trans. Med. Imaging **24**(4), 457–467 (2005)
3. Ford, M.D., Alperin, N., Lee, S.H., Holdsworth, D.W., Steinman, D.A.: Characterization of volumetric flow rate waveforms in the normal internal carotid and vertebral arteries. Physiol. Meas. **26**(4), 477 (2005)
4. Gooya, A., Lekadir, K., Alba, X., Swift, A.J., Wild, J.M., Frangi, A.F.: Joint clustering and component analysis of correspondenceless point sets: application to cardiac statistical modeling. In: Ourselin, S., Alexander, D.C., Westin, C.-F., Cardoso, M.J. (eds.) IPMI 2015. LNCS, vol. 9123, pp. 98–109. Springer, Heidelberg (2015)
5. Schiavazzi, D., Hsia, T., Marsden, A.: On a sparse pressure-flow rate condensation of rigid circulation models. J. Biomech. **49**(11), 2174–2186 (2015)
6. Tipping, M.E., Bishop, C.M.: Mixtures of probabilistic principal component analyzers. Neural Comput. **11**(2), 443–482 (1999)

7. Villa-Uriol, M., Berti, G., Hose, D., Marzo, A., Chiarini, A., Penrose, J., Pozo, J., Schmidt, J., Singh, P., Lycett, R., et al.: @ neurist complex information processing toolchain for the integrated management of cerebral aneurysms. Interface Focus **1**(3), 308–319 (2011). rsfs20100033
8. Xiang, J., Siddiqui, A., Meng, H.: The effect of inlet waveforms on computational hemodynamics of patient-specific intracranial aneurysms. J. Biomech. **47**(16), 3882–3890 (2014)

Multi-task Shape Regression
for Medical Image Segmentation

Xiantong Zhen[1,2(✉)], Yilong Yin[3], Mousumi Bhaduri[4], Ilanit Ben Nachum[1,2],
David Laidley[4], and Shuo Li[1,2]

[1] Digital Imaging Group (DIG), London, ON, Canada
[2] The University of Western Ontario, London, ON, Canada
xzhen7@uwo.ca
[3] Shandong University, Shandong, China
[4] London Health Sciences Centre, London, ON, Canada

Abstract. In this paper, we propose a general segmentation framework of *Multi-Task Shape Regression* (MTSR) which formulates segmentation as multi-task learning to leverage its strength of jointly solving multiple tasks enhanced by capturing task correlations. The MTSR entirely estimates coordinates of all points on shape contours by multi-task regression, where estimation of each coordinate corresponds to a regression task; the MTSR can jointly handle nonlinear relationships between image appearance and shapes while capturing holistic shape information by encoding coordinate correlations, which enables estimation of highly variable shapes, even with vague edge or region inhomogeneity. The MTSR achieves a long-desired general framework without relying on any specific assumptions or initialization, which enables flexible and fully automatic segmentation of multiple objects simultaneously, for different applications irrespective of modalities. The MTSR is validated on six representative applications of diverse images, achieves consistently high performance with dice similarity coefficient (DSC) up to 0.93 and largely outperforms state of the arts in each application, which demonstrates its effectiveness and generality for medical image segmentation.

1 Introduction

Segmentation plays a fundamental role in medical image analysis, which however has long been regarded as a challenging task due to great diversity of applications in multiple modalities, huge appearance variations of images with multiple objects and high shape variabilities of objects with complex anatomical structures. However, conventional segmentation methods cannot handle all these challenges in one framework due to the lack of generality, which are usually application specific in a certain modality, designed for images with one single object and cannot segment multiple objects simultaneously. Moreover, they usually need initialization and rely on the assumption that shape contours are supported by clear edges and region homogeneity [1], which does not always hold due to overlapping of anatomical structures, complex image textures and appearances, especially with the presence of pathology.

© Springer International Publishing AG 2016
S. Ourselin et al. (Eds.): MICCAI 2016, Part III, LNCS 9902, pp. 210–218, 2016.
DOI: 10.1007/978-3-319-46726-9_25

Shape regression has recently shown great effectiveness for medical image segmentation with significantly better performance than conventional methods [2]. The central idea is to directly estimate point coordinates on shape contours by regression, that is, to find a nonlinear regressor to associate nonrigid shape with image appearance. Compared to traditional segmentation methods, shape regression enables leveraging the advanced machine learning techniques to extract knowledge from annotated database to tackle huge shape variabilities. Moreover, shape regression removes manual interaction and initialization in conventional segmentation methods, and is computationally more efficient. However, it remains unaddressed to explicitly model coordinate correlations resulting in shapes with outlier points falling off the contour, especially with vague edge or region inhomogeneity, which leaves a theoretical deficiency to be a general model for shape regression.

A general shape regression is desired to jointly model inherent correlations among point coordinates and highly complicated relationships between image appearance and variable shapes. The points on the shape contour are spatially coherent and statistically correlated, which should be explored to capture holistic shape information to recover contours not supported by edges or region homogeneity for robust shape regression; meanwhile, the relationship between image appearance and the associated shape is highly complex and nonlinear due to great variations of image appearance and huge shape variabilities of objects, which cannot be handled by linear regression models.

In this paper, to tackle these challenges, we propose a general segmentation framework of *Multi-Task Shape Regression* (MTSR) by formulating segmentation as multi-task learning, which leverages its strength of jointly solving multiple tasks, i.e., estimating point coordinates directly and simultaneously, while enhanced by modeling their relationships, i.e., coordinate correlations. By incorporating a latent space associated with a structure matrix, the MTSR is able to simultaneously encode holistic shape information by modeling coordinate correlations via sparse learning and disentangle nonlinear relationships between image appearance and variable shapes by kernel regression.

The major contribution of this work lies in that we for the first time achieve a general segmentation framework of shape regression by multi-task learning. Compared to previous methods, the MTSR offers multiple advantages.

- By formulating as a multi-task learning problem, the MTSR achieves a general shape regression framework without relying on specific assumptions and initialization, which enables segmentation of images with multiple objects from diverse applications irrespective of imaging modalities.
- By explicitly modeling correlations between coordinates via sparse learning, the MTSR can capture holistic shape information by reliably and accurately estimating each coordinate, which enables to recover contours not supported by edges and region homogeneity.
- By seamlessly working with the kernel trick, the MTSR achieves nonlinear regression, which enables disentangling highly complicated relationships between image appearance of great variations and shapes of huge variabilities.

2   Multi-task Shape Regression

The proposed MTSR formulates segmentation as multi-task regression to directly and simultaneously estimates the coordinates of the points on shape contours, where estimation of each coordinate is a regression task. By incorporating a latent space, the MTSR explicitly models coordinate correlations in a structure matrix S via the $\ell_{2,1}$-norm based sparse learning to capture the holistic information of shapes (Sect. 2.2); by kernelization, the MTSR achieves kernel regression to effectively tackle complicated nonlinear relationships between image appearance and variable shapes (Sect. 2.3).

2.1   Shape Regression by Multi-task Regression

Shape regression is to directly estimate point coordinates on the shape contour of the object by regression from input images, where the shape is represented by $\mathbf{y} = [h_1, \ldots, h_i, \ldots, h_{\mathcal{P}}, v_1, \ldots, v_i, \ldots, v_{\mathcal{P}}]^\top \in \mathbb{R}^Q$, $Q(= 2\mathcal{P})$ is the number of coordinates of the $\mathcal{P}$ points on the shape contour, h_i and v_i are the horizontal and vertical axises of the i-the point, respectively. The associated image is represented by a feature descriptor $\mathbf{x} \in \mathbb{R}^d$, e.g., the histogram of oriented gradient (HOG) [3], where d is the dimensionality.

The proposed MTSR realizes shape regression by multi-task regression to directly and simultaneously estimates coordinates while jointly capturing coordinate correlations to capture holistic shape information; and it is derived based on the widely-used fundamental multi-task regression model $\mathbf{y} = W\mathbf{x} + \mathbf{b}$, where $W = [\mathbf{w}_1, \ldots, \mathbf{w}_i, \ldots, \mathbf{w}_Q]^\top \in \mathbb{R}^{Q \times d}$ is the regression coefficient, $\mathbf{w}_i \in \mathbb{R}^d$ is the task parameter for y_i, and $\mathbf{b} \in \mathbb{R}^Q$ is the bias.

2.2   Modeling Correlation by Sparse Learning

We propose modeling the inherent correlations between point coordinates by sparse learning to learn shared features for correlated point coordinates. Since the points on the shape contour are spatially coherent and statistically correlated, encoding correlations enables to capture the holistic shape information to recover contours not supported by edges or region homogeneity.

Rather than directly imposing regularization on regression matrix W as widely explored in existing multi-task learning algorithms, we propose incorporating a latent space. On top of the latent variables, a structure matrix S is deployed to explicitly model coordinate correlations via the $\ell_{2,1}$-norm based sparse learning. Based on the least square loss function and ℓ_2 regularization, we have the following objective function w.r.t. W and S

$$\min_{W,S} \frac{1}{\mathcal{N}} ||Y - SZ||_F^2 + \lambda ||W||_F^2 + \beta ||S^\top||_{2,1},$$

$$s.t. \ Z = WX \tag{1}$$

where $X = [\mathbf{x}_1, \mathbf{x}_2, \ldots, \mathbf{x}_{\mathcal{N}}]$, $Y = [\mathbf{y}_1, \mathbf{y}_2, \ldots, \mathbf{y}_{\mathcal{N}}]$, $Z = [\mathbf{z}_1, \ldots, \mathbf{z}_i, \ldots, \mathbf{z}_{\mathcal{N}}] \in \mathbb{R}^{Q \times \mathcal{N}}$, $\mathbf{z}_i \in \mathbb{R}^Q$ is a variable in the latent space and $S \in \mathbb{R}^{Q \times Q}$ is named as the structure matrix; the $\ell_{2,1}$-norm constraint on the structure matrix S in (1) encourages to learn an S that is prone to be column sparsity [4]; the parameter β controls the column sparsity of S and a larger β induces higher sparsity; the bias is omitted since it is proven that the bias can be absorbed into the regression coefficient W [4].

Thanks to the $\ell_{2,1}$-norm based sparse learning, regressors of correlated coordinates on the shape contour are encouraged to share similar parameter sparsity patterns to capture a common set of features from the latent space, which enables to encode the inherent correlations between coordinates. Therefore, holistic shape information is effectively captured, which enables to recover the coordinates that are not supported by clear edges or region homogeneity to achieve more accurate and robust shape estimation. Moreover, the performance of all regressors can be improved by leveraging knowledge across correlated coordinates that share common features. By deploying a structure matrix S to explicitly model coordinate correlations, our MTSR can automatically learn the inherence of coordinates on the shape contour from data to cater different applications, which further improves the generality.

We highlight that due to the incorporation of the latent space associated with the structure matrix S, the proposed MTSR brings multiple attractive merits:

- The latent space decouples inputs and outputs with W and S, which enables effectively handling high image appearance variations and huge shape variability to disentangle their complex relationships.
- The structure matrix allows to explicitly encode inherent correlations between coordinates to capture the holistic shape information, which enables recovering contours not supported by clear edges or region homogeneity.

Due to the huge appearance variations of images and the high shape variabilities of objects to be segmented, the relationship between image appearance and variable shapes is complicated and highly nonlinear, which cannot be handled by linear regression and demands more powerful nonlinear regressors.

2.3   Kernelization for Nonlinear Regression

Although the objective function (1) is not guaranteed to be jointly convex with W and S, it is easy to show that kernelization can be derived with respect to W with a fixed S thanks to the incorporation of the latent space according to the Representer Theorem [5]. This enables kernel regression to handle nonlinear relationship between image appearance and shapes, while being able to encode coordinate correlations by S.

The linear representer theorem [5] is particularly useful when $\mathcal{H}$ is a reproducing kernel Hilbert space (RKHS), which simplifies the empirical risk minimization problem from an infinite dimensional to a finite dimensional optimization problem [5]. Assume that we map $\mathbf{x}_i$ to $\phi(\mathbf{x}_i)$ in some RKHS of infinite dimensionality where $\phi(\cdot)$ denotes the feature map of $\mathbf{x}_i$; the mapping serves as a nonlinear feature extraction that enables to disentangle complicated relationships between image appearance and variable shapes. The corresponding kernel

Table 1. The statistics of the six datasets.

Dataset \ Information	Task	Subjects	Images	Modalities
SKI12 [7]	Knee	20	1438	MR
CRASS12 [8]	Clavicle	20	548	CT
PROMISE12 [9]	Prostate	50	778	MR
Cardiac Bi-Ventricles (CBV) [10]	LV/RV	145	8700	MR
Cardiac 4 Chambers (C4C-MR) [6]	LV/LA/RV/RA	125	3125	MR
Cardiac 4 Chambers (C4C-CT)	LV/LA/RV/RA	101	3920	CT

function $k(\cdot, \cdot)$ satisfies $k(\mathbf{x}_i, \mathbf{x}_j) = \phi(\mathbf{x}_i)^\top \phi(\mathbf{x}_j)$. To facilitate the derivation of kernelization, we rewrite (1) in term of traces as follows:

$$\min_{W,S} \frac{1}{\mathcal{N}} tr((Y - SWX)^\top (Y - SWX)) + \lambda tr(W^\top W) + \beta ||S^\top||_{2,1}. \qquad (2)$$

According to the linear representer theorem, we can obtain W by

$$W = \boldsymbol{\alpha}\Phi(X)^\top \qquad (3)$$

where $\Phi(X) = [\phi(\mathbf{x}_1), \ldots, \phi(\mathbf{x}_i), \ldots, \phi(\mathbf{x}_\mathcal{N})]$ and $\boldsymbol{\alpha} \in \mathbb{R}^{Q \times \mathcal{N}}$. Substituting (3) into (2) gives rise to the objective function w.r.t $\boldsymbol{\alpha}$ and S:

$$\min_{\boldsymbol{\alpha},S} \frac{1}{\mathcal{N}} tr((Y - S\boldsymbol{\alpha}K)^\top (Y - S\boldsymbol{\alpha}K)) + \lambda tr(\boldsymbol{\alpha}K\boldsymbol{\alpha}^\top) + \beta ||S^\top||_{2,1} \qquad (4)$$

where $K = \Phi(X)^\top \Phi(X)$ is the kernel matrix in the RKHS. The latent space spanned by $Z = \boldsymbol{\alpha}K$ is obtained by the linear transformation $\boldsymbol{\alpha}$ via the Representer Theorem from the KRHS induced by a nonlinear kernel K. As a result, higher-level concepts are extracted to fill the semantic gap between image representations of low-level feature descriptors and variable shapes, which enables efficient linear $\ell_{2,1}$-based sparse learning of S to explicitly model inherent correlations of coordinates to capture the holistic shape information. The objective function in (4) is non-convex jointly with $\boldsymbol{\alpha}$ and S, which fortunately can be efficiently solved by alternating optimization [6].

2.4   Training and Prediction

In the training stage, the MTSR is trained on annotated data with ground truth of contours; in the prediction stage, given a new input $\mathbf{x}_t$, the point coordinates on the shape contour of objects to be segmented can efficiently be predicted by $\hat{\mathbf{y}}_t = S\boldsymbol{\alpha}K_t$, where $K_t = \Phi(X)^\top \phi(\mathbf{x}_t)$. Segmentation is then obtained based on the predicted shape contours.

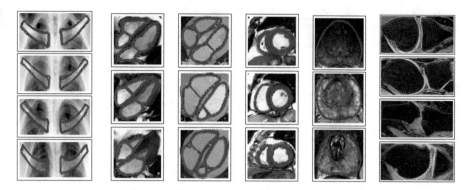

Fig. 1. Segmentation results: (from left to right) clavicle, cardiac four chambers MR/CT, bi-ventricles, prostate, knee (red: MTSR and blue: ground truth). (Color figure online)

3   Experiments

Our method has been validated by extensive experiments on six representative applications for clinical image segmentation and achieves high performance on all six applications with a dice similarity coefficient (DSC) [11] up to 0.93 and consistently outperforms state of the arts in each application.

3.1   Datasets and Implementation Details

The six datasets contain three public datasets from Grand Challenges for prostate, knee and clavicle, and three newly collected cardiac MR/CT datasets for bi-ventricles and four chambers. The statistics of the six datasets are reported in Table 1. Following [2], contours are represented by the coordinates of a set of $\mathcal{P}$ (=100) points on the shape of an object $\{p_i = (h_i, v_i)|_{i=1:\mathcal{P}}\}$ sampled evenly along the manually annotated contour from a fixed point. In cardiac four chambers, four landmark points are indicated during manual annotation to segment atrium and ventricle, respectively. The histogram of oriented gradient (HOG) descriptor [3] is used due to its computational efficiency for image representation. To benchmark with existing methods, we measure the performance using the DSC [7,9,11] obtained using leave-one-subject-out cross validation. We compare the two shape regression models fulfilled by the MSVR [2] and adaptive k-cluster regression forests (AKRF) [12]. The multi-target kernel ridge regression (mKRR) is regarded as a baseline of multi-task learning for comparison. The parameter β is obtained by cross validation on the training set.

3.2   Results

The MTSR yields high performance in comparison to ground truth on all six applications, which demonstrates its effectiveness and generality for medical

Table 2. The dice similarity coefficients (DSC) for six different applications.

Method \ Task	Clavicle	Prostate	Knee	C4C-MR	C4C-CT	CBV
MTSR	**0.857**	**0.930**	**0.894**	**0.885**	**0.886**	**0.892**
mKRR	0.829	0.906	0.861	0.826	0.824	0.843
mSVR [2]	0.851	0.924	0.889	0.849	0.836	0.868
AKRF [12]	0.842	0.921	0.879	0.847	0.841	0.869
State of Arts	0.80 [8]	0.89 [9]	0.857 [11]	-	-	-

image segmentation. We show qualitative results in Fig. 1 and the quantitative comparison to state-of-the-art algorithms are reported in Table 2.

Effectiveness. The effectiveness of the MTSR is shown by overcoming great image variations and huge shape variabilities caused by region inhomogeneity, vague edges, illumination change, low intensity contrast and spatial/temporal nonrigid deformations. As shown in Fig. 1, *Clavicle:* the medial part of the clavicle is heavily obscured by other anatomical structures such as the mediastinum and large vessels [8], and both femoral and tibial cartilages demonstrate high anatomical shape variations; *Knee:* The contours are discontinuous and not consistently visible due to the poor intensity contrast, and shapes vary greatly across spatial slices. *Prostate:* The contours are not supported by region intensity homogeneity because of the complex texture and illumination. *Cardiac:* Both four chambers and bi-ventricles demonstrate high variabilities caused by the large spatial and temporal deformations. However, as shown in Fig. 1 the MTSR produces contours (red) very close to ground truth (blue) on all six applications, which demonstrates its effectiveness of jointly modeling coordinate correlation and nonlinear relationship between image appearance and variable shapes.

Generality. The generality of the MTSR is shown by conquering the diversity of images with multiple objects, from a large variety of applications and in multiple imaging modalities. These images from six tasks cover a broad range of medical applications, contains varied numbers of objects from one prostate to four chambers, and are obtained in multiple modalities, i.e., MT and CT, both of which are widely used in clinical routines. However, the MTSR is able to consistently and successfully produce accurate shape contours with high performance up to 0.93 of DSC on all six applications as shown in Table 2, which validates its generality for medical image segmentation by shape regression, indicating its great potential in clinical use.

Comparison. As shown in Table 2, the MTSR achieves consistently higher performance on all applications, and substantially outperforms state-of-the-art methods with large margins up to 4.5 %. The MTSR performs much better than the MSVR/AKRF and the baseline mKRR on all six tasks, which demonstrates the strength of modeling coordinate correlations by the proposed $\ell_{2,1}$-norm based sparse learning.

4   Conclusion

In this paper, we proposed a general segmentation method, multi-target shape regression (MTSR), which formulates the segmentation of shapes as a multi-task learning problem. The MTSR is able to simultaneously capture the holistic shape information and handle highly nonlinear relationships between image appearance and variable shapes in one single framework, which enables more accurate and reliable shape regression for image segmentation with multiple varied numbers of objects, irrespective of modalities. Experiments on six diverse segmentation tasks show that the MTSR achieves consistently high performance and significantly outperforms state-of-the-art algorithms, which demonstrates its effectiveness and generality for medical image segmentation.

Acknowledgement. This work was supported by the NSFC Joint Fund with Guangdong under Key Project (Grant No. U1201258) and NSFC (Grant No. 61571147).

References

1. Cootes, T.F., Edwards, G.J., Taylor, C.J.: Active appearance models. TPAMI **23**(6), 681–685 (2001)
2. Wang, Z., Zhen, X., Tay, K., Osman, S., Romano, W., Li, S.: Regression segmentation for M^3 spinal images. TMI **34**(8), 1640–1648 (2015)
3. Dalal, N., Triggs, B.: Histograms of oriented gradients for human detection. In: CVPR, vol. 1, pp. 886–893 (2005)
4. Nie, F., Huang, H., Cai, X., Ding, C.H.: Efficient, robust feature selection via joint $\ell_{2,1}$-norms minimization. In: NIPS, pp. 1813–1821 (2010)
5. Kimeldorf, G.S., Wahba, G.: A correspondence between Bayesian estimation on stochastic processes and smoothing by splines. Ann. Math. Stat. **41**(2), 495–502 (1970)
6. Zhen, X., Islam, A., Bhaduri, M., Chan, I., Li, S.: Direct and simultaneous four-chamber volume estimation by multi-output regression. In: Navab, N., Hornegger, J., Wells, W.M., Frangi, A.F. (eds.) MICCAI 2015. LNCS, vol. 9349, pp. 669–676. Springer, Heidelberg (2015). doi:10.1007/978-3-319-24553-9_82
7. Heimann, T., Morrison, B.J., Styner, M.A., Niethammer, M., Warfield, S.: Segmentation of knee images: a grand challenge. In: Proceedings of MICCAI Workshop on Medical Image Analysis for the Clinic, pp. 207–214 (2010)
8. Hogeweg, L., Sánchez, C.I., de Jong, P.A., Maduskar, P., van Ginneken, B.: Clavicle segmentation in chest radiographs. Med. Image Anal. **16**(8), 1490–1502 (2012)
9. Litjens, G., Toth, R., van de Ven, W., Hoeks, C., Kerkstra, S., van Ginneken, B., Vincent, G., Guillard, G., Birbeck, N., Zhang, J., et al.: Evaluation of prostate segmentation algorithms for MRI: the promise12 challenge. Med. Image Anal. **18**(2), 359–373 (2014)
10. Zhen, X., Wang, Z., Islam, A., Bhaduri, M., Chan, I., Li, S.: Multi-scale deep networks and regression forests for direct bi-ventricular volume estimation. Med. Image Anal. **30**, 120–129 (2016)

11. Shan, L., Zach, C., Charles, C., Niethammer, M.: Automatic atlas-based three-label cartilage segmentation from MR knee images. Med. Image Anal. **18**(7), 1233–1246 (2014)
12. Hara, K., Chellappa, R.: Growing regression forests by classification: applications to object pose estimation. In: Fleet, D., Pajdla, T., Schiele, B., Tuytelaars, T. (eds.) ECCV 2014, Part II. LNCS, vol. 8690, pp. 552–567. Springer, Heidelberg (2014)

Soft Multi-organ Shape Models via Generalized PCA: A General Framework

Juan J. Cerrolaza[1(✉)], Ronald M. Summers[2],
and Marius George Linguraru[1,3]

[1] Sheikh Zayed Institute for Pediatric Surgical Innovation,
Children's National Health System, Washington, D.C., USA
{JCerrola, MLingura}@cnmc.org
[2] Department of Radiology and Imaging Sciences,
National Institute of Health, Bethesda, MD, USA
[3] School of Medicine and Health Sciences, George Washington University,
Washington, D.C., USA

Abstract. This paper addresses the efficient statistical modeling of multi-organ structures, one of the most challenging scenarios in the medical imaging field due to the frequently limited availability of data. Unlike typical approaches where organs are considered either as single objects or as part of predefined groups, we introduce a more general and natural approach in which all the organs are inter-related inspired by the rhizome theory. Combining canonical correlation analysis with a generalized version of principal component analysis, we propose a new general and flexible framework for multi-organ shape modeling to efficiently characterize the individual organ variability and the relationships between different organs. This new framework called SOMOS can be easily parameterized to mimic a wide variety of alternative statistical shape modeling approaches, including the classic point distribution model, and its more recent multi-resolution variants. The significant superiority of SOMOS over alternative approaches was successfully verified for two different multi-organ databases: six subcortical structures of the brain, and seven abdominal organs. Finally, the organ-prediction capability of the model also significantly outperformed a partial least squared regression-based approach.

Keywords: Shape models · Generalized PCA · Multi-organ · Hierarchical model

1 Introduction

Organ modeling and shape analysis are of crucial importance in the development of robust diagnostic tools, treatment planning, and patient follow-up. However, most statistical shape models have focused on single organ-based applications, proven inefficient when dealing with the variability of the shape and position of some challenging anatomical structures (e.g. the pancreas). Shifting from organ-based to organism-based approaches, there has been growing interest in the development of comprehensive and holistic computational anatomical models in recent years [1–3]. However, as the complexity and detail of anatomical models increase, there are new

© Springer International Publishing AG 2016
S. Ourselin et al. (Eds.): MICCAI 2016, Part III, LNCS 9902, pp. 219–228, 2016.
DOI: 10.1007/978-3-319-46726-9_26

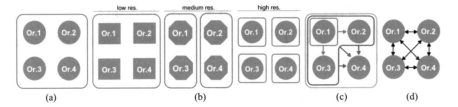

Fig. 1. Multi-organ shape modeling strategies. (a) Classic PDM: all the organs (Or.) are modeled together as a single object. (b) Multi-resolution hierarchical model [1]: all the organs are modeled together at coarser resolutions, modeling smaller groups as we move toward finer resolutions. In the picture, square, octagons, and circles, represent low, intermediate, and high resolution of the organs, respectively. (c) Sequential organ modeling [2]: Or.1 is used to estimate Or.2 and Or.3. Or.1, Or.2, and Or.3 will be used to estimate Or.4. (d) Rhizomatic structure: all the inter-organ relationships are considered in the model.

technical challenges that hinder the use of traditional shape modeling methods, such as the limited availability of data. While a limited number of examples may be sufficient to model relatively simple organs, such as the kidneys, an adequately large training set is not always available as the dimensionality and complexity of the structures increase. This issue is known as the high-dimension-low-sample-size (HDLSS) problem.

One of the most popular shape modeling techniques is the Point Distribution Model (PDM) proposed by Cootes et al. [4]. Despite the inherent capability of PDMs to model multi-organ structures by performing global statistics on all the objects (see Fig. 1(a)), these models are particularly sensitive to the HDLSS issue. Moreover, PDMs do not represent object-based scale level, which limits their ability to describe the local geometry information of organs. More recently, Cerrolaza et al. [1] proposed a new generalized multi-resolution hierarchical variant of PDM (GEM-PDM). Based on a multi-resolution decomposition of the shapes, GEM-PDM defines clusters of organs that are modeled together at each resolution (see Fig. 1(b)), providing an efficient characterization of the inter-organs relations, as well as the particular locality of each organ. Although GEM-PDM is robust for general multi-organ modeling, the hierarchical configuration may be affected by some design parameters of the model. The inter-organ relations were also explored by Okada et al. [2], presenting an automated framework for the modeling and segmentation of multiple abdominal organs in CT images (Fig. 1(c)). Based on a predefined ranking of organ stability, the authors defined a sequential modeling of the organs designed to improve the analysis of challenging structures, such as the pancreas, using information from neighboring stable organs, such as the liver and spleen.

Unlike the classic rigid organization of the information as a unified structure ruled by hierarchy [1] or linearity [2], the rhizomatic structure developed by Deleuzed and Guattari [5] proposes an alternative organization of the information units (e.g., organs) as an interconnected, non-linear network. Inspired by this new concept, we propose a new general framework for SOft Multi-Organ Shape models (SOMOS). In SOMOS, a multi-organ structure is modeled by a graph (see Fig. 1(d)), whose nodes and edges represent the organs and the relationships between them, respectively. Based on generalized principal component analysis (G-PCA), the flexibility of the SOMOS also allows to replicate previous approaches (e.g. PDM, GEM-PDM) by defining particular parameterizations of the model (i.e., imposing hard inter-organ constraints). However, the rhizomatic nature of SOMOS assumes the general scenario where all the inter-organ relationships are considered in the model, bringing together the advantages of all those alternative approaches in a common flexible framework.

2 Shape Models

Let $\{x_1, \ldots, x_M\}$ be the set of $M \in \mathbb{N}$ organs in a d-dimensional ($d = 2$ or 3) space. Each x_j ($1 \leq j \leq M$) represents the vector form of a single-object structure defined by the concatenation of the $K_j \in \mathbb{N}$ landmarks that define each organ (i.e., $x_j = (x_{j(1)}, \ldots, x_{j(d \cdot K_j)})^T$). In the same way, x is defined as the $(d \cdot K \times 1)$ vector resulting from the concatenation of the M organs, $x = (x_1; \ldots; x_M)^T$, and $K = \sum K_j$. Unlike the classic PDM, where a single global shape model is built for x, SOMOS creates M individual models, one for each organ of interest. The goal of each individual model is, not only to characterize the particular anatomical variability of a particular organ (i.e. a node in the graph), but also its relationships with any other structure in the model. The creation of these individual shape models is detailed below.

2.1 Organ-Based Shape Models via Generalized PCA

Consider the creation of the statistical model for the i-th organ, x_i. The relationship between x_i and the remaining organs is defined by means of the $(M \times 1)$ vector, w_i, whose j-th component, $w_{ij} \in [0, 1]$, represents the correlation between x_i and x_j. A factor of 1 means perfect correlation (e.g. $w_{ii} = 1$), while 0 represents the absence of relationship between both organs. An efficient statistical model should be able to model the variability of the organ of interest, x_i, as well as those significant inter-organ relationships (i.e. with high values of w_{ij}). Based on the G-PCA formulation proposed by Greenancre [6] we formulate the problem as a weighted variant of PCA.

Let X represents the $(N \times d \cdot K)$ centered data matrix (i.e. zero mean) containing the vector form of the $N \in \mathbb{N}$ training cases. Using the generalized singular value decomposition (G-SVD) [6] of X, this matrix can be de written as $X = VDB^T$, where V and B are $(N \times r)$ and $(d \cdot K \times r)$ matrices respectively (r is the rank of X), and D is a $(r \times r)$ diagonal matrix. However, unlike classic SVD, V and B are not necessarily orthonormal. In G-SVD, V and B satisfy $V^T \Phi V = I_r$, and $B^T \Omega B = I_r$, with Φ and Ω being specified positive-definite symmetric matrices, and I_r the identity matrix of order r. G-SVD finds the ordinary SVD of $\tilde{X} = \Phi^{1/2} X \Omega^{1/2}$. In the particular case in which Φ and Ω are diagonal, $\tilde{X}$ can be considered as a weighted version of X, where different observations and variables can have different weights. Assuming all the observations are treated identically, we can define $\phi_{11} = \ldots = \phi_{NN} = 1$. SVD of $\tilde{X}$ can be written as $\tilde{X} = UEC^T$, where E is a diagonal matrix and $U^T U = C^T C = I_r$. Then, $X = \tilde{X} \Omega^{-1/2} = UEC^T \Omega^{-1/2}$, and thus $V = U$, $D = E$, and $B = \Omega^{-1/2} C$.

G-PCA is defined by P, the $(d \cdot K \times m)$ matrix formed by the first $m \leq r$ columns of B. Like in the classic PCA-based PDM [4], each shape can be now modeled as $x \approx \tilde{x} = \bar{x} + P \cdot b$, where b is the $(m \times 1)$ coordinate vector of x in the space defined by P. It can be demonstrated that among all possible rank m approximations, $\tilde{x}$ minimizes $\sum_{k=1}^{K} \omega_k (\tilde{x}_{(k)} - x_{(k)})^2$. That is, the shape model provides a weighted least square approximation where the contribution of each variable is weighted by $\omega_k \in \mathbb{R}^+$, the diagonal components of $\mathbf{\Omega}$. In SOMOS, $\mathbf{\Omega}$ is defined by w_i as follow: $\omega_k = w_{ij}$ s.t. $x_{(k)} \in x_j$. Therefore, the resulting shape model for organ x_i not only prioritizes the variability of that organ (which reduces the HDLSS effect in x_i), but also considers the context of the organ thanks to its inherent rhizomatic structure.

To define w_{ij}, the correlation factor between two organs, x_i and x_j, we use canonical correlation analysis (CCA) between these two sets of variables. CCA determines the linear combinations of the components in x_i that are maximally correlated with linear combinations of the components in x_j. The strength of these correlations is described by the corresponding correlation coefficients with values between 0 and 1 (see Fig. 2). The capacity of CCA was previously studied by Rao et al. [7] and Okada et al. [2] to define inter-organ relationships of sub-cortical brain structures. In SOMOS, the overall inter-organ correlation factor, w_{ij}, is defined automatically as the average correlation coefficient over all calculated canonical modes of $CCA(x_i, x_j)$.

2.2 Shape Modeling Using SOMOS

Let $y = (y_1; \ldots; y_M)^T$ be the vector form of any d-dimensional multi-organ structure we want to model using the new SOMOS framework, i.e. finding $\tilde{y} = (\tilde{y}_1; \ldots; \tilde{y}_M)^T$, the best approximation of y in the subspace of valid shapes defined by the set of M statistical models created in Sect. 2.1. For each of these models, y can be approximated as $(\tilde{y}_j; \ldots; \tilde{y}_{jM})^T = \bar{x} + P_j \cdot b_j$, where the vector of coefficients b_j is obtained as $b_j = P_j^T \Omega_j^{1/2}(y - \bar{x})$. Thus, the j-th organ in $\tilde{y}$, $\tilde{y}_j$, is modeled by $\tilde{y}_{jj}$.

3 SOMOS: General Framework for Shape Modeling

SOMOS can be considered as a generalization of the traditional shape models able to integrate alternative methods in a common framework. In the particular case in which $\mathbf{\Omega} = \mathbf{I}$ (i.e., $w_{ij} = 1$, $\forall i, j$) SOMOS becomes equivalent to the original PDM [4] (and thus, suffering from HDLSS). On the other hand, defining $w_{ij} = \delta_{ij}$, where δ_{ij} is the Kronecker delta function, the model becomes equivalent to an independent modeling of each organ (and thus, not integrating into the model relevant inter-organ relationships). Other interesting applications of the SOMOS framework are presented below.

3.1   Multi-resolution Hierarchical Multi-organ Shape Modeling

Suppose now $\{x^r\}_{r=0,\ldots,R}$ represents the multi-resolution (MR) decomposition of the shape x, where x^0 and x^R represent the finest and the coarsest level of resolution, respectively. The detail information missed from x^r to x^{r-1} is represented by the corresponding high-frequency vector z^r. From x^0, $\{x^r\}_{r=0,\ldots,R}$ and $\{z^r\}_{r=1,\ldots,R}$ can be obtained using the corresponding analysis equations: $x^r = A^r x^{r-1}$, and $z^r = H^r x^{r-1}$, respectively, where A and H are the analysis filters (see [8] for details). Similarly to the work proposed by Cerrolaza et al. [1], SOMOS can incorporate MR shape analysis as follows. Imposing the initial condition that $\Omega^R = I$ (i.e. a global model of the entire multi-organ structure is built at the coarsest resolution to guarantee the coherent disposition of the elements), G-PCA is used at each level of resolution obtaining $\{\bar{x}^r, P^r_j, \Omega^r_j\}_{j=1,\ldots,M;r=0,\ldots R}$. However, unlike the original framework proposed in [1] where a hard separation of organs was required at each resolution (i.e., $w^r_{ij} = 0$ or 1) (see Fig. 1(b)), we propose the use of new inter-organ correlation factors defined as $\hat{\Omega}^r_j = \prod_{k=r}^{R} \Omega^k_j$, where Ω^k_j are the correlation factors at resolution k obtained via CCA, as described in Sect. 2.1. Since $w^r_{ij} \in (0,1)$, the inter-organ information incorporated by the model, $\hat{\Omega}^r_j$, decreases as we move towards finer level or resolution, and thus, reducing the HDLSS effect. Starting from the finest resolution, the fitting of a new shape y is obtained by applying the modeling process described in Sect. 2.2 at each resolution, $\{y^r\}_{r=0,\ldots,R}$. The high frequency component of the new constrained shape $\tilde{y}^r$, $\tilde{z}^r$, is used to recover the original resolution at the end of the process using the corresponding synthesis filters: $\tilde{y}^{r-1} = F^r \tilde{y}^r + G^r \tilde{z}^r$ (see [8]).

3.2   Sequential Multi-organ Shape Modeling

Suppose now $\{x_1, x_2, x_3, x_4\}$ represents an ordered sequence of organs from highest to lowest stability, as the one depicted in Fig. 1(c) and presented by Okada et al. [2] for the segmentation of abdominal organs (in this example x_1: liver, x_2: spleen, x_3: left kidney and x_4: pancreas; the extension to a more general scenario with K organs is straighforward). In their original work, Okada et al. used partial least square regression (PLSR) to obtain an initial estimation of the organs using the previous ones (i.e., the more stable organs) as predictors (see Fig. 1(c)). This initial segmentation was further refined via probability atlas and a shape model of the residuals. This sequential modeling of organs can be easily modeled in SOMOS as follows. Starting with the most stable organ, x_1, the elements of Ω_1 are defined as $w_{ij} = \delta_{1j}$, thereby preventing the propagation of errors from less table organs. Having modeled x_1, Ω_2 and Ω_3 are defined as $w_{ij} = \delta_{\{1,2\}j}$ and $w_{ij} = \delta_{\{1,3\}j}$, respectively, where $\delta_{\{i,k\}j} = 1$ if $j \in \{i,k\}$, and 0 otherwise. Similarly, Ω_4 is defined as $w_{ij} = \delta_{\{1,2,3\}j}$, i.e. all the previous organs will be used to model the least stable organ, the pancreas. When modeling the less stable structures in a new shape $y = (y_1; y_2; y_3; y_4)^T$, the influence of these organs estimating b_j can be controlled by means of the classic weighted PDM formulation [9]

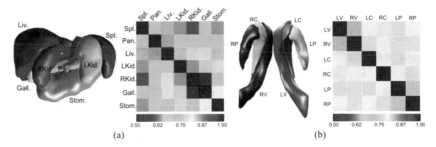

Fig. 2. Canonical Correlation Analysis (CCA) of the organs. (a) CCA of 7 abdominal organs: Spleen (Spl.), pancreas (Pan.), liver (Liv.), left kidney (LKid), right kidney (RKid), gallblader (Gall.) and stomach (Stom.). (b) CCA of 6 subcortical structures: left and right lateral ventricles (LV, RV), left and right caudate nuclei (LC, RC), and left and right putamens (LP,RP).

$b_j = \left(\mathbf{P}_j^T \mathbf{\Psi}_j \mathbf{P}_j\right)^{-1} \mathbf{P}_j^T \mathbf{\Omega}_j^{1/2} (y - \bar{x})$. In particular, $\mathbf{\Psi}_j$ is a $(d \cdot K \times d \cdot K)$ diagonal matrix with corresponding weight value (i.e., reliability) for each landmark. Thus, $diag(\mathbf{\Psi}_1) = (1_{K_1}, 0_{K_2}, 0_{K_3}, 0_{K_4})$, $diag(\mathbf{\Psi}_2) = (1_{K_1}, \psi_2 \cdot 1_{K_2}, 0_{K_3}, 0_{K_4})$, $diag(\mathbf{\Psi}_3) = (1_{K_1}, 0_{K_2}, \psi_3 \cdot 1_{K_3}, 0_{K_4})$, and $diag(\mathbf{\Psi}_2) = (1_{K_1}, \psi_2, 1_{K_2}, \psi_3 \cdot 1_{K_3}, \psi_4, 1_{K_4})$, where 1_k and 0_k represent $(1 \times d \cdot K)$ vectors of 1's and 0's respectively, and $\psi_j \in [0, 1]$ are constants indicating the stability of each organ (and thus, $1 = \psi_1 > \psi_2 \geq \psi_3 > \psi_4$). Similarly to the method proposed by Okada et al. [2], this SOMOS-based sequential shape model can turn into a predictive model for the particular case in which $\psi_2 = \psi_3 = \psi_4 = 0$ (i.e., x_2, x_3, and x_4 are estimated by x_1).

4   Results and Discussion

We use two different datasets to evaluate the ability of SOMOS to model multi-organ structures: a database of 18 CT abdominal studies (voxel resolution: 0.58×0.58 1.00 mm; volume: $512 \times 512 \times 360$) including seven organs (see Fig. 2(a)), and a public database of 18 T1-weighted brain MRI volumes [10] (voxel resolution: $0.94 \times 0.94 \times 1.50$ mm; volume: $256 \times 256 \times 256$ with six subcortical structures (see Fig. 2 (b)).

The most general multi-resolution version of SOMOS (MR-SOMOS) described in Sect. 3.1 is compared with two alternative approaches: GEM-PDM [1], and PDM [4]. Thanks to the flexibility of SOMOS, both approaches, PDM and GEM-PDM, were implemented using the same common framework, to which we refer to as SOMOS-PDM and SOMOS-GEM, respectively. Thus, we define $R = 0$ and $\mathbf{\Omega}^0 = I$ to generate SOMOS-PDM. In SOMOS-GEM we define hard separations between groups of organs at each level of resolution (i.e., $w_{ij}^r = 0$ or 1), following the configuration detailed in [1]. The number of resolution levels is set to 5 (i.e., R = 4) for both, MR-SOMOS and SOMOS-GEM. To characterize the accuracy of the three methods to model new instances we compute the symmetric landmark-to-surface distance (L2S) and Dice coefficient (DC), using leave-one-out cross-validation.

Table 1. Abdominal database – shape modeling accuracy of 7 abdominal structures; * marks statistically significant improvement over PDM; ● marks statistically significant improvement over PDM and GEM (p-value < 0.01).

DC	Spl.	Pan.	Liv.	LKid.	RKid.	Gall.	Stom.	Avg.
MR-SOMOS	●0.85±0.05	*0.82±0.08	*0.86±0.03	●0.87±0.03	*0.87±0.04	●0.74±0.11	*0.83±0.03	●0.82±0.08
SOMOS-GEM	0.82±0.08	0.83±0.05	0.86±0.03	0.74±0.09	0.87±0.04	0.69±0.10	0.82±0.04	0.80±0.09
SOMOS-PDM	0.77±0.08	0.78±0.07	0.82±0.04	0.73±0.14	0.76±0.07	0.60±0.13	0.74±0.06	0.73±0.12

L2S(mm)	Spl.	Pan.	Liv.	LKid.	RKid.	Gall.	Stom.	Avg.
SOMOS	●2.76±0.88	*2.78±0.94	*4.74±1.05	●2.43±0.70	*2.53±0.70	*2.71±1.00	*3.75±1.10	*3.10±1.20
SOMOS-GEM	4.41±0.66	2.74±0.88	3.20±1.30	3.49±1.18	4.05±1.14	3.18±0.99	2.36±0.80	3.35±1.19
SOMOS-PDM	5.60±1.07	3.90±1.33	4.68±1.47	4.57±1.65	5.96±1.81	4.18±1.50	4.50±1.30	4.77±1.59

The results obtained for the abdominal database are shown in Table 1. The new MR-SOMOS (avg. DC: 0.82 ± 0.08; avg. L2S: 3.10 ± 1.20 mm) provides statistically significant improvement (Wilcoxon signed rank test with p-value < 0.01) over both, SOMOS-GEM (avg. DC: 0.80 ± 0.09; avg. L2S: 3.35 ± 1.19 mm) and SOMOS-PDM (avg. DC: 0.73 ± 0.12; avg. L2S: 4.77 ± 1.59 mm). The superiority of the new framework is also proven in the brain database (Table 2). The average DC are 0.93 ± 0.05, 0.87 ± 0.04 and 0.85 ± 0.05, and the average L2S are 0.61 ± 0.13, 0.68 ± 0.11 and 0.78 ± 0.25 mm, for MR-SOMOS, SOMOS-PDM, and SOMOS-GEM, respectively.

Next, we also evaluate the predictive capability of the new framework to estimate a sequence of organs. In particular, we use the four-organ sequence proposed by Okada et al. [2]. Starting with an initial model of the liver, the authors of [2] estimated the spleen and the left kidney via PLSR. The pancreas was finally estimated using the previous three organs as predictors. This PLSR-based approach is compared with the SOMOS predictive model (Sect. 3.2); results are shown in Table 3. The shape of the liver obtained in the previous experiment is used in both cases. It can be observed how the G-PCA-based estimation provided by SOMOS significantly outperforms PLSR-based models ($p < 0.01$) in terms of DC and L2S metric for all the analyzed organs. The ultimate goal is not to provide a final shape, but to generate a shape model-based initial estimation of challenging organs, such as the pancreas, from more stable organs, that will be refined later by other methods (e.g., probabilistic atlas or texture models). Therefore, the metrics shown in Table 1 are better than those shown in Table 3, where only the liver is used to estimate the spleen, left kidney, and spleen.

The computational cost of SOMOS (~ 2 min.) is slightly higher than alternative approaches (PDM: ~ 30 s.; GEM: ~ 1 min.) due to the iterative modeling over each organ (Matlab® R2015a, 64-bits 2.80 GHz Intel® Xeon® with 16 GB or RAM).

Table 2. Brain database – shape modeling accuracy of 6 subcortical structures.

DC	LV	RV	LC	RC	LP	RP	Avg.
SOMOS	*0.86 ±0.06	●0.92 ±0.04	●0.92 ±0.03	●0.93 ±0.01	*0.93 ±0.01	●0.97 ±0.02	●0.93 ±0.05
SOMOS-GEM	0.84 ±0.05	0.84 ±0.04	0.88 ±0.02	0.87 ±0.03	0.90 ±0.01	0.91 ±0.01	0.87 ±0.04
SOMOS-PDM	0.81 ±0.05	0.80 ±0.05	0.87 ±0.03	0.86 ±0.03	0.89 ±0.03	0.98 ±0.02	0.85 ±0.05
L2S(mm)	LV	RV	LC	RC	LP	RP	Avg.
SOMOS	●0.77 ±0.18	●0.76 ±0.20	●0.51 ±0.15	●0.56 ±0.14	●0.55 ±0.08	●0.50 ±0.14	●0.61 ±0.13
SOMOS-GEM	0.82 ±0.19	0.81 ±0.20	0.60 ±0.09	0.68 ±0.14	0.60 ±0.0.09	0.59 ±0.0.06	0.68 ±0.11
SOMOS-PDM	0.99 ±0.21	1.04 ±0.32	0.66 ±0.14	0.70 ±0.14	0.66 ±0.15	0.66 ±0.11	0.78 ±0.25

Table 3. Organ Prediction Model; ● marks statistically significant improvement (p-val. < 0.01).

DC	Liv.	Spl.	LKid.	Pan.
SOMOS	0.87±0.03	●0.66±0.12	●0.79±0.06	●0.51±0.10
PLSR	0.87±0.03	0.43±0.18	0.51±0.12	0.38±0.14
L2S(mm)	Liver	Spleen	L Kidney	Pancreas
SOMOS	2.27±0.68	●5.60±1.62	●3.77±0.92	●5.40±1.64
PLSR	2.27±0.68	12.46±8.20	9.78±3.20	7.77±3.00

5 Conclusions

We presented SOMOS, a new general framework for multi-organ shape modeling. Unlike typical multi-organ approaches where hard divisions between organs are defined, we adopt a more flexible and natural model: a rhizomatic structure in which all the objects are inter-connected. Using CCA to parameterize the model automatically, we propose a new set of weighted statistical shape models able to characterize efficiently the relationships of each organ with the surrounding structures, as well as its own individual variability. Based on a generalization of PCA, the formulation proposed here integrates easily and naturally not only the SOMOS framework, but also previous approaches in the literature, such as the classic PDM, or the most recent GEM-PDM. Experiments with two different databases (abdomen and brain) demonstrate that the new method significantly outperforms alternative approaches in terms of model accuracy, and organ estimation capabilities. Finally, we also evaluated the prediction capability of SOMOS showing a significant improvement over the alternative PLSR-based approach. In the near future we plan to continue expanding the new framework to integrate temporal variability of organs, and non-linear PDM.

Acknowledgment. This project was supported by a philanthropic gift from the Government of Abu Dhabi to Children's National Health System.

References

1. Cerrolaza, J.J., et al.: Automatic multi-resolution shape modeling of multi-organ structures. Med. Image Anal. **25**(1), 11–21 (2015)
2. Okada, T., et al.: Abdominal multi-organ segmentation from ct images using conditional shape-location and unsupervised intensity priors. Med. Image Anal. **26**(1), 1–18 (2015)
3. Wolz, R., et al.: Automated abdominal multi-organ segmentation with subject-specific atlas generation. IEEE Trans. Med. Image **32**(9), 1723–1730 (2013)
4. Cootes, T.F., et al.: Active shape models their training and application. Comput. Vis. Image Underst. **61**(1), 38–59 (1995)
5. Deleuze, G., Guattari, F.: A Thousand Plateaus. Les Editions de Minuit, Paris (1980)
6. Greenacre, M.J.: Theory and Applications of Correspondence Analysis. Academic Press, New York (1984)

7. Rao, A., et al.: Hierarchical statistical shape analysis and prediction of sub-cortical brain structures. Med. Image Anal. **12**(1), 55–68 (2008)
8. Lounsbery, M., et al.: Multiresolution analysis for surfaces of arbitrary topological type. ACM Trans. Graph. **16**(1), 34–73 (1997)
9. Cootes, T.F., Taylor, C.J.: Active shape model search using local grey-level models: a quantitative evaluation. In: BMVC (1993)
10. IBSR. The Internet Brain Segmentation Repository (IBSR). http://www.cma.mgh.harvard.edu/ibsr/

An Artificial Agent for Anatomical Landmark Detection in Medical Images

Florin C. Ghesu[1,2]([✉]), Bogdan Georgescu[1], Tommaso Mansi[1],
Dominik Neumann[1], Joachim Hornegger[2], and Dorin Comaniciu[1]

[1] Medical Imaging Technologies, Siemens Healthineers, Princeton, NJ, USA
florin.c.ghesu@fau.de
[2] Pattern Recognition Lab, Friedrich-Alexander-Universität, Erlangen, Germany

Abstract. Fast and robust detection of anatomical structures or pathologies represents a fundamental task in medical image analysis. Most of the current solutions are however suboptimal and unconstrained by learning an appearance model and exhaustively scanning the space of parameters to detect a specific anatomical structure. In addition, typical feature computation or estimation of meta-parameters related to the appearance model or the search strategy, is based on local criteria or predefined approximation schemes. We propose a new learning method following a fundamentally different paradigm by simultaneously modeling both the object appearance and the parameter search strategy as a unified behavioral task for an artificial agent. The method combines the advantages of behavior learning achieved through reinforcement learning with effective hierarchical feature extraction achieved through deep learning. We show that given only a sequence of annotated images, the agent can automatically and strategically learn optimal paths that converge to the sought anatomical landmark location as opposed to exhaustively scanning the entire solution space. The method significantly outperforms state-of-the-art machine learning and deep learning approaches both in terms of accuracy and speed on 2D magnetic resonance images, 2D ultrasound and 3D CT images, achieving average detection errors of 1-2 pixels, while also recognizing the absence of an object from the image.

1 Introduction

At the core of artificial intelligence is the concept of knowledge-driven computational models which are able to emulate human intelligence. The textbook [8] defines intelligence as the ability of an individual or artificial entity to explore, learn and understand tasks, as opposed to following predefined solution steps.

Machine learning is a fundamental technique used in the context of medical image parsing. The robust detection, segmentation and tracking of the anatomy are essential in both the diagnostic and interventional suite, enabling real-time guidance, quantification and processing in the operating room. Typical

© Springer International Publishing AG 2016
S. Ourselin et al. (Eds.): MICCAI 2016, Part III, LNCS 9902, pp. 229–237, 2016.
DOI: 10.1007/978-3-319-46726-9_27

machine learning models are learned from given data examples using suboptimal, handcrafted features and unconstrained optimization techniques. In addition, any method-related meta-parameters, e.g. ranges, scales, are hand-picked or tuned according to predefined criteria, also in state-of-the-art deep learning solutions [3,11]. As a result, such methods often suffer from computational limitations, sub-optimal parameter optimization or weak generalization due to overfitting, as a consequence of their inability to incorporate or discover intrinsic knowledge about the task at hand [1,5,6]. All aspects related to understanding the given problem and ensuring the generality of the algorithm are the responsibility of the engineer, while the machine, completely decoupled from this higher level of understanding, blindly executes the solution [8].

In this paper we make a step towards self-taught virtual agents for image understanding and demonstrate the new technique in the context of medical image parsing by formulating the landmark detection problem as a generic learning task for an artificial agent. Inspired by the work of Mnih et al. [7], we leverage state-of-the-art representation learning techniques through deep learning [1] and powerful solutions for generic behavior learning through reinforcement learning [10] to create a model encapsulating a cognitive-like learning process to discover strategies, i.e. optimal search paths for localizing arbitrary landmarks. In other words, we enable the machine to learn how to optimally search for a target as opposed to following time-consuming exhaustive search schemes. In parallel to our work, similar ideas have been exploited also in the context of 2D object detection [2].

2   Background

Building powerful artificial agents that can emulate or even surpass human performance at given tasks requires the use of an automatic, generic learning model inspired from human cognitive models [8]. The artificial agent needs to be equipped with at least two fundamental capabilities to achieve intelligence. At perceptual level is the automatic capturing and disentangling of high-dimensional signal data describing the environment, while on cognitive level is the ability to reach decisions and act upon the observed information [8]. Deep learning and reinforcement learning provide the tools to build such capabilities.

2.1   Deep Representation Learning

Inspired by the feed-forward type of information processing observable in the early visual cortex, the deep convolutional neural network (CNN) represents a powerful representation learning mechanism with an automated feature design, closely emulating the principles of the animal and human receptive fields [1]. The architecture is composed of hierarchical layers of translation-invariant convolutional filters based on local spatial correlations observable in images. Denoting the l-th convolutional filter kernel in the layer k by $\boldsymbol{w}^{(k,l)}$, we can write the representation map generated by this filter as: $o_{i,j} = \sigma((\boldsymbol{w}^{(k,l)} * \boldsymbol{x})_{i,j} + b^{(k,l)})$,

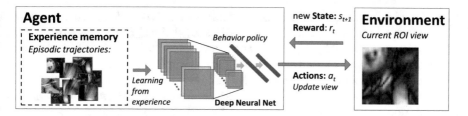

Fig. 1. System diagram showing the interaction of the artificial agent with the environment for landmark detection. The state s_t at time t is defined by the current view, given as an image window. The actions of the agent directly impact the environment, resulting in a new state and a quantitative feedback: (s_{t+1}, r_t). The experience memory stores the visited states, which are periodically sampled to learn the behavior policy.

where x denotes the representation map from the previous layer (used as input), (i, j) define the evaluation location of the filter and $b^{(k,l)}$ represents the neuron bias. The function σ represents the activation function used to synthesize the input information. In our experiments we use rectified linear unit activations (ReLU) given their excellent performance. In a supervised setup, i.e. given a set of independent observations as input patches $\boldsymbol{X}$ with corresponding value assignments $\boldsymbol{y}$, we can define the network response function as $\mathcal{R}(\,\cdot\,; \boldsymbol{w}, \boldsymbol{b})$ and use Maximum Likelihood Estimation to estimate the optimal network parameters: $\hat{\boldsymbol{w}}, \hat{\boldsymbol{b}} = \arg\min_{\boldsymbol{w},\boldsymbol{b}} \|\mathcal{R}(\boldsymbol{X}; \boldsymbol{w}, \boldsymbol{b}) - \boldsymbol{y}\|_2^2$. We solve this optimization problem with a stochastic gradient descent (SGD) approach combined with the backpropagation algorithm to compute the network gradients.

2.2 Cognitive Modeling Using Reinforcement Learning

Reinforcement learning (RL) is a technique aimed at effectively describing learning as an end-to-end cognitive process [9]. A typical RL setting involves an artificial agent that can interact with an uncertain environment, thereby aiming to reach predefined goals. The agent can observe the state of the environment and choose to act on it, similar to a trial-and-error search [9], maximizing the future reward signal received as a supervised response from the environment (see Fig. 1). This reward-based decision process is modeled in RL theory as a *Markov Decision Process* (MDP) [9] $\mathcal{M} := (\mathcal{S}, \mathcal{A}, \mathcal{T}, \mathcal{R}, \gamma)$, where: $\mathcal{S}$ represents a finite set of states over time, $\mathcal{A}$ represents a finite set of actions allowing the agent to interact with the environment, $\mathcal{T} : \mathcal{S} \times \mathcal{A} \times \mathcal{S} \to [0; 1]$ is a stochastic transition function, where $\mathcal{T}_{s,a}^{s'}$ describes the probability of arriving in state s' after performing action a in state s, $\mathcal{R} : \mathcal{S} \times \mathcal{A} \times \mathcal{S} \to \mathbb{R}$ is a scalar reward function, where $\mathcal{R}_{s,a}^{s'}$ denotes the expected reward after a state transition, and γ is the discount factor controlling future versus immediate rewards.

Formally, the future discounted reward of an agent at time $\hat{t}$ can be written as $R_{\hat{t}} = \sum_{t=\hat{t}}^{T} \gamma^{t-\hat{t}} r_t$, with T marking the end of a learning episode and r_t defining the immediate reward the agent receives at time t. Especially in model-free reinforcement learning, the target is to find the optimal so called action-value function, denoting the maximum expected future discounted reward when starting in state s and performing action a: $Q^*(s,a) = \max_\pi \mathbb{E}[R_t | s_t = s, a_t = a, \pi]$, where π is an action policy, in other words a probability distribution over actions in each given state. Once the optimal action-value function is estimated the optimal action policy, determining the behavior of the agent, can be directly computed in each state: $\forall s \in \mathcal{S} : \pi^*(s) = \arg\max_{a \in \mathcal{A}} Q^*(s,a)$. One important relation satisfied by the optimal action-value function Q^* is the Bellman optimality equation [9]. This is defined as:

$$Q^*(s,a) = \sum_{s'} \mathcal{T}_{s,a}^{s'} \left(\mathcal{R}_{s,a}^{s'} + \gamma \max_{a'} Q^*(s',a') \right) = \mathbb{E}_{s'} \left(r + \gamma \max_{a'} Q^*(s',a') \right), \quad (1)$$

where s' defines a possible state visited after s, a' the corresponding action and $r = \mathcal{R}_{s,a}^{s'}$ represents a compact notation for the current, immediate reward. Viewed as an operator τ, the Bellman equation defines a contraction mapping. Strong theoretical results [9] show that by iteratively applying $Q_{i+1} = \tau(Q_i), \forall (s,a)$, the function Q_i converges to Q^* at infinity. This standard, model-based policy iteration approach is however not always feasible in practice. An alternative is the use of model-free temporal difference methods, typically Q-Learning [10], which exploit correlations of consecutive states. A step further towards a higher computational efficiency is the use of parametric functions to approximate the Q-function. Considering the expected non-linear structure of the Q-function [10], neural networks represent a potentially powerful solution for policy approximation [7]. In the following we leverage these techniques in an effort to make a step towards machine-driven intelligence for image parsing.

3   Proposed Method

We propose to formulate the image parsing problem as a deep-learning-driven behavior policy encoding automatic, intelligent paths in parametric space towards the correct solution. Let us consider the example of landmark detection. The optimal search policy in this case represents a trajectory in image space converging to the landmark location $p \in \mathbb{R}^d$ (d is the image dimensionality).

3.1   Agent Learning Model

As previously motivated, we model this new paradigm with an MDP $\mathcal{M}$. While the system dynamics $\mathcal{T}$ are implicitly modeled through our deep-learning-based policy approximation, the state space $\mathcal{S}$, the action space $\mathcal{A}$ and reward/feedback scheme $\mathcal{R}$ need to be explicitly designed:

- **States** describe the surrounding environment - in our context we model this as a focus of attention, a region of interest in the image with its center representing the current position of the agent.

- **Actions** denote the moves of the agent in the parametric space. We select a discrete action-scheme allowing the agent to move one pixel in all directions: *up, down, left, right* - corresponding to a shift of the image patch. This allows the agent to explore the entire image space.
- **Rewards** encode the supervised feedback received by the agent. Opposed to typical choices [7], we propose to follow more closely a standard human learning environment, where rewards are scaled according to the quality of a specific move. We select the reward to be δd, the supervised relative distance-change to the landmark location after executing a move.

3.2   Deep Reinforcement Learning for Image Parsing

Given the model definition, the goal of the agent is to select actions by inter-acting with the environment in order to maximize cumulative future reward. The optimal behavior is defined by the optimal policy π^* and implicitly optimal action-value function Q^*. In this work we propose a model-free, temporal difference approach introduced in the context of game learning by Mnih *et al.* [7], using a deep CNN to approximate the optimal action-value function Q^*. Defining the parameters of a deep CNN as θ, we use this architecture as a generic, non-linear function approximator $Q(s, a; \theta) \approx Q^*(s, a)$ called deep Q network (DQN). A deep Q network can be trained in this context using an iterative approach to minimize the mean squared error based on the Bellman optimality criterion (see Eq. 1). At any learning iteration i, we can approximate the optimal expected target values using a set of reference parameters $\theta_i^{ref} := \theta_j$ from a previous iteration $j < i$: $y = r + \gamma \max_{a'} Q(s', a'; \theta_i^{ref})$. As such we obtain a sequence of well-defined optimization problems driving the evolution of the network parameters. The error function at each step i is defined as:

$$\hat{\theta}_i = \arg\min_{\theta_i} \mathbb{E}_{s,a,r,s'}\left[(y - Q(s, a; \theta_i))^2\right] + \mathbb{E}_{s,a,r}\left[\mathbb{V}_{s'}[y]\right]. \qquad (2)$$

This is a standard, supervised setup for DL in both 2D and 3D (see Sect. 2).

Reference Update-Delay. Using a different network to compute the reference values for training brings robustness to the algorithm. In such a setup, changes to the current parameters θ_i and implicitly to the current approximator $Q(\cdot\,; \theta_i)$ cannot directly impact the reference output y, introducing an update-delay and thereby reducing the probability to diverge and oscillate in suboptimal regions of the optimization space [7].

Experience Replay. To ensure the robustness of the parameter updates and train more efficiently, we propose to use the concept of experience replay [4]. In experience replay, the agent stores a limited memory of previously visited states as a set of explored trajectories: $\mathcal{E} = [t_1, t_2, \cdots, t_P]$. This memory is constantly sampled randomly to generate mini-batches guiding the robust training of the CNN and implicitly of the agent behavior policy.

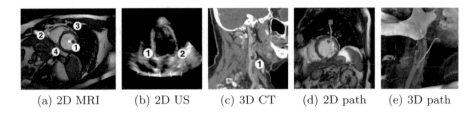

| (a) 2D MRI | (b) 2D US | (c) 3D CT | (d) 2D path | (e) 3D path |

Fig. 2. Figures depicting the landmarks considered in the experiments. Figure (a) shows the LV-center (1), RV-extreme (2) and the anterior / posterior RV-insertion points (3) / (4) in a short-axis cardiac MR image. Figure (b) highlights the mitral septal annulus (1) and the mitral lateral annulus points (2) in a cardiac ultrasound image and figure (c) the right carotid artery bifurcation (1) in a head-neck CT scan. Figures (d) and (e) depict trajectories/optimal paths followed by the agent for detection, blue denotes the random starting point, red the groundtruth and green the optimal path. (Color figure online)

4   Experiments

Accurate landmark detection is a fundamental prerequisite for medical image analysis. We developed a research prototype to demonstrate the performance of the proposed approach on this type of application for 2D magnetic resonance (MR), ultrasound (US) and 3D computed tomography (CT) images.

4.1   Datasets

We use three datasets containing 891 short-axis view MR images from 338 patients, 1186 cardiac ultrasound apical four-chamber view images from 361 patients and 455 head-neck CT scans from 455 patients. The landmarks selected for testing are presented in Fig. 2. The train/cross-validation/test dataset split is performed randomly at patient level, for the MR dataset 711/90/90 images, for the US dataset 991/99/96 images and for the CT dataset 341/56/58 images. The results on the MR dataset are compared to the state-of-the art results achieved in [5,6] with methods combining context modeling with machine-learning for robust landmark detection. Please note that we use the same dataset as [5,6], but a different train/test split. On the CT dataset we compare to [11], a state-of-the-art deep learning solution combined with exhaustive hypotheses scanning. Here we use the same dataset and data split. In terms of preprocessing we resample the images to isotropic resolution, $2\,mm$ in 2D and $1\,mm$ in 3D.

4.2   Learning How to Find Landmarks

The learning occurs in episodes in which the agent explores random paths in random training images, constantly updating the experience memory and implicitly the search policy modeled by the deep CNN. Based on the cross-validation set we systematically select the meta-parameters and number of training rounds

Table 1. Table showing the detection error on the test sets with superior results highlighted in bold. The error is quantified as the distance to the ground-truth, measured in *mm*. With * we signify that the results are reported on the same dataset, but on a different training/test data-split than ours.

	Detection error [mm]											
	2D-MRI								2D-US		3D-CT	
	LV-center		RV-ext		RV-post			RV-ant	M-sep	M-lat	Bifurc.	
	Our	[6]	Our	[5]	Our	[6]	[5]	Our	Our	Our	Our	[11]
Mean	**1.8**	6.2*	**4.9**	8.4*	**2.2**	7.9*	5.9*	**3.7**	**1.3**	**1.6**	**1.8**	2.6
Median	**1.7**	5.4*	**4.2**	5.9*	**1.8**	4.7*	3.9*	**3.0**	**1.2**	**1.3**	**0.8**	1.2
STD	**2.2**	4.0*	**3.6**	16.5*	**1.5**	11.5*	16.0*	**2.3**	**0.8**	**1.4**	**2.9**	5.0

following a grid search: $\gamma = 0.9$, replay memory size $P = 100000$, learning rate $\eta = 0.00025$ and ROI 60^2 pixels, respectively 26^3 voxels. The network topology is composed of 3 convolution+pooling layers followed by 3 fully-connected layers with dropout. We emphasize that except for the adaptation of the CNN to use 3D kernels on 3D data, the meta-parameters are kept fixed for all experiments.

Policy Evaluation. During the evaluation the agent starts in a random state and follows the optimal policy with *no* knowledge about the groundtruth, navigating through the image space until an oscillation occurs - an infinite loop between two neighboring states, indicating the location of the sought landmark. The location is considered a high-confidence landmark detection if the expected reward from this location $\max_a Q^*(s_{target}, a) < 1$, i.e. the agent is closer than one pixel. This means the policy is consistent, rejecting the possibility of a local optimum and giving a powerful confidence measure about the detection. Table 1 shows the results on the test sets for all modalities and landmarks.

Object not in the Image? Using this property we not only detect diverging trajectories, but can also recognize if the landmark is not contained in the image. For example we evaluated trained agents on 100 long-axis cardiac MR images from different patients, observing that in such cases the oscillation occurs at points where $\max_a Q^*(s_{target}, a) > 4$. This suggests the ability of our algorithm to detect when the anatomical landmark is absent. (see Fig. 3(c–d)).

Convergence. We observed in random test images that typically more than 90 % of the possible start points converge to the solution (see Fig. 3(a–b)).

Speed Performance. While typical state-of-the-art methods [3,11] exhaustively scan solution hypotheses in large 2D or 3D spaces, the agent follows a simple path (see Fig. 2(d-e)). The average speed-up to scanning with a similar network (see for example [11]) is around **80× in 2D** and **3100×** in **3D**. The very fast detection in 3D in less than 0.05 seconds highlights the potential of this technology for real-time applications, such as tracking of anatomical objects.

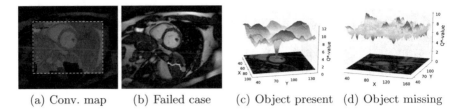

(a) Conv. map   (b) Failed case   (c) Object present   (d) Object missing

Fig. 3. Figure (a) highlights in transparent red all the starting positions converging to the landmark location (the border is due to the window-based search). Figure (b) shows an example of a failed case. Figures (c) and (d) visualize the optimal action-value function Q^* for two images, the latter not containing the landmark. For this image there is no clear global minimum, indicating the absence of the landmark.

5   Conclusion

In conclusion, in this paper we presented a new learning paradigm in the context of medical image parsing, training intelligent agents that overcome the limitations of standard machine learning approaches. Based on a Q-Learning inspired framework, we used state-of-the-art deep learning techniques to directly approximate the optimal behavior of the agent in a trial-and-error environment. We evaluated our approach on various landmarks from different image modalities showing that the agent can automatically discover and efficiently evaluate strategies for landmark detection at high accuracy.

References

1. Bengio, Y., Courville, A.C., Vincent, P.: Unsupervised Feature Learning and Deep Learning: A Review and New Perspectives. CoRR abs/1206.5538 (2012)
2. Caicedo, J.C., Lazebnik, S.: Active object localization with deep reinforcement learning. In: IEEE ICCV, pp. 2488–2496 (2015)
3. Ghesu, F.C., Krubasik, E., Georgescu, B., Singh, V., Zheng, Y., Hornegger, J., Comaniciu, D.: Marginal space deep learning: efficient architecture for volumetric image parsing. IEEE TMI **35**(5), 1217–1228 (2016)
4. Lin, L.J.: Reinforcement Learning for Robots Using Neural Networks. Ph.D. thesis, Carnegie Mellon University, Pittsburgh, PA, USA (1992)
5. Lu, X., Georgescu, B., Jolly, M.-P., Guehring, J., Young, A., Cowan, B., Littmann, A., Comaniciu, D.: Cardiac anchoring in MRI through context modeling. In: Jiang, T., Navab, N., Pluim, J.P.W., Viergever, M.A. (eds.) MICCAI 2010, Part I. LNCS, vol. 6361, pp. 383–390. Springer, Heidelberg (2010)
6. Lu, X., Jolly, M.-P.: Discriminative context modeling using auxiliary markers for LV landmark detection from a single MR image. In: Camara, O., Mansi, T., Pop, M., Rhode, K., Sermesant, M., Young, A. (eds.) STACOM 2012. LNCS, vol. 7746, pp. 105–114. Springer, Heidelberg (2013)
7. Mnih, V., Kavukcuoglu, K., Silver, D., Rusu, A.A., Veness, J., Bellemare, M.G., Graves, A., Riedmiller, M., Fidjeland, A.K., Ostrovski, G., Petersen, S., Beattie, C., Sadik, A., Antonoglou, I., King, H., Kumaran, D., Wierstra, D., Legg, S., Hassabis, D.: Human-level control through deep reinforcement learning. Nature **518**(7540), 529–533 (2015)

8. Russell, S.J., Norvig, P.: Artificial Intelligence: A Modern Approach, 2nd edn. Pearson Education, Upper Saddle River (2003)
9. Sutton, R.S., Barto, A.G.: Introduction to Reinforcement Learning, 1st edn. MIT Press, Cambridge (1998)
10. Watkins, C.J.C.H., Dayan, P.: Q-learning. Mach. Learn. **8**(3), 279–292 (1992)
11. Zheng, Y., Liu, D., Georgescu, B., Nguyen, H., Comaniciu, D.: 3D deep learning for efficient and robust landmark detection in volumetric data. In: Navab, N., Hornegger, J., Wells, W.M., Frangi, A.F. (eds.) MICCAI 2015. LNCS, vol. 9349, pp. 565–572. Springer, Heidelberg (2015). doi:10.1007/978-3-319-24553-9_69

Identifying Patients at Risk for Aortic Stenosis Through Learning from Multimodal Data

Tanveer Syeda-Mahmood[(✉)], Yufan Guo, Mehdi Moradi, D. Beymer,
D. Rajan, Yu Cao, Yaniv Gur, and Mohammadreza Negahdar

IBM Almaden Research Center, San Jose, CA, USA
stf@us.ibm.com

Abstract. In this paper we present a new method of uncovering patients with aortic valve diseases in large electronic health record systems through learning with multimodal data. The method automatically extracts clinically-relevant valvular disease features from five multimodal sources of information including structured diagnosis, echocardiogram reports, and echocardiogram imaging studies. It combines these partial evidence features in a random forests learning framework to predict patients likely to have the disease. Results of a retrospective clinical study from a 1000 patient dataset are presented that indicate that over 25 % new patients with moderate to severe aortic stenosis can be automatically discovered by our method that were previously missed from the records.

1 Introduction

With the growth of big data through large electronic health records (EHR), there is an opportunity to leverage medical image analysis in combination with other modality data in EHR to impact the quality of care to patients in a significant way. In this paper, we present one such clinical study in uncovering patients likely to have aortic stenosis. Aortic stenosis (AS) is a common heart disease that can result in sudden death. It can be diagnosed through the Doppler patterns in echocardiogram studies as shown in Fig. 1b. Although the disease can be treated through surgery or transcatheter aortic valve replacements (AVR), it often goes untreated for several reasons. The absence of chest pain and other symptoms may make the disease asymptomatic and not a candidate for detection in echocardiographer's instructions. This together with echocardiographer's skill errors can cause a

---

The original version of this chapter was revised: Correct name of the author "Yufan Guo" has now been updated. The correction to this chapter is available at https://doi.org/10.1007/978-3-319-46726-9_73

Electronic supplementary material The online version of this chapter (https://doi.org/10.1007/978-3-319-46726-9_28) contains supplementary material, which is available to authorized users.

© Springer International Publishing AG 2016
S. Ourselin et al. (Eds.): MICCAI 2016, Part III, LNCS 9902, pp. 238–245, 2016.
DOI: 10.1007/978-3-319-46726-9_28

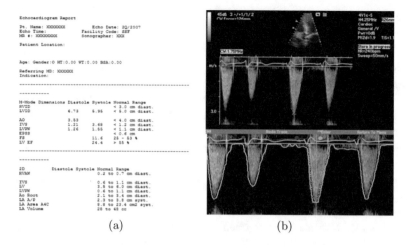

(a)   (b)

Fig. 1. Illustration of missed diagnosis from echocardiogram (a) reports and (b) images

Doppler pattern depicting the disease to be missed entirely. Figure 1b (top) shows one such case where the echocardiographer missed the evidence for moderate aortic stenosis in the Doppler spectrum. When the relevant measurements are made by the echocardiographer and inserted into the study screens, they may still fail to make it into the overall report. Finally, even if the pattern is detected and makes it into the echocardiogram report, pure data entry errors in EHR can leave out the evidence of the disease from a patient record. With thousands of echocardiography studies taken annually, manual peer review is costly and rarely performed, with the result that many patients are going untreated.

The goal of this work is to develop an automated method for retrospectively predicting patients likely to have aortic stenosis by combining medical image analysis of Doppler patterns with textual content analysis of imaging and reports in a multimodal learning framework. Specifically, we extract evidence of aortic stenosis from 5 sources, namely, (a) billable diagnosis, (b) significant problems from EHR, (c) echocardiogram reports, (d) measurements shown on echocardiography video frames, and (e) CW Doppler patterns in echocardiography videos. Disease concepts are identified in echocardiogram reports using a concept extraction algorithm to detect UMLS concept vocabularies and their relevant associated measurements. Measurements captured by echocardiographers are reliably extracted through selective image processing and optical character recognition in tabular regions on echocardiogram video frames. Finally, diagnostically relevant measurements for aortic stenosis are automatically extracted from Doppler envelopes using a three step process of relevant Doppler frame identification, envelope tracing and measurement extraction. The frame identification involved classification of convolutional neural network (CNN)-based learned features from Doppler regions. The envelop extraction was made robust by incorporating echocardiographer's tracings. Finally the disease-specific features extracted from each multimodal source of information are combined using a random forest learning formulation to predict patients that are likely to have aortic valve disease.

2   Related Work

To our knowledge, this is the first work on identifying patients at risk that combines medical text and image analysis of echocardiogram studies. While previous studies have argued for the use of multimodal information for cohort identification [7], the primary information leveraged was either structured or textual data. The work reported here, however, overlaps three inter-disciplinary fields of text analysis, optical character recognition (OCR), and medical image analysis each of which is rich in literature. Several algorithms for extraction of clinical concepts from text have been reported in [9]. However, measurements must be extracted in addition to disease name mentions for aortic stenosis detection, which has not been addressed previously. Similarly, while there is considerable work in OCR in general, extracting clinical measurements from text screens of echocardiogram studies has not been well-addressed with the reported methods relying on manual creation of templates for various manufacturer's echo screens [8]. Finally, reliable extraction of Doppler envelopes has proved to be notoriously challenging particularly in the presence of electrocardiogram (ECG) fluctuations during arrhythmia and overlay artifacts in Doppler spectra [3,5,9]. Lastly, the automatic selection of Doppler frames depicting aortic valves has not been previously reported in literature.

3   Disease Evidence Extraction from Multimodal Data

Disease Extraction from Reports. To extract evidence of aortic stenosis from echocardiogram reports, we generated a large knowledge graph of over 5.6 million concept terms by combining over 70 reference vocabularies such as SNOMED CT, ICD9, ICD10, RadLex, RxNorm, and LOINC and used its concept nodes as vocabulary phrases. The occurrences of clinical concepts within sentences of the clinical reports uses the longest common subfix (LCF) algorithm as described in [9]. To detect evidence of stenosis, we find tuples of $< D_i, S_j, A_k, V_l >$, where D_i are disease name indicators (e.g. "aortic valve disorders", "aortic valve stenosis", etc.), S_j are specific symptoms associated with the disease such as "chest pain", A_k are anatomical abnormalities such as "thickened", "calcified", and V_l are qualifiers such as "mild, moderate, severe". These detections are done within neighboring sentences in selected paragraphs where the aortic valve is described in echocardiogram reports.

Next, we selected key measurement names indicating aortic stenosis as per AHA guidelines, namely, peak velocity, mean pressure gradient, and aortic valve area. Using their values ranges and units, as per guidelines, we developed a measurement name-value pair detector. As the spoken utterances of these names vary in echocardiograms, we did a n-gram analysis of a corpus of over 50,000 reports in our data collection to identify all such significant variants of the measurement names. To detect occurrences of measurement names and their associated values within the context of a detected sentence, we analyze the pattern of their occurrences in a sentence using part-of-speech (POS) tagging, and dependency graph parsing [4]. For each root concept (e.g. 'gradient'), a chain of its modifiers

Table 1. False discovery rate (FDR) of disease (AS) and measurement (peak velocity and mean gradient) detection.

	FDR	False positives
AS	2/191	Indication/Hx: EVAL FOR MS/MR, **AS**/AI
		De-Identified **AS** SMOKER
Peak velocity	1/364	aortic stenosis is present. The **aortic valve peak velocity** is 2.6 ↩ **9 m/s**, the peak gradient is 28.9 mmHg,
Mean gradient	0/410	-

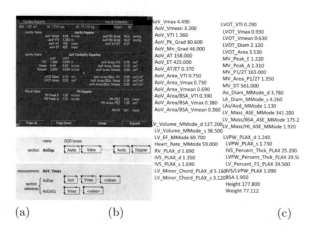

(a)   (b)   (c)

Fig. 2. Illustration of measurement extraction from echocardiography screens.

(in the form of nouns or adjectives, e.g. 'mean trans aortic') were automatically identified from a sentence using the Stanford POS tagger [4]. By analyzing thousands of sentences containing the occurrences of measurement vocabulary terms in connection with measurement values and units, we formed regular expression patterns, such a pattern "$< A >< B >< C >$" where "A" is any disease indicating phrase A: {aorta, aortic, AV, AS}, "B" is any measurement term {gradient, velocity, area}, and C is no negation terms of the kind {no, not, without, neither, none}. Once the pattern was matched, we looked for numeric values following the measurement names in the same sentence that were juxtaposed with names of relevant units. An example of aortic stenosis measurement extraction is illustrated below in bold.

Aortic Valve: The **aortic valve** is thickened and calcified. Severe **aortic stenosis** is present. The **aortic valve peak velocity** is **6.18 m/s**, the peak gradient is 152.8 mmHg, and the **mean gradient** is **84.9 mmHg**. The **aortic valve area** is estimated to be **0.28 cm2**.

In general, the text-based aortic stenosis detection is fairly stable with very few false positives as indicated in Table 1. Only 3 errors were observed after a thorough analysis of the detected cases, as listed in the third column.

Table 2. Accuracy of Doppler envelop extraction and measurement calculation.

Measurement made	Images tested	Error
V_{max}	1054	$0.29 \pm 0.78\,\mathrm{m/s}$
M_g	785	$0.08 \pm 10.05\,\mathrm{mmHg}$
+		

Extracting Echocardiographer Measurements. The evidence for aortic stenosis can be extracted from the measurements made by the echocardiographer captured as text-only screens such as the one shown in Fig. 2a. To extract the measurements, we select the frames depicting the measurements and apply relevant tabular template to identify the semantic names of the measurements. An optical character recognition algorithm is then used to extract text. Unlike the approach in [8], we use a different OCR engine (DataCap) and learn the document layout templates of device manufacturer's screens automatically. The template learning is focused per anatomical region and exploits the invariance in topological layout of the measurement name value pairs in the tabular regions. Once the templates are learned, they are matched to any given text only screen to read off the expected measurement names. Following the approach in [8], we process the images within the text regions through an image enhancement process to increase the robustness of OCR. Figure 2c shows the text extracted from measurement screen of Fig. 2a using our video text detection algorithm. The OCR-based measurement extraction module was tested on 114 text-only frames across 114 patients, and a total of 1719 measurements were verified. For this validation set, our system extracted 99.7 % of the measurements correctly, with the remaining errors caused by the numeric values being split by the OCR engine.

Disease Extraction from Doppler Image Analysis. In Doppler echocardiography images, the clinically relevant region is known to be within the Doppler spectrum, contained in a rectangular region of interest as shown in Fig. 1b. To ensure the measurement extraction is attempted on relevant frames depicting the aortic valve, we developed a classifier using features derived from the region depicting Doppler patterns in images. This image region was fed to a pre-trained convolutional neural network (CNN) consisting of 5 convolution layers, two fully connected layers and a SoftMax layer with 1000 output nodes [2]. The CNN is being used as a feature generator here as has been reported in other literature [6]. Even though the CNN was trained in another imaging domain, the earlier layers of the neural network capture generic features such as edges which are also applicable in our domain. For our task of feature generation, we harvest a feature vector of size 4096 at the output of the first fully connected layer of the network and classify the images using a support vector machine (SVM) classifier. To train the SVM, we created an expert reviewed dataset of 496 CW Doppler patterns, each labeled with one of the four valve types. A set consisting of 100 of these images was randomly isolated as a test set. The SVM was optimized for kernel type and slack and kernel variables on the remaining 396 images using five-fold cross validation. Using the CNN derived features, the SVM achieved an accuracy of 92 % across all valves with all aortic valve CW Doppler frames being labeled correctly. The tricuspid stenosis valve pattern accounted for nearly half the errors as it is similar to the aortic stenosis valve pattern.

Extraction of Doppler Patterns. Our method of extracting Doppler spectrum uses similar pre-processing steps of region of interest detection, ECG extraction, and periodicity detection as described in [9], but adds a major enhancement exploiting the tracings of echocardiographers as shown in Fig. 3. To extract echocardiographer's envelope annotation, we exclude the calculated Doppler velocity profile from the ROI and apply Otsu's thresholding algorithm on the remaining image to highlight the manual delineation which is connected to the baseline. Then, we add the extracted annotation to the filled up largest region, as shown in Fig. 3 and trace the boundary pixels. The Doppler envelop extraction was tested on over 7000 images during training, and the results of the various stages of processing are indicated in Table 2.

Measurement Extraction from Doppler Patterns. Using the AHA guidelines, the maximum jet velocity (V_{max}) is defined as the peak velocity in the negative direction for the Doppler pattern for aortic stenosis. Since the Doppler envelope traces are available, the pixel value of the negative peak in the Doppler spectra can be easily noted. To convert the imaging-based measurement to a physical velocity value, we analyze the text calibration markers on the vertical axis in the ROI using OCR engine to read off the velocity value. The maximum value of velocity during systole within each cycle is a candidate for the V_{max}. The second measurement indicative of aortic stenosis is mean pressure gradient (MPG). MPG is calculated from velocity information following the estimation reported in [1] as $M_g \approx \sum_V \frac{4V^2}{N}$ where N is the number of pixels within the QT interval of ECG, and V is the velocity.

Disease Prediction using Multimodal Learning. Collecting all the measurements derived from each modality processing, we form a feature vector as follows.

$$F_p = \{V_{1b}, V_{2s}, V_{3t}, V_{4t}, V_{5t}, V_{6o}, V_{7o}, V_{8i}, V_{9i}\} \tag{1}$$

where the 'b' is for billable diagnosis, 's' for significant problems, 't' for textual reports, 'o' for video text, and 'i' for image analysis features. The first 3 features are binary while the rest are actual measurements made in the respective modalities. To train the predictor, we use a set of patients with known aortic stenosis (confirmed diagnosis in EHR), and learn the correlation between feature values and the disease label (aortic stenosis) using a random forests learner. The random forests were constructed with 100 trees, with each tree having a minimum node size of 10, and maximum depth of 10.

4   Clinical Study Results

We conducted a retrospective clinical study on a large patient data set acquired from a nearby hospital. The experimental context was to evaluate if there were missed diagnosis of aortic stenosis in their records when in fact evidence could be

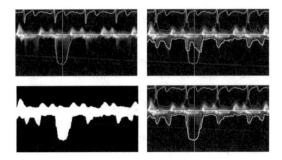

Fig. 3. Illustration of Doppler envelop extraction using echocardiographer annotations.

Table 3. Comparative performance of rule-based baseline and random forest with features extracted from structured information, reports, images, and OCR text. min(I,O) refers to the fusion of image and OCR features by taking the minimum of the two for each individual feature/parameter.

	Features					Performance			
	Structured	Report	Image	OCR	min(I,O)	Precision	Recall	F-score	Accuracy
Baseline	x	x	x	x		0.84	1.00	0.93	0.92
	x					1.00	0.53	0.70	0.81
		x				0.96	0.55	0.70	0.81
			x			0.80	0.50	0.62	0.75
				x		0.94	0.50	0.66	0.79
Random					x	0.94	0.56	0.70	0.81
Forest			x	x		0.78	0.59	0.67	0.77
		x			x	0.93	0.73	0.82	0.87
		x	x	x		0.82	0.71	0.77	0.83
	x	x			x	**0.96**	**0.89**	**0.92**	**0.94**
	x	x	x	x		0.87	0.89	0.88	0.90

found from the underlying clinical data. Specifically, we restricted the analysis to patients for which all 4 modalities of information were available, namely, billable diagnosis, significant problems, and echocardiogram reports and imaging studies giving rise to a total of 991 patients with 1,226 reports and 121,811 Doppler images. These studies were independently validated clinically and 395 patients were found to have aortic stenosis serving as the ground truth.

A 10 fold cross-validation was done by randomly splitting the data into 10 folds, 9 for training and 1 for testing. Table 3 shows the precision, recall, F-score, and overall accuracy of the baseline and random forests with different combinations of features, including a fusion of image and OCR features – referred to as min(I,O). Selecting the minimum of these two values gave a more conservative estimate of the severity of the disease. Out of the 395 patients manually identified by experts, 99 were newly discovered patients from our multimodal analysis giving rise to over 25 % new discoveries.

Comparison Against Baseline. Our baseline was a rule-based model, which returned all patients with at least one piece of evidence from any of the five sources. Here the evidence was either the presence of disease mentions or exceeding the normal ranges for V_{max} and M_g according to the AHA guidelines. The best-performing model was a random forest with features from all the different sources, achieving 96 % precision that is 12 % higher than the baseline. Combining features using random forests compensates for potential errors in individual modality detections, making its precision higher than the baseline method. The higher precision will reduce unnecessarily flagging of patients which would have otherwise have lowered the confidence in such prediction system for practical uses.

5 Conclusions

In this paper we have presented a new use of medical image analysis in combination with textual and other multimodal data analysis for purposes of identifying patient cohorts at risk for serious diseases such as aortic stenosis. While the textual detection method can be easily generalized for other diseases, future work will focus on developing disease detectors in imaging modalities to augment the decision making.

References

1. Baumgartner, H., Hung, J., Bermejo, J., Chambers, J.B., Evangelista, A., Griffin, B.P., Iung, B., Otto, C.M., Pellikka, P.A., Quiñones, M.: Echocardiographic assessment of valve stenosis: EAE/ASE recommendations for clinical practice. Eur. Heart J. Cardiovasc. Imaging **10**(1), 1–25 (2009)
2. Chatfield, K., Simonyan, K., Vedaldi, A., Zisserman, A.: Return of the devil in the details: delving deep into convolutional nets. In: British Machine Vision Conference (2014)
3. Chen, T., Kumar, R., Troianowski, G., Syeda-Mahmood, T., Beymer, D., Brannon, K.: PSAR: predictive space aggregated regression and its application in valvular heart disease classification. In: ISBI, pp. 1122–1125 (2013)
4. Manning, C.D., Surdeanu, M., Bauer, J., Finkel, J., Bethard, S.J., McClosky, D.: The Stanford CoreNLP natural language processing toolkit. In: Association for Computational Linguistics (ACL) System Demonstrations, pp. 55–60 (2014)
5. Shechner, O., Sheinovitz, M., Feinberg, M., Greenspan, H.: Image analysis of doppler echocardiography for patients with atrial fibrillation. In: ISBI, pp. 488–491 (2004)
6. Shin, H.C., Roth, H.R., Gao, M., Lu, L., Xu, Z., Nogues, I., Yao, J., Mollura, D., Summers, R.M.: Deep convolutional neural networks for computer-aided detection: CNN architectures, dataset characteristics and transfer learning. IEEE Trans. Med. Imaging **35**(5), 1285–1298 (2016)
7. Shivade, C., Raghavan, P., Fosler-Lussier, E., Embi, P.J., Elhadad, N., Johnson, S.B., Lai, A.M.: A review of approaches to identifying patient phenotype cohorts using electronic health records. J. Am. Med. Inform. Assoc. **21**(2), 221–230 (2014)
8. Syeda-Mahmood, T., Beymer, D., Amir, A.: Disease-specific extraction of text from cardiac echo videos for decision support. In: ICDAR, pp. 1290–1294 (2009)
9. Syeda-Mahmood, T., Kumar, R., Compas, C.: Learning the correlation between images and disease labels using ambiguous learning. In: Navab, N., Hornegger, J., Wells, W.M., Frangi, A.F. (eds.) MICCAI 2015. LNCS, vol. 9350, pp. 185–193. Springer, Heidelberg (2015). https://doi.org/10.1007/978-3-319-24571-3_23

Multi-input Cardiac Image Super-Resolution Using Convolutional Neural Networks

Ozan Oktay[1]([✉]), Wenjia Bai[1], Matthew Lee[1], Ricardo Guerrero[1],
Konstantinos Kamnitsas[1], Jose Caballero[3], Antonio de Marvao[2], Stuart Cook[2],
Declan O'Regan[2], and Daniel Rueckert[1]

[1] Biomedical Image Analysis Group, Imperial College London, London, UK
o.oktay13@imperial.ac.uk
[2] Institute of Clinical Science, Imperial College London, London, UK
[3] Magic Pony Technology, London, UK

Abstract. 3D cardiac MR imaging enables accurate analysis of cardiac morphology and physiology. However, due to the requirements for long acquisition and breath-hold, the clinical routine is still dominated by multi-slice 2D imaging, which hamper the visualization of anatomy and quantitative measurements as relatively thick slices are acquired. As a solution, we propose a novel image super-resolution (SR) approach that is based on a residual convolutional neural network (CNN) model. It reconstructs high resolution 3D volumes from 2D image stacks for more accurate image analysis. The proposed model allows the use of multiple input data acquired from different viewing planes for improved performance. Experimental results on 1233 cardiac short and long-axis MR image stacks show that the CNN model outperforms state-of-the-art SR methods in terms of image quality while being computationally efficient. Also, we show that image segmentation and motion tracking benefits more from SR-CNN when it is used as an initial upscaling method than conventional interpolation methods for the subsequent analysis.

1 Introduction

3D magnetic resonance (MR) imaging with near isotropic resolution provides a good visualization of cardiac morphology, and enables accurate assessment of cardiovascular physiology. However, 3D MR sequences usually require long breath-hold and repetition times, which leads to scan times that are infeasible in clinical routine, and 2D multi-slice imaging is used instead. Due to limitations on signal-to-noise ratio (SNR), the acquired slices are usually thick compared to the in-plane resolution and thus negatively affect the visualization of anatomy and hamper further analysis. Attempts to improve image resolution are typically carried out either during the acquisition stage (sparse k-space filling) or retrospectively through super resolution (SR) of single/multiple image acquisitions.

Related work: Most of the SR methods recover the missing information through the examples observed in training images, which are used as a prior

© Springer International Publishing AG 2016
S. Ourselin et al. (Eds.): MICCAI 2016, Part III, LNCS 9902, pp. 246–254, 2016.
DOI: 10.1007/978-3-319-46726-9_29

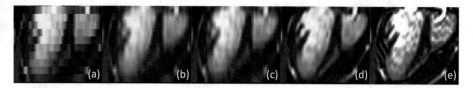

Fig. 1. The low resolution image (a) is upscaled using linear (b) and cubic spline (c) interpolations, and the proposed method (d) which shows a high correlation with the ground-truth high resolution image (e) shown on the rightmost.

to link low and high resolution (LR-HR) image patches. Single image SR methods, based on the way they utilize training data, fall into two categories: non-parametric and parametric. The former aims to recover HR patches from LR ones via a co-occurrence prior between the target image and external training data. Atlas-based approaches such as the patch-match method [15] and non-local means based single image SR [10] methods are two examples of this category. These approaches are computationally demanding as the candidate patches have to be searched in the training dataset to find the most suitable HR candidate. Instead, compact and generative models can be learned from the training data to define the mapping between LR and HR patches. Parametric generative models, such as coupled-dictionary learning based approaches, have been proposed to upscale MR brain [14] and cardiac [3] images. These methods benefit from sparsity constraint to express the link between LR and HR. Similarly, random forest based non-linear regressors have been proposed to predict HR patches from LR data and have been successfully applied on diffusion tensor images [1]. Recently, convolutional neural network (CNN) models [5,6] have been put forward to replace the inference step as they have enough capacity to perform complex nonlinear regression tasks. Even by using a shallow network composed of a few layers, these models [6] achieved superior results over other state-of-the-art SR methods.

Contributions: In the work presented here, we extend the SR-CNN proposed by [5,6] with an improved layer design and training objective function, and show its application to cardiac MR images. In particular, the proposed approach simplifies the LR-HR mapping problem through residual learning and allows training a deeper network to achieve improved performance. Additionally, the new model can be considered more data-adaptive since the initial upscaling is performed by learning a deconvolution layer instead of a fixed kernel [6]. More importantly, a multi-input image extension of the SR-CNN model is proposed and exploited to achieve a better SR image quality. By making use of multiple images acquired from different slice directions one can further improve and constrain the HR image reconstruction. Similar multi-image SR approaches have been proposed in [11,12] to synthesize HR cardiac images; however, these approaches did not make use of available large training datasets to learn the appearance of anatomical structures in HR. Compared to the state-of-the-art image SR approaches [6,15], the proposed method shows improved performance in terms of peak

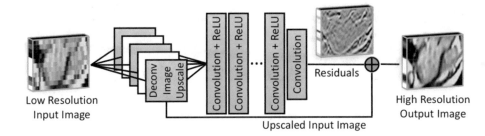

Fig. 2. The proposed single image super resolution network model

signal-to-noise-ratio (PSNR) and structural similarity index measure (SSIM) [18]. We show that cardiac image segmentation can benefit from SR-CNN as the segmentations generated from super-resolved images are shown to be similar to the manual segmentations on HR images in terms of volume measures and surface distances. Lastly, we show that cardiac motion tracking results can be improved using SR-CNN as it visualizes the basal and apical parts of the myocardium more clearly compared to the conventional interpolation methods (see Fig. 1).

2   Methodology

The SR image generation is formulated as an inverse problem that recovers the high dimensional data through the MR image acquisition model [7], which has been the starting point of approaches in [3,11,15]. The model links the HR volume $y \in \mathbb{R}^M$ to the low dimensional observation $x \in \mathbb{R}^N$ ($N \ll M$) through the application of a series of operators as: $x = DBSMy + \eta$ where M defines the spatial displacements caused due to respiratory and cardiac motion, S is the slice selection operator, B is a point-spread function (PSF) used to blur the selected slice, D is a decimation operator, and η is the Rician noise model. The solution to this inverse problem estimates a conditional distribution $p(y|x)$ that minimizes the cost function Ψ defined by y and its estimate $\Phi(x, \Theta)$ obtained from LR input data. The estimate is obtained through a CNN parameterized by Θ that models the distribution $p(y|x)$ via a collection of hidden variables. For the smooth ℓ_1 norm case, the loss function is defined as $\min_{\Theta} \sum_i \Psi_{\ell_1} (\Phi(x_i, \Theta) - y_i)$, where $\Psi_{\ell_1}(r) = \{0.5\,r^2$ if $|r| < 1$, $|r| - 0.5$ otherwise$\}$ and (x_i, y_i) denote the training samples. The next section describes the proposed CNN model.

Single Image Network: The proposed model, shown in Fig. 2, is formed by concatenating a series of convolutional layers (Conv) and rectified linear units (ReLU) [8] to estimate the non-linear mapping Φ, as proposed in [6] to upscale natural images. The intermediate feature maps $h_j^{(n)}$ at layer n are computed through Conv kernels (hidden units) w_{kj}^n as $\max\left(0, \sum_{k=1}^K h_k^{(n-1)} * w_{kj}^n\right) = h_j^n$

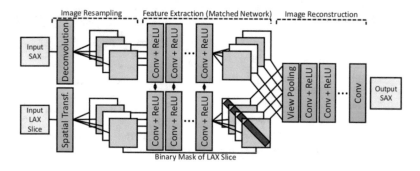

Fig. 3. The proposed Siamese multi-image super resolution network model.

where $*$ is the convolution operator. As suggested by [16], in order to obtain better non-linear estimations, the proposed architecture uses small Conv kernels $(3 \times 3 \times 3)$ and a large number of Conv+ReLU layers. Such approach allows training of a deeper network. Different to the models proposed in [5,6], we include an initial upscaling operation within the model as a deconvolution layer (Deconv) $(\boldsymbol{x} \uparrow U) * w_j = h_j^0$ where $\uparrow$ is a zero-padding upscaling operator and $U = M/N$ is the upscaling factor. In this way, upsampling filters can be optimized for SR applications by training the network in an end-to-end manner. This improves the image signal quality in image regions closer to the boundaries. Instead of learning to synthesize a HR image, the CNN model is trained to predict the residuals between the LR input data and HR ground-truth information. These residuals are later summed up with the linearly upscaled input image (output of Deconv layer) to reconstruct the output HR image. In this way, a simplified regression function Φ is learned where mostly high frequency signal components, such as edges and texture, are predicted (see Fig. 2). At training time, the correctness of reconstructed HR images is evaluated based on the $\Psi_{\ell_1}(.)$ function, and the model weights are updated by back-propagating the error defined by that function. In [19] the ℓ_1 norm was shown to be a better metric than the ℓ_2 norm for image restoration and SR problems. This is attributed to the fact that the weight updates are not dominated by the large prediction errors.

Multi-image Network: The single image model is extended to multi-input image SR by creating multiple input channels (MC) from given images which are resampled to the same spatial grid and visualize the same anatomy. In this way, the SR performance is enhanced by merging multiple image stacks, e.g. long-axis (LAX) and short axis (SAX) stacks, acquired from different imaging planes into a single SR volume. However, when only a few slices are acquired, a mask or distance map is required as input to the network to identify the missing information. Additionally, the number of parameters is supposed to be increased so that the model can learn to extract in image regions where the masks are defined, which increases the training time accordingly. For this reason, a Siamese network [4] is proposed as a third model (see Fig. 3) for comparison purposes, which was used in similar problems such as shape recognition from multiple

Table 1. Quantitative comparison of different image upsampling methods.

Exp (a)	PSNR (dB)	SSIM	# Filter/ Atlas
Linear	20.83±1.10	.70±.03	–
CSpline	22.38±1.13	.73±.03	–
MAPM	22.75±1.22	.73±.03	350
sh-CNN	23.67±1.18	.74±.02	64,64,32,1
CNN	24.12±1.18	.76±.02	64,64,32,16,8,4,1
de-CNN	**24.45±1.20**	**.77±.02**	64,64,32,16,8,4,1

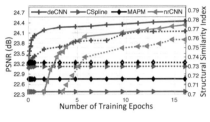

Fig. 4. Results on the testing data, PSNR (solid) and SSIM (dashed)

images [17]. The first stage of the network resamples the input images into a fixed HR spatial grid. In the second stage the same type of image features are extracted from each channel which are sharing the same filter weights. In the final stage, the features are pooled and passed to another Conv network to reconstruct the output HR image. The view pooling layer averages the corresponding features from all channels over the areas where the images are overlapping. The proposed models are initially pre-trained with small number of layers to better initialize the final deeper network training, which improves the network performance [5].

3   Results

The models are evaluated on end-diastolic frames of cine cardiac MR images acquired from 1233 healthy adult subjects. The images are upscaled in the direction orthogonal to the SAX plane. The proposed method is compared against linear, cubic spline, and multi-atlas patchmatch (MAPM) [15] upscaling methods in four different experiments: image quality assessment for (a–b) single and multi-input cases, (c) left-ventricle (LV) segmentation, (d) LV motion tracking.

Experimental details: In the first experiment, an image dataset containing 1080 3D SAX cardiac volumes with voxel size $1.25 \times 1.25 \times 2.00\,\text{mm}$, is randomly split into two subsets and used for single-image model training (930) and testing (150). The images are intensity normalized and cropped around the heart. Synthetic LR images are generated using the acquisition model given in Sect. 2, which are resampled to a fixed resolution $1.25 \times 1.25 \times 10.00\,\text{mm}$. The PSF is set to be a Gaussian kernel with a full-width at half-maximum equal to the slice thickness [7]. For the LR/HR pairs, multiple acquisitions could be used as well, but an unbalanced bias would be introduced near sharp edges due to spatial misalignments. For the evaluation of multi-input models, a separate clinical dataset of 153 image pairs of LAX cardiac image slices and SAX image stacks are used, of which 10 pairs are split for evaluation. Spatial misalignment between SAX and LAX images are corrected using image registration [9]. For the single/multi image model, seven consecutive Conv layers are used after the upscaling layer. In the Siamese model, the channels are merged after the fourth Conv layer.

Table 2. Image quality results obtained with three different models: single-image de-CNN, Siamese, and multi-channel (MC) that uses multiple input images.

Exp (b)	de-CNN (SAX)	Siamese (SAX/4CH)	MC (SAX/4CH)	MC (SAX/2/4CH)
PSNR (dB)	24.76±0.48	25.13±0.48	25.15±0.47	**25.26±0.37**
SSIM	.807±.009	.814±.013	.814±.012	**.818±.012**
p - values	0.005	0.016	0.017	-

Table 3. Segmentation results for different upsampling methods, CSpline ($p = .007$) and MAPM ($p = .009$). They are compared in terms of mean and Hausdorff distances (MYO) and LV cavity volume differences (w.r.t. manual annotations).

Exp (c)	Linear	CSpline	MAPM	de-CNN	High Res
LV Vol Diff (ml)	11.72±6.96	10.80±6.46	9.55±5.42	**9.09±5.36**	8.24±5.47
Mean Dist (mm)	1.49±0.30	1.45±0.29	1.40±0.29	**1.38±0.29**	1.38±0.28
Haus Dist (mm)	7.74±1.73	7.29±1.63	6.83±1.61	**6.67±1.77**	6.70±1.85

Image Quality Assessment: The upscaled images are compared with the ground-truth HR 3D volumes in terms of PSNR and SSIM [18]. The latter measure assesses the correlation of local structures and is less sensitive to image noise. The results in Table 1 show that learning the initial upscaling kernels (de-CNN) can improve ($p = .007$) the quality of generated HR image compared to convolution only network (CNN) using the same number of trainable parameters. Additionally, the performance of 7-layer network is compared against the 4-layer shallow network from [6] (sh-CNN). Addition of extra Conv layers to the 7-layer model is found to be ineffective due to increased training time and negligible performance improvement. In Fig. 4, we see that CNN based methods can learn better HR synthesis models even after a small number of training epochs. On the same figure, it can be seen that the model without the residual learning (nrCNN) underperforms and requires a large number of training iterations.

Multi-input Model: In the second experiment, we show that the single image SR model can be enhanced by providing additional information from two and four chamber (2/4CH) LAX images. The results given in Table 2 show that by including LAX information in the model, a modest improvement in image visual quality can be achieved. The improvement is mostly observed in image regions closer to areas where the SAX-LAX slices overlap, as can be seen in Fig. 5 (a–d). Also, the results show that the multi-channel (MC) model performs slightly better than Siamese model as it is given more degrees-of-freedom, whereas the latter is more practical as it trains faster and requires fewer trainable parameters.

Segmentation Evaluation: As a subsequent image analysis, 18 SAX SR images are segmented using a state-of-the-art multi-atlas method [2]. The SR images generated from clinical 2D stack data with different upscaling

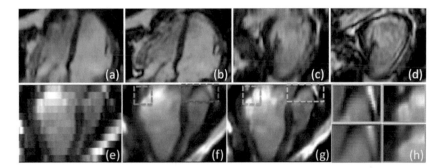

Fig. 5. The LV is better visualized by using multi-input images (b,d) compared to single image SR (a,c). Also, the proposed method (g) performs better than MAPM [15] (f) in areas where uncommon shapes are over-smoothed by atlases.

methods are automatically segmented and those segmentations are compared with the manual annotations performed on ground-truth HR 3D images. Additionally, the HR images are segmented with the same method to show the lower error bound. The quality of segmentations are evaluated based on the LV cavity volume measure and surface-to-surface distances for myocardium (MYO). The results in Table 3 show that CNN upscaled images can produce segmentation results similar to the ones obtained from HR images. The main result difference between the SR methods is observed in image areas where thin and detailed boundaries are observed (e.g. apex). As can be seen in Fig. 5 (e–h), the MAPM over-smooths areas closer to image boundaries. Inference of the proposed model is not as computationally demanding as brute-force searching (MAPM), which requires hours for a single image, whereas SR-CNN can be executed in 6.8 s on GPU or 5.8 min CPU on average per image. The shorter runtime makes the SR methods more applicable to subsequent analysis, as they can replace the standard interpolation methods.

Motion Tracking: The clinical applications of SR can be extended to MYO tracking as it can benefit from SR as a preprocessing stage to better highlight the ventricle boundaries. End-diastolic MYO segmentations are propagated to end-systolic (ES) phase using B-Spline FFD registrations [13]. ES meshes generated with CNN and linear upscaling methods are compared with tracking results obtained with 10 3D-SAX HR images based on Hausdorff distance. The proposed SR method produces tracking results (4.73 ± 1.03 mm) more accurate ($p = 0.01$) than the linear interpolation (5.50 ± 1.08 mm). We observe that the images upscaled with the CNN model follow the apical boundaries more accurately, which is shown in the supplementary material: www.doc.ic.ac.uk/~oo2113/M16

4   Discussion and Conclusion

The results show that the proposed SR approach outperforms conventional upscaling methods both in terms of image quality metrics and subsequent image analysis accuracy. Also, it is computationally efficient and can be applied to image analysis tasks such as segmentation and tracking. The experiments show that these applications can benefit from SR images since 2D stack image analysis with SR-CNN can achieve similar quantitative results as the analysis on isotropic volumes without requiring long acquisition time. We also show that the proposed model can be easily extended to multiple image input scenarios to obtain better SR results. SR-CNN's applicability is not only limited to cardiac images but to other anatomical structures as well. In the proposed approach, inter-slice and stack spatial misalignments due to motion are handled using a registration method. However, we observe that large slice misplacements can degrade SR accuracy. Future research will focus on that aspect of the problem.

References

1. Alexander, D.C., Zikic, D., Zhang, J., Zhang, H., Criminisi, A.: Image quality transfer via random forest regression: applications in diffusion MRI. In: Golland, P., Hata, N., Barillot, C., Hornegger, J., Howe, R. (eds.) MICCAI 2014, Part III. LNCS, vol. 8675, pp. 225–232. Springer, Heidelberg (2014)
2. Bai, W., Shi, W., O'Regan, D.P., Tong, T., Wang, H., Jamil-Copley, S., Peters, N.S., Rueckert, D.: A probabilistic patch-based label fusion model for multi-atlas segmentation with registration refinement: application to cardiac MR images. IEEE TMI **32**(7), 1302–1315 (2013)
3. Bhatia, K.K., Price, A.N., Shi, W., Rueckert, D.: Super-resolution reconstruction of cardiac MRI using coupled dictionary learning. In: IEEE ISBI, pp. 947–950 (2014)
4. Bromley, J., Guyon, I., Lecun, Y., Sckinger, E., Shah, R.: Signature verification using a "Siamese" time delay neural network. In: NIPS, pp. 737–744 (1994)
5. Dong, C., Deng, Y., Change Loy, C., Tang, X.: Compression artifacts reduction by a deep convolutional network. In: IEEE CVPR, pp. 576–584 (2015)
6. Dong, C., Loy, C.C., He, K., Tang, X.: Image super-resolution using deep convolutional networks. IEEE PAMI **38**(2), 295–307 (2016)
7. Greenspan, H.: Super-resolution in medical imaging. Comput. J. **52**(1), 43–63 (2009)
8. LeCun, Y., Bottou, L., Bengio, Y., Haffner, P.: Gradient-based learning applied to document recognition. Proc. IEEE **86**(11), 2278–2324 (1998)
9. Lötjönen, J., Pollari, M., Kivistö, S., Lauerma, K.: Correction of movement artifacts from 4-D cardiac short- and long-axis MR data. In: Barillot, C., Haynor, D.R., Hellier, P. (eds.) MICCAI 2004. LNCS, vol. 3217, pp. 405–412. Springer, Heidelberg (2004)
10. Manjón, J.V., Coupé, P., Buades, A., Fonov, V., Collins, D.L., Robles, M.: Non-local MRI upsampling. MedIA **14**(6), 784–792 (2010)
11. Odille, F., Bustin, A., Chen, B., Vuissoz, P.-A., Felblinger, J.: Motion-corrected, super-resolution reconstruction for high-resolution 3D cardiac cine MRI. In: Navab, N., Hornegger, J., Wells, W.M., Frangi, A.F. (eds.) MICCAI 2015. LNCS, vol. 9351, pp. 435–442. Springer, Heidelberg (2015). doi:10.1007/978-3-319-24574-4_52

12. Plenge, E., Poot, D.H.J., Niessen, W.J., Meijering, E.: Super-resolution reconstruction using cross-scale self-similarity in multi-slice MRI. In: Mori, K., Sakuma, I., Sato, Y., Barillot, C., Navab, N. (eds.) MICCAI 2013, Part III. LNCS, vol. 8151, pp. 123–130. Springer, Heidelberg (2013)
13. Rueckert, D., Sonoda, L.I., Hayes, C., Hill, D.L., Leach, M.O., Hawkes, D.J.: Nonrigid registration using free-form deformations: application to breast MR images. IEEE TMI **18**(8), 712–721 (1999)
14. Rueda, A., Malpica, N., Romero, E.: Single-image super-resolution of brain MR images using overcomplete dictionaries. MedIA **17**(1), 113–132 (2013)
15. Shi, W., Caballero, J., Ledig, C., Zhuang, X., Bai, W., Bhatia, K., de Marvao, A.M.S.M., Dawes, T., O'Regan, D., Rueckert, D.: Cardiac image super-resolution with global correspondence using multi-atlas patchmatch. In: Mori, K., Sakuma, I., Sato, Y., Barillot, C., Navab, N. (eds.) MICCAI 2013, Part III. LNCS, vol. 8151, pp. 9–16. Springer, Heidelberg (2013)
16. Simonyan, K., Zisserman, A.: Very deep convolutional networks for large-scale image recognition. arXiv preprint arXiv:1409.1556 (2014)
17. Su, H., Maji, S., Kalogerakis, E., Learned-Miller, E.: Multi-view convolutional neural networks for 3D shape recognition. In: IEEE CVPR, pp. 945–953 (2015)
18. Wang, Z., Bovik, A.C., Sheikh, H.R., Simoncelli, E.P.: Image quality assessment: from error visibility to structural similarity. IEEE TIP **13**(4), 600–612 (2004)
19. Zhao, H., Gallo, O., Frosio, I., Kautz, J.: Is L2 a good loss function for neural networks for image processing? arXiv preprint arXiv:1511.08861 (2015)

GPNLPerf: Robust 4d Non-rigid Motion Correction for Myocardial Perfusion Analysis

S. Thiruvenkadam[1](✉), K. S. Shriram[1], B. Patil[1], G. Nicolas[2], M. Teisseire[2], C. Cardon[2], J. Knoplioch[2], N. Subramanian[1], S. Kaushik[1], and R. Mullick[1]

[1] GE Global Research, Bangalore, India
sheshadri.thiruvenkadam@ge.com
[2] GE Healthcare, Buc, France

Abstract. Since the introduction of wide cone detector systems, CT myocardial perfusion has been an area of increased interest, for which non-rigid registration [NRR] is a key step to further analysis. We propose a novel motion management pipeline for perfusion data, GPNLPerf (*Group-wise, non-local, NRR for perfusion analysis*) centering on group-wise NRR using non-local spatio-temporal constraints. The proposed pipeline deals with the NRR challenges for 4D perfusion data and results in generating clinically relevant perfusion parameters. We demonstrate results on 9 dynamic perfusion exams comparing results quantitatively with ANTs NRR and also show qualitative results on perfusion maps.

1 Introduction

Full coverage dynamic CT contrast scans are key to quantify myocardial perfusion parameters such as blood flow which are key to the diagnosis of cardiac disease [1]. An important challenge that needs to be addressed for computing reliable perfusion maps is motion induced by repiration and cardiac movement. Such respiratory/cardiac motion would result in gross errors in the estimated perfusion maps. In this work, we propose a fully automatic end-end solution for addressing the motion challenges of 4D CT perfusion studies. In order to deduce clinically meaningful perfusion parameters, any NRR approach has to handle challenges of large motion, intensity variations due to contrast dynamics, and presence of small structures like vessels. Further, it is important for NRR to preserve the inherent contrast dynamics, and work in a feasible compute time. Although there have been several works for NRR of perfusion data in the context of dynamic CT perfusion ([2,3]) and for DCE MR ([4,5]), previous works have not fully handled the above challenges to offer a viable clinical solution.

Two broad categories of aligning 4D data are '*reference*' based methods and *groupwise* NRR (see [6]). Unlike reference based methods, groupwise NRR is not biased by the choice of the reference image. In general, for cardiac contrast data, there are dramatic changes in intensity that vary spatially, with structures becoming visible at different time points. Thus, large differences in NRR results could occur depending on the choice of the reference image. Hence, groupwise NRR could prove quite useful for dynamic cardiac perfusion data.

© Springer International Publishing AG 2016
S. Ourselin et al. (Eds.): MICCAI 2016, Part III, LNCS 9902, pp. 255–263, 2016.
DOI: 10.1007/978-3-319-46726-9_30

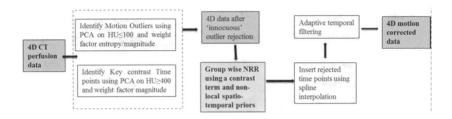

Fig. 1. GPNLPerf: pipeline composed of (a) Outlier Rejection and interpolation (b) Group-wise NRR (c) Adaptive temporal filtering.

However, a challenge for groupwise NRR is to handle small populations of data with large motion in the absence of a good initial guess for both the evolving reference image and the transforms. Previous groupwise NRR methods for perfusion data, [4,5], have been for 2D DCE MRI data where typically several timepoints [TPs] are available giving a good initial guess for the groupwise mean. Secondly, schemes such as breaking the data into groups of pre- and post-contrast as in [4] may not be feasible for CT cardiac perfusion given that there might be very few TPs (e.g. 12–15) with large regions peaking with contrast at different times. In [7], the issue of large motion for small populations within groupwise NRR is handled for PET data using non-local spatio-temporal penalties. In our work, we address groupwise NRR for CT dynamic perfusion data, adapting and extending the framework in [7]. As a result, compared to previous groupwise NRR works for perfusion, we can effectively handle the challenge of large motion of small number of TPs.

Our proposed solution GPNLPerf is a generic pipeline composed of (a) Outlier Rejection and interpolation (b) Robust group-wise NRR using non-local spatio-temporal constraints, and (c) Adaptive temporal filtering. Firstly, we call out 'innocuous' TPs with extreme motion as outliers and drop them from 4D NRR. These TPs are later interpolated from neighbouring registered TPs. Next, in the core of the algorithm, we propose a metric that models the contrast dynamics seen in perfusion studies, within the groupwise NRR approach [7]. Lastly, to meet computational feasibility for clinically deployment, we run NRR at a manageable lower resolution and later arrest the jitter due to interpolation effects using an adaptive temporal filtering approach. Results are analyzed on 9 dynamic perfusion exams. We quantitatively compare our performance to a pairwise approach using the ANTs package. Finally, a qualitative assessment of reconstructed perfusion maps is presented using standard visualization.

2   Methods

Here, we describe the proposed GPNLPerf pipeline. Firstly, we drop out TPs with extreme motion especially if they would play no role in the final perfusion map computation. Typically, in breathhold acquisitions, when the patient starts to free breathe, there is extreme motion in 1 or 2 transition TPs. If these extreme

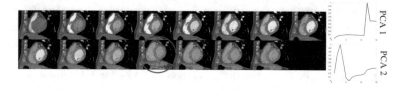

Fig. 2. Outlier Rejection for a 4D CT case with 15 TPs: An 'innocuous' outlier time-point (highlighted in Red) is rejected because the resulting PCA weight factors are large (first plot). The timepoint is innocuous since it does not have peak contrast activity and this is seen in the weight factors of the 2nd PCA step (second plot).

TPs lie in 'innocuous' locations from a contrast dynamics point of view, these volumes can be safely dropped without the risk of altering the end perfusion maps. After NRR, these rejected temporal positions can be re-inserted using interpolation. The algorithm flow is shown in Fig. 1.

2.1 PCA Based Outlier Rejection

The objective here is to conservatively reject one or two time points as motion outliers and also make sure that they are not key time points for the contrast dynamics. Here, we use a simple two stage technique based on Principal Component Analysis (PCA) to achieve the above. Firstly, motion outliers are identified by limiting the dynamic range of the data to air and soft tissue, Hounsfield Unit $HU \leq 200$. This data, after spatial down sampling is passed through PCA to get the principal eigenvectors (restricted to the first two) that quantify large motion directions. Projecting the eigen vectors back to the data gives the weight factors that quantifies the motion of each timepoint in the direction of the eigenvectors. Motion outliers (not more than two TPs) if any, are then identified by looking at entropy and magnitude of these temporal weight factors. Entropy is a key feature here to distinguish cases with large motion in several time points (e.g. data from a free breathing protocol), for which an outlier rejection step would not make sense. Next, to make sure that only 'innocuous' time points are rejected, we perform one more round of PCA in a higher range $HU \geq 400$, to consider only contrast induced intensity changes across time points. Now, large weight factors corresponding to first two eigen vectors would tell us the interesting TPs from a contrast dynamics perspective. If the motion outliers do not fall in the set of interesting TPs, we can safely reject them as 'innocuous' TPs (example of utility of the two PCA steps are shown in Fig. 2). Post NRR, these rejected TPs are inserted using standard spline interpolation using neighboring TPs.

2.2 Non-local Group-Wise NRR for Perfusion Data

In this discussion, we address the main contribution of the paper; NRR of the outlier rejected data. We propose a group-wise NRR energy in a variational framework with non-local spatio temporal penalties on the transforms. We adapt the mono-modal groupwise formulation from [7] proposed for gated PET data, to handle intensity variations seen in CT perfusion. To do this, we add an additional contrast term to distinguish intensity changes due to motion from intensity changes due to contrast flow. Assume we are given N volumes $\{I_k^o\}_{k=1}^N$ defined on Ω. Firstly, the input volumes are preprocessed to lie in the HU range $[-200,400]$ where we would see minimal contrast dynamics, to give N preprocessed volumes $\{J_k\}_{k=1}^N$. We seek a reference volume μ_{med} and deformation fields $\{w_k\}_{k=1}^N$, $\mathbf{w} = [w_1, w_2, ..., w_N]$, which minimizes:

$$L[\mu_{med}, \mathbf{w}] = \sum_{k=1}^N \int_\Omega |J_k(. + w_k) - \mu_{med}| dx + \alpha \int_\Omega |(Id - VV^T)(I_{\mathbf{w}}^o - \mu_{I_o})|^2 dx$$

$$+ \beta \sum_{k=1}^N \int_\Omega \int_\Omega m(x,y)|w_k(x) - w_k(y)|^2 dx dy$$

$$+ \beta_1 \sum_{k=1}^N \int_\Omega \int_\Omega \hat{m}(x,y)|v_k(x) - v_k(y)|^2 dx dy$$

This is a groupwise formulation with the data term tuned to handle contrast dynamics. The first term minimizes the voxel wise median deviation of the 4D data. The above term can be minimized by iteratively solving for the median of the data, μ_{med}, and the transforms $\mathbf{w}$. The second term seeks transforms so that the registered 4D data (i.e. the transforms $\mathbf{w}$ applied to the original data I^o) conforms to learnt contrast trends. Here, we utilize a contrast model term which uses contrast trends learnt from coarse resolutions. We use PCA once again to learn principal directions of variation in contrast, V and mean trend, μ_{I_o}. The contrast term is useful in finer resolutions to align smaller structures better and reduce artefacts due to intensity variations induced by contrast dynamics.

Similar to [7], the regularization terms on the transforms $\mathbf{w}$ consist of a non-local [NL] spatial term, and a NL temporal term seeking spatial coherence of velocity $v_k = w_{k+1} - w_k$. The NL penalties are critical in robustly handling large motion, residual intensity variations (inspite of pre-processing and the contrast term), and maintaining integrity of key structures such as myocardium and coronories. Scalars α, β, β_1 balance the terms; $m(x,y), \hat{m}(x,y)$ are spatial weight functions defined by Gaussians. We minimize the above equation using steepest descent, in a multi-resolution framework. In the coarse resolutions, the contrast term is turned off, i.e. $\alpha = 0$. The contrast trends V, μ_{I_o} learnt at the end of coarse resolutions are then applied in finer resolutions. A brief illustration and importance of contributions of the NL terms and the contrast term is shown in a synthetic experiment, Fig. 3. As seen, the contrast term handles NRR better under contrast dynamics (thus distinguishing our work from [7] which is susceptible to intensity variations, third row, Fig. 3.

2.3   Adaptive Temporal Filtering

Lastly, given that we want a computationally tractable solution, the deformation fields are at a finest resolution of 1.5 mm^3 while the original data is typically

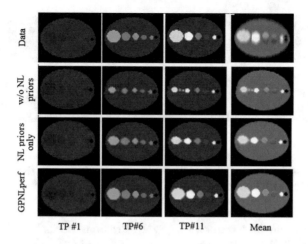

Fig. 3. Contribution of the NL priors and the contrast term: the synthetic data (first row) has 11 TPs, results for 3 TPs are shown in columns 1 to 3. The last column is the mean across TPs. The second row is Eq. 1 w/o any priors. The contrast dynamics combined with motion creates artefacts (e.g. shrinking of bright structures) in the registered images. The third row shows slightly improved results with only the NL priors (as in [7]). The last row shows the best results with the contrast term and the NL priors (GPNLPerf).

at higher resolution. For visualizing the perfusion maps and the registered data, the deformation fields are upsampled and applied to the original data at native resolution. The resulting jitter artifacts due to this interpolation step is handled using a simple temporal filtering step. A moving temporal median filter is employed at each voxel location. The median filter is also made adaptive to work only in non-contrast regions (defined using a smooth sigmoid cutoff on a suitable HU range ≤ 400).The above adaptive filter ensures that interpolation artifacts are arrested and contrast activity is preserved for the perfusion maps.

3 Experiments

We show a qualitative example in Fig. 4 with large motion. The proposed algorithm has resulted in a motion corrected result (as seen by the good agreement of the red ellipse marker with the inner boundary of the myocardium) which is reasonable for myocardial perfusion analysis. Next we show quantitative results on 9 dynamic perfusion exams acquired with a wide axial coverage (16 cm). Each exam consisted 15 cardiac volumes acquired at different time points with an average acquisition time of 35s. The end-end computational time of GPNLPerf was ≈ 6 min for processing a 4D dataset of dimensions ($512 \times 512 \times 224 \times 15$), voxel size ($0.45 \times 0.45 \times 0.625$), on a 8 core HP Z-800 workstation.

Here, for comparison, we choose ANTs [8] with a combination of Mutual Information [MI] and Local Cross Correlation [CC] as the metric posed in a

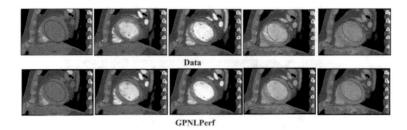

Fig. 4. GPNLPerf result on a 4D CT perfusion large motion case with 15 TPs. 5 TPs are shown in this figure. The alignment quality is visually seen in the red ellipse which lies very close to inner boundary of the myocardium post NRR.

symmetric diffeomorphic framework (SyN). Previous works in CT dynamic cardiac perfusion NRR ([2,3]) have mainly used MI and CC as registration metrics and posed in a reference based framework. Given that ANTs SyN has been quite successful in registration/segmentation competitions, we have used ANTs since it is similar in flavour to the above perfusion NRR works. The middle TP of each exam was picked as the reference volume for ANTs NRR. The pre-process steps and the deformation resolution ($1.5\ mm^3$) are the same for GPNLPerf and ANTs. Below, we consider two validation metrics based on expert given LMs.

3.1   Spatial Alignment

To quantify motion correction achieved by NRR, an expert marked 4 different locations on the edge of the myocardium and at bifurcation points in most of the TPs of each exam. Each of the expert-marked landmarks formed a temporal cluster due to motion across TPs. To evaluate the efficacy of registration, distance of every landmark from its temporal cluster center is calculated. NRR should give improved temporal alignment resulting in lower distance values.

Figure 5 shows results after consolidating landmarks across datasets (9 exams, 4 landmarks, 294 landmarks in total), shows both ANTs and GPNLPerf reducing error compared to before registration. It can also be seen from the Scatter plot and error Histogram that GPNLPerf has resulted in *lesser, tighter* errors. It is also observed that the fine accuracy of GPNLPerf is better than ANTs resulting in a significant number of LMs having error $\leq 1.5\ mm$ (deformation field resolution) as seen from the histogram. A paired t-test between ANTs and GPNLPerf was done. The p-value was less than 0.001 and the 95 % confidence interval for the difference between ANTs and GPNLPerf results was 0.072 to 0.24 showing statistically significant improvement in alignment using GPNLPerf.

3.2   Intensity Trend Error

Another metric that we use to quantify registration accuracy is to compare intensity trends observed post NRR to Ground Truth [GT] trends. This metric would

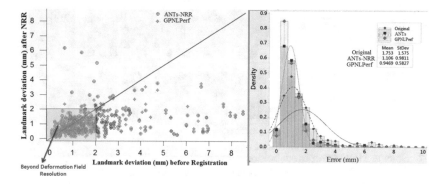

Fig. 5. Effect of registration at landmark locations (9 datasets: 4 landmarks, 294 landmarks in total). **Scatter Plot**: ANTs and GPNLPerf have brought about greater spatial coherence around landmark locations after registration. It can be seen that ANTs (red circles) has resulted in gross errors in a few cases. **Histogram**: a consolidated histogram of errors with a Gaussian fit for before NRR, ANTs, GPNLPerf errors is shown. GPNLPerf has resulted in lesser, tighter errors compared to ANTs.

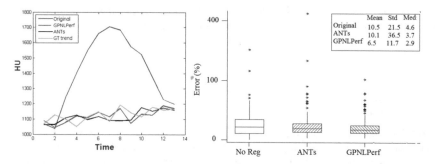

Fig. 6. Intensity trend compared to GT trend. For an example case, we see that the temporal intensity profile in the homogenous region closely matches the GT profile after registration (Left). The bar plot (on 9 cases, 15 TPs, 2 LMs) and statistics shows that GPNLPerf trend has matched well with the GT trend compared to ANTs.

additionally catch distortions introduced to the contrast dynamics. We evaluated the error between expert marked intensity profile (LM in homogeneous regions tracked by the expert over time) and profile post NRR at the LM location. On 9 datasets with two LMs each in the homogenous myocardium, the error with respect to the GT profile is seen to have reduced post NRR (Fig. 6, bar plot on the Right). GPNLPerf shows clearly better alignment ($\mu = 6.5, \sigma = 11.7$) (on 9 cases, 15 TPs, 2 LMs) with the GT intensity profile compared to ANTs.

3.3   Perfusion Maps

Here, we do a qualitative assessment of the resulting perfusion maps. The perfusion maps were derived using a deconvolution algorithm based on the

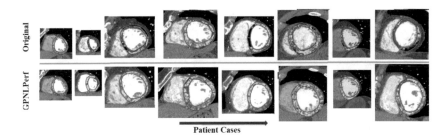

Fig. 7. Shown MBF computed before (Top row) and with GPNLPerf (Bottom row) for a few studies. MBFs after GPNLPerf seem more clinically relevant. (Color figure online)

Lawrence-Lee tissue model [9]. In Fig. 7, Myocardial blood flow (MBF) LUT of all screen captures have same color code (rainbow) and same threshold (0–250). GPNLPerf images show much better uniformity within the MBF whereas original images due to motion, show much wider values: very high values - red - due to cardiac cavity (both left and right ventricles) contamination and very low values - dark blue - because of pericardiac fat contamination. Thus, MBF estimations provided after GPNLPerf maps seem more clinically realistic and relevant.

4   Conclusion

In GPNLPerf, a fully automatic end-end solution for addressing the motion challenges of 4D CT perfusion studies is proposed. Quantitative landmark based comparison is done with ANTs and better NRR is demonstrated in terms of alignment and artifacts. Finally, the resulting perfusion maps are seen to be more clinically realistic after registration.

References

1. Varga-Szemes, A., Meinel, F.G., et al.: CT myocardial perfusion imaging. Am. J. Roentgenol. **204**, 487–497 (2015)
2. Fahmi, R., Eck, B.L., et al.: Dynamic CT myocardial perfusion imaging: detection of ischemia in a porcine model with FFR verification. In: Proceedings of SPIE (2014)
3. Isola, A.A., Schmitt, H., et al.: Image registration and perfusion imaging: application to dynamic circular cardiac CT. In: IEEE NSS/MIC 2010 (2010)
4. Kim, M., Wu, G., Shen, D.: Groupwise registration of breast DCE-MR images for accurate tumor measurement. In: ISBI (2011)
5. Mahapatra, D.: Joint segmentation and groupwise registration of cardiac perfusion images using temporal information. ISRN Mach. Vis. (2012)
6. Metz, C.T., Klein, S., et al.: Nonrigid registration of dynamic medical imaging data using nD+t B-splines. MIA **15**, 238–249 (2010)

7. Thiruvenkadam, S., Shriram, K., Manjeshwar, R., Wollenweber, S.: Robust PET motion correction using non-local spatio-temporal priors. In: Navab, N., Hornegger, J., Wells, W.M., Frangi, A.F. (eds.) MICCAI 2015. LNCS, vol. 9350, pp. 643–650. Springer, Heidelberg (2015). doi:10.1007/978-3-319-24571-3_77
8. Avants, B.B., Tustison, N.J., Song, G., Gee, J.C.: Ants: advanced open-source normalization tools for neuroanatomy. In: PICSL (2009)
9. Lawrence, K.S.S., Lee, T.Y.: An adiabatic approximation to the tissue homogeneity model for water exchange in the brain: a theoretical derivation. Nature **359**, 843–845 (1998)

Recognizing End-Diastole and End-Systole Frames via Deep Temporal Regression Network

Bin Kong[1], Yiqiang Zhan[2], Min Shin[1], Thomas Denny[3],
and Shaoting Zhang[1(✉)]

[1] Department of Computer Science, UNC Charlotte, Charlotte, NC, USA
szhang16@uncc.edu
[2] Siemens Healthcare, Malvern, PA, USA
[3] MRI Research Center, Auburn University, Auburn, AL, USA

Abstract. Accurate measurement of left ventricular volumes and Ejection Fraction from cine MRI is of paramount importance to the evaluation of cardiovascular functions, yet it usually requires laborious and tedious work of trained experts to interpret them. To facilitate this procedure, numerous computer aided diagnosis (CAD) methods and tools have been proposed, most of which focus on the left or right ventricle segmentation. However, the identification of ES and ED frames from cardiac sequences is largely ignored, which is a key procedure in the automated workflow. This seemingly easy task is quite challenging, due to the requirement of high accuracy (*i.e.*, precisely identifying specific frames from a sequence) and subtle differences among consecutive frames. Recently, with the rapid growth of annotated data and the increasing computational power, deep learning methods have been widely exploited in medical image analysis. In this paper, we propose a novel deep learning architecture, named as temporal regression network (TempReg-Net), to accurately identify specific frames from MRI sequences, by integrating the Convolutional Neural Network (CNN) with the Recurrent Neural Network (RNN). Specifically, a CNN encodes the spatial information of a cardiac sequence, and a RNN decodes the temporal information. In addition, we design a new loss function in our network to constrain the structure of predicted labels, which further improves the performance. Our approach is extensively validated on thousands of cardiac sequences and the average difference is merely 0.4 frames, comparing favorably with previous systems.

1 Introduction

Stroke volume (SV) and left ventricle ejection fraction, defined by the unnormalized and normalized difference between End-Diastole (ED) and End-Systole (ES) volumes respectively, are the most commonly used clinical diagnostic parameters for cardiac systolic funtion. This is because it reflects the contractile function of myocardium. However, current practice to calculate these parameters is mostly done manually by experts. Many previous methods have been devoted to automating this process, and the majority of them focus on left

S. Ourselin et al. (Eds.): MICCAI 2016, Part III, LNCS 9902, pp. 264–272, 2016.
DOI: 10.1007/978-3-319-46726-9_31

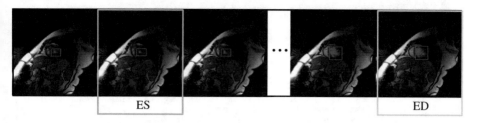

Fig. 1. A typical example of cardiac sequences (bright areas in red rectangles are left ventricles, the green and yellow rectangles indicate ES and ED frames respectively). (Color figure online)

ventricle segmentation [9,17]. However, the very first step of this automation, recognizing the ES and ED frames is largely ignored, while it is also an important process in the automatic system. In addition, even when SV and EF are computed manually or semi-automatically, reliably automating this step could reduce both inter and intra observer errors. Although the identification of ES and ED frames seems to be relatively easy, at least for human experts, the main challenges are the following: (1) the semantic gap between the high-level ES and ED concepts and low-level cardiac image sequence images, (2) the complex temporal relationships in cardiac cycles and subtle differences among consecutive cardiac frames (demonstrated in Fig. 1), and (3) the requirement of high accuracy since mislabeling even one frame may affect the diagnosis results. Therefore, determining ES and ED frames still remains a manual or semi-automatic task in many scenarios. Currently, this process could be time-consuming and error-prone, especially when dealing with large-scale datasets. It becomes a road block of a fully automatic solution.

Several attempts have been made to automate this process. A pioneer work [4] took advantage of rapid mitral opening in early diastole. However, it requires the identification by the user of three important landmarks: the apex and each angle of the mitral annulus, indicating a semi-automatic approach. Saeed Darvishi *et al.* [3] used a segmentation paradigm. In particular, they segmented every left ventricle region of the cardiac sequence by using level set. The frames corresponding to the largest ventricular area are the ED frames and the smallest ventricular area the ES frames. Since the initial contour has to be placed by the user, this method still remains semi-automatic. In addition, the final result largely relies on the quality of the initial contour. Another widely used method [6] tackled this problem with unsupervised learning. For this method, every frame of the cardiac sequence is embedded on a low-dimensional manifold, and a Euclidean distance between every two consecutive points in the manifold is computed to determine the ED and ES frames. However, a cardiac cycle is extremely complex and one individual's cardiac cycle may differ greatly from another's. Thus, this simple distance rule may not be applicable to other special patients, *e.g.*, those with cardiac diseases.

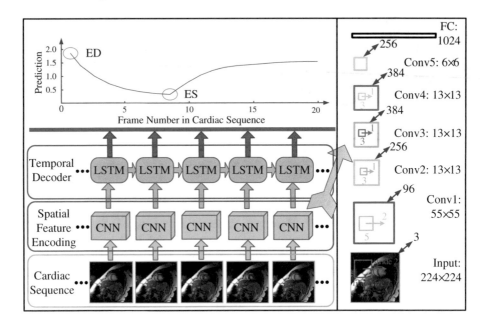

Fig. 2. An overview of the proposed framework, temporal regression network (TempReg-Net). Note that only convolutional layers are shown and Conv1 and Conv2 and Conv5 layers are followed by Pooling layers of size 3 × 3 and stride 2.

To overcome the above drawbacks, a joint network which combines Convolutional Neural Networks (CNN) and Recurrent Neural Network (RNN) has been designed to automate the whole detection process. Specifically, our framework has two phases, *i.e.*, encoding and decoding. During the first phase, the CNN acts as an encoder to encode the spatial pattern of the cardiac image sequence, transforming every frame of the sequence into a fixed-length feature vector to facilitate the decoding phase. During the second phase, the RNN is used to decode the temporal information of the above mentioned feature vectors. The joint network can be trained to learn the complex spatial and temporal patterns of the cardiac sequences, and give predictions for the ED and ES frames during testing. The contribution of our work is twofold: (1) A deep temporal regression network is designed to recognize the ED and ES frames; and (2) A temporal structured loss is proposed to improve the accuracy of the network. Although deep learning has been widely used for medical image analysis [2, 7, 12, 16], our network architecture is novel and carefully designed for this use case. This approach has several advantages compared to the previous methods: (1) No prior information or interaction is needed in the detection framework, since our system automatically learns everything from the patterns of the data. (2) Since RNN is able to learn long-term patterns, our framework can detect the complex and long temporal dynamics in the cardiac sequence.

2   Methodology

In this section, we provide an overview of our TempReg-Net framework. Then, we show that our framework can be trained end-to-end by jointly optimizing the regression and temporal structured constraints.

2.1   TempReg-Net Architectures

Figure 2 shows an overview of the proposed TempReg-Net framework, combining CNN and RNN (more specifically, the Long Short Term Memory (LSTM)). First, a feature encoder based on CNN is trained to encode the input into vectors. Then, the LSTM model takes over by exploring the temporal information sequentially. Finally, the ES and ED frames are detected according to the predictions from the LSTM model. At the training time, instead of using classification to identify the ES and ED frames, the network is trained to regress the location of the ES and ED frame numbers. During the testing phase, we examine the output sequence from TempReg-Net, where the ED frame is the local maximum and the ES frame is the local minimum.

Cardiac Frame Encoding with CNN: To fully capture the spatial information relevant to the left ventricle in every frame, we employ a CNN as the feature extractor in order to efficiently encode the spatial information. Recent years have witnessed numerous different kinds of CNN architectures. The Zeiler-Fergus (ZF) model is employed in our framework. The architecture of ZF model is illustrated in Fig. 2 (right). The reason of our choice is twofold: (1) Leveraging transferred knowledge across similar tasks is very useful when the labeled data is not adequate [14] and the architecture proposed in [5] achieved intriguing results in several image sequence analysis tasks; (2) the ZF model is reasonably deep and produces prominent results so we have a balance between computational complexity and the results. Essentially, a CNN acts as a feature transformer $\psi(S; V)$ parametrized by V to map cardiac sequence S to fixed-length vector sequence representations $< x_1, x_2, ..., x_T >$, in which V is the learnt weights of the CNN model and $x_t \in \mathbb{R}^q$ ($t = 1, 2, ..T$ and $q = 1024$ in our experiments).

Recognizing ED and ES Frames via RNN: Temporal information in cardiac sequence provides contextual clues regarding left ventricle volume changes. We tap into the temporal dimension by passing the above mentioned feature vector sequence into a RNN model. Instead of using traditional vanilla RNN, the LSTM model is adopted to avoid the vanishing or exploding gradients problem during back-propagation. The difference between a LSTM model

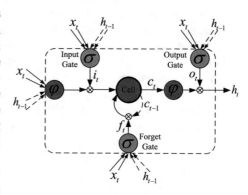

Fig. 3. A diagram of a LSTM memory block.

and a vanilla RNN is that a LSTM contains memory blocks instead of regular network units. A slightly simplified LSTM memory block [15] is used in this article, shown in Fig. 3. Benefited from the memory blocks, a LSTM learns when to forget previous hidden states h_{t-1} and when to update them given new information, shown as:

$$i_t = \sigma(W_{xi}x_t + W_{hi}h_{t-1} + b_i)$$
$$f_t = \sigma(W_{xf}x_t + W_{hf}h_{t-1} + b_f)$$
$$o_t = \sigma(W_{xo}x_t + W_{ho}h_{t-1} + b_o)$$
$$c_t = f_t \odot c_{t-1} + i_t \odot \varphi(W_{xi}x_t + W_{hi}h_{t-1} + b_i)$$
$$h_t = o_t \odot \varphi(c_t) \tag{1}$$

where $\varphi(x) = \frac{e^x - e^{-x}}{e^x + e^{-x}}$ and $\sigma(x) = (1 + e^{-x})^{-1}$ are nonlinear functions which squash its inputs to $[-1, 1]$. i_t, f_t, o_t are input gate, forget gate and output gate respectively. $\odot$ denotes element-wise product.

The memory cell c_t is a function of the previous memory cell c_{t-1} and the current input x_t and the previous hidden state h_{t-1}. i_t and f_t enable the memory cell to selectively forget its previous memory or consider new input. These additional units enable the LSTM to learn very complex temporal dynamics.

The final step in estimating a regression at time t is to take a fully-connected layer over the output of the RNN. The sequential weights W are reused at every frame, forcing the model to learn generic time-to-time cardiac motion dynamics and preventing the parameter size from growing linearly with respect to the sequence length T.

2.2   Jointly Optimize the Regression and Temporal Structured Constraints

Essentially, TempReg-Net gives a prediction for every single frame in a cardiac sequence and there is no constraint among the prediction sequences. However, TempReg-Net is designed to model the left ventricle volumes in a cardiac cycle, *i.e.*, the predictions for a cardiac sequence should decrease during the systole phase and increase during the diastole phase. Solely doing a regression cannot ensure such a structured output. In order to address this problem, we explicitly model this sequential constraint by penalizing predictions with wrong structures. Suppose that we are given the ground truth label y, which will be discussed later, and the TempReg-Net regressor η. Ideally, given two consecutive ground truth labels y_{k-1} and y_k and $y_{k-1} < y_k$, *i.e.*, the kth frame is in a systole phase, we expect that the predictions for these two frames should subject to $\eta_{k-1} < \eta_k$ as well, and vice versa. To enforce this constraint in TempReg-Net, a new loss function which we name as temporal structured loss is defined:

$$L_{temp} = \tfrac{1}{2}(L_{inc} + L_{dec})$$
$$L_{inc} = \tfrac{1}{T} \sum_{k=2}^{T} \mathbb{1}(y_k > y_{k-1}) \max(0, \eta_{k-1} - \eta_k)$$
$$L_{dec} = \tfrac{1}{T} \sum_{k=2}^{T} \mathbb{1}(y_k < y_{k-1}) \max(0, \eta_k - \eta_{k-1})$$
$$(2)$$

where $\mathbb{1}(\cdot)$ is the indicator function. L_{inc} penalizes the decreasing predictions during a diastole phase, $i.e.$, the left ventricle volume is increasing. L_{dec} penalizes the increasing predictions during a systole phase, $i.e.$, the left ventricle volume is decreasing.

Having defined the temporal structured loss, the training criteria for TempReg-Net can be further explored. We denote the training example as (S, N_{es}, N_{ed}), where N_{es} and N_{ed} stand for the ES and ED frame numbers respectively in the sequence S. Given the training data $\mathbb{S} = \{S, N_{es}, N_{ed}\}$, the training objective becomes the task of estimating the network weights $\lambda = (U, V)$ (U and V are the parameters for the CNN and RNN, respectively):

$$\lambda = \arg\min_{\lambda} \{ \sum_{S \in \mathbb{S}} \sum_{k} ||y_k - \eta_k(S, \lambda)||^2 + \alpha L_{reg}(\lambda) + \beta L_{temp} \}$$
$$L_{reg}(\lambda) = \tfrac{1}{2}(||U||_2^2 + ||V||_2^2)$$
$$(3)$$

where k is the kth frame of training sequence S. L_{reg} is the regularization penalty term which ensures the learnt weights are sparse. α and β are hyper-parameters which are cross-validated in our experiments. At training stage, the ground truth label y_k is synthesised to imitate the left ventricle volume changes during a typical cardiac cycle [3]:

$$y_k = \begin{cases} \left| \frac{k - N_{es}}{N_{es} - N_{ed}} \right|^{\delta}, & \text{if } N_{ed} < k \leq N_{es} \\ \left| \frac{k - N_{es}}{N_{es} - N_{ed}} \right|^{v}, & \text{otherwise} \end{cases}$$
$$(4)$$

where δ and v are hyper-parameters, set as 3 and $\tfrac{1}{3}$ respectively to imitate the typical left ventricle volume changes in cardiac cycle.

3   Experiments

Experimental Setting and Implementations: Our experiments are conducted on MRI sequences, acquired from our collaborative hospital and labeled by experts. Specifically, this dataset comprises of cardiac sequences (consists of around $113,000$ cardiac frames) gathered from 420 patients, from different imaging views and different positions, including long-axis, short-axis, four-chamber and two-chamber views. There are about 18 cardiac sequences for each patient (around 15 for short-axis view, and one for long-axis, four-chamber and two-chamber views, respectively). Every sequence has 20 frames with 256×256 pixels. ED and ES frames are carefully identified by cardiologists. Four-fold cross-validation is performed to obtain quantitative results.

Regarding implementation, TempReg-Net's implementation is based on Caffe [8]. In order to fully utilize the CNN architecture and make use of transferred knowledge, we squash all gray-scale cardiac frames to the range of [0, 255], and these single-channel cardiac frames are replicated for three times, resulting in three-channel images. In order to get a reasonable initialization and avoid over-fitting, we fine-tune our TempReg-Net on a pre-trained model based on the 1.2M ImageNet [10]. In our experiment, the learning rate for the last fully-connected layer is set to be 1×10^{-3}, which is 10 times larger than the rest layers. Regarding the RNN, the LSTM is used to avoid vanishing and exploding gradient problems. All the parameters of the LSTM are randomly initialized within $[-0.01, 0.01]$. Since each cardiac sequence in our dataset contains 20 frames, the LSTM is unrolled to 20 time steps. All the hyper-parameters of the proposed TempReg-Net are cross-validated for the best results. During the training stage, we augment our datasets by randomly cropping the resized cardiac images. The whole network is trained end-to-end with back propagation.

Results and Analysis: To quantitatively evaluate our method, we use average Frame Difference (aFD) to quantify the error of the prediction, following the convention [6,11]. Assuming that the frame label for the mth patient is N_m and the predicted frame label is $\hat{N}_m$, aFD can be defined as:

$$aFD = \frac{1}{M} \sum_{m=1}^{M} |\hat{N}_m - N_m|, \tag{5}$$

where M is the total number of examples in the testing set.

Table 1 shows the evaluation of our framework. Even without using the temporal structured constraints (TSC), our TempReg-Net is already a competitive solution to detect ED and ES from MRI. It has achieved good performance, *i.e.*, aFD 0.47 and 0.52 for identifying ED and ES, respectively, meaning that the error is within one frame. This is a promising result considering that our framework is end-to-end and automatic, with no requirement for interactions. After adding the temporal structured constraints, the aFD is improved to 0.38 and 0.44 for ED and ES, reducing the errors by around 15 %. This shows that the structures enforced upon the predictions contribute positively to the network. Regarding the computational efficiency, this framework takes merely 1.4 seconds to process one sequence. Therefore, it has the potential to be integrated with cardiac analysis systems owing to the small overhead.

We also compare our method with other types of systems or algorithms. For example, the system in [1] first segments the left ventricle, and then identifies the ED and ES by measuring areas of segmented regions. We have developed a similar system, using variations of level set (used in [3]) or graph cut (used in [13]) to segment the left ventricle. This type of segmentation-based system is very intuitive and widely used. However, compared to our solution, it has several limitations, including the computational efficiency, human interactions, and the segmentation errors. In our experiments, the system takes 2.9 and 3.5 seconds to segment the left ventricle from one sequence using level set and graph

Table 1. Average frame differences, standard deviation and running time of different methods.

Methods		Seg-based: Level Set [3]	Seg-based: Graph Cut [13]	Reg-based: CNN + Reg	TmpReg-Net (without TSC)	TempReg-Net
aFD	ED	1.54	2.27	1.30	0.47	**0.38**
	ES	1.24	1.65	1.97	0.52	**0.44**
STD	ED	1.93	2.89	1.77	0.49	**0.39**
	ES	1.64	1.96	2.42	0.53	**0.46**
Time (s)		2.9	3.5	1.5	1.4	**1.4**

cut, respectively, which are slower than our method. Note that we do not count the time of human interactions to initialize the segmentation procedure (e.g., graph cut method needs to specify foreground and/or background), which could take extra time. The aFD is 1.54 for ED and 1.24 for ES when using level set, and 2.27 as well as 1.65 when using graph cut, both of which are much worse than ours. The reason is that these segmentation algorithms cannot perfectly segment left ventricles in all frames, while even small errors adversely affect the prediction results based on the subtle difference of areas. Moreover, a similar regression framework is implemented. In this framework, The only difference is that logistic regression is used to predict the ventricle volumes. The aFD is 1.30 for ED and 1.97 for ES when using this method, still worse than the proposed method. Note that [13] is a recently proposed method and it has achieved sound accuracy for the segmentation of myocardium. The standard deviation is 0.39 and 0.46 for ED and ES respectively when using the proposed methods, which compares favorably against other methods. This further proves its effectiveness. Therefore, our end-to-end deep learning solution is more competitive in this task.

4   Conclusion

In this paper, we proposed a novel deep neural network, TempReg-Net, by integrating the CNN and RNN to identify specific frames in a cardiac sequence. In our method, a CNN and RNN tap into the spatial and temporal information respectively. Since the predictions should be temporally ordered, we explicitly model this constraint by adding a novel loss function in our framework. Extensive experiments on cardiac sequences demonstrate the efficacy of the proposed method. As deep learning methods have advanced segmentation tasks as well, future work will be devoted to develop a segmentation framework to fully automate the calculation of cardiac functional parameters.

References

1. Abboud, A.A., et al.: Automatic detection of the end-diastolic and end-systolic from 4d echocardiographic images. JCS **11**(1), 230 (2015)

2. Chen, H., Dou, Q., Ni, D., Cheng, J.-Z., Qin, J., Li, S., Heng, P.-A.: Automatic fetal ultrasound standard plane detection using knowledge transferred recurrent neural networks. In: Navab, N., Hornegger, J., Wells, W.M., Frangi, A.F. (eds.) MICCAI 2015. LNCS, vol. 9349, pp. 507–514. Springer, Heidelberg (2015). doi:10.1007/978-3-319-24553-9_62

3. Darvishi, S., et al.: Measuring left ventricular volumes in two-dimensional echocardiography image sequence using level-set method for automatic detection of end-diastole and end-systole frames. Res. Cardiocvasc. Med. 2(1), 39 (2013)

4. Dominguez, C.R., Kachenoura, N., Mulé, S., Tenenhaus, A., Delouche, A., Nardi, O., Gérard, O., Diebold, B., Herment, A., Frouin, F.: Classification of segmental wall motion in echocardiography using quantified parametric images. In: Frangi, A.F., Radeva, P., Santos, A., Hernandez, M. (eds.) FIMH 2005. LNCS, vol. 3504, pp. 477–486. Springer, Heidelberg (2005)

5. Donahue, J., et al.: Long-term recurrent convolutional networks for visual recognition and description. In: CVPR, pp. 2625–2634 (2015)

6. Gifani, P., et al.: Automatic detection of end-diastole and end-systole from echocardiography images using manifold learning. PMEA 31(9), 1091 (2010)

7. Greenspan, H., et al.: Guest editorial deep learning in medical imaging: overview and future promise of an exciting new technique. IEEE TMI 35(5), 1153–1159 (2016)

8. Jia, Y., et al.: Caffe: convolutional architecture for fast feature embedding. In: ACMMM, pp. 675–678. ACM (2014)

9. Marino, M., et al.: Fully automated assessment of left ventricular volumes, function and mass from cardiac MRI. In: CinC, pp. 109–112. IEEE (2014)

10. Russakovsky, O., et al.: Imagenet large scale visual recognition challenge. IJCV 115(3), 211–252 (2015)

11. Shalbaf, A., et al.: Automatic detection of end systole and end diastole within a sequence of 2-d echocardiographic images using modified isomap algorithm. In: MECBME, pp. 217–220. IEEE (2011)

12. Shin, H.C., et al.: Interleaved text/image deep mining on a very large-scale radiology database. In: CVPR, pp. 1090–1099 (2015)

13. Uzunbaş, M.G., et al.: Segmentation of myocardium using deformable regions and graph cuts. In: ISBI, pp. 254–257. IEEE (2012)

14. Yosinski, J., et al.: How transferable are features in deep neural networks? In: NIPS, pp. 3320–3328 (2014)

15. Zaremba, W., et al.: Learning to execute. CoRR abs/1410.4615 (2014)

16. Zhang, W., et al.: Deep convolutional neural networks for multi-modality isointense infant brain image segmentation. NeuroImage 108, 214–224 (2015)

17. Zhen, X., et al.: Multi-scale deep networks and regression forests for direct biventricular volume estimation. MedIA 30, 120–129 (2015)

Basal Slice Detection Using Long-Axis Segmentation for Cardiac Analysis

Mahsa Paknezhad[1]([⊠]), Michael S. Brown[2], and Stephanie Marchesseau[3]

[1] National University of Singapore (NUS), Singapore, Singapore
mahsa@u.nus.edu
[2] York University, York, Canada
[3] Clinical Imaging Research Centre, A*STAR-NUS, Singapore, Singapore

Abstract. Estimating blood volume of the left ventricle (LV) in the end-diastolic and end-systolic phases is important in diagnosing cardiovascular diseases. Proper estimation of the volume requires knowledge of which MRI slice contains the topmost basal region of the LV. Automatic basal slice detection has proved challenging; as a result, basal slice detection remains a manual task which is prone to inter-observer variability. This paper presents a novel method that is able to track the basal slice over the whole cardiac cycle. The method was tested on 56 healthy and pathological cases and was able to identify the basal slices similar to experts' selection for 80 % and 85 % of the cases for end-diastole and end-systole, respectively. This provides a significant improvement over the leading state-of-the-art approach that obtained 59 % and 44 % agreement with experts on the same input.

Keywords: Basal slice · Long-axis motion · Two-chamber view · Long-axis view · Cardiac analysis · MRI

1 Introduction and Related Work

Analysis of the cardiac function is routinely performed using magnetic resonance imaging (MRI). In a standard cardiovascular MRI scan, three different views of the heart are acquired: a single two-chamber view, a four-chamber view, and a stack of 12–15 short-axis slices covering the whole left ventricle (LV). Important cardiac pathology determinants are stroke volume (SV), ejection fraction (EF), and LV mass which are measured by finding the volume of the LV in the end-systolic and the end-diastolic phases of the cardiac cycle. In order to compute the LV volume, significant progress has been made in developing short-axis segmentation algorithms (e.g. [1]). While these methods give good segmentation accuracy, given the cardiac motion, they often ignore the basal slices which do not have full myocardium around the blood pool. In order to provide an accurate estimate of the LV volume, the most basal slice in the LV must be specified. This can be an issue since manual basal slice specification has been found prone to inter- and intra-observer variability which significantly impacts measured clinical parameters [2,3].

© Springer International Publishing AG 2016
S. Ourselin et al. (Eds.): MICCAI 2016, Part III, LNCS 9902, pp. 273–281, 2016.
DOI: 10.1007/978-3-319-46726-9_32

Efforts have been made for automatic basal slice detection. In a recent study, Tufvesson et al. [4] proposed a method to automatically segment the basal short-axis slices considering the long-axis motion of the heart. The approach works by segmenting the basal short-axis slices by considering 24 circumferential sectors over the LV which are analysed individually and removed in case no myocardium is detected. This method is motivated by recently published guidelines by the society for cardiovascular magnetic resonance [5] which indicate that the basal slice is the topmost short-axis slice that has more than 50 % myocardium around the blood cavity. In this approach, the long-axis motion of the heart is also estimated by deforming an LV model based on the segmentations helping to find a more accurate estimation of the volume in the end-systole and end-diastole according to the same guidelines. The algorithm is implemented in the freely available cardiac image analysis software Segment [6] and represents the current state-of-the-art for basal slice detection.

Other methods often exploit the availability of the long-axis views. Notable examples include Lu and Jolly [7] and Mahapatra [8], who proposed methods that train a model by intensity, texture, and contextual features extracted from a bounding box around manually annotated landmarks around the mitral valve in the long-axis view. These methods, however, need further improvement to provide a reliable estimation. There are also trained models of the heart in the literature for segmentation of the left ventricle from different views including the two-chamber view such as the works by Zhuang et al. [9] and Paknezhad et al. [10]. However, these models usually need considerable amounts of training data.

This paper presents a model-free method that relies on the long-axis view to find the basal slice. The long-axis view was chosen as it provides useful information about the base of the LV given the poor quality of the short-axis slices around the base due to heavy blood flow in this area. The proposed approach works by segmenting the LV walls in each slice of the long-axis view and using this segmentation to estimate the basal slice. Consequently, the method is able to provide basal slice identification and long-axis motion estimation over the entire cardiac cycle.

2 Segmenting the Base of the Left Ventricle

The proposed method works by segmenting the basal myocardium walls for the whole time-sequence in the two-chamber view. This is achieved via a two-pass segmentation approach. The first pass is a multi-phase level set that provides an initial segmentation. From the level-set segmentation, seed points are extracted that are used in a random-walk segmentation. The results from these two segmentations are fused to obtain the final basal myocardium wall segmentation. This information is then used to determine the basal slice as described in Sect. 3. The two-pass segmentation approach is described in the following.

User-Input and Pre-processing. The long-axis two-chamber view is selected for segmentation as it provides the clearest view of the LV walls around the

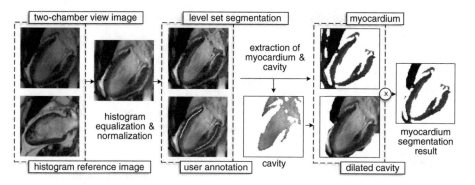

Fig. 1. Steps taken before and after applying the multiphase level set segmentation algorithm on the user-annotated two-chamber view image of the LV.

base. The user is asked to locate the LV walls on an arbitrary two-chamber CINE image by drawing two lines on the LV walls. A 101×101 box is considered around the LV and the histogram of each CINE image is adjusted to a reference image sequence to normalize the contrast.

Multi-phase Level Set. We obtain an initial segmentation using the multi-phase level set algorithm proposed by Li et al. [11]. This segmentation method is deployed since it is capable of following highly varying structures while capturing detailed edges within the image. The algorithm takes intensity inhomogeneity, typical of MRI scans, into account by modeling the relationship between a real-world image I and the true image J as $I = bJ + n$ in which b is a slow-varying bias field that accounts for the intensity inhomogeneities, and n is an additive noise. The final segmentation partitions the true image into N disjoint regions $\Omega_1, \Omega_2, \cdots, \Omega_N$. To estimate the bias field, a circular neighborhood around each pixel y (specified as O_y) is considered. Due to the slow-varying property assumed for the bias field b, the value $b(x)$ for each pixel $x \in O_y$ is approximated to $b(y)$. Since segmentation of the whole image domain Ω into multiple regions $\{\Omega_i\}_{i=1}^N$ partitions the neighborhood O_y, the intensities in the neighborhood of O_y were classified into N clusters with centers $b(y)c_i$ by minimizing the following clustering criterion:

$$\varepsilon_y = \sum_{i=1}^{N} \int_{\Omega_i \cap O_y} K(y - x)|I(x) - b(y)c_i|^2 \, dx, \tag{1}$$

The N disjoint regions take N constant values $c_1, c_2, \cdots, c_N$ that minimize the energy function. $K(y - x)$ was chosen to be a truncated gaussian function with scale parameter of σ and $K(y - x) = 0$ for $x \notin O_y$. Consequently, The best segmentation was one such that the clustering criterion ε_y was minimized for all $y \in \Omega$. The energy function for the level set was defined as the sum of the clustering criterion ε_y and two regularization terms with μ as the coefficient for the distance regularization term. The algorithm is applied on the user annotated

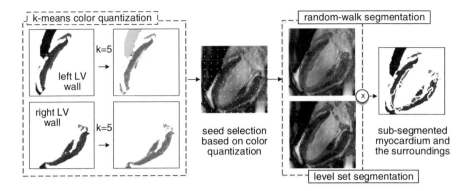

Fig. 2. Selection of seeds for initialization of the random-walk segmentation algorithm by applying k-means color quantization on each wall from the level set segmentation result. The final result is the combination of both segmentation results.

image and the final segments are labeled as left or right wall depending on the user annotation. From this information, the blood cavity of the LV can be estimated and segments that have an average intensity close to the average intensity of the blood cavity are removed. Figure 1 overviews the user annotation and level set segmentation.

Random Walk Segmentation. While the level set segmentation provides a good starting point, we found that it is necessary to further refine the segmentation by integrating the results with the random-walk segmentation algorithm proposed by Grady [12]. The random-walk segmentation algorithm is able to improve the segmentation by subdividing the level set segmentation result into areas with similar intensities and weak edges. This is mainly because the random-walk segmentation is robust to noise and low contrast or absent of boundaries, which make up many of the regions for which level set fails. The drawback of random walk is that it requires user-defined seeds which assign unlabeled pixels to one of the m regions in the image. To this end, we leverage the initial level set results. In particular, the extracted segments from the level set segmentation are smooth and k seed colors are estimated using the color quantization proposed by Verevka [13] as shown in Fig. 2. Areas with similar intensity values are sampled uniformly and assigned the same labels. Samples from the cluster with cluster center close to zero, if any, are assigned similar label as the label for the areas out of the region of interest.

Random walk segmentation works by assigning a label to an unlabeled pixel as the one most likely reached first if a random walker starts from a labeled pixel. This can be treated as a graph problem where the random walker path is biased by assigning weights to the edges which connect the nodes in the graph using the gaussian weighting function $w_{ij} = exp(-\beta(g_i - g_j)^2)$, where w_{ij} is the weight defined for the edge e_{ij} which connects the nodes v_i and v_j and g_i is the image intensity at pixel i. The intensity-related weights prevents the random walker from crossing sharp intensity gradients while moving from one node to

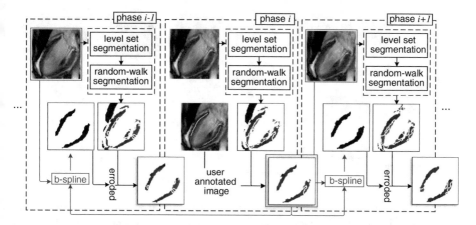

Fig. 3. The segmentation result for the user-annotated (ith) phase is registered to the $(i + 1)th$ phase $((i - 1)th$ phase) and used as a mask to select segments from the segmentation result for that phase. The registered mask in the $(i+1)th$ phase $((i-1)th$ phase) is then registered to the $(i + 2)nd$ phase $((i - 2)nd$ phase) and so on.

the other. This algorithm is applied to the two-chamber view image using the assigned labels and the segments which touched the user's annotations were selected and regarded as the final segmentation for the user-annotated image.

Segmentation Propagation. Once the two-pass segmentation is obtained for the user-annotated image, the result is propagated to the other slices in the two-chamber view for segment selection. This is done by using b-spline registration [14] of the initial image to the other images. Segmentation for the other frames is carried out using the same two-pass segmentation approach, however, the warped initial segmentation by the b-spline is used instead of user annotation. This procedure is shown in Fig. 3. The segmentation for each frame is later corrected by incorporating the segmentation results from the two frames before and after the current frame. This temporal consideration helps ameliorate the effects of the noisy segmentation. The top row in Fig. 4 shows the final LV segmentation after this procedure.

3   Estimating the Basal Slice and the Long-Axis Motion

Having segmented the two-chamber view image sequence, the SCMR guidelines [5] are used for basal slice selection. Considering the facts that the line connecting the mitral valve points may not be parallel to the short-axis slices and that multiple short-axis slices may intersect this line, the slice featured by the SCMR guidelines can be approximated to be the topmost short-axis slice below the middle of the line connecting the mitral valve points in the long-axis view. This is mainly because the two-chamber view provides an overview of two opposite walls of LV which are close to the center of the blood cavity. The long-axis motion is also estimated by tracking the relative movement of the mitral

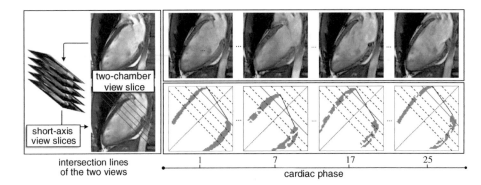

Fig. 4. (Left) Intersections lines between the two-chamber view slice and the short-axis view slices. (Top right) Final segmentation results after correction for a few phases in the cardiac cycle. (Bottom right) Basal slice for each phase. (Color figure online)

valve points along the LV. The bottom row in Fig. 4 shows the position of the basal short-axis slices (dashed lines), the line connecting the mitral valve points (black solid line), and the basal slice (blue line) for several phases for a sample LV. Once the end-diastolic and end-systolic phases are known, the basal slice for those phases can be retrieved and the long-axis motion can be estimated.

4   Evaluation and Results

The method was applied to clinical data from 56 cases, including 30 MRI scans of patients with degenerative mitral valve regurgitation acquired on a Siemens 3T Biograph mMR scanner, 19 MRI scans of healthy subjects acquired on a Siemens 3T Magnetom Trio, and 7 MRI scans of patients with myocardial infarction acquired on a Siemens 3T Magnetom Prisma scanner. The two-chamber cine CMR sequences comprised of 25 phases and the images were 256×232, 192×192, 256×216 pixels in size respectively with resolutions in the range of 1.32–1.56 mm. All 25 images of the two-chamber view were segmented using the proposed method. The number of iterations for the level set segmentation algorithm was set to 10, with scale parameter (σ) of 4, and distance regularization coefficient (μ) of 1. For k-means color quantization, k was set to 5 for all test cases. The weighting parameter (β) for the random-walk segmentation algorithm was set to 30. For images with 1.56 mm resolution, 1.5 times more seeds were sampled for random-walk segmentation. Three hierarchical levels were defined for the b-spline registration algorithm and the mesh window size was set to 10.

For each test case, the basal slice for the end-systole and the end-diastole were retrieved and the long-axis motion was estimated. The results were compared to the manual selections done by consensus between two experts prior to this work. The automatic basal slice selections and long-axis motion estimations by the Segment software [6], as the state-of-the-art approach, were also compared to the manual selections. In order to compare accuracy of the long-axis motion estimation, the short-axis slices for each test case were segmented using the Segment software [6] and EF, SV, and LV mass were extracted for each case. While using the same short-axis slice segmentations, experts' estimated long-axis motion was input to the Segment manually, so was the long-axis motion measured by the proposed algorithm and the ED, SV, and LV mass were extracted.

Table 1. Comparison of the measured EF, SV and LV mass (LVM) by the Segment tool, our experts and the proposed algorithm. Mean difference error and Pearson's R2 correlation between the two methods and the experts results are also shown. Stars (*) indicate significant differences (p-value<0.001).

		Segment	Experts	Proposed Alg.
	mean ± std (%)	62.5 ± 6.8	65.5 ± 6.0	65.2 ± 6.8
EF	mean diff. error ± std	-2.96 ± 4.55		**-0.22 ± 2.66** *
	R^2 corr.	0.515		**0.702**
	mean ± std(ml)	89.7 ± 25.1	96.4 ± 25.3	95.6 ± 27.8
SV	mean diff. error ± std	-6.63 ± 7.83		**-0.75 ± 6.25** *
	R^2 corr.	0.855		**0.929**
	mean ± std(g)	85.4 ± 25.0	84.1 ± 24.6	84.3 ± 24.6
LVM	mean diff. error ± std	1.34 ± 1.27		**0.15 ± 1.10** *
	R^2 corr.	0.904		**0.975**

From the 56 tested MRI scans, 80 % and 85 % of basal slice selections were found to be identical to the experts' selections for end-diastole and end-systole, respectively. This is while the Segment tool [6] selected the same basal slices as the experts' selected slices for 59 % of the cases in end-diastole and 44 % of the cases in end-systole. The EF, SV, and the LV mass for the proposed algorithm and the Segment tool were compared with those of experts' results using Pearson's R^2 correlation parameter. Table 1 shows the mean and standard deviation for the analysis done by the proposed approach, the Segment tool, and our experts. As can be seen, the mean values for the measured EF, SV, and LV mass by the proposed algorithm are closer to those of experts' measurements. It also shows the Pearson's R^2 correlation values for both methods. For all three parameters, the proposed algorithm provided more similar results to experts' analysis results. The average execution time for the proposed algorithm was 30 s for a non-optimized Matlab code with user input time of 9 s.

5   Discussion and Conclusion

Due to the high anatomical variability of the heart as well as the resolution and contrast limitations of MR scans, landmark-based approaches have not been able to accurately distinguish and locate mitral valve points using feature extraction methods. Model-based segmentation approaches also require considerable amount of training data. Consequently, an image-driven segmentation approach for basal LV segmentation was proposed in this paper providing accurate segmentation of the area around the mitral valve points. The proposed method does not require model training. The proposed approach is able to detect the basal slice through the whole cardiac cycle as well as estimate the long-axis motion of the heart which are essential to provide a robust and accurate method for cardiac analysis. Although our method is semi-automatic, the required user input has minimum influence on the final results since it only guides selection of the cluster of segments to include for volume measurement. Future work will remove the currently required user input.

References

1. Ben Ayed, I., Punithakumar, K., Li, S., Islam, A., Chong, J.: Left ventricle segmentation via graph cut distribution matching. In: Yang, G.-Z., Hawkes, D., Rueckert, D., Noble, A., Taylor, C. (eds.) MICCAI 2009, Part II. LNCS, vol. 5762, pp. 901–909. Springer, Heidelberg (2009)
2. Marcus, J.T., Gtte, M.J.W., DeWaal, L.K., Stam, M.R., Van der Geest, R.J., Heethaar, R.M., Van Rossum, A.C.: The influence of through-plane motion on left ventricular volumes measured by magnetic resonance imaging: implications for image acquisition and analysis. J. Cardiovasc. Magn. Reson. 1(1), 1–6 (1999)
3. Marchesseau, S., Ho, J.X.M., Totman, J.J.: Influence of the short-axis cine acquisition protocol on the cardiac function evaluation: a reproducibility study. Eur. J. Radiol. 3, 60–66 (2016)
4. Tufvesson, J., Hedstrm, E., Steding-Ehrenborg, K., Carlsson, M., Arheden, H., Heiberg, E.: Validation and development of a new automatic algorithm for time-resolved segmentation of the left ventricle in magnetic resonance imaging. BioMed Res. Int. 970357 (2015)
5. Schulz-Menger, J., Bluemke, D.A., Bremerich, J., Flamm, S.D., Fogel, M.A., Friedrich, M.G., Nagel, E.: Standardized image interpretation and post processing in cardiovascular magnetic resonance: society for cardiovascular magnetic resonance (SCMR). J. Cardiovasc. Magn. Reson. 15(35), 1167–1186 (2013)
6. Heiberg, E., Sjgren, J., Ugander, M., Carlsson, M., Engblom, H., Arheden, H.: Design and validation of segment a freely available software for cardiovascular image analysis. BMC Med. Imaging 10(1) (2010)
7. Lu, X., Jolly, M.-P.: Discriminative context modeling using auxiliary markers for LV landmark detection from a single MR image. In: Camara, O., Mansi, T., Pop, M., Rhode, K., Sermesant, M., Young, A. (eds.) STACOM 2012. LNCS, vol. 7746, pp. 105–114. Springer, Heidelberg (2013). doi:10.1007/978-3-642-36961-2_13
8. Mahapatra, D.: Landmark detection in cardiac MRI using learned local image statistics. In: Camara, O., Mansi, T., Pop, M., Rhode, K., Sermesant, M., Young, A. (eds.) STACOM 2012. LNCS, vol. 7746, pp. 115–124. Springer, Heidelberg (2013). doi:10.1007/978-3-642-36961-2_14
9. Zhuang, X., Rhode, K.S., Razavi, R.S., Hawkes, D.J., Ourselin, S.: A registration-based propagation framework for automatic whole heart segmentation of cardiac MRI. IEEE TMI 29(9), 1612–1625 (2010)
10. Paknezhad, M., Marchesseau, S., Brown, M.S.: Automatic basal slice detection for cardiac analysis. In: SPIE 9784, Medical Imaging: Image Processing (2016)

11. Li, C., Huang, R., Ding, Z., Gatenby, J.C., Metaxas, D.N., Gore, J.C.: A level set method for image segmentation in the presence of intensity inhomogeneities with application to MRI. IEEE TIP **20**(7), 2007–2016 (2011)
12. Grady, L.: Random walks for image segmentation. IEEE PAMI **28**(11), 1768–1783 (2006)
13. Verevka, O.: The Local K-means Algorithm for Colour Image Quantization. ProQuest Dissertation Publishing (1995)
14. Myronenko, A., Song, X.: Intensity-based image registration by minimizing residual complexity. IEEE PAMI **29**(11), 1882–1891 (2010)

Spatially-Adaptive Multi-scale Optimization for Local Parameter Estimation: Application in Cardiac Electrophysiological Models

Jwala Dhamala[1(✉)], John L. Sapp[2], Milan Horacek[2], and Linwei Wang[1]

[1] Rochester Institute of Technology, Rochester, NY 14623, USA
jd1336@rit.edu
[2] Dalhousie University, Halifax, Canada

Abstract. The estimation of local parameter values for a 3D cardiac model is important for revealing abnormal tissues with altered material properties and for building patient-specific models. Existing works in local parameter estimation typically represent the heart with a small number of pre-defined segments to reduce the dimension of unknowns. Such low-resolution approaches have limited ability to estimate tissues with varying sizes, locations, and distributions. We present a novel optimization framework to achieve a higher-resolution parameter estimation without using a high number of unknowns. It has two central elements: (1) a multi-scale coarse-to-fine optimization that uses low-resolution solutions to facilitate the higher-resolution optimization; and (2) a spatially-adaptive scheme that dedicates higher resolution to regions of heterogeneous tissue properties whereas retaining low resolution in homogeneous regions. Synthetic and real-data experiments demonstrate the ability of the presented framework to improve the accuracy of local parameter estimation in comparison to optimization based on fixed-segment models.

Keywords: Parameter estimation · Cardiac electrophysiological model · Multi-scale optimization · Gaussian process

1 Introduction

Many cardiac diseases stem from abnormal myocardial tissues with altered material properties. The quantitative knowledge about these abnormal tissues is paramount to the diagnosis, treatment, and prevention of relevant cardiac diseases. Since it is difficult to directly measure the material property of cardiac tissues, one effective way to quantify pathological tissue properties is to estimate the three-dimensionally distributed parameters of a cardiac model using indirect measurement data. This will in addition provide a patient-specific model useful for personalized treatment planning and prognosis [4].

Much effort has been reported on parameter estimation for complex physiological models. For example, derivative-free optimization methods [9] are shown

© Springer International Publishing AG 2016
S. Ourselin et al. (Eds.): MICCAI 2016, Part III, LNCS 9902, pp. 282–290, 2016.
DOI: 10.1007/978-3-319-46726-9_33

to be effective in handling the complex objective functions. Alternatively, surrogate models such as spectral representation based on polynomial chaos [4], multivariate polynomial regression [10], and Gaussian processes [5] have gained increasing interest in recent years.

Nevertheless, progress has been limited in estimating local parameters that are three-dimensionally distributed in space. Many previous works focus on the estimation of global parameters [5] by assuming uniform tissue property throughout the myocardium. Although it provides a fast calibration of a model, global parameter estimation does not reveal the local change of tissue properties. Toward local parameter estimation, a commonly-used approach is to divide the myocardium into a set of pre-defined segments and assume the parameter to be uniform within each segment. This substantially reduces the dimension of unknowns (to a range of 3 to 27) [9,10], yet the resolution is too low to capture abnormal tissues with different sizes, locations, and distributions. Moreover, as the number of segments increases, a good initialization becomes critical [9] which typically requires additional data to delineate diseased regions *a priori*. A critical gap remains between the need for a high-resolution local parameter estimation and the difficulty to accommodate high-dimensional optimization.

To bridge this gap, we propose a novel framework that goes beyond fixed low-resolution parameter estimation without invoking an infeasible number of unknowns. This is achieved via two primary elements. First, a multi-scale hierarchy is used to progressively use low-resolution results to facilitate higher-resolution optimization, thereby alleviating the issue of identifiability. Second, instead of uniform resolution, an adaptive scheme is used to selectively allocate higher resolution in heterogeneous regions whereas retaining lower resolution in homogeneous regions. It shares an important intuition with [1] where non-uniform mesh is used, although with fundamental differences in the coarser-to-finer transition of information and the motivation (heterogeneity) for adaptive resolution.

The proposed framework is applied to local parameter estimation for a 3D cardiac electrophysiological (EP) model using non-invasive electrocardiographic (ECG) data. It is noteworthy that the remote global ECG data increase the difficulty in identifying local tissue properties in comparison to local direct mapping data. The presented method is tested on a set of synthetic and real-data experiments. In comparison to the derivative-free BOBYQA [6] method carried out on a predefined 18-segment model, the presented method demonstrates higher accuracy using a similar or even fewer unknowns. While this framework is reported with GP based optimization, it can be used with other optimization methods. It is also applicable to local parameter estimation beyond cardiac EP models.

2   Cardiac Electrophysiology and ECG

2.1   Cardiac Electrophysiological Model

The spatiotemporal evolution of cardiac action potential can be described by a set of differential equations, ranging from complex ionic models with tens of hundreds of parameters to simpler models with a few parameters [2]. As an initial demonstration of feasibility for the proposed framework, we consider parameter estimation for the *Aliev-Panfilov* (AP) [2] model because of its ability to simulate electrical dynamics with fewer parameters and reasonable computation.

$$\partial u/\partial t = \partial/\partial x_i d_{ij} \partial u/\partial x_j - ku(u-a)(u-1) - uv$$
$$\partial v/\partial t = \varepsilon(u,v)(-v - ku(u-a-1)). \tag{1}$$

where, u is the transmembrane action potential and v is the recovery current. Parameter d_{ij} is the spatial conductivity, ε controls the coupling between the recovery current and action potential, k controls the repolarization, and a controls the excitability of a cell. In this study, we focus on a as it is one of the most sensitive model parameter and its value is associated to the ischemic severity of the myocardial tissue [2]. The meshfree method is used to discretize and solve (1) on the 3D myocardium [8], with a resolution of $\sim$6-mm ($\sim 10^3$ nodes).

2.2 ECG Measurement Model

Cardiac action potential produces potential on the body surface that is measured as time-varying ECG signals. This measurement process can be described by the quasi-static approximation of the electromagnetic theory [8]. Solving this governing equation on the discrete mesh of heart and torso models specific to an individual, a linear model between ECG data $\mathbf{\Phi}$ and transmural action potential $\mathbf{u}$ can be obtained as: $\mathbf{\Phi} = \mathbf{Hu}$ [8].

3 Spatially-Adaptive, Multi-scale Optimization

Estimation of the three-dimensionally distributed tissue excitability $\boldsymbol{\theta}$ from ECG data $\mathbf{y}$ can be formulated as a bounded global maximization problem:

$$\max_{1 \le \boldsymbol{\theta} \le \mathbf{u}} G(\boldsymbol{\theta}) = \max_{1 \le \boldsymbol{\theta} \le \mathbf{u}} \sum_{i=1}^{L} \left(\frac{\sum_{t=1}^{M}(y_{it} - \bar{y}_i)(\Phi_{it} - \bar{\Phi}_i)}{L\sqrt{\sum_{t=1}^{M}(y_{it} - \bar{y}_i)^2 \sum_{t=1}^{M}(\Phi_{it} - \bar{\Phi}_i)^2}} - \lambda \sum_{t=1}^{M}(\Phi_{it} - y_{it})^2 \right). \tag{2}$$

where $\mathbf{\Phi} = f(\boldsymbol{\theta})$ is a composite of the measurement an AP models (see Sect. 2). The objective function (2) includes both a correlation coefficient and a squared error to balance the morphology and magnitude similarity between the ECG data and the model output. L is the number of ECG leads.

The direct estimation of $\boldsymbol{\theta}$ requires a high-dimensional optimization (order of 10^3) that is not feasible due to both un-identifiability and high computation. To achieve higher-resolution local parameter estimation, the optimization framework described below includes two key components: (1) a hierarchical coarse-to-fine estimation, and (2) a spatially-adaptive resolution that is refined at regions of heterogeneity. This framework is developed with GP-based optimization.

3.1   Multi-scale Hierarchy

A coarse-to-fine optimization has the advantage to use lower-resolution solution to reduce the search during higher-resolution optimizations. To facilitate this, we construct a multi-scale representation of the cardiac mesh using Agglomerative Hierarchical Clustering [3], exploiting the spatial smoothness of tissue properties. A partial tree structure of this multi-scale model can be seen in Fig. 1. The clustering starts with each node in the cardiac mesh as a separate cluster. Every two closest clusters, based on the Euclidean distance and average linkage metric, are then merged until the entire ventricular mesh belongs to a single cluster. On this hierarchy model, the optimization starts at the root as a global estimation, and progressively moves to a higher level of resolution. Each level of optimization consists of two primary tasks: (1) optimization exploiting the lower-level solution (Sect. 3.3); and (2) determination of the spatial resolution for the next level of optimization (Sect. 3.2).

3.2   Adaptive Spatial Refinement

Instead of uniform resolution, we aim for a spatially-adaptive resolution so that higher resolution is used at regions of heterogeneity. In other words, after each level of optimization, instead of splitting all leaf nodes selective splitting and retraction is done to generate a skewed tree.

The key task is to identify the heterogeneous versus homogeneous clusters in tissue properties. Intuitively, if a cluster is homogeneous, its split is expected to yield children clusters with similar parameter values; *i.e.*, there will be minimal gain in the objective function (2). The contrary is true for heterogeneous clusters. Therefore, we propose a criterion based on gains in the objective function value.

Specifically, after obtaining an optimal solution $\boldsymbol{\theta}^k$ at level k, we examine two types of leaf nodes. First, we examine each pair of sibling nodes $(\theta_{i,c1}^k, \theta_{i,c2}^k)$ that share same parent node $\boldsymbol{\theta}_i^{k-1}$. For each pair of $(\theta_{i,c1}^k, \theta_{i,c2}^k)$, we evaluate the gain of splitting them from their parent as the difference in objective function evaluated on $\boldsymbol{\theta}^k$ versus replacing $(\theta_{i,c1}^k, \theta_{i,c2}^k)$ with their parent θ_i^{k-1}:

$$r_{k,i} = G(\boldsymbol{\theta}^k) - G(\mathbf{s}^k), \quad \text{where} \quad \mathbf{s}^k = (\boldsymbol{\theta}^k \setminus (\theta_{i,c1}^k, \theta_{i,c2}^k), \boldsymbol{\theta}_i^{k-1}) \tag{3}$$

Second, for leaf nodes that do not any sibling, no resolution change has occurred but their values may have been changed as a result of resolution change else-where. For such a node $\boldsymbol{\theta}_i^k$, the gain $r_{k,i}$ equals the change in the objective function due to the change in $\boldsymbol{\theta}_i^k$ before and after the optimization.

Based on $r_{k,i}$, we take two actions on tree structure before the next level of optimization: (1) for a leaf node or a pair of leaf nodes with maximum gain $r_{k,i}$, we consider them to be most heterogeneous and warrant a higher-resolution representation (*i.e.*, a split); and (2) for those that bring negligible or negative gain ($r_{k,i} < \delta$, δ is the same tolerance in the improvement of global optimum used for the convergence of overall framework), the split suggested by the previous level was not beneficial and retract it. The rest of nodes are unchanged.

3.3   Optimization via Surrogate Models

The proposed framework can be used in combination with any optimization method suitable for handling a complex objective function like (2). In this paper, a GP surrogate model based method is used [7]. In brief, the optimization assumes a prior distribution, in the form of a GP $\sim \mathcal{N}(\mu(\boldsymbol{\theta}), \sigma(\boldsymbol{\theta}))$, to denote the belief over the objective function (2) and sequentially updates the prior based on new data to better approximate the objective function, especially in the region of global optimum. Here, we elaborate the three main steps of the optimization at each level of resolution:

1. Initialize the GP: We start with a GP with zero mean and "Matern 5/2" covariance function [7] to impose a minimal assumption of smoothness over the objective function (2). While the GP-based optimization is gaining increasing attention for optimizing highly expensive cost functions, it suffers from an inability to scale in high dimension (≤ 15) [7]. Here, we utilize the low-resolution optimum to facilitate the higher-resolution GP optimization. In the proposed framework, a set of higher-resolution points are generated from the previous lower-resolution optimum through a convolution operator and parameter bounds. These points serve to quickly obtain an initial higher-resolution GP surrogate.

2. Determine the next query point: To update the GP, the best point to query should both exploit the solution space of the current GP where the predictive mean $\mu(\boldsymbol{\theta})$ is high and explore the solution space where the predictive uncertainty $\sigma(\boldsymbol{\theta})$ is high. This is done by finding the point that maximizes the upper confidence bound $\mu(\boldsymbol{\theta}) + \kappa\sigma(\boldsymbol{\theta})$ of the current GP [7], using the BOBYQA [6] optimization. The parameter κ balances the exploitation and exploration.

3. Update the GP: On the new query point obtained from step 2, the objective function (2) is evaluated and the posterior distribution of the GP is updated [7]. Steps 2 and 3 run in iteration until convergence of the GP based optimization.

4   Experiments

Synthetic Experiments: In a set of 22 synthetic experiments conducted on 3 image-derived realistic human heart-torso models, we test the proposed method in estimating the excitability of cardiac tissue in presence of infarct of varying locations and sizes. The parameter "a" of the AP model (1) is set to be 0.15 ± 0.01 and 0.45 ± 0.01, respectively, for normal and infarction tissues. 120-lead ECG are simulated and corrupted with 20 dB Gaussian noise. Infarct covering 1 % to 40 % of the LV/RV is set at different locations using various combinations of the AHA segments and random initializations with sizes smaller than one segment.

The presented method is compared with the BOBYQA method [6] carried out on a fixed 18-segment model (17 LV AHA segments + 1 RV segment) [9]. Because GP-based optimization did not scale well to 18-dimensional optimization in our

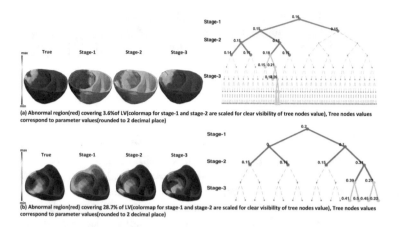

(a) Abnormal region(red) covering 3.6%of LV(colormap for stage-1 and stage-2 are scaled for clear visibility of tree nodes value), Tree nodes values correspond to parameter values(rounded to 2 decimal place)

(b) Abnormal region(red) covering 28.7% of LV(colormap for stage-1 and stage-2 are scaled for clear visibility of tree nodes value), Tree nodes values correspond to parameter values(rounded to 2 decimal place)

Fig. 1. Examples of the progression of the multi-scale optimization. Left: true parameter settings *vs.* estimation results over 3 successive stages of the optimization. Right: the corresponding growth of the tree at each stage. The gray, dotted structure shows the full hierarchy, whereas the colored line show the path taken by the presented method. (Color figure online)

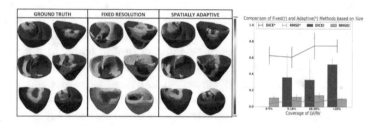

Fig. 2. Comparison of the presented method with BOBYQA on a 18-segment model. Left: examples of different infarcts. Right: quantitative comparison in DC and RMSE.

experiments, it is not included in this paper. We evaluate the estimated parameters using two metrics: (1) root mean square error (RMSE) between the true and estimated parameters; and (2) dice coefficient DC $= \frac{2(S_1 \cap S_2)}{S_1 \cup S_2}$, where S_1 and S_2 are the sets of cardiac nodes in the true and estimated regions of infarct; these regions are defined from the final tree in the presented method, and by thresholding parameter values in the BOBYQA method. Both metrics are evaluated at the resolution of the cardiac mesh.

Figure 1 demonstrates how the presented adaptive coarse-to-fine optimization progresses: the left panel shows the improvement in estimation at 3 successive stages, with the corresponding growth of the tree in the right panel. Figure 1a shows an example on a small infarct (3 %). The tree shows that since stage 1, the optimization split only along the heterogeneous region that contains the abnormality. It continued narrowing down the infarct with higher resolution, generating a narrow yet deep tree. The estimation shown in stage 3 of Fig. 1b

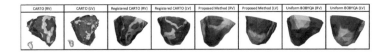

Fig. 3. Real-data experiment: comparison with *in-vivo* voltage maps of scar. (Color figure online)

was achieved with only 13 unknowns. In comparison, if a uniform resolution is used, a dimension of 128 is needed to achieve estimation at the same resolution. Figure 1b shows an example with a larger infarct (29 %). Because abnormal tissues span a larger number of clusters compared to a small infarct, it is not until stage 2 before the tree can be split along major branch. In addition, because both normal and abnormal tissues are large enough to be represented by low-resolution, homogeneous regions, an overall lower-resolution solution is obtained with a wider yet shallow tree. Similarly, in this case the presented method converged at a dimension of 7 whereas a uniform resolution of 16 is required.

Figure 2 summarizes the comparison between the presented method and the BOBYQA method directly on the fixed 18-segment. The improvement of the presented method is statistically significant in both DC and RMSE (paired-t tests, $p < 0.001$). More specifically, the performance of the presented method is much more robust to the size and shape of the infarct. While optimization on fixed segments has trouble handling infarcts of size equal to a single AHA segment, the presented method could provide an accurate estimation using only 12–14 unknowns. Furthermore, optimization on fixed segments tends to show false-positives across multiple segments, falling short to reveal the spatial distribution of an infarct. The presented method improves this accuracy by adaptively allocating higher-resolution on the heterogeneous regions. Depending on the type of the infarct, the computational cost of the presented method is comparable or higher than direct optimization on 18 uniform divisions. For medium sized infarcts (5–25 % of LV), the tree is shallower (Fig. 1b) and requires fewer coarse to fine optimizations. For small infarcts (≤ 5 % of LV), the tree is deeper with many leaf nodes (Fig. 1a) and requires larger coarse to fine optimizations. In such cases, the number of model evaluations for presented method was at most 1.5 times that needed for direct optimization on 18 segments. Although for such size, direct optimization has trouble in estimation mainly due to un-identifiability.

Real-Data Experiment: As a feasibility test, we conducted a case study on a patient who underwent catheter ablation of ventricular tachycardia due to prior tissue infarction. Tissue excitability was estimated from 120-lead ECG on the patient-specific heart-torso geometry obtained from CT images. Bipolar voltage data from *in-vivo* CARTO mapping were used as reference: as illustrated in Fig. 3, they reveal low-voltage regions at both lateral LV and RV (red: dense scar ≤ 0.5 mV; green: scar border $= 0.5$–1.5 mV; blue: normal > 1.5 mV). Excitability estimated from the presented framework successfully captured abnormal tissues at both locations whereas estimation from direct BOBYQA optimization using pre-defined 23 segments (17-LV, 6-RV) captured the abnormal tissue located on RV only. Interestingly, during post-processing of CARTO, the clinician marked that the low-voltage region at middle-apical lateral RV was caused by poor catheter contact rather than scar tissue. The estimated excitability values on RV, reflected this tissue property on RV. Overall, the core and border of abnormal tissues as revealed by the estimated excitability appear to co-locate with CARTO maps. It should be noted that, because CARTO maps show voltage data whereas the estimated parameter map shows tissue excitability, they are not expected to appear identical; further caution is needed in interpreting the results.

5   Conclusion

This paper presents a novel framework to achieve a higher-resolution local parameter estimation using a small number of unknowns. This is enabled by a multi-scale optimization, and a spatially-adaptive scheme that allocates higher resolution only at heterogeneous regions. Theoretically, the proposed method has the potential to reach the resolution of mesh. Experiments show that at the current stage, the accuracy is limited around the infarct border. One main future work is to improve the ability to go deeper along the tree, overcoming the issues of computation and observability. Additionally, it is desired to incorporate probabilistic estimation to handle the uncertainties in real data.

Acknowledgment. This work is supported by the National Science Foundation under CAREER Award ACI-1350374 and the National Institute of Heart, Lung, and Blood of the National Institutes of Health under Award R21Hl125998.

References

1. Chinchapatnam, P., Rhode, K.S., Ginks, M., Rinaldi, C.A., Lambiase, P., Razavi, R., Arridge, S., Sermesant, M.: Model-based imaging of cardiac apparent conductivity and local conduction velocity for diagnosis and planning of therapy. IEEE Trans. Med. Imaging **27**(11), 1631–1642 (2008)
2. Clayton, R., Panfilov, A.: A guide to modelling cardiac electrical activity in anatomically detailed ventricles. Prog. Biophys. Mol. Biol. **96**(1), 19–43 (2008)
3. Hastie, T., Tibshirani, R., Friedman, J.: Unsupervised Learning. Springer, New York (2009)
4. Konukoglu, E., Relan, J., Cilingir, U., Menze, B.H., Chinchapatnam, P., Jadidi, A., Cochet, H., Hocini, M., Delingette, H., Jaïs, P., et al.: Efficient probabilistic model personalization integrating uncertainty on data and parameters: application to eikonal-diffusion models in cardiac electrophysiology. Prog. Biophys. Mol. Biol. **107**(1), 134–146 (2011)
5. Lê, M., Delingette, H., Kalpathy-Cramer, J., Gerstner, E.R., Batchelor, T., Unkelbach, J., Ayache, N.: Bayesian personalization of brain tumor growth model. In: Navab, N., Hornegger, J., Wells, W.M., Frangi, A.F. (eds.) MICCAI 2015, Part II. LNCS, vol. 9350, pp. 424–432. Springer, Heidelberg (2015). doi:10.1007/978-3-319-24571-3_51

6. Powell, M.J.: The bobyqa algorithm for bound constrained optimization without derivatives. Cambridge NA report NA2009/06, University of Cambridge, Cambridge (2009)

7. Shahriari, B., Swersky, K., Wang, Z., Adams, R.P., Freitas, N.: Taking the human out of the loop: a review of bayesian optimization. Proc. IEEE **104**(1), 148–175 (2016)

8. Wang, L., Zhang, H., Wong, K.C., Liu, H., Shi, P.: Physiological-model-constrained noninvasive reconstruction of volumetric myocardial transmembrane potentials. IEEE Trans. Biomed. Eng. **57**(2), 296–315 (2010)

9. Wong, K.C., Sermesant, M., Rhode, K., Ginks, M., Rinaldi, C.A., Razavi, R., Delingette, H., Ayache, N.: Velocity-based cardiac contractility personalization from images using derivative-free optimization. J. Mech. Behav. Biomed. Mater. **43**, 35–52 (2015)

10. Zettinig, O., et al.: Fast data-driven calibration of a cardiac electrophysiology model from images and ECG. In: Mori, K., Sakuma, I., Sato, Y., Barillot, C., Navab, N. (eds.) MICCAI 2013, Part I. LNCS, vol. 8149, pp. 1–8. Springer, Heidelberg (2013)

Reconstruction of Coronary Artery Centrelines from X-Ray Angiography Using a Mixture of Student's t-Distributions

Serkan Çimen[1,2(✉)], Ali Gooya[1,2], Nishant Ravikumar[1,3], Zeike A. Taylor[1,3], and Alejandro F. Frangi[1,2]

[1] Center for Computational Imaging
and Simulation Technologies in Biomedicine, Sheffield, UK
s.cimen@sheffield.ac.uk
[2] Department of Electronic and Electrical Engineering,
University of Sheffield, Sheffield, UK
[3] Department of Mechanical Engineering, University of Sheffield, Sheffield, UK

Abstract. Three-dimensional reconstructions of coronary arteries can overcome some of the limitations of 2D X-ray angiography, namely artery overlap/foreshortening and lack of depth information. Model-based arterial reconstruction algorithms usually rely on 2D coronary artery segmentations and require good robustness to outliers. In this paper, we propose a novel probabilistic method to reconstruct coronary artery centrelines from retrospectively gated X-ray images based on a probabilistic mixture model. Specifically, 3D coronary artery centrelines are described by a mixture of Student's t-distributions, and the reconstruction is formulated as maximum-likelihood estimation of the mixture model parameters, given the 2D segmentations of arteries from 2D X-ray images. Our method provides robustness against the erroneously segmented parts in the 2D segmentations by taking advantage of the inherent robustness of t-distributions. We validate our reconstruction results using synthetic phantom and clinical X-ray angiography data. The results show that the proposed method can cope with imperfect and noisy segmentation data.

1 Introduction

X-ray coronary angiography is one of the commonly utilized imaging modalities in the assessment of coronary artery disease. However, this modality is known to be limited, since it can only deliver 2D X-ray images to visualise 3D moving coronary arteries. To overcome this limitation, 3D description of the coronary arteries can be reconstructed from X-ray angiography images [1]. However, inverse problem of reconstruction remains a challenging task due to intensity inhomogeneities, artery overlap/foreshortening, and cardiac/respiratory motion.

Numerous methods have been proposed to reconstruct coronary artery trees from X-ray angiography. Among these methods, model-based reconstruction methods try to reconstruct a 3D representation of the coronary arteries that comprises of artery centrelines and, occasionally, the arterial lumen surface.

© Springer International Publishing AG 2016
S. Ourselin et al. (Eds.): MICCAI 2016, Part III, LNCS 9902, pp. 291–299, 2016.
DOI: 10.1007/978-3-319-46726-9_34

Most of the existing model-based reconstruction methods require clean segmentations of arteries from 2D X-ray angiography images [1]. However, segmentation of coronary arteries from X-ray angiography is still a challenging task because of inhomogeneous intensities and artery overlap/foreshortening, thus prone to errors. Therefore, the reconstruction methods should be devised in a way that they become robust to possible errors in the 2D coronary artery segmentations (such as over-segmentations due to the other structures that are also visible in the X-ray angiography images).

In this paper, we propose a novel method to reconstruct coronary artery centrelines from retrospectively gated X-ray angiography images acquired via a calibrated X-ray angiography system. Our method employs a novel probabilistic formulation based on a mixture of Student's t-distributions that describes the coronary artery centrelines in 3D space. Given the 2D over-segmentations of arteries from 2D X-ray images, we formulate the reconstruction problem as maximum-likelihood (ML) estimation of mixture model parameters. The t-distributions are known to be inherently robust to the outliers in the data. The utilization of t-distributions as the components of the mixture model allows us to significantly reduce the burden of manual inspecting the segmented arteries. This opens the possibility to use the results from semi/automatic 2D vascular segmentation algorithms, facilitating the reconstruction process. To the best of our knowledge, this is the first paper proposing that the reconstruction problem can be alternatively viewed as the task of a Student's t-mixture model fitting. Apart from robustness, the proposed method is a versatile framework that can handle complex arterial geometries, and requires no point-to-point correspondences.

2   Method

Our method assumes that the X-ray images and a simultaneous ECG are collected using a calibrated angiography system. Coronary artery segmentations, possibly containing erroneously segmented parts, are extracted from retrospectively gated 2D X-ray images. Coronary arteries are represented by a mixture of Student's t-distributions in 3D, from which the points in the 2D segmentations are considered to be generated. Reconstruction is formulated as a ML estimation of the parameters of the mixture model.

X-ray Image Acquisition and Retrospective ECG Gating: Our method requires an X-ray acquisition by a calibrated angiography system, i.e. the system geometry is known for each X-ray projection. This information can be exploited to define the projection between the patient and X-ray detector coordinate systems, which can be modelled by weak-perspective or perspective camera models [3]. Weak-perspective camera model provides a linear approximation of perspective camera model, when the depth of the object is small compared to distance from camera and the field of view is small [3], which are valid for X-ray angiography. Linearity of weak-perspective approximation yields closed form solutions for the estimation of mixture model parameters. Our method benefits from both camera models, starting with a weak-perspective model and, upon convergence, switching to perspective model for refinement.

Respiratory motion can be reduced by collecting X-ray images during a breath hold. Following image acquisition, a subset of X-ray images are selected via retrospective ECG gating in order to compensate for the cardiac motion. We select frames that are closest to a cardiac phase with minimal motion.

Segmentation of X-ray Images: The coronary arteries are segmented from 2D X-ray images using an automatic segmentation algorithm such as the ones proposed in [5,8]. The resulting segmentation may include some parts, which are erroneously segmented due to noise or other structures such as catheter, spine and diaphragm. We refer to these erroneous parts of the segmentation as outliers. Next, the segmented arteries are converted to point sets and further processed by our algorithm.

Reconstruction Based on Mixture of Student's t-distributions: To formulate the reconstruction, we represent 3D coronary artery centrelines by a probabilistic mixture model. Specifically, the 3D centrelines can be described by a set of points in 3D space. Furthermore, spatial locations of these points can be defined by the mean values of mixture model components. As a result, the points describing the 3D coronary artery centrelines form a mixture distribution in 3D space. We opt for Student's t-distribution as the component distribution of the mixture model, which is known to be a robust alternative to Gaussian distribution in the presence of outlier samples, owing to its heavier tails [6].

Segmented 2D artery points on X-ray images are considered to be the projections of samples generated from mixture model distribution. Therefore, reconstruction problem can be formulated as the estimation of the mean values of the mixture components and other mixture model parameters, given the 2D points describing the artery segmentations in the X-ray images.

Let $\boldsymbol{X}^f = \{\boldsymbol{x}_n^f \in \mathbb{R}^2\}_{n=1}^{N^f}$ be the set of 2D segmented artery points for the fth X-ray image of F retrospectively gated images. Similarly, let $\boldsymbol{Y} = \{\boldsymbol{y}_m \in \mathbb{R}^3\}_{m=1}^M$ denotes the set of M 3D points corresponding to the mean values of the t-distributions. A multivariate t-distribution with mean $\boldsymbol{\mu}$, covariance $\boldsymbol{\Sigma}$ and degrees of freedom ν can be written as an infinite mixture of scaled Gaussians

$$S(\boldsymbol{x}|\boldsymbol{\mu}, \boldsymbol{\Sigma}, \nu) = \int_0^\infty \mathcal{N}(\boldsymbol{x}|\boldsymbol{\mu}, \boldsymbol{\Sigma}/u)\mathcal{G}(u|\nu/2, \nu/2)du, \tag{1}$$

where $\mathcal{N}(\cdot)$ and $\mathcal{G}(\cdot)$ denote the Gaussian and Gamma distributions, respectively [6]. To compute the maximum-likelihood (ML) solution, u can be considered as an implicit latent variable introduced for each observation [6]. In our formulation, these latent variables are denoted by $\boldsymbol{U}^f = \{u_n^f \in \mathbb{R}\}_{n=1}^{N^f}$ for the 2D points in fth X-ray image. Similarly, let $\boldsymbol{Z}^f = \{\boldsymbol{z}_n^f \in \mathbb{R}^M\}_{n=1}^{N^f}$ be the set of latent variables for the 2D points in fth X-ray image, where $\boldsymbol{z}_n^f$ is an M-dimensional binary vector that has only one non-zero entry. These vectors specify from which mixture component that the 2D segmentation point is generated. Finally, we can write the complete data probability for our mixture model as

$$P(\mathbb{X}, \mathbb{Z}, \mathbb{U}|\boldsymbol{\theta}) = \prod_{f=1}^{F} \prod_{n=1}^{N^f} \prod_{m=1}^{M} \left[\pi_m \mathcal{N}(\boldsymbol{x}_n^f|\mathcal{H}^f(\boldsymbol{y}_m), \sigma^2/u_n^f) \mathcal{G}(u_n^f|\nu_m/2, \nu_m/2) \right]^{z_{nm}^f}$$

(2)

where $\mathbb{X} = \{\boldsymbol{X}^f\}_{f=1}^{F}$, $\mathbb{Z} = \{\boldsymbol{Z}^f\}_{f=1}^{F}$ and $\mathbb{U} = \{\boldsymbol{U}^f\}_{f=1}^{F}$. In addition, $\mathcal{H}^f$: $\mathbb{R}^3 \rightarrow \mathbb{R}^2$ is the projection function for the fth frame, which is modelled by a weak-perspective or a perspective camera model. Furthermore, mixture model parameters are given by $\boldsymbol{\theta} = \{\{\pi_m\}_{m=1}^{M}, \boldsymbol{Y}, \sigma^2, \{\nu_m\}_{m=1}^{M}\}$, where π_m and ν_m are the mixing coefficient and degrees of freedom for mth component, respectively, and σ^2 is the isotropic variance for the mixture model components.

Given the 2D points segmented from X-ray images, $\mathbb{X}$, the goal is to find the mixture model parameters that maximize the complete data log-likelihood function, i.e. $\hat{\boldsymbol{\theta}} = \arg \max_{\boldsymbol{\theta}} \ln P(\mathbb{X}, \mathbb{Z}, \mathbb{U}|\boldsymbol{\theta})$. The final 3D reconstruction of the coronary artery centreline points is given by the estimated mean values of the mixture model components, $\hat{\boldsymbol{Y}} \in \hat{\boldsymbol{\theta}}$.

The ML estimation of the parameters $\hat{\boldsymbol{\theta}}$ can be found using expectation-conditional-maximization (ECM) algorithm [6]. In the E-step at iteration (t), we compute expectations $E_{z_{nm}^f}(z_{nm}^f|\boldsymbol{x}_n^f, \boldsymbol{\theta}^{(t)}) = (\gamma_{nm}^f)^{(t)}$, $E_{u_n^f}(u_n^f|\boldsymbol{x}_n^f, \boldsymbol{\theta}^{(t)}, z_{nm}^f = 1) = (\tau_{nm}^f)^{(t)}$ and $E_{u_n^f}(\ln u_n^f|\boldsymbol{x}_n^f, \boldsymbol{\theta}^{(t)}, z_{nm}^f = 1)$. In the M-step, the parameters are updated from $\boldsymbol{\theta}^{(t)}$ to $\boldsymbol{\theta}^{(t+1)}$ using the expectations computed in E-step, such that the expectation of the log-likelihood function is maximized. After some algebra, it can be shown that the mean values of the t-distribution components can be computed by solving

$$\sum_{f=1}^{F} \sum_{n=1}^{N^f} (\gamma_{nm}^f)^{(t)} (\tau_{nm}^f)^{(t)} \left(\boldsymbol{x}_n^f - \mathcal{H}^f(\boldsymbol{y}_m)\right)^T \frac{\partial \mathcal{H}^f(\boldsymbol{y}_m)}{\partial \boldsymbol{y}_m} = \boldsymbol{0}.$$

(3)

For weak-perspective camera model, the Jacobian of the projection function is given by a linear projection operation which does not depend on $\boldsymbol{y}_m$. On the other hand, Jacobian is a function of $\boldsymbol{y}_m$ for the perspective camera model. Therefore, we obtain a closed form solution for weak-perspective model, and use numerical optimization for the perspective model to compute the reconstruction, which is defined by the mean values of the t-distribution components.

We obtain coronary artery centrelines from the set of reconstructed points by computing minimum spanning arborescence of a directed graph, whose vertices are the reconstructed points and edges are the possible connections between the neighbouring points. To this end, we select one of the reconstructed point as root of the graph based on our prior knowledge about the patient coordinate system. The graph is generated by connecting the root to all the remaining points, and each point to its neighbours inside 10 mm neighbourhood. The edge weights of the graph are determined by the Euclidean distance between the connecting points. After minimum spanning arborescence is computed using Edmonds algorithm [10], we apply some automatic pruning steps to obtain the final coronary arterial tree. First, we discard the reconstructed points that are located far from the remaining reconstructed points. Second, we remove the short branches that consist of less than 3 points. Finally, we fit a cubic spline to each branch of the coronary arterial tree (Fig. 1c and d).

3   Experiments and Results

Results on Synthetic Data: Due to the lack of ground truth information for validation, the quantitative validations of coronary artery reconstruction methods are typically based on synthetic data experiments. To this end, we generated two synthetic X-ray rotational angiography sequences and corresponding artery centreline segmentations using left coronary artery geometry of 4D XCAT phantom [9] (Fig. 1a). For both of the X-ray sequences, information related to acquisition, namely number of images (117), frame rate (30 fps), angular coverage (60° RAO to 60° LAO with 25° CRA angulation), and the parameters defining the acquisition geometry model, was derived from a clinical dataset. In the first sequence, we employed the static geometry of the coronary arteries at end-diastole to generate the synthetic sequence. In the second sequence, we simulated cardiac motion where we set the heart beat rate to 70 beats per minute. Finally, we performed ECG gating on this sequence via a gating window of width 10 % of the cardiac cycle. Effectively, a total of 11 images were selected that are close to end-diastolic phase, but still at different cardiac phases. For the experiments involving the static sequence, we selected the corresponding subset of X-ray images, which were acquired from the same viewpoints as the gated X-ray images from the dynamic sequence. We refer to the sets of X-ray images selected from the first and second sequence as *StaticSet* and *CardiacSet*, respectively.

In the synthetic data experiments, we assess: (i) the effect of erroneously segmented structures in the 2D segmentations (outliers), (ii) the effect of residual cardiac motion between the X-ray images, and (iii) the effect of number of 3D points describing the mixture model representation of the coronary arteries, on the coronary artery centreline reconstruction accuracy.

To study the effect of outliers, we generated random 2D points and added these points to the corresponding 2D coronary artery segmentations. Specifically, we generated random 2D curves using a trajectory of a particle subject to Brownian motion, and sampled outlier points from these curves (Fig. 1a). The number of additional outlier points for each X-ray image was varied from 0 % to 40 % of the number of points in the 2D coronary artery segmentations for the same X-ray image with 10 % increments. This procedure is carried out for all X-ray images in *StaticSet* and *CardiacSet*, so that we can additionally study the effect of residual motion. To initialize both the number and the spatial locations of the mixture model components, we assumed that points are located on a regular grid in spherical coordinates centred at the origin of the patient coordinate system. By changing the radial sampling rate of the grid, we adjusted M to 168 and 210 points (Fig. 1b).

In all of the experiments, the reconstruction accuracy measured in terms of two 3D centreline to centreline scores, namely overlap (OV_{3D}) and accuracy (AC_{3D}) scores, which were introduced as a part of the standardized evaluation framework described in [7]. Briefly, the overlap score measures how the

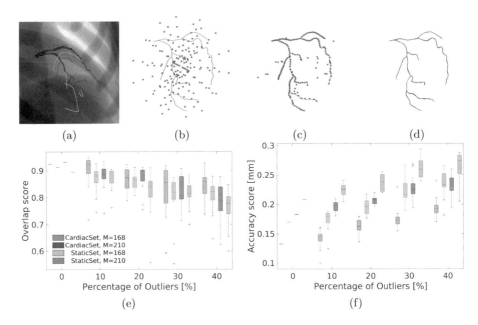

Fig. 1. (a)–(d) Qualitative results on synthetic data with 40 % outliers: (a) An example synthetic X-ray angiogram and the corresponding 2D segmentations (dark green) with outliers (light green) are shown. (b) The method is initialized using model points located on a regular spherical grid. (c) Reconstructed points are shown. (d) The final reconstruction output after pruning. In (b)–(d), the ground truth centrelines are shown in green, whereas reconstructed points or centrelines are shown in red. (e)–(f) Quantitative results with cardiac motion, different number of model components, and varying levels of outliers are presented using overlap and accuracy scores. (Color figure online)

reconstructed centreline agrees with the ground truth, based on the labelling of correspondences between reconstructed points and the ground truth centreline points as false positive, negative and true positive. On the other hand, the accuracy score measures the mean 3D Euclidean distance between the true positive correspondences.

We repeated the reconstruction experiments 15 times with different random outlier points in each outlier level. The qualitative and quantitative results of the synthetic data experiments are shown in Fig. 1. Results indicate that the performance of our method does not decrease drastically, even in the presence of high level of outlier points. As expected, the scores for *CardiacSet*, generated under cardiac motion, are lower, but comparable to the results from *StaticSet*.

As shown in Fig. 1c, the reconstructed points may contain some scattered points as we increase the outlier level. This can be explained as follows: when there is a significant number of outliers, the possibility of consistent point correspondences between various projection frames increases. As a result, some mixture model components are displaced towards those outliers. However, with lower outlier level, the heavy tails of t-distribution mixture components

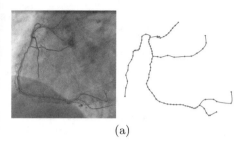

	AC$_{3D}$	RPE$_{2D}$
	(synthetic)	(clinical)
Jandt et al. [4]	0.19	NA
Liao et al. [5]	0.38	1.02
Yang et al. [11]	0.48	0.34
Cong et al. [2]	0.57	0.35
Proposed	0.13	0.39

(a)   (b)

Fig. 2. Results on clinical data: (a) Projection of the reconstructed coronary arteries (red) is overlaid on top of the segmented coronary arteries (green) on the left, and the corresponding 3D reconstruction result is shown on the right. (b) The results of the proposed algorithm for both synthetic and clinical experiments are compared with the relevant literature. These results were obtained using different synthetic and clinical datasets, but nonetheless show the accuracies of the various techniques. (Color figure online)

sufficiently explain those points. Therefore, no significant displacement of the mixture components is observed. Additionally, the situation is also aggravated when we increase the number of mixture model components as reflected by the increased dispersion of the overlap scores.

Results on Clinical Data: We reconstructed centrelines from 2 RCA and 1 LCA rotational angiography studies. The angular coverage of the acquisitions was 120° (60° RAO to 60° LAO with 25° CRA/CAU angulation). From each study, 4 images (one from each cardiac cycle) were selected via ECG gating.

Coronary artery segmentations from X-ray angiograms are carried out by the automatic algorithm given in [8]. Because the ground truth is not available for the clinical data, we present qualitative 3D reconstruction result and its back-projection onto the X-ray images (Fig. 2a). These results underscore the robustness of the algorithm in the presence of outliers. Although using TMM makes our reconstruction robust to outliers, reconstructed centrelines can be further improved if better segmentations (free from obvious errors or missing parts) are provided. To this end, we segmented centrelines using a workflow similar to the one proposed in [5], and cleaned the resulting segmentations. To facilitate quantitative evaluation, we computed 2D reprojection error (RPE$_{2D}$), which is defined as the average 2D Euclidean distance between 2D ground truth points and 2D projections of the reconstructed centrelines. The results are shown in Fig. 2b in comparison with the results from the relevant literature.

There is a trade-off between target accuracy (associated with M), and the computation time. Mean computation time for the clinical dataset was 21.8 min with $M = 168$ points describing the arteries.

4 Conclusion

In this paper, we propose a novel probabilistic framework to reconstruct coronary artery centrelines from retrospectively gated X-ray angiography images using a mixture of Student's t distributions. Given 2D segmentations of coronary arteries from X-ray images, we formulate the reconstruction problem as ML estimation of mixture model parameters. The framework is highly versatile and does not require point correspondences across various projections. The heavy tail of Student's t-distribution allows robust reconstruction and good handling of outliers. The quantitative validation on synthetic data indicates that our method can cope with reasonable level of erroneously segmented parts in the 2D coronary artery segmentations. As demonstrated in the experiments using clinical X-ray angiography images, this aspect enables using coronary segmentation algorithms which may produce some level of outliers. Proposed method provides a convenient framework to incorporate prior information (e.g. Bayesian priors enforcing linearity of local structures, and sparsity of mixture components), owing to its probabilistic formulation. This topic will be the focus of our future research.

Acknowledgements. This project was partly supported by the Marie Curie Individual Fellowship (625745, A. Gooya).

References

1. Çimen, S., Gooya, A., Grass, M., Frangi, A.F.: Reconstruction of coronary arteries from X-ray angiography: a review. Med. Image Anal. **32**, 46–68 (2016)
2. Cong, W., Yang, J., Ai, D., Chen, Y., Liu, Y., Wang, Y.: Quantitative analysis of deformable model-based 3-D reconstruction of coronary artery from multiple angiograms. IEEE Trans. Biomed. Eng. **62**(8), 2079–2090 (2015)
3. Hartley, R., Zisserman, A.: Multiple View Geometry in Computer Vision, 2nd edn. Cambridge University Press, Cambridge (2004)
4. Jandt, U., Schäfer, D., Grass, M., Rasche, V.: Automatic generation of 3D coronary artery centerlines using rotational X-ray angiography. Med. Image Anal. **13**(6), 846–858 (2009)
5. Liao, R., Luc, D., Sun, Y., Kirchberg, K.: 3-D reconstruction of the coronary artery tree from multiple views of a rotational X-ray angiography. Int. J. Cardiovasc. Imaging **26**(7), 733–749 (2010)
6. Peel, D., McLachlan, G.J.: Robust mixture modelling using the t distribution. Stat. Comput. **10**(4), 339–348 (2000)
7. Schaap, M., Metz, C.T., van Walsum, T., van der Giessen, A.G., Weustink, A.C., Mollet, N.R., Bauer, C., Bogunović, H., Castro, C., Deng, X., Dikici, E., O'Donnell, T., Frenay, M., Friman, O., Hernández Hoyos, M., Kitslaar, P.H., Krissian, K., Kühnel, C., Luengo-Oroz, M.A., Orkisz, M., Smedby, O., Styner, M., Szymczak, A., Tek, H., Wang, C., Warfield, S.K., Zambal, S., Zhang, Y., Krestin, G.P., Niessen, W.J.: Standardized evaluation methodology and reference database for evaluating coronary artery centerline extraction algorithms. Med. Image Anal. **13**(5), 701–714 (2009)

8. Schneider, M., Sundar, H.: Automatic global vessel segmentation and catheter removal using local geometry information and vector field integration. In: Proceedings IEEE ISBI, pp. 45–48. IEEE (2010)

9. Segars, W.P., Sturgeon, G., Mendonca, S., Grimes, J., Tsui, B.M.W.: 4D XCAT phantom for multimodality imaging research. Med. Phys. **37**(9), 4902–4915 (2010)

10. Tarjan, R.E.: Finding optimum branchings. Networks **7**(1), 25–35 (1977)

11. Yang, J., Cong, W., Chen, Y., Fan, J., Liu, Y., Wang, Y.: External force back-projective composition and globally deformable optimization for 3-D coronary artery reconstruction. Phys. Med. Biol. **59**(4), 975–1003 (2014)

Barycentric Subspace Analysis: A New Symmetric Group-Wise Paradigm for Cardiac Motion Tracking

Marc-Michel Rohé, Maxime Sermesant, and Xavier Pennec[✉]

Université Côte d' Azur, Inria, Asclepios Research Group, Antibes, France
{marc-michel.rohe,xavier.pennec}@inria.fr

Abstract. In this paper, we propose a novel approach to study cardiac motion in 4D image sequences. Whereas traditional approaches rely on the registration of the whole sequence with respect to the first frame usually corresponding to the end-diastole (ED) image, we define a more generic basis using the barycentric subspace spanned by a number of references images of the sequence. These subspaces are implicitly defined as the locus of points which are weighted Karcher means of $k + 1$ references images. We build such subspace on the cardiac motion images, to get a Barycentric Template that is no longer defined by a single image but parametrized by coefficients: the barycentric coordinates. We first show that the barycentric coordinates - the coefficients of the projection of the motion during a cardiac sequence - define a meaningful signature for group-wise analysis of dynamics and can efficiently separate two populations. Then, we use the barycentric template as a prior for regularization in cardiac motion tracking, efficiently reducing the error of tracking between end-systole and end-diastole by almost 40 % as well as the error of the evaluation of the ejection fraction. Finally, to best exploit the fact that multiple reference images allow to reduce the registration displacement, we derived a symmetric and transitive registration that can be used both for frame-to-frame and frame-to-reference registration and further improves the accuracy of the registration.

1 Introduction

Understanding and analyzing the cardiac motion pattern in a patient is an important task in many clinical applications. It can give insight into a pathology, by evaluating for example how the cardiac function is affected by a cardiovascular disease and if a therapy is needed or not. On top of traditional simple parameters such as the ejection fraction (EF), it can also be used to compute more complex parameters - such as strains in different directions - giving deeper insight to the efficiency of the heart motion and function. The cardiac motion is usually studied by finding correspondences - the registration step - between each of the frame of the sequence and the first frame corresponding to the end-diastole (ED) image, yielding a dense displacement field that tracks the motion of the myocardium. Taking the ED image as a reference is natural as it is the starting

© Springer International Publishing AG 2016
S. Ourselin et al. (Eds.): MICCAI 2016, Part III, LNCS 9902, pp. 300–307, 2016.
DOI: 10.1007/978-3-319-46726-9_35

point of the contraction of the heart which is the most important phase in evaluating the efficiency of the cardiac function but this specific choice can lead to important biases in quantifying the motion especialy at end-systole (ES) where the deformations to be evaluated are large [8].

In this paper, we propose a novel approach to study cardiac motion. Instead of taking an unique image as the reference to evaluate the motion, we build affine subspaces on the manifold of deformations encoding cardiac motion. There are different ways to extend the concept of principal affine spaces from an Euclidian space to something defined on manifolds. The simplest generalization is tangeant PCA, where a covariance matrix is build on the tangeant space of the Karcher or Frechet mean. In Principle Geodesic Analysys (PGA) [2], subspaces are spanned by the geodesics going through a point and the tangent vector is restricted to belong to a linear space of the tangent space. In this paper, we use more general type of family of subspaces on manifolds called Barycentric Subspaces which were first introduced in [4]. With respect to the method previously mentioned, it has the benefit not to be controlled by the central value. This gives a more consistent framework to study data in the case the underlying distribution is either multimodal or simply not sufficiently centered.

In the context of deformation analysis in medical imaging, the points of the manifold corresponds to 3D images whereas the geodesic are deformations mapping two images together. Optimal paths (geodesics) are represented by the initial velocity field at the geodesic path resulting from the registration of images. In the first part of this article, we define the barycentric subspaces of manifold and introduce the way to compute the barycentric coefficients and the projection of an image on a Barycentric Subspace of dimension k based on $k+1$ images. Instead of performing registration with respect to a single template, we build a subspace based on multiple references images and take advantage of the information of group-wise registration [10], by building a Barycentric Template of dimension 2 parametrized by the barycentric coefficients. Experiments are conducted on sequences of healthy and pathological patients and show that the barycentric coefficients of both populations present significant differences and two clear clusters appear. Then, we improve the registration of cardiac motion by relaxing the regularization within the 2-dimensional barycentric template representing a cardiac sequence. Finally, we further improve the methodology by deriving a formula leading to symmetric and transitive registration.

2   Barycentric Subspaces in Deformation Manifolds

In this section, we introduce barycentric subspaces following the notation described in [4]. In order to adapt the framework from Riemaniann Manifolds to the context of computational anatomy (image deformation analysis), we follows the framework of [3]. Working in the space of images $\mathcal{M}$, we define I as a point of this space, which can be for example an image of a cardiac sequence and we identify paths to deformations. In the following, we will use $(k+1)$ points R_j, the *references images*, on this Manifold as well as $(k+1)$ coefficients λ_j the *barycentric coefficients*. The *Barycentric Subspace* of dimension k

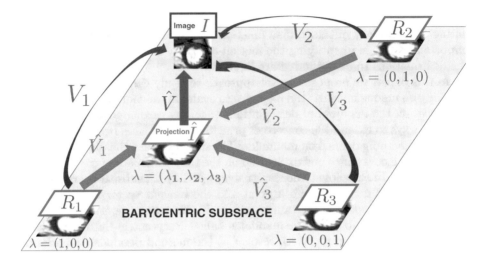

Fig. 1. Barycentric subspace of dimension 2 built from 3 references images (R_1, R_2, R_3). $\hat{I}$ is the projection of the image I within the barycentric subspace such that $\| \hat{v} \|^2$ is minimum under the conditions $\sum_j \lambda_j \hat{v}_j = 0$ and $\hat{v} + \hat{v}_j = v_j$.

spanned by these points is then defined as the set of points (images) $\hat{I}$ in $\mathcal{M}$ such that: $\sum_{j=1}^{k+1} \lambda_j \overrightarrow{\hat{I}R_j} = 0$, where $\overrightarrow{\hat{I}R_j} = \log_{\hat{I}}(R_j)$ is the smallest velocity field that registers I to R_j. Contrary to the Riemaniann setting where we would have exactly $R_j = \exp_{\hat{I}}(\overrightarrow{\hat{I}R_j})$, we obtain through registration an inexact matching that approximates the log vector. This is the tangeant vector of the geodesic shooting I to R_j. In the following, we will place ourselves in stationary velocity fields (SVF) framework [9] which gives a simple and yet effective way to parametrize smooth deformations along geodesics using one-parameter sub-group. In this case, the tangent vector $\overrightarrow{\hat{I}R_j}$ will be parametrized by the SVF $\hat{v}_j$ and the condition simply becomes $\sum_{j=1}^{k+1} \lambda_j \hat{v}_j = 0$. The notation are summed up in Fig. 1.

2.1 Projection on Barycentric Subspace

Having defined the barycentric subspace spanned by a set of $k + 1$ references R_j, we are looking to find the projection $\hat{I}$ of any image I in $\mathcal{M}$ on this subspace together with the coefficient λ_j representing the coordinates of $\hat{I}$ within the barycentric template. The projection $\hat{I}$ of I is the closest point to I that belongs to the barycentric subspace. We define the SVF $\hat{v}$ which parametrizes the projection of I such that $\overrightarrow{\hat{I}I} = \hat{v}$ as well as the SVFs $(v_i)_{i=1,\dots,k+1}$ such that $\overrightarrow{R_iI} = v_i$ as shown in Fig. 1. The distance between I and $\hat{I}$ is represented by the norm of the SVF $\| \hat{v} \|^2$. As seen previously, the constraint that $\hat{I}$ belongs to the barycentric subspace can be written as $\sum_j \lambda_j \hat{v}_j = 0$. Using the Baker-Campbell-Hausdorff (BCH) [9] formula, we get a first order development of $v_i = \hat{v} + \hat{v}_i$.

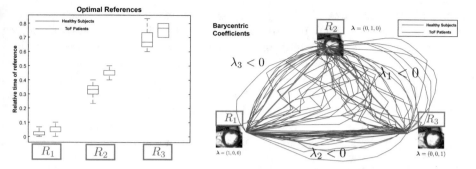

Fig. 2. (Left): Optimal references for the two group for each of the 3 references. (Right): Barycentric coefficient curves λ projected on the 2D-plan $\sum_i \lambda_i = 1$.

The problem can now be written as:

$$\min_{\hat{v}} \| \hat{v} \|^2, \quad \text{subject to} \sum_i \lambda_i(v_i - \hat{v}) = 0, \quad \sum_i \lambda_i \neq 0$$

whose set of solutions is:

$$\lambda = \alpha A^{-1}\mathbf{1}, \quad \alpha \in \mathbb{R}^*, \quad A = \langle v_i | v_j \rangle_{i,j}.$$

With the additional constraint $\sum_j \lambda_j = 1$, we get the unique solution by normalizing the λ.

Finally, given a set of N images I_n, we can define the distance of a barycentric subspace spanned by the references $(R_j)_{j=1,...,M}$ to the set of images $(I_n)_{n=1,...,N}$ as the sum of the error over all the residual projection vector $\hat{v}_n$ such that:

$$\mathcal{E}((R_j)_{j=1,...,M}) = \sum_{n=1,...,N} \| \hat{v}_n \|^2, \tag{1}$$

and find the closest subspace with respect to the cardiac sequence by minimizing this distance over all set of references.

2.2 Cardiac Motion Signature for Group-Wise Analysis of Dynamics

We applied the previously defined methodology to compare the cardiac motion signature of two different populations. The first group consists of 15 healthy subjects from the STACOM 2011 cardiac motion tracking challenge dataset [8]: an openly available data-set, and the second group is made of 10 Tetralogy of Fallot (ToF) patients. Short axis cine MRI sequences were acquired with $T = 15$ to 30 frames. The methodology described was applied by projecting each of the T frame of the cardiac motion to a barycentric subspace of dimension 2 spanned by 3 references. This set of 3 references is chosen by building the optimal barycentric subspace as induced by the distance defined in Eq. 1. Significant differences in the frame for the optimal references can be seen between the two populations (Fig. 2, left). In particular, the second reference - corresponding the end-systole - is significantly higher for the ToF patients showing that this population has on average longer systolic contraction. Then we project the whole cardiac motion on the barycentric subspace made of these three references to compute the barycentric coefficients (Fig. 2, right). We see significant differences between both group of curves, especially in the region $\lambda_1 < 0$ showing that this signature of the motion is encoding relevant features and classical machine learning algorithms can separate the two populations using this representation.

3   Registration Using Barycentric Subspaces

In this section, we show how the use of barycentric subspaces as a prior on the cardiac motion can improve the registration by relaxing the regularization. Most of the registration methods rely on a trade-off between a fidelity-to-data term - capturing how well the registration matches the intensities of the voxels of the images - and a smoothness regularization term - encoding our prior information about the regularity of the deformations we are looking. It is standard practice in registration algorithms to consider slowly varying deformation as our prior knowledge of the transformation (either by constraining the deformation to be within a small subspace of all diffeomorphisms or by penalizing large deformations). While this methodology works well to find small deformations, the regularization often leads to an underestimation of the large deformations as the one happening between the ED and ES frame. To overcome this drawback, solutions usually rely on performing the registration in a group-wise manner: a group of images are considered simultaneously and an additional criteria is added to ensure temporal-consistency [1,5]. In this paper, we propose to use the barycentric template defined by 3 frames of the sequence as an additional prior on the transformations by considering that only the distance to the closest image within this barycentric subspace should be minimized. In the regularization step, we no longer consider the whole velocity field v but we run the regularization only with respect to $\hat{v}$ which encodes the distance of the current image to the closest image within the barycentric template representing the cardiac motion.

3.1   Barycentric Log-Demons Algorithm

We apply this methodology to the *Symmetric Log-Domain Diffeomorphic Demons* algorithm [9] which successively updates the velocity field to match the data, then smooths the velocity field with a gaussian filter. Instead of performing the regularization on the complete velocity field (the "standard" method), we decompose the velocity field v_i as the sum of $\hat{v}_i$ mapping the reference R_i to the projection $\hat{I}$ inside the template and the residual velocity field $\hat{v}$ of the projection (see Fig. 1) and we regularize only the residual $\hat{v}$ with the gaussian filter. The barycentric template is therefore used as a prior on the cardiac motion for which we do not perform regularization. The method was evaluated using a

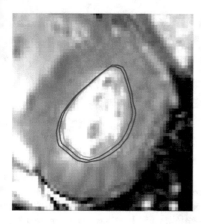
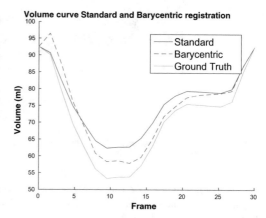

Fig. 3. (Left): Image of heart at end-systole, the contour of the warped mesh of the initial frame 1 (ED) using barycentric (red), standard (blue) registrations are shown together with the ground truth (green). Using barycentric regularization, the registration is less constrained and we manage to get a more accurate contours for the end-systolic endocardium. (Middle): Error of the registration with respect to 3 reference images using the two methods, barycentric (dotted lines) and standard (plain lines). (Right): volume curves induced by the registration and comparison with the ground truth volume. (Color figure online)

synthetic time serie of $T = 30$ cardiac image frames [6], so that we have ground truth meshes along the sequence allowing us to estimate the accuracy of the registration. First, we find the optimal references by minimizing the energy in Eq. 1 giving us the frames 1, 11 and 21 which will be the three references spanning the barycentric subspace. Then we register each frame i of the sequence using the method described above to get the deformations from each of the three references to the current images. We deform the ground truth meshes at the references frames with these deformations and compare the results with classical registration. As can be seen in Fig. 3, barycentric registration performs better at catching the end-systolic deformation with the contour of the warped mesh at end-systole matching better the ground truth. The estimation of the ejection fraction from the volume curve is also improved, going from 32 % with the standard method to 38 %, closer to the ground truth (43 %), reducing the estimation error by half. Finally, the average point-to-point error for both methods shows (in Fig. 4, right) that, while barycentric registration has largest error for small deformations close to each reference, it has around 30 % smaller error for largest deformations as between ED and ES.

3.2 Towards Symmetric Transitive Registration

In this last section, we quickly introduce a way to derive approximately consistent transitive (at the first-order of the BCH approximation) registration from the barycentric SVFs computed in the previous section. Symmetry and transitivity

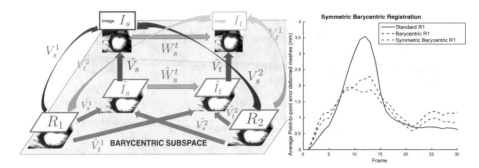

Fig. 4. (Left): Schematic representation of the symmetric multi-references barycentric registration in the case of a 1-D barycentric subspace spanned by 2 references. I_t and I_s are two frames of the sequence and $\hat{I}_t, \hat{I}_s$ corresponds to the respective projection to the barycentric subspace. (Right): comparaison of the error between the standard registration (blue plain), the barycentric method presented in Sect. 3.2 (blue dotted) and the symmetric-barycentric extension presented in Sect. 3.1 (red dotted). (Color figure online)

are two important properties for registration methods to improve robustness and reduce the unpredictability of the results [7]. A registration method is said to be symmetric if it associates two points regardless of the order of images that are registered together (in the SVF setting it is equivalent to $v_i^j = -v_j^i$). Transitivity requires that the deformation given by the registration between two images should be equal whether it is done directly or by the composition of the result of the registration with an intermediate image (in the SVF setting it can be stated as $v_i^j = BCH(v_i^k, v_k^j) \simeq v_i^k + v_k^j$ with the BCH at the first order). Most registration methods fail to be transitive due to the accumulation of the registration errors at each step of the registration. Using Barycentric Subspaces as a basis for the registration at each step, we define the symmetric registration using the following formula which is schematically represented in Fig. 4:

$$W_s^t = \hat{v}_t - \hat{v}_s + \frac{1}{2}\sum_i (\lambda_s^i \hat{v}_t^{\ i} - \lambda_t^i \hat{v}_s^{\ i}). \tag{2}$$

In this formula, the first two SVFs on the left represent the residual transformations from the barycentric subspace to the two time points, and the sum on the right is a symmetric estimation of the SVF $\hat{W}_t^s$ within the barycentric subspace by going through each reference image forward and backward. This formula defines registrations that are both symmetric and transitive up to higher orders of the BCH in the compositions. It can be used for frame-to-frame as well as for frame-to-reference registration. In the former case, setting the reference to the first frame ($s = 1$ in the above formula) leads to improved results as shown in Fig. 4: the maximum error over the sequence is reduced by approx. 10 % with respect to barycentric registration.

4   Conclusion

A new symmetric group-wise paradigm to study cardiac motion was proposed. Our approach relies on building subspaces as the reference for registration instead of choosing a specific arbitrary single image which can introduce bias. These subspaces represent the cardiac motion by meaningful parameters showing different clear patterns between two populations. Using these subspace as a prior, thereby relaxing the regularization on a 2-dimensional subspace, we achieve a better evaluation of the deformation between ED and ES frames and in particular we improve the estimation of the ejection fraction. Finally, the methodology can also be used to perform symmetric transitive registration, for better tracking along the sequence.

Ackowledgements. The authors acknowledge the partial funding by the EU FP7-funded project MD-Paedigree (Grant Agreement 600932).

References

1. Balci, S.K., Golland, P., Wells, W.: Non-rigid groupwise registration using b-spline deformation model. In: Open Source and Open Data for MICCAI, pp. 105–121 (2007)
2. Fletcher, P.T., Lu, C., Pizer, S.M., Joshi, S.: Principal geodesic analysis for the study of nonlinear statistics of shape. IEEE Trans. Med. Imaging 995–1005 (2004)
3. Joshi, S., Davis, B., Jomier, M., Gerig, G.: Unbiased diffeomorphic atlas construction for computational anatomy. NeuroImage 151–160 (2004)
4. Pennec, X.: Barycentric subspaces and affine spans in manifolds. In: Nielsen, F., Barbaresco, F. (eds.) GSI 2015. LNCS, vol. 9389, pp. 12–21. Springer, Heidelberg (2015). doi:10.1007/978-3-319-25040-3_2
5. Perperidis, D., Mohiaddin, R.H., Rueckert, D.: Spatio-temporal free-form registration of cardiac MR image sequences. Med. Image Anal. **9**(5), 441–456 (2005)
6. Prakosa, A., et al.: Generation of synthetic but visually realistic time series of cardiac images combining a biophysical model and clinical images. IEEE Trans. Med. Imaging 99–109 (2013)
7. Škrinjar, O., Bistoquet, A., Tagare, H.: Symmetric and transitive registration of image sequences. J. Biomed. Imaging 1–9 (2008)
8. Tobon-Gomez, C., et al.: Benchmarking framework for myocardial tracking and deformation algorithms: an open access database. Med. Image Anal. 632–648 (2013)
9. Vercauteren, T., Pennec, X., Perchant, A., Ayache, N.: Symmetric log-domain diffeomorphic registration: a demons-based approach. In: Metaxas, D., Axel, L., Fichtinger, G., Székely, G. (eds.) MICCAI 2008, Part I. LNCS, vol. 5241, pp. 754–761. Springer, Heidelberg (2008). doi:10.1007/978-3-540-85988-8_90
10. Yigitsoy, M., Wachinger, C., Navab, N.: Temporal groupwise registration for motion modeling. In: Székely, G., Hahn, H.K. (eds.) IPMI 2011. LNCS, vol. 6801, pp. 648–659. Springer, Heidelberg (2011). doi:10.1007/978-3-642-22092-0_53

Extraction of Coronary Vessels in Fluoroscopic X-Ray Sequences Using Vessel Correspondence Optimization

Seung Yeon Shin[1], Soochahn Lee[2(✉)], Kyoung Jin Noh[2], Il Dong Yun[3], and Kyoung Mu Lee[1]

[1] Department of ECE, ASRI, Seoul National University, Seoul, Republic of Korea
syshin@snu.ac.kr
[2] Department of Electronic Engineering,
Soonchunhyang University, Asan, Republic of Korea
sclsch@sch.ac.kr
[3] Division of Computer and Electronic Systems Engineering,
Hankuk University of Foreign Studies, Yongin, Republic of Korea

Abstract. We present a method to extract coronary vessels from fluoroscopic x-ray sequences. Given the vessel structure for the source frame, vessel correspondence candidates in the subsequent frame are generated by a novel hierarchical search scheme to overcome the aperture problem. Optimal correspondences are determined within a Markov random field optimization framework. Post-processing is performed to extract vessel branches newly visible due to the inflow of contrast agent. Quantitative and qualitative evaluation conducted on a dataset of 18 sequences demonstrate the effectiveness of the proposed method.

Keywords: Vessel extraction · MRF optimization · Vessel registration · Motion estimation · Fluoroscopic X-ray sequence

1 Introduction

Fluoroscopic X-ray angiograms (XRA, Fig. 1) are used to evaluate stenosis in coronary arteries and provide guidance for percutaneous coronary intervention. Here, vessel extraction enables registration of pre-operative CT angiograms (CTA) for visualization of 3-D arterial structure. For chronic total occlusion, this can visualize otherwise invisible arteries due to blockage of contrast agent.

Many works focus on vessel extraction from a single image. Pixelwise enhancement [1], and segmentation methods with sophisticated optimization [2,3] or learning [4] are some examples. While these methods are applicable to

This work was supported by the Institute for Information & communications Technology Promotion (IITP) Grant (No. R0101-16-0171) and by the National Research Foundation (NRF) Grant (2015R1A5A7036384), both funded by the Korean Government (MSIP).

© Springer International Publishing AG 2016
S. Ourselin et al. (Eds.): MICCAI 2016, Part III, LNCS 9902, pp. 308–316, 2016.
DOI: 10.1007/978-3-319-46726-9_36

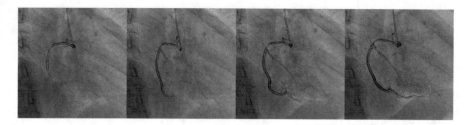

Fig. 1. A fluoroscopic XRA sequence with vessels extracted by the proposed method overlaid (green). Frames (13, 18, 24, and 31, respectively) are sparsely sampled to clearly show dynamics. (Color figure online)

a wide variety of vessels, they do not consider temporal continuity and thus may give inconsistent results for a sequence. Many works use an accurate vessel structure extracted from a detailed 3D CTA to extract an accurate and consistent vessel structure for XRA sequences [5,6]. Relatively few works have been proposed that do not require 3D CTA to detect and track curvilinear structures such as vessels [7] or guide-wires [8] from fluoroscopic image sequences.

Thus, we present a method, which we term vessel correspondence optimization (VCO), to extract coronary vessels from fluoroscopic x-ray angiogram sequences. Given the vessel structure of a source frame (obtained by manual annotation or automatic methods [2–4]), the detailed global and local motion is estimated by determining the optimal correspondence for vessel points in the subsequent frame. Local appearance similarity and structural consistency are enforced within a Markov random field (MRF) optimization framework. Essentially, VCO performs registration of the vessel structure. Post-processing is performed to deal with vessel branches newly visible due to the inflow of contrast agent. The proposed method is summarized in Fig. 2.

The main contributions are the development of (i) an MRF optimization method for optimal registration of the vessel structure, and (ii) an accurate vessel extraction method for XRA sequences based on accurate motion estimation. Experiments show that VCO is robust to complicated vessel structures and abrupt motions. We believe that VCO can be used to provide analytic visual information to the clinician without CTA acquisition. It can also be used in the automatic registration of vessels between 2D XRA sequences and 3D CTA.

2   Vessel Correspondence Optimization

2.1   Markov Random Field Representation

A pairwise MRF graph is constructed from the vessel centerlines of the source frame. Nodes correspond to sampled points from the centerlines and edges represent connectivities between the vessel points. The MRF energy is defined as follows:

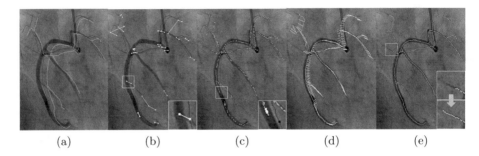

Fig. 2. Illustration of overall framework. Vessel centerlines of the destination frame are extracted based on the centerlines of the source frame, which we assume to be given. (a) Global search by chamfer matching. Source (green) and translated (red) vessel centerlines are overlaid. (b) Vessel branch search by keypoint correspondence (white). (c) Correspondence candidates (green) by vessel point search. White points in zoomed box show candidates for the black vessel point. (d) Optimal point correspondences (white) from MRF optimization. (e) Extraction of newly visible vessel branches. (a)-(c) Comprise a hierarchical search scheme. (Color figure online)

$$E(\mathbf{x}) = \sum_i \varphi(x_i) + \sum_{(i,j)\in\varepsilon} \psi(x_i, x_j), \tag{1}$$

where $\mathbf{x}$ is the vector comprising the set of all random variables x_i at each node with index i. Each x_i can be labeled by N_p+1 different values, and the optimal $\mathbf{x}$ is determined by minimizing (1). The N_p+1 labels comprise N_p correspondence candidates and 1 dummy label which will be assigned to a node when there are no candidates with consistent local shape or appearance. If the dummy label is found to be optimal, that node is excluded from the resulting VCO point set.

The unary cost function $\varphi(x_i)$ depends on the similarity between the local appearance of the ith node and the x_ith correspondence candidate. Since we seek corresponding points with similar appearance, we define $\varphi(x_i)$ to decrease as local appearance similarity increases as:

$$\varphi(x_i) = \min(\|D(F_{src}, p_i) - D(F_{dst}, \pi_i(x_i))\|, T_\varphi). \tag{2}$$

F_{src} and F_{dst} denote the source and destination frames, p_i and $\pi_i(x_i)$ denote the coordinate of the ith node of the source vessel structure and the x_ith correspondence candidate from the destination frame, respectively. D is a function for a local feature descriptor. Note that $\varphi(x_i)$ is truncated by T_φ to ensure robustness to outliers. Outliers may occur when there is no corresponding point due to severe local deformations.

The pairwise cost $\psi(x_i, x_j)$ enforces similar displacement vectors between neighboring points, and thus consistent local shape. It is defined similar to that of [9], as follows:

$$\psi(x_i, x_j) = \lambda \min(\|(p_i - \pi_i(x_i)) - (p_j - \pi_j(x_j))\|, T_\psi), \tag{3}$$

where p_i and p_j are coordinates of the ith and jth source node, while $\pi_i(x_i)$ and $\pi_j(x_j)$ are coordinates in the destination frame of the correspondence candidates of x_i and x_j, respectively. $p_i - \pi_i(x_i)$ is the displacement vector of the ith source node. Again, truncation is included based on threshold T_ψ. The parameter λ controls the amount of this regularization in (1).

2.2   Hierarchical Search of Vessel Correspondence Candidates

The tubular shapes of vessels, together with the aperture problem, make it very challenging to distinguish different local regions. We thus propose a hierarchical correspondence search scheme comprising global, branch, and point searches.

We define vessel junctions, including bifurcations and crossings from 3D-2D projection, and endpoints, both of which have distinctive appearances, as vessel keypoints. A vessel branch refers to the line connecting two vessel keypoints. In the following, we denote the αth keypoint as p^α, with a superscript, to distinguish it from general vessel point p_i. The mth branch is denoted as b_m.

Global Search by Chamfer Matching: We perform chamfer matching [10] to estimate large global translational motion from heart beating, breathing, or viewpoint change. The template shape is the set of source vessel points. The target shape is constructed by sequentially applying vessel enhancement [1], thresholding, and skeletonization to the destination frame. We find the global displacement vector that minimizes the sum of distances between each template point and target shape by brute force search on the distance transform (DT) of the target shape. Figure 2(a) shows an example result of this step.

Branch Search by Vessel Keypoint Correspondence: We search for corresponding points π^α and π^β for both keypoints p^α and p^β of a branch b_m, each within a local search region of size $w_k \times h_k$. Correspondences are determined by similarity of local appearance, measured using (2). Non-max suppression is applied to avoid nearby matches, and up to N_k possible correspondences are obtained for both p^α and p^β. The set of candidate branches is generated for b_m by simply applying all displacement vectors $\delta_1^\alpha = \pi_1^\alpha - p^\alpha, ..., \delta_{N_k}^\alpha = \pi_{N_k}^\alpha - p^\alpha$ and $\delta_1^\beta = \pi_1^\beta - p^\beta, ..., \delta_{N_k}^\beta = \pi_{N_k}^\beta - p^\beta$ to b_m. We note that there can be up to $N_k \times 2$ candidate branches, depending on the number of keypoint correspondences. We also include the branch with no displacement, in case all keypoint matches are unreliable, which results in at most $N_k \times 2 + 1$ branch candidates.

Correspondence Candidate Generation by Vessel Point Search: For a vessel point $p_i \in b_m$, the set of corresponding points based on candidate branches are $\{p_i + \delta_1^\alpha, ..., p_i + \delta_{N_k}^\alpha, p_i + \delta_1^\beta, ..., p_i + \delta_{N_k}^\beta, p_i\}$. We define local search regions of size $w_p \times h_p$ at each of these points and determine the N_l best corresponding points, again, based on (2). Figure 3 shows an example where the correspondence candidates are greatly improved with a smaller local search range based on the prior branch search.

The resulting maximum number of candidates is $N_p = N_l \times (N_k \times 2 + 1)$. Due to non-max suppression, the actual candidate number N_c can be less than N_p depending on the image, which can complicate implementation. Thus, we fix the number of labels to N_p for all vessel points, but nullify labels larger than N_c without an actual corresponding candidate by assigning an infinite unary cost.

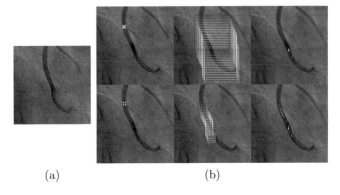

(a)   (b)

Fig. 3. Effect of hierarchical branch-point search. (a) Example vessel branch in source frame. (b) Each column shows (left) the positioned vessel branch in the destination frame, (mid) local search regions at branch vessel points, and (right) obtained correspondence candidates. Top/bottom rows compare the local point search without and with hierarchical search. Branch alignment enables reduction of local search range. Search regions and candidate points color-coded for clarity. (Color figure online)

2.3   Post-processing for Complete Centerline Extraction

After VCO, obtained vessel points are connected to construct vessel centerline structure $\mathcal{V}$ by the fast marching method [11]. To extract newly visible branches, a binary segmentation mask is first obtained by thresholding vesselness [1], and regions not connected to the vessel centerlines are excluded. The DT is computed for this mask, with the non-vessel regions as seeds. Based on the mask and the DT, the following is iterated until no branch longer than the maximum vessel radius is found: (i) perform fast marching method, with $\mathcal{V}$ as the seeds and the DT values as marching speed; (ii) find the shortest path from the pixel with the latest arrival time to $\mathcal{V}$, and add to $\mathcal{V}$. This method is adopted from [12].

3   Experimental Results

Evaluation Details: The dataset comprises 18 XRA sequences of total 617 frames from 5 different patients. All sequences were acquired by Philips digital fluoroscopic systems at 512×512 resolution, 8 bit depth, and 15 fps frame rate. Parameter values were manually selected and fixed to $N_k = 2$, $w_k = 101$, $h_k = 101$, $N_l = 5$, $w_p = 21$, $h_p = 21$, and $N_p = N_l \times (N_k \times 2 + 1) = 25$. Source vessel points are sampled from the centerline at a 5 pixel interval. The VLFeat [13] library for SIFT [14] is used for D in (2). TRW-S is used for MRF optimization [15]. VCO without post-processing took a few minutes by an unoptimized Matlab implementation on a Intel Zeon processor with over 80 % of computation on SIFT matching. Ground truth vessel centerlines and corresponding bifurcation point coordinates in frame pairs were obtained by expert annotation. For centerlines, the semi-automatic method of [2] was used.

Table 1. Quantitative results of **Exp1**, where vessel extraction is performed for 599 frame pairs using the ground truth source vessel structure. Higher is better for precision, recall, and F-measure, and lower is better for TRE.

	OF+ACM [7]	CM+ACM	VCO-HS	VCO-DL	VCO
Precision	0.832	0.860	0.900	0.901	0.905
Recall	0.733	0.719	0.840	0.841	0.841
F-measure	0.779	0.783	0.869	0.870	0.872
TRE	6.321	6.418	-	-	5.018

Comparisons are made with two relevant methods: (1) that by Fallavollita et al. [7], which combines optical flow (OF) and an active contour model (ACM), modified to handle whole vessel structures, denoted as **OF+ACM**, and (2) a variant of **OF+ACM** where OF is substituted with global chamfer matching, denoted as **CM+ACM**. Further comparisons are made with two variants of VCO: (3) **VCO-HS** VCO without hierarchical search, with enlarged search regions instead, and (4) **VCO-DL**, VCO without dummy labels.

Quantitative Evaluation: We perform two different experiments. In **Exp1**, vessel extraction is performed for all source-destination frame pairs, using the ground truth source vessel structure. The average precision, recall, F-measure, along with the target registration error (TRE) for bifurcation points, of 599 sequential frame pairs are presented in Table 1. TRE is defined as the average distance between the estimated and ground truth point coordinate. A vessel point is true positive if there is a ground truth point within a two pixel radius. VCO achieves the highest accuracy, with additional improvement from hierarchical search and dummy labels. Here, post-processing is applied only up to point connection to exclusively evaluate the VCO accuracy.

In **Exp2**, we evaluate the average number of consecutive frames with *sufficient* vessel extraction when iteratively applying all methods for a single initial frame. Here, *sufficient* is defined as F-measure higher than 0.7. Evaluation on the 18 sequences showed that *sufficient* vessel extraction was obtained for 2.0, 5.3, and 8.6 subsequent frames, by the **OF+ACM**, **CM+ACM**, and **VCO** methods, respectively. This demonstrates the practical usefulness of VCO.

Qualitative Evaluation: Figure 4 presents representative sample results of **Exp1**. Significant improvements compared to previous methods are visible. Figure 1 presents results of **Exp2** for a sample sequence. Both figures highlight the effectiveness of the proposed method. Figure 5 shows one limitation of VCO, where VCO is not able to handle the topology change due to vessel superimposition.

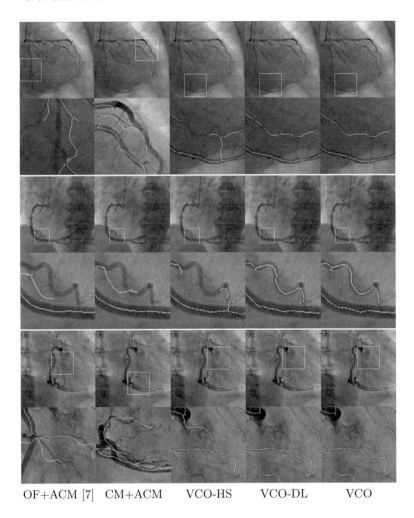

OF+ACM [7]   CM+ACM   VCO-HS   VCO-DL   VCO

Fig. 4. Qualitative results. Odd and even rows show sample frames and their corresponding enlarged views of erroneous regions, from different sequences, respecitively. Red points in column 3–5 are resulting vessel points of VCO. (Color figure online)

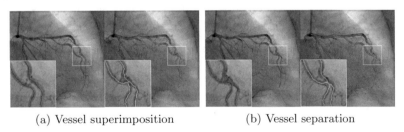

(a) Vessel superimposition   (b) Vessel separation

Fig. 5. Limitations of VCO. Subsequent frame pairs showing (a) success and (b) failure. Left/right show source/destination frame pairs. Ground truth (red) and VCO result vessel structures (green) are overlaid. (Color figure online)

4 Conclusion

We have proposed a method to determine optimal vessel correspondences for registration and extraction of vessel structures from fluoroscopic x-ray sequences. Experiments show promising results on complicated structures. In future work, we plan to investigate optimization measures including GPU implementation for real-time performance as well as other measures required for actual clinical application such as overlaying the extracted vessel structure to sequences acquired without the use of contrast agents.

References

1. Frangi, A.F., Niessen, W.J., Vincken, K.L., Viergever, M.A.: Multiscale vessel enhancement filtering. In: Wells, W.M., Colchester, A.C.F., Delp, S.L. (eds.) MICCAI 1998. LNCS, vol. 1496, pp. 130–137. Springer, Heidelberg (1998)
2. Poon, K., Hamarneh, G., Abugharbieh, R.: Live-vessel: extending livewire for simultaneous extraction of optimal medial and boundary paths in vascular images. In: Ayache, N., Ourselin, S., Maeder, A. (eds.) MICCAI 2007, Part II. LNCS, vol. 4792, pp. 444–451. Springer, Heidelberg (2007)
3. Honnorat, N., Vaillant, R., Duncan, J.S., Paragios, N.: Curvilinear structures extraction in cluttered bioimaging data with discrete optimization methods. In: ISBI, pp. 1353–1357 (2011)
4. Becker, C., Rigamonti, R., Lepetit, V., Fua, P.: Supervised feature learning for curvilinear structure segmentation. In: Mori, K., Sakuma, I., Sato, Y., Barillot, C., Navab, N. (eds.) MICCAI 2013, Part I. LNCS, vol. 8149, pp. 526–533. Springer, Heidelberg (2013)
5. Rivest-Henault, D., Sundar, H., Cheriet, M.: Nonrigid 2D/3D registration of coronary artery models with live fluoroscopy for guidance of cardiac interventions. IEEE Trans. Med. Imaging $31(8)$, 1557–1572 (2012)
6. Sun, S.-Y., Wang, P., Sun, S., Chen, T.: Model-guided extraction of coronary vessel structures in 2D X-Ray angiograms. In: Golland, P., Hata, N., Barillot, C., Hornegger, J., Howe, R. (eds.) MICCAI 2014, Part II. LNCS, vol. 8674, pp. 594–602. Springer, Heidelberg (2014)
7. Fallavollita, P., Cheriet, F.: Robust coronary artery tracking from fluoroscopic image sequences. In: Kamel, M.S., Campilho, A. (eds.) ICIAR 2007. LNCS, vol. 4633, pp. 889–898. Springer, Heidelberg (2007)
8. Honnorat, N., Vaillant, R., Paragios, N.: Graph-based geometric-iconic guide-wire tracking. In: Fichtinger, G., Martel, A., Peters, T. (eds.) MICCAI 2011, Part I. LNCS, vol. 6891, pp. 9–16. Springer, Heidelberg (2011)
9. Glocker, B., Komodakis, N., Paragios, N., Tziritas, G., Navab, N.: Inter and intra-modal deformable registration: continuous deformations meet efficient optimal linear programming. In: Karssemeijer, N., Lelieveldt, B. (eds.) IPMI 2007. LNCS, vol. 4584, pp. 408–420. Springer, Heidelberg (2007)
10. Barrow, H., Tenenbaum, J., Bolles, R., Wolf, H.: Parametric correspondence and chamfer matching: two new techniques for image matching. In: Proceedings of International Joint Conference on Artificial Intelligence, vol. 2, pp. 659–663 (1977)
11. Yatziv, L., Bartesaghi, A., Sapiro, G.: O(N) implementation of the fast marching algorithm. J. Comput. Phys. $212(2)$, 393–399 (2005)

12. Van Uitert, R., Bitter, I.: Subvoxel precise skeletons of volumetric data based on fast marching methods. Med. Phys. **34**(2), 627–638 (2007)
13. Vedaldi, A., Fulkerson, B.: VLFeat: an open and portable library of computer vision algorithms (2008). http://www.vlfeat.org/
14. Lowe, D.G.: Distinctive image features from scale-invariant keypoints. Int. J. Comput. Vision **60**(2), 91–110 (2004)
15. Kolmogorov, V.: Convergent tree-reweighted message passing for energy minimization. IEEE Trans. Pattern Anal. Mach. Intell. **28**(10), 1568–1583 (2006)

Coronary Centerline Extraction via Optimal Flow Paths and CNN Path Pruning

Mehmet A. Gülsün[✉], Gareth Funka-Lea, Puneet Sharma, Saikiran Rapaka, and Yefeng Zheng

Medical Imaging Technologies, Siemens Medical Solutions USA, Inc., Princeton, USA
akif.gulsun@siemens.com

Abstract. We present a novel method for the automated extraction of blood vessel centerlines. There are two major contributions. First, in order to avoid the shortcuts to which minimal path methods are prone, we find optimal paths in a computed flow field. We solve for a steady state porous media flow inside a region of interest and trace centerlines as maximum flow paths. We explain how to estimate anisotropic orientation tensors which are used as permeability tensors in our flow field computation. Second, we introduce a convolutional neural network (CNN) classifier for removing extraneous paths in the detected centerlines. We apply our method to the extraction of coronary artery centerlines found in Computed Tomography Angiography (CTA). The robustness and stability of our method are enhanced by using a model-based detection of coronary specific territories and main branches to constrain the search space [15]. Validation against 20 comprehensively annotated datasets had a sensitivity and specificity at or above 90 %. Validation against 106 clinically annotated coronary arteries showed a sensitivity above 97 %.

1 Motivation and Overview

The automatic segmentation of coronary arteries in Computed Tomography Angiography (CTA) facilitates the diagnosis, treatment and monitoring of coronary artery diseases. An important step in coronary segmentation is to extract a centerline representation that supports visualizations such as curved planar reformatting or that supports lumen segmentation methods for quantitative assessments such as stenosis grading. In this work, our focus is to detect the full coronary tree of centerlines including the distal part of side branches for better visualization and quantification of the coronary anatomy.

Coronary arteries constitute only a small portion of a large CTA volume because of their thin tubular geometry. Their centerline extraction is not an easy task due to nearby heart structures or coronary veins. The majority of existing centerline extraction techniques compute centerline paths by minimizing a vesselness or medialness cost metric such as Hessian based vesselness [6], flux based medialness [2,8] or other tubularity measures [9] along the paths. However, the cumulative cost nature of these methods makes them very sensitive to the underlying cost metric causing them to easily make shortcuts through nearby

© Springer International Publishing AG 2016
S. Ourselin et al. (Eds.): MICCAI 2016, Part III, LNCS 9902, pp. 317–325, 2016.
DOI: 10.1007/978-3-319-46726-9_37

non-coronary structures, especially when there are pathologies, large contrast variations, bifurcations or imaging artifacts along the true path. In addition, these methods are sensitive to length and curvature of the vessel.

Vessel centerlines have frequently been found through minimum paths, minimum spanning trees or tracking algorithms such as Kalman filtering. These are generally run on hand-crafted vesselness measures computed from the image data. A review of 3D vessel segmentation can be found in [9]. More recent work evaluates consistency among multiple minimum paths [11] or considers multiple hypothesis tracking [7]. Constraints on possible paths have been applied through constrained optimization including a term for the conservation of network flow in [13] or through prior shape models [15].

The main contributions of this paper are

(1) a formulation of centerline extraction as finding the maximum flow paths in a steady state porous media flow,
(2) a learning based estimation of anisotropic vessel orientation tensors and their use as permeability for a flow computation,
(3) a CNN based branch classifier for distinguishing true centerlines from leakages, and
(4) the use of model-based coronary specific territories and main branches for robustness and efficiency.

2   Method

Figure 1 shows the workflow of our method. In each step, we aim to reduce the search space while keeping the detection sensitivity very high. In outline, we first compute coronary specific regions to constrain the detection and then extract the main coronary branches in order to handle gaps due to severe occlusions or motion artifacts. [15] builds models of the main coronary arteries (Right Coronary Artery (RCA), Left Anterior Descending (LAD) and Left Circumflex (LCX)) learned from a training set. In this work, we build a region around the right and left coronary trees, Fig. 1a. Our approach constrains the detection to voxels inside these regions in order to eliminate false positive voxels and significantly speed up the runtime. We compute a rough coronary mask from a vesselness based region growing algorithm seeded with the detected ostia and main branches. We then estimate voxel-wise orientation tensors which are fed into our steady state flow computation as permeability tensors. We extract centerlines of the paths carrying maximum flow from the ostia to distal locations. Finally, we prune false positive centerlines by using the branch classification scores assigned to each centerline point. Detailed explanation of each step is provided below. For training and testing our method, we use annotated CTA datasets with left (LCA) and right (RCA) coronary artery centerlines which consist of densely sampled centerline points with a rough estimate of cross-sectional radius.

We compute a rough coronary mask by performing a region growing algorithm that visits voxels based on their vesselness scores predicted by [14]. Specifically, we use a vesselness threshold that produces high detection sensitivity

($> 98\,\%$) in our training set. We use the detected main branches of [15] together with a local neighborhood ($5\,mm$) of detected coronary ostia points for seeding our region growing approach. Figure 1b and c show detected main branches and the coronary mask for a test dataset.

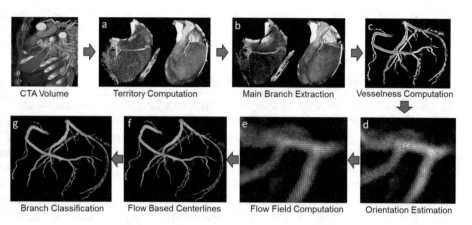

Fig. 1. Complete workflow of the proposed method. (a) Coronary specific territories, (b) Detected main branches (red), (c) Detected coronary mask, (d) Principal component of the estimated orientation tensors around the LAD second diagonal bifurcation (red → blue is high → low), (e) Computed flow field, (f) Flow based centerlines. Overlaps with annotation are shown in green. (g) Final centerlines obtained after leakage pruning. (Color figure online)

2.1   Estimation of Anisotropic Vessel Orientation Tensors

Traditional vesselness measurements [9] estimate a single measure of the principle local orientation. More recent work makes use of multiple estimates of the local orientation as a vector [1] or tensor [4]. This provides better information at bifurcations or where vessels touch. We present a classification based approach for predicting an anisotropic vessel orientation tensor at an image voxel that can be used to compute the likelihood of a particular vessel orientation.

At a given image voxel, our method first predicts classification scores for 13 non-symmetric discrete orientations and constructs a tensor from these scores. Previous work [14] estimated vesselness scores using a sample patch aligned with the image axis. In this work, we use the same classifier but with a sample patch oriented along discrete orientations. Therefore, our training examples are sampled to learn both location and orientation instead of only location as in [14]. We sample positive examples for every voxel within half a radius range of the annotated coronary centerlines. Each positive example is assigned a discrete orientation that makes the smallest angle with the true orientation. For negative examples, we consider all voxels inside the coronary lumen and a $2\,mm$ band around it and assign the following orientations. If the voxel is inside the band, all discrete orientations are used. Otherwise, discrete orientations that make an angle of more than 45° with the true vessel orientation are used in order to avoid confusing the classifier. We use the predicted orientation scores to scale each corresponding discrete orientation unit vector including their symmetric counterparts and compute a tensor K as the covariance matrix of these vectors. Note that our orientation tensor K is both symmetric and positive semi-definite. Figure 1d illustrates the estimated orientation tensors.

2.2   Flow Constrained Centerline Extraction

We use the analogy of fluid flowing from regions of high pressure to those of low pressure by setting up a fluid flow problem where the coronary ostia are the high pressure region. For each coronary tree, our approach first computes an incompressible inviscid steady state porous media flow inside the detected vesselness mask with boundary conditions on the pressure. Each voxel of the porous material is assigned a tensor of permeability. The permeability can be understood as an inverse resistance to flow in the voxel. The principal directions of the tensor and its eigenvalues relate the ease of flow along each direction in the voxel giving a local anisotropic structure. The voxels in the vicinity (5 mm) of the automatically detected ostia points are considered as inlet points with high permeability. However, outlet points corresponding to coronary distal points are not known *a priori*. Therefore, we consider all voxels along the mask boundary as outlet points with low permeability, or equivalently, high resistance to ensure that most of the flow stays in the vascular structures. The pressure is forced to be unit for inlet voxels and zero outside the mask. We use the estimated coronary orientation tensors as permeability tensors. The flow can be efficiently computed by solving a tensor weighted Laplacian model $\nabla \cdot (K \nabla p) = 0$ where p is the pressure. Figure 1e illustrates the computed flow field.

Using the estimated local orientation tensor as permeability has several advantages. First, since the orientation tensor is lower along directions that are not aligned with true coronary orientation, the computed flow is forced to be low between coronaries and touching structures. Consequently centerlines at bifurcations are improved and the number of leaks is reduced, Fig. 2a. Second, the magnitude of the orientation tensor is higher in the coronary center and gradually decreases towards the background which is ideal for centerline tracking. Finally, anisotropy of the orientation tensors yields natural flow fields at bifurcation where common centerline metrics are not well-defined [4], Fig. 2b.

We extract the centerlines from the detected ostia to locations inside the coronary mask based on the path that carries maximum flow. Let $G = (V, E)$ be a directed 26-connected graph with vertices V corresponding to image voxels and directed edges E connecting vertices from high pressure to low pressure. Each edge is assigned a weight based on the cross-sectional flow rate computed inside a disc oriented along that edge and scaled with maximum diameter that fits to coronary mask. The maximum flow path between two vertices in this directed graph can be computed by finding the widest path defined as the path

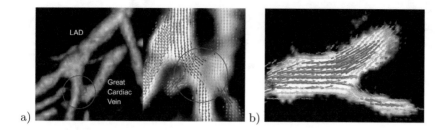

Fig. 2. (a) Computed flow is low between the touching Great Cardiac Vein and LAD second diagonal branch. Red is high flow from the ostia. (b) Flow inside a bifurcation.

which maximizes the weight of the minimum-weight edge along the path. Single source widest path in a directed graph can be solved efficiently by a modified Dijkstra's algorithm [10]. To obtain a centerline tree, we consider widest paths to all vertices in the graph and iteratively pick the path that has maximum flow volume, i.e., the integral of flow-rate along the path. Paths that are below a saliency measure defined by the length-scale ratio are pruned away. Figures 1f and 5c show the detected centerlines for a test dataset.

2.3 Branch Classification

Our flow based centerlines have very high sensitivity but at the expense of false branches, Table 1. We developed a classification approach to distinguish true coronary centerlines from leaks. Existing learning based methods [3,13] that remove false branches use support vector machines, probabilistic boosting trees or random forest classifiers with a set of hand-crafted features such as simple statistics or histograms of intensity, gradient, diameter and curvature along the branch. However, statistical or histogram features cannot accurately capture when the coronary artery makes a leak into a touching vein, Fig. 3.

We propose to use a CNN to learn a branch classifier using multi-channel 1D input. The CNN input channels consist of various profiles sampled along the branch such as vessel scale, image intensity, centerline curvature, tubularity measure, intensity and gradient statistics (mean, standard deviation) along

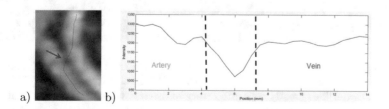

Fig. 3. (a) Curved MPR visualization of a centerline leaking into a touching vein. Non-vessel region is depicted with red arrow. (b) Intensity signal along the branch segment.

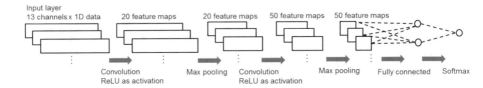

Fig. 4. Our convolutional neural network for branch classification.

and inside a cross-sectional circular boundary, and distance to the most proximal point in the branch. Our aim is to learn the best discriminative features from these profiles rather than extracting hand-crafted features. Figure 4 shows our CNN. Since CNNs can learn global features from local features inside sub regions, the method can capture small non-vessel regions along the branch which is difficult to achieve with statistical or histogram based features. Because of the translation invariant property of CNNs, by means of weight sharing and pooling layers, the approach is robust to the location of the false section along the branch. The use of multi-channel 1D input makes the training less prone to over-fitting. Our method assigns probabilistic scores to overlapping fixed length branch segments sampled along from the ostia to distal endpoints. For training, our positive and negative examples are sampled based on the overlap between hand annotated and automatically detected centerlines.

In order to obtain the final tree, each point is assigned a final score based on the maximum score among branch segments containing that point. We apply median filtering with a small kernel along the branches in order to remove noisy detections. The final centerline tree is obtained by pruning downstream of points that have scores below a threshold, Figs. 1g and 5d. In order to make our pruning step robust to occlusions due to pathologies or image artifacts, we do not prune along the detected main branches because of their clinical significance.

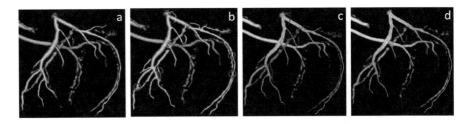

Fig. 5. (a) VRT rendering of detected vesselness with LCA annotation (yellow). (b) Minimal path centerlines frequently leak into touching veins (red circles). (c) Proposed flow based centerlines mostly separate artery and veins. Overlaps with annotation are depicted in green, false positives in red. (d) Results after proposed leakage pruning. (Color figure online)

3   Results

We have 110 comprehensively annotated CTA coronary datasets which were acquired from patients known or suspected to have coronary artery disease. The annotations were carefully done such that all coronary artery branches visible in the CTA data were included. Among 110 datasets, we randomly picked 90 for training purpose and used the remaining 20 for our first evaluation. The training data originated from 5 clinical sites and contained 17 low kV datasets. The testing data were from 4 clinical sites and contained 4 low kV datasets.

The testing sensitivity for the computed coronary territories were 100 % and for the vesselness masks were 95 %. The three main coronary arteries (RCA, LAD, LCX) were found in our model-based [15] first stage with a success rate of 95 %. We evaluated the detected centerlines based on point-wise overlap with annotations. In order to better assess shortcuts, we provide an up-to-first-error evaluation which counts all the points downstream of the first error as a false detection. Table 1 shows that after pruning the sensitivity slightly drops but there is a significant improvement in the specificity. The small difference in the up-to-first error results also shows that the flow constrained centerline extraction is very robust to shortcut issues. Figure 5b and c compare the flow based centerlines with a minimal path approach on a sample dataset. Note that the minimal path approach makes frequent jumps between arteries and veins.

Table 1. Evaluation of LCA and RCA centerline detections on 20 test cases.

	OV [12]	$\frac{|Overlap|}{|Annotation|}$ %	$\frac{|Overlap|}{|Detection|}$ %	$\frac{|OverlapUpTo1stError|}{|Annotation|}$ %	$\frac{|OverlapUpTo1stError|}{|Detection|}$ %
	Before leakage pruning				
LCA	70.2	94.6	51.7	91.7	50.2
RCA	84.1	91.1	80.4	89.7	77.1
	After leakage pruning				
LCA	90.8	91.6	90.6	90.0	90.0
RCA	92.7	90.0	95.0	88.0	91.0

We evaluated our approach against the ground truth annotations from the MICCAI Grand Challenge [12]. For the 8 datasets made available for *training* but which are unseen for us, the overall sensitivity is 94.5 % for the LCA and 95.7 % for the RCA. The up-to-first error sensitivity is 92.7 % for the LCA and 95.7 % for the RCA. Most errors occur distally. Since our approach attempts to find all coronary arteries and for the challenge only the three main arteries and one random side branch were annotated, it is not useful to report specificity.

We evaluated our approach on 106 clinically annotated datasets used in another study [5] where coronary arteries that have a diameter greater than 2 mm were annotated by radiologists. Overall sensitivity is 98 % for the LCA and 97.4 % for the RCA. Up-to-first-error sensitivity is 94.2 % for LCA and 95.1 % for RCA.

The average computation for all coronaries takes about 1 min on an Intel Core i7 2.8 GHz processor and 32 GB RAM (5 s for territory computation, 10 s for main branch extraction, 8 s for vesselness computation, 19 s for orientation estimation, 17 s for centerline extraction and 1 s for branch classification).

4   Conclusion

In this work, we have presented a novel method for coronary centerline extraction in CTA. Our method addresses commonly seen shortcut problems by finding optimal paths in computational flow fields. Our learning based anisotropic vessel orientation tensors are used as permeability in a flow formulation. We propose a CNN classier to prune false centerlines leaking into non-coronary structures. The accuracy and runtime of our approach are further improved by the use of model-based coronary territories and main branches. We report a sensitivity and specificity at or above 90 % for 20 comprehensively annotated datasets, and report a sensitivity above 97 % for 106 clinically annotated datasets.

Acknowledgment. The authors thank Adriaan Coenen, MD at Erasmus Univ. Medical Center for processing and making available the clinical data set.

References

1. Bekkers, E., Duits, R., Berendschot, T., Ter Haar Romeny, B.: A multi-orientation analysis approach to retinal vessel tracking. J. Math. Imaging Vis. **49**(3), 583–610 (2014)
2. Bouix, S., Siddiqi, K., Tannenbaum, A.: Flux driven automatic centerline extraction. MedIA **9**(3), 209–221 (2005)
3. Breitenreicher, D., Sofka, M., Britzen, S., Zhou, S.K.: Hierarchical discriminative framework for detecting tubular structures in 3D images. In: Gee, J.C., Joshi, S., Pohl, K.M., Wells, W.M., Zöllei, L. (eds.) IPMI 2013. LNCS, vol. 7917, pp. 328–339. Springer, Heidelberg (2013)
4. Cetin, S., Demir, A., Yezzi, A., Degertekin, M., Unal, G.: Vessel tractography using an intensity based tensor model with branch detection. IEEE T-MI. **32**(2), 348–363 (2013)
5. Coenen, A., et al.: Fractional flow reserve computed from noninvasive CT angiography data: diagnostic performance of an on-site clinician-operated computational fluid dynamics algorithm. Radiology **274**(3), 674–683 (2015)
6. Frangi, A.F., Niessen, W.J., Vincken, K.L., Viergever, M.A.: Multiscale vessel enhancement filtering. In: Wells, W.M., Colchester, A.C.F., Delp, S.L. (eds.) MICCAI 1998. LNCS, vol. 1496, p. 130. Springer, Heidelberg (1998). doi:10.1007/BFb0056195
7. Friman, O., Hindennach, M., Kühnel, C., Peitgen, H.-O.: Multiple hypothesis template tracking of small 3D vessel structures. MedIA **14**(2), 160–171 (2010)
8. Law, M., Chung, A.: Efficient implementation for spherical flux computation and its application to vascular segmentation. IEEE T-IP **18**(3), 596–612 (2009)
9. Lesage, D., Angelini, E., Bloch, I., Funka-Lea, G.: A review of 3D vessel lumen segmentation techniques: models, featuers and extraction schemes. MedIA **13**(6), 819–845 (2009)

10. Pollack, M.: The maximum capacity through a network. Oper. Res. **8**(5), 733–736 (1960)
11. Rouchdy, Y., Cohen, L.: Geodesic voting for the automatic extraction of tree structures. Methods and applications. CVIU **117**, 1453–1467 (2013)
12. Schaap, M., et al.: Standardized evaluation methodology and reference database for evaulating coronary artery centerline extraction algorithms. MedIA **13**(5), 701–714 (2009)
13. Türetken, E., Benmansour, F. Fua, P.: Automated reconstruction of tree structures using path classifiers and mixed integer programming. In: CVPR, pp. 566–573, June 2012
14. Zheng, Y., Loziczonek, M., Georgescu, B., Zhou, S., Vega-Higuera, F. Comaniciu, D.: Machine learning based vesselness measurement for coronary artery segmentation in cardiac CT volumes. In: SPIE Medical Imaging (2011)
15. Zheng, Y., Tek, H., Funka-Lea, G.: Robust and accurate coronary artery centerline extraction in CTA by combining model-driven and data-driven approaches. In: Mori, K., Sakuma, I., Sato, Y., Barillot, C., Navab, N. (eds.) MICCAI 2013, Part III. LNCS, vol. 8151, pp. 74–81. Springer, Heidelberg (2013)

Vascular Registration in Photoacoustic Imaging by Low-Rank Alignment via Foreground, Background and Complement Decomposition

Ryoma Bise[1(✉)], Yingqiang Zheng[1], Imari Sato[1], and Masakazu Toi[2]

[1] National Institute of Informatics, Chiyoda, Japan
{bise-r,yqzheng,imari}@nii.ac.jp
[2] Kyoto University Hospital, Kyoto, Japan
toi@kuhp.kyoto-u.ac.jp

Abstract. Photoacoustic (PA) imaging has been gaining attention as a new imaging modality that can non-invasively visualize blood vessels inside biological tissues. In the process of imaging large body parts through multi-scan fusion, alignment turns out to be an important issue, since body motion degrades image quality. In this paper, we carefully examine the characteristics of PA images and propose a novel registration method that achieves better alignment while effectively decomposing the shot volumes into low-rank foreground (blood vessels), dense background (noise), and sparse complement (corruption) components on the basis of the PA characteristics. The results of experiments using a challenging real data-set demonstrate the efficacy of the proposed method, which significantly improved image quality, and had the best alignment accuracy among the state-of-the-art methods tested.

1 Introduction

Photoacoustic (PA) imaging is a promising new technology for early clinical diagnosis of cancer, tumor angiogenesis, and many other diseases [1]. PA takes advantage of the thermoacoustic effect; that is, objects (*i.e.*, blood vessels) absorb short-pulsed near-infrared irradiation and emit ultrasonic waves thereafter. 3D structures of objects can be reconstructed by sensing the thermoacoustic waves [2]. This technique can non-invasively visualize blood vessels in vivo with high spatial resolution without any contrast media. In order for PA imaging to capture entire portions of the human body, multi-scan and registration systems [3] have been developed that separately scan local areas of the sample and merge them. A single-shot volume reconstructed by PA technology usually suffers from severe noise caused by sound and light scattering and sensor layout limitations (Fig. 1). The goal of this study is to generate high-quality 3D volumes from these noisy shot volumes, in which vessels become clearly visible.

To reduce such noise, image averaging techniques have often been used, where the average of the random noise in the background becomes a small constant, and the linearly correlated foreground becomes apparent. Image averaging is

© Springer International Publishing AG 2016
S. Ourselin et al. (Eds.): MICCAI 2016, Part III, LNCS 9902, pp. 326–334, 2016.
DOI: 10.1007/978-3-319-46726-9_38

effective as long as the sample is static or the size of the target is much larger than the motion. However, in the case of PA images reconstructed by merging shot-volumes of local scans, the patient often moves during scanning, and this assumption rarely holds true. It should be easy to imagine that even small motions adversely affect the image quality, considering the fact that blood vessels are thin (0.5 mm). What is required, therefore, is an accurate alignment of multiple shot volumes that can cope with such body motion.

A low-rank based alignment framework has a potential to address aligning such challenging data that contain severe dense noise and small foreground area. In the low-rank based alignment framework, an observation matrix D is first generated from given multiple images, where the i-th row indicates the i-th vectorized image. If we successfully make images well-aligned and eliminate the differences among aligned images, this results in making the data matrix low-rank. The low-rank based alignment framework achieves this by searching for the transform function τ and the difference component α that convert D into a low-rank component as $D \circ \tau - \alpha$. Since this optimization problem is basically ill-posed, it is usually required to introduce some assumptions for the difference components in the optimization.

Contribution: The main contribution of this work is designing the difference component and the optimization method for aligning multiple PA volumes that contain small foreground, severe dense noise, and corrupted foregrounds based on the characteristics of PA images. To achieve this goal, we propose a coarse-to-fine approach to correctly extract the small blood vessel area without falling into a local minimum. For coarse-alignment, Frangi-filter [4] is first applied to the PA volumes to reduce the background noise and enhance blood vessels. A multi-scale pyramid scheme is then used for optimizing the transform function that converts the aligned data into low-rank. Given the initial estimate of transformation function at the previous step, we further align the data by decomposing it into a low-rank foreground (blood vessels), dense background (severe noise), and sparse complement components (complementary parts of the foreground) based on characteristics of PA imaging. A key novelty here is effective use of a statistical prior of PA imaging for optimization, in which the average of the dense noise background at each spatial voxel is forced to be a constant. Experimental results using real PA data demonstrate that the propose approach is effective for aligning and finding blood vessels without suffering from severe dense noise and corruption, and yields high quality 3D volumes with clear vascular structures.

Related works: Many registration methods have been proposed for aligning multiple images in medical imaging [5–7]. Since it is difficult to segment blood vessels in PA shot-volumes because of severe noise and corruption, modeling-and-alignment methods [8] do not work well. Blood vessels observed in PA images tend to be sparsely distributed throughout a dense noisy background, and it is difficult to align such images by using these alignment methods that rely on image similarities computed from both foreground and background. To reduce the influence of image corruption, a robust alignment method (RASL) [9] has been proposed, and successfully applied to registration problems in medical imaging [10,11]. RASL optimizes an image transformation while separating an image into a low-rank foreground and sparse error components, where they assume that the differences among aligned images are caused from sparse corruptions. Compared with the images handled by RASL, the area of blood vessels is small with severe noise in vascular images in PA imaging. The error component becomes no longer sparse in this case, and RASL does not work properly; the low-rank component is optimized by adjusting the error component instead of properly transforming the data. To relax this sparse assumption, new decomposition methods have been proposed for recovering low-rank, sparse, and Gaussian noise components from the input data [12]. These methods assume that the foreground area is not small and the magnitude of the Gaussian noise is small. Thus, they are not suitable for PA images that contain heavy dense noise and the small area of blood vessels. In addition, these decomposition methods consider images that are well aligned and thus alignment problems were not considered before. In this paper, we propose a unified framework which simultaneously estimates the transformation and three-component decomposition.

2   Characteristics of PA Image

Figure 1 shows examples of x-y MIPs of PA shot volumes obtained from the same position, where the intensity range of each volume is −1 to 1. Let us first define the three components in these images. The first component is the *foreground* that represents blood vessels with high intensities. The second component is the *background* that represents noise that is in parts other than the blood vessels. The third is the *complement* that represents parts where foreground corruption occurs; in PA images, parts of vessels are corrupted by inhomogeneous light irradiation in vivo. For instance, in Fig. 1, the blood vessel in the red circle of the right image is not visible, while the corresponding vessel is visible in the left image. This missing portion corresponds to the complement. By examining real PA data, we found a statistical prior wherein the intensity distribution of the background is close to a Gaussian distribution with a large standard deviation (0.249), and the distribution of the averages of the aligned background at each spatial voxel is close to a Gaussian distribution with a constant mean (−0.001)

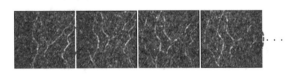

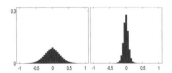

Fig. 1. Examples of x-y maximum intensity projection (MIP) of shot volume data in PA, where high-intensity curves are blood vessels. (Color figure online)

Fig. 2. Left: intensity distribution of background, Right: that of each spatial voxel averages.

and a small standard deviation (0.081), as shown in Fig. 2. By contrast, the average intensity in the vessels has a high value since the vessels are linearly correlated among well-aligned shot volumes. Note that this statistical prior is often true not only in our PA imaging system but also in many applications since the traditional image averaging techniques, which are widely used for reducing noise, use this prior implicitly. We effectively use these characteristics for simultaneously estimating the transform and the three-component decomposition.

3   Coarse-to-Fine Low-Rank-Based Alignment

In the case of PA images that contain dense noise and small foreground area, the current low-rank based methods tend to optimize the low-rank component by adjusting the difference component. To avoid this problem, we take a coarse-to-fine approach. For coarse alignment, we use a multi-scale pyramid scheme for optimizing the transformation using the noise-reduced data, without considering any difference components. This helps to find a proper transformation without falling into a such local minimum. To further refine the alignment, we optimize the transform function while decomposing the properly aligned data into three components, i.e., the low-rank foreground, dense noisy background, and sparse complement on the basis of the characteristics of PA imaging. The details of this procedure are described in the following sections.

3.1   Coarse Alignment by Low-Rank Minimization with Pyramid

Suppose we are given m volume data $I_1^0, ..., I_m^0 \in \mathcal{R}^{n=w \times h \times d}$ of a certain specimen, which might have moved during scanning. This step roughly aligns these volumes by using preprocessed foreground data, in which the background noise is reduced by enhancing the blood vessels with a Frangi filter [4], which uses the eigenvectors of the Hessian to compute the likeliness of tubular structures. The filtered data still include false positives in the background, and the vessels are corrupted. Yet, it is good enough for coarse alignment.

To find a proper transform function instead of adjusting the difference components, we only optimize the transform function τ to convert the preprocessed data matrix D into a low-rank component, $A = D \circ \tau$, without considering any difference components. $D \in \mathcal{R}^{m \times n}$ is the observation data matrix, and n is the number of voxels in each shot volume. τ denotes a certain transformation, such as the affine transform. According to [9], when the change in τ is small, $D \circ \tau = A$ can be approximated by linearizing about the current estimate of τ, and the rank minimization is relaxed into minimizing the nuclear norm $\|A\|_*$.

$$\min_{A, \Delta\tau} \|A\|_* \quad \text{s.t.} \quad D \circ \tau + \sum_i J_i \Delta\tau \epsilon_i \epsilon_i^T = A \tag{1}$$

where $\Delta\tau$ denotes the variance of τ in each iteration, $J_i \doteq \frac{\delta}{\delta\zeta}(I_i \circ \zeta) \mid_{\zeta=\tau_i} \in \mathcal{R}^{n \times p}$ is the Jacobian of the i-th data, and ϵ_i denotes the standard basis for $\mathcal{R}^m$. Equation (1) can be efficiently solved using augmented Lagrange multiplier

---

Algorithm 1. fine alignment by decomposing data into three components

---

1: Input: vectorized 3D volume data $I_1, ..., I_m \in \mathcal{R}^n$, initial transformations $\tau_1, ..., \tau_m$.

2: **while** not converged **do**
3:      (1) compute the Jacobian matrices
4:      $J_i \leftarrow \frac{\delta}{\delta\zeta}(\frac{I_i \circ \zeta}{\|I_i \circ \zeta\|_2}) |_{\zeta = \tau_i}$, $i = 1, ..., m$
5:      (2) warp and normalize the images:
6:      $D \circ \tau \leftarrow [\frac{I_1 \circ \tau_1}{\|I_1 \circ \tau_1\|}, ..., \frac{I_m \circ \tau_m}{\|I_m \circ \tau_m\|}]$, $i = 1, ..., m$
7:      (3) (inner loop): solve the linearized convex optimization:
8:      $(A^*, B^*, C^*, \Delta\tau^*) \leftarrow \arg\min_{A,B,C,\Delta\tau} \|A\|_* + \lambda_1 \|aB - b\|^2 + \lambda_2 \|C\|_1$
9:                s.t. $D \circ \tau + \sum_i J_i \Delta\tau \epsilon_i \epsilon_i^T = A + B + C$ use Eq. (4)
10:      (4) update transformation: $\tau \leftarrow \tau + \Delta\tau^*$:
11: **end while**
12: OUTPUT: solution A^*, B^*, C^*, τ^*

(ALM) algorithm [13], in a similar manner to [9]. This optimization is applied with a multi-scale pyramid scheme, which successively aligns data with finer Gaussian pyramids.

3.2   Fine Alignment via Three Components Decomposition

The aforementioned preprocessed data may include false-positive and false-negative noise, which lead to small alignment errors because the optimization in the previous step does not consider noise. We further refine the results from the coarse alignment by using original volumes considering noise. To handle images that contains dense noise, we introduce a dense-noise term in the alignment, wherein our method aligns the data while decomposing it into a low-rank foreground A, dense noisy background B, and sparse complement C, by using characteristics of the dense noisy background. Specifically, the distribution of the averages of the aligned dense noise at the same positions becomes a Gaussian distribution with a constant mean and small variance. We introduce this statistical prior into the formulation of the decomposition problem as follows:

$$\min_{A,B,C,\Delta\tau} \|A\|_* + \lambda_1 \|aB - b\|^2 + \lambda_2 \|C\|_1 \quad \text{s.t. } D \circ \tau + \sum_i J_i \Delta\tau \epsilon_i \epsilon_i^T = A + B + C \quad (2)$$

where A and B denote the aligned foreground and background data matrix respectively, and C denotes the complement matrix. The sum of A, B, and C equals the aligned data $D \circ \tau$. a denotes a $1 \times m$ vector whose elements are all 1. b denotes a $1 \times n$ vector whose elements are all constant value b that is the mean of the Gaussian. We set b to 0 on the basis of our observations of real PA data. The term $\lambda_1 \|aB - b\|^2$ penalizes the optimization function when the mean of the aligned backgrounds in the same positions stays away from the mean of the Gaussian. We set the weighting parameters λ_1 as $\kappa_1/(m \times d \times \sqrt{n})$, and λ_2 as $\kappa_2/\sqrt{n}$, where $\kappa_1 = 1$, $\kappa_2 = 3$ in all our experiments.

Algorithm 1 shows the complete procedure. At each iteration of the outer loop, we need to solve a linearized optimization problem by linearizing the transformation at the current estimate of τ. This optimization problem is convex and thus solvable via ALM. Specifically, the optimization problem to minimize the augmented Lagrange function is as follows:

$$\min_{A,B,C,\Delta\tau,Y} \|A\|_* + \lambda_1\|aB - b\|^2 + \lambda_2\|C\|_1 + \langle Y, D \circ \tau + \sum_i J_i \Delta\tau\epsilon_i\epsilon_i^T - A - B - C\rangle$$

$$+ \frac{\mu}{2}\|D \circ \tau + \sum_i J_i \Delta\tau\epsilon_i\epsilon_i^T - A - B - C\|^2 \tag{3}$$

where $Y \in \mathcal{R}^{m \times n}$ is a Lagrange multiplier matrix, μ is a positive scalar, and $\langle \cdot, \cdot \rangle$ denotes the matrix inner product. This problem is iteratively minimized as follows:

$$A_{k+1} = US_{\frac{1}{\mu_k}}[\Sigma]V, \quad (U, \Sigma, V) = \text{svd}(D \circ \tau + \sum_i J_i \Delta\tau_k\epsilon_i\epsilon_i^T - B_k - C_k + \frac{1}{\mu_k}Y_k),$$

$$B_{k+1} = \frac{\mu_k}{\mu_k + 2\lambda_1 m}(D \circ \tau + \sum_i J_i \Delta\tau_k\epsilon_i\epsilon_i^T - A_{k+1} - C_k + \frac{1}{\mu_k}Y_k),$$

$$C_{k+1} = S_{\frac{\lambda_2}{\mu_k}}[D \circ \tau + \sum_i J_i \Delta\tau_k\epsilon_i\epsilon_i^T - A_{k+1} - B_{k+1} + \frac{1}{\mu_k}Y_k],$$

$$\Delta\tau_{k+1} = \sum_i J_i^\dagger(A_{k+1} + B_{k+1} + C_{k+1} - D \circ \tau - \frac{1}{\mu_k}Y_k)\epsilon_i\epsilon_i^T,$$

$$Y_{k+1} = Y_k + \mu_k[D \circ \tau + \sum_i J_i \Delta\tau_{k+1}\epsilon_i\epsilon_i^T - A_{k+1} - B_{k+1} - C_{k+1}] \tag{4}$$

where svd($\cdot$) denotes the singular value decomposition operator, and shrinkage operator $S_\beta[\cdot] = sign(x) \cdot \max\{|x| - \beta, 0\}$ is for the singular value thresholding algorithm to optimize the nuclear norm. μ_k is a monotonically increasing positive sequence. We set $\mu_k = (1.25)^k/\|D\|$, according to [9].

4   Experimental Evaluation

First, we evaluated the robustness and accuracy of the proposed method on shot volumes of real 3D PA data. We created five ground-truth data-sets by fixing the body during the scanning so that, there would be no pixel-level misalignment. We synthetically added different levels of position gaps to the shot volumes of the ground-truth, wherein the original volumes were randomly displaced with a uniformly distributed pseudorandom number $[-d\,d]$ of voxels along each axis (x, y, z). The voxel size was $[0.25\ 0.25\ 0.25]$ mm, and the thickness of a vessel was 0.5 to 2 mm. We set the misalignment level d from 1 to 10. In total, we generated 10×5 data-set, in which each data-set included 21 to 36 shot volumes.

For comparison, we compared our results with those obtained by the following state-of-the-art methods: B-spline free-form deformation(B-FFD) [6] which optimizes the control points while minimizing the similarity function; spectral log demon registration [7], which finds the pointwise correspondence between images with simple nearest-neighbor searches (called Log-demon); and RASL [9] with the pyramid scheme. These methods were applied to vessel-enhanced data for a fair comparison. Figure 4 shows the results for each method, where a small value on the vertical axis indicates that the method successfully aligned the data-set. It shows that the proposed method works well until misalignment level 7; it should be good enough for dealing with real body motions. The other

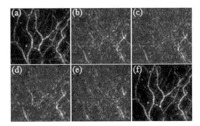

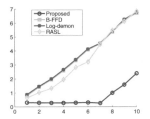

Fig. 3. Examples of averaging images for (a) ground-truth, (b) synthetic misaligned, (c) B-FFD, (d) Log-demon, (e) RASL, (f) Proposed.

Fig. 4. Evaluation results, where the horizontal axis indicates the misalignment level, the vertical axis indicates the metrics of the position gaps (voxels).

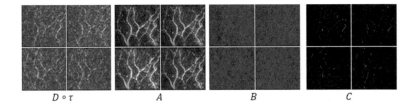

Fig. 5. Examples of the decomposition results. The images are x-y MIPs of the input data, decomposed foreground (A), background (B), and complement (C) respectively.

methods could not align the data so well, even with very low misalignment levels. Figure 3 shows examples of the x-y MIPs of the average images of the aligned results obtained by each method at misalignment level 6. The computational time of the proposed method is comparable with that of the other methods.

Figure 3(a) shows the ground-truth, in which the vessels are clearly visible. The synthetic misalignment makes the image quality significantly worse (Fig. 3(b)). The result of the proposed method (Fig. 3(f)) shows clear vessels, and the image is similar to the ground-truth. This indicates that the proposed method properly aligned the shot volumes. By contrast, vessels are still hard to identify in the results of the other methods (Figs. 3(c), (d), and (e)).

Now let us examine how well the proposed method decomposes real PA data into three components. For example, Fig. 5 shows the results at misalign level 6. The background noise is correctly decomposed in B, all vessels clearly appear in the low-rank component A, and the sparse corruptions of the vessels appear in the complement component C. This results show that the proposed method successfully decomposed the original noisy and misaligned PA data into three meaningful components.

Next, let us examine the robustness of the proposed method against real body motion. To get the real data, a hand was scanned using a wide-field range PA imaging system that scans local areas multiple times with a spiral pattern, and real body motions were added during scanning. The total number of shot

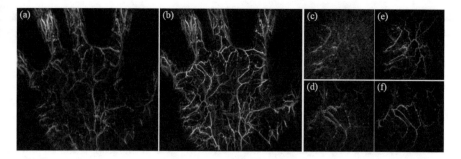

Fig. 6. Examples of registration results. x-y MIP of (a) average data without alignment, (b) from our method, (c), (d) enlarged images of (a), and (e), (f) results of using the proposed method on (c), (d). (Color figure online)

volumes was 2048, and the total scanning time was about 2 min. Successive local shot volumes were overlaid over 85 %. The entire data was $512 \times 512 \times 100$. Since each shot volume is a peace of local-area data, we first generated the data-sets of the local areas ($168 \times 168 \times 100$), which included 16 to 59 shot volumes. Next, we aligned the shot volumes in each data-set, then stitched together the aligned average volumes in order to generate the entire data. For comparison, an image averaging technique without alignment was applied to the data.

Figures 6(a), (c), and (d) show the average data without alignment. In the images, the contrast of the vessels is low, and some vessels are blurry because of body motion. Figures 6(b), (e), and (f) show the registration results from the proposed method. Here, the vessels are obviously clearer than in the original image and some vessels that are hard to see in the averages data without alignment become visible. Here, we should note that the vessels that appear thrice in the red box in Fig. 6(b), where two veins run side-by-side with artery, are not blurry. These image features were confirmed by a doctor of anatomy. The results show that our method significantly improved the image quality of PA imaging.

5   Conclusions

We examined the characteristics of PA images and proposed a registration method for PA imaging to generate high-quality 3D volumes in which vessels become clearly visible. By introducing the statistical prior, in which the mean of the values in the same position of the aligned background data tends to be a constant, our alignment method is capable of handling challenging PA data with strong noise and large misalignments. The experimental results on real data-sets demonstrate the effectiveness of our method; it significantly improved image quality and achieved the best alignment accuracy in the comparison. Currently, our method can only handle one global domain transformation per image, such as affine transformation. We will address the deformable transformation problems in future work. Besides PA imaging, the proposed method has the potential to be applied to many other sorts of medical imaging; these will be explored in our future work.

Acknowledgments. This work was funded by ImPACT Program of Council for Science, Technology and Innovation (Cabinet Office, Government of Japan).

References

1. Kitai, T., Torii, M., Sugie, T., et al.: Photoacoustic mammography: initial clinical results. Breast Cancer **21**, 146–153 (2014)
2. Li, C., Wang, L.V.: Photoacoustic tomography and sensing in biomedicine. Phys. Med. Biol. **54**(19), 5997 (2009)
3. Kruger, R.A., Kuzmiak, C.M., Lam, R.B., et al.: Dedicated 3D photoacoustic breast imaging. Med. Phys. **40**(11), 1–8 (2013). 113301
4. Frangi, A.F., Niessen, W.J., Vincken, K.L., Viergever, M.A.: Multiscale vessel enhancement filtering. In: Wells, W.M., Colchester, A.C.F., Delp, S.L. (eds.) MICCAI 1998. LNCS, vol. 1496, pp. 130–137. Springer, Heidelberg (1998)
5. Sotiras, A., Davatzikos, C., Paragios, N.: Deformable medical image registration: a survey. IEEE Trans. Med. Imaging **32**, 1153–1190 (2013)
6. Rueckert, D., Sonoda, L.I., Hayes, C., Hill, D.L.G., Leach, M.O., Hawkes, D.J.: Nonrigid registration using free-form deformations: application to breast MR images. IEEE Trans. Med. Imaging **8**, 712–721 (1999)
7. Lombaert, H., Grady, L., Pennec, X., et al.: Spectral log-demons: diffeomorphic image registration with very large deformations. IJCV **107**, 254–271 (2014)
8. Aylward, S.R., Jomier, J., Weeks, S., Bullitt, E.: Registration and analysis of vascular images. IJCV **55**(2/3), 123–138 (2003)
9. Peng, Y., Ganesh, A., Wright, J., et al.: RASL: robust alignment by sparse and low-rank decomposition for linearly correlated images. IEEE Trans. PAMI **34**(11), 2233–2246 (2012)
10. Liu, X., Niethammer, M., Kwitt, R., McCormick, M., Aylward, S.: Low-rank to the rescue – atlas-based analyses in the presence of pathologies. In: Golland, P., Hata, N., Barillot, C., Hornegger, J., Howe, R. (eds.) MICCAI 2014, Part III. LNCS, vol. 8675, pp. 97–104. Springer, Heidelberg (2014)
11. Baghaie, A., D'souza, R.M., Yu, Z.: Sparse and low rank decomposition based batch image alignment for speckle reduction of retinal oct images, ISBI, pp. 226–230 (2015)
12. Tao, M., Yuan, X.: Recovering low-rank and sparse components of matrices from incomplete and noisy observations. SIAM J. Optim. **21**(1), 57–81 (2011)
13. Lin, Z., Chen, M., Wu, L., Ma, Y.: The augmented Lagrange multiplier method for exact recovery of corrupted low-rank matrices, UIUC Technical report UILU-ENG-09-2215 (2009)

From Real MRA to Virtual MRA: Towards an Open-Source Framework

N. Passat[1]([✉]), S. Salmon[1], J.-P. Armspach[2], B. Naegel[2], C. Prud'homme[2],
H. Talbot[3], A. Fortin[1], S. Garnotel[1,4], O. Merveille[1,3], O. Miraucourt[1,3],
R. Tarabay[1,2], V. Chabannes[5], A. Dufour[2], A. Jezierska[3], O. Balédent[4],
E. Durand[2], L. Najman[3], M. Szopos[2], A. Ancel[2], J. Baruthio[2], M. Delbany[2],
S. Fall[2,4], G. Pagé[4], O. Génevaux[2], M. Ismail[5], P. Loureiro de Sousa[2],
M. Thiriet[6], and J. Jomier[7,8]

[1] Université de Reims Champagne-Ardenne, CReSTIC and LMR, Reims, France
nicolas.passat@univ-reims.fr
[2] Université de Strasbourg, CNRS, ICube and IRMA, Strasbourg, France
[3] Université Paris-Est, ESIEE, CNRS, LIGM, Paris, France
[4] Université Picardie Jules Verne, BioFlow Image, Amiens, France
[5] Université de Grenoble, CNRS, LJK and LIPhy, Grenoble, France
[6] Université Paris 6, CNRS, INRIA, LJLL, Paris, France
[7] Kitware SAS, Villeurbanne, France
[8] Kitware SAS, New York, USA

Abstract. Angiographic imaging is a crucial domain of medical imaging. In particular, Magnetic Resonance Angiography (MRA) is used for both clinical and research purposes. This article presents the first framework geared toward the design of virtual MRA images from real MRA images. It relies on a pipeline that involves image processing, vascular modeling, computational fluid dynamics and MR image simulation, with several purposes. It aims to provide to the whole scientific community (1) software tools for MRA analysis and blood flow simulation; and (2) data (computational meshes, virtual MRAs with associated ground truth), in an open-source/open-data paradigm. Beyond these purposes, it constitutes a versatile tool for progressing in the understanding of vascular networks, especially in the brain, and the associated imaging technologies.

1 Introduction

Angiographic imaging constitutes a crucial area of medical imaging. It led, in particular, to the development of devoted acquisition protocols in Magnetic Resonance Imaging, X-ray Computed Tomography, or Ultra-Sound imaging. Within this wide spectrum of modalities and specific sequences, Magnetic Resonance

This research was funded by the Agence Nationale de la Recherche (Grant Agreement ANR-12-MONU-0010) and Régions Champagne-Ardenne and Picardie. MRI images were provided by the In Vivo Imaging Platform (Univ. Strasbourg) and Institut Faire Faces (Univ. Picardie).

© Springer International Publishing AG 2016
S. Ourselin et al. (Eds.): MICCAI 2016, Part III, LNCS 9902, pp. 335–343, 2016.
DOI: 10.1007/978-3-319-46726-9_39

Angiography (MRA) is particularly used, for instance in the case of detection and diagnosis of vascular alterations (e.g., stenoses, aneurysms, thromboses, . . .), and patient follow-up after treatment (e.g., by stents, coils, . . .). MRA is also an effective tool for clinical research devoted to the understanding of human macro and mesovascular physiology, since it provides non-invasive/non-ionising modalities (e.g., Phase Contrast (PC) or Time-of-Flight (TOF) MRA), available in 2D, 3D, and even 3D+time.

Due to the nature of structures visualized in MRA, namely thin, elongated, curvy vessels, the development of specific image analysis tools has been an active research area during the last decades [1]. However, contrary to other morphological structures (e.g., brain tissues and structures, with BrainWeb [2]), there does not exist any common framework to facilitate the development and validation of related image analysis methods. In particular, despite a few attempts (such as MICCAI challenges [3]), that rely on datasets equiped with manual ground truth, there does not exist any "vascular analogue" of BrainWeb, i.e., a framework for generating efficiently virtual MRA images naturally equiped with a ground-truth and/or associated to a real MRA.

Stemming on this fact, we have been working, in the context of the VIVABRAIN Project[1] with the final goal to tackle this issue by providing an efficient and versatile methodological framework allowing for the generation of virtual MRAs from real MRAs. The notion of virtual angiography is not new, and was already developed for CT Angiography simulation [4]. However, the case of MRA was not intensively considered, in particular via the efficient coupling of CFD and MRI simulation.

This article presents our framework. In Sect. 2, we present the proposed methodological pipeline. In Sect. 3, we focus on the most challenging issues raised by the instanciation of this pipeline, and some of our approaches for tackling them. In Sect. 4, we describe experimental results that validate and/or illustrate our main contributions.

2   Overview of the Framework

Our framework relies on a pipeline composed of five main steps, going from real MRA to virtual MRA. Four of these steps require to tackle methodological issues, and are related to three main disciplinary fields, namely computer science (image processing and analysis), mathematics (CFD), and physics (MRI simulation). The first step is devoted to MRA acquisition. The second aims at segmenting vascular volumes from such data, in order to further define mixed 2D/3D computational meshes of vascular structures. The third step consists of designing a vascular model, in particular by exp- licitly

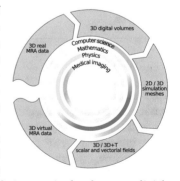

---

[1] URL: http://vivabrain.fr.

modeling anatomical and physiological features. The fourth step aims to simulate the flowing blood in the designed vascular model, leading to velocity and pressure fields. The fifth step consists of generating MRA images based on the previously computed information, in order to produce virtual MRA data.

This methodological pipeline is materialized by a software framework, namely AngioTk[2], which can embed plug-ins implementing some of the above methodological steps. The data flowchart associated to this pipeline is the following: 3D real MRAs $\rightarrow$ 3D digital volumes $\rightarrow$ 2D/3D computational meshes $\rightarrow$ 3D / 3D+T scalar and vectorial fields $\rightarrow$ 3D virtual MRAs. Providing some of them as open-data is a complementary purpose of the software framework, itself developed in an open-source way.

3 Challenges and Principal Contributions

In this section, we discuss some of the principal contributions within the proposed framework, in relation with the four aforementioned methodological steps.

3.1 Segmentation of Vascular Volumes

The very first issue raised by the instanciation of the proposed framework is related to the efficient extraction of vascular volumes from 3D MRA images, i.e., the segmentation of vessels. Many approaches have been developed so far, for this specific topic. In particular, deformable model paradigms (e.g., level-sets) have been widely investigated. These approaches were mainly motivated by the dual handling of data-driven information (namely the hypersignal of blood) and a regularization term (related to the geometry of vessels). However, the use of a 2D model (either implicit or explicit) for handling structures mainly 1-dimensional generally tends to decrease the robustness of such approaches.

Considering the relevance of the dual handling of two, data- and feature-based terms, we propose to express the problem of vessel segmentation as a variational problem. As for deformable models, this leads to minimize a two-term energy; however, this formulation no longer consists of mapping a geometric model onto the sought vascular structures. In particular, we developed a Chan-Vese formulation [5], in which the regularization term is directly driven by a vesselness measure.

In this context, we investigated two kinds of vesselness measures, namely Frangi Vesselness, and an alternative morphological feature, namely RORPO[3] [6], proved to present complementary properties in terms of accuracy and precision. In addition, such an approach can be enhanced with directional information in the regularization term. Results of filtering with RORPO and segmentation with our Chan-Vese approach are provided in Sect. 4.1.

---

[2] URL: http://angiotk.org.
[3] URL: http://path-openings.github.io/RORPO.

3.2   Modeling of Vascular Networks

The digital vascular volumes can be processed to design 2D/3D computational mesh models. Many works have been devoted to this issue, and we did not investigate alternative approaches. In particular, we rely on freely available existing tools[4]. We focus here on the issue of accurately modeling the physiological hypotheses associated to the considered vascular networks. To illustrate our modus operandi, we consider the case study of the cerebral venous network. At the macroscopic scale, it is composed by input veins (7–11) draining the blood into sinuses (2,3) until their confluence (4). The blood then passes into lateral sinuses (5,6) and reaches an extracranial area, composed of the internal jugular veins (1).

We assume that: (i) the blood density is constant; (ii) the flow is incompressible and isothermal; (iii) the Newtonian model is used for blood flow. The latter assumption consists of neglecting shear thinning and viscoelastic effects [7]. The cranium is considered as a rigid closed box, and the brain tissues and cerebrospinal fluid contain mainly water, thus constituting an incompressible tissue. We then suppose that vessel walls are rigid. Patient-specific blood flow data are usually not collected from routine clinical examinations. Hence, 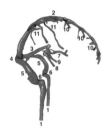 scarce literature data are used for the velocity magnitude in cerebral veins [8]. The above hypotheses and the governing parameters computed from the literature (Reynold: 75 → 1055; Stokes: 1.10 → 3.84; Strouhal: 0.013 → 0.030) lead to model the venous blood flow dynamics by the Navier-Stokes (NS) equations

$$\begin{cases} \rho(\partial_t\mathbf{u} + (\mathbf{u} \cdot \nabla)\mathbf{u}) - \mu\Delta\mathbf{u} + \nabla p = \mathbf{f} & \text{in } \Omega \times [0,T] \\ \text{div } \mathbf{u} = 0 & \text{in } \Omega \times [0,T] \\ \mathbf{u}|_{t=0} = \mathbf{u_0} \text{ in } \Omega \end{cases} \quad (1)$$

where $\mathbf{u}$: fluid velocity, p: pressure, ρ: density, μ: dynamic viscosity, $\mathbf{f}$: an applied body force. For boundary conditions, we use a constant velocity of small magnitude at the inflow (coming from microcirculation), and free traction boundary condition for the outflow. The no-slip condition is imposed on the wall boundaries, assumed to be rigid.

3.3   Simulation of Flowing Blood

In order to simulate flowing blood in complex networks, reduced order models are often considered [9]. However, this is not sufficient to accurately capture subtle behaviours, in particular for MRA simulation. Then, we aim to generalize the 3D CFD approaches generally considered for vessel samples [10] to the case of more complete networks.

The two numerical methods we use to compute an approximate solution to the NS equations are finite element methods. Both are available as open-source

---

[4] See, e.g., http://www.ann.jussieu.fr/frey/software.html.

(FreeFem++/Feel++)[5]. FreeFem++ uses characteristics method to handle the non-linear term, while Feel++ uses the Oseen linearization. Both methods were validated[6] with analytical solutions, e.g., Ethier-Steinman. The finite element spaces used to discretize the velocity and the pressure are the Inf-Sup stable Taylor-Hood finite elements P2P1. In order to speed-up the resolution, this method is coupled with an iterative Uzawa conjuguate gradient algorithm with a Cahouet-Chabart preconditionner. For Feel++ simulations, we used a second order finite difference scheme to approximate the time derivative and a second order extrapolation of the nonlinear convective term. The resolution in the latter is handled by a LU solver. The discretized NS equations were supplemented for both Feel++ and Freefem++ simulations by a no-slip boundary conditions on the lateral surface of the computational domain, since we are dealing with viscous fluid. At the inflow and the outflow, we imposed a Dirichlet and a Neumann boundary conditions.

3.4   MRA Simulation

From the 3D geometry of the vascular network, and the velocity field obtained from the NS equations resolution, MRA can finally be simulated. The sample to be imaged is divided into equal subvolumes called isochromats, assumed to possess uniform physical properties (spin relaxation times T1, T2, T2*, equilibrium magnetization $\mathbf{M_0}$, ...). The measurable signal emitted by one isochromat is obtained by numerically solving the Bloch equations, that give the temporal evolution of tissue magnetization for one isochromat

$$\frac{d\mathbf{M}}{dt} = \gamma \mathbf{M} \times \mathbf{B} - \hat{\mathbf{R}}(\mathbf{M} - \mathbf{M_0}) \tag{2}$$

with $\mathbf{M}$ the magnetization vector of the tissue, γ the gyromagnetic ratio of hydrogen, $\mathbf{B}$ the external magnetic field, $\hat{\mathbf{R}}$ the relaxation matrix containing T1 and T2. The whole MR signal is obtained by summing the contribution of each isochromat over the sample.

To handle movement of spins over the time, we consider the Lagrangian approach. This requires to determine each individual spin trajectory. While solving Bloch equations, we need not use a different treatment for static tissues and flowing particles. We vary the position of the spin over time, which changes the field value seen by the particle

$$\mathbf{B}(\mathbf{r}, t) = [\mathbf{G}(t).\mathbf{r}(t) + \Delta B(\mathbf{r}, t)].\mathbf{e_z} + \mathbf{B_1}(\mathbf{r}, t) \tag{3}$$

where the magnetic field term $\mathbf{B}$ contains all the MR sequence elements (gradients and RF pulses): $\mathbf{G}$ the gradient sequence, $\mathbf{r}$ the isochromat position, ΔB the field inhomogeneities, $\mathbf{B_1}$ the RF pulses sequence.

Specific software packages have been designed for MRI simulation, including JEMRIS[7], which is an advanced MRI simulator software written in C++, open-source and freely modifiable. Natively, Bloch equation solving in JEMRIS is only

---

[5] FreeFem++: http://www.freefem.org and Feel++: http://www.feelpp.org.

[6] Results and algorithms are freely available at http://numtourcfd.univ-reims.fr.

[7] http://www.jemris.org.

dedicated to simulate static tissues; indeed, JEMRIS only allows to specify one trajectory for all spins. Then, we added a specific class to the C++ code to allow users to specify a different trajectory for each spin, thus implementing an MRA simulation functionality [11].

4   Experiments and Results

4.1   Validation of Image Processing Methods

In terms of image processing and analysis, two validations were carried out. The first is devoted to RORPO by comparing the efficiency of the associated vesselness feature vs. the gold standard of Frangi vesselness, in terms of image filtering (namely, vessel enhancement). Some qualitative results for filtering of a 3D MRA of brain vasculature are illustrated in Fig. 1. The efficiency of RORPO vs. Frangi vesselness, was also emphasised by a comparative threshold-based segmentation study, whose results are provided in the ROC curves, on the right (mean value and standard deviation).

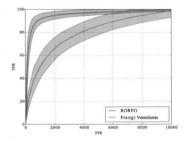

The second validations are devoted to the Chan-Vese segmentation method embedding a vesselness measure as regularization term. In order to quantitatively assess the robustness of this approach on complex vascular networks, we applied this method on the DRIVE database [12], that is composed of 2D images (our approach is valid both for 2D and 3D), and comes with accurate ground truths. The results obtained on this database present an accuracy score of 0.9434, compared to 0.9442 for the state of the art [12] and 0.9479 for Human observer. These results, very close to the state of the art, prove the relevance of the approach, in particular for a method that was neither designed nor parametrically tuned for this application.

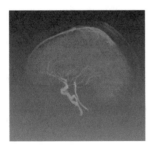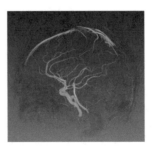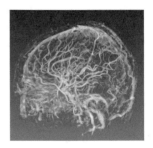

Fig. 1. Left: TOF MRA volume rendering (from low intensities, in red, to high intensities, in yellow). Center: RORPO filtering. Right: Frangi Vesselness. (Color figure online)

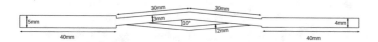

Fig. 2. Physical phantom, designed as a double bifurcation fluid circuit, to reproduce acceleration, deceleration and recirculation all of which can be encountered in real vascular networks.

4.2 Validation of CFD Methods

Various experiments were performed to assess the relevance of the proposed CFD methods. First, the numerical results were compared to those actually measured from MRA images of a physical phantom (Fig. 2). A pulsatile flow, obtained with MRA measurements, was used to impose the

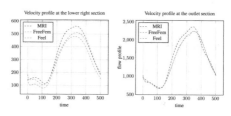

velocity at the inlet of the phantom. In order to carry out a cross-validation of the two finite elements methods, we compared velocity (and pressure) profiles at six different radial sections previously defined, and along the centerline. Two of these six profiles are presented on the right. Most of the results are equivalent in this Feel++–Freefem++ comparison. The input and output flows are very similar, both between the two simulations and between simulations and experiment. Branches flow are equally similar for the two simulations, while MRA measurements are slightly higher. These differences can be explained by the fact that MRA images were segmented beforehand, and this process tends to overestimate the real conditions of the experiment. In a more qualitative way, we also run a simplified NS problem on a realistic cerebral venous network with both Feel++ and Freefem++. The results very close from each other are illustrated in Fig. 3.

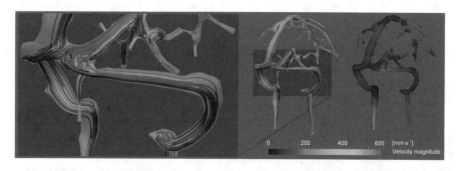

Fig. 3. Blood flow simulation in a cerebral venous network: streamlines and velocity fields.

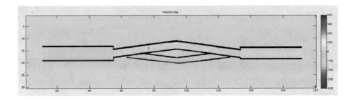

Fig. 4. Virtual MRA obtained from the velocity field computed by the CFD methods, and the MRA simulation implemented in JEMRIS. (Phantom geometry superimposed, in black.)

4.3   Validation of MRA Simulation Methods

MRI simulations were performed using JEMRIS with constant flows computed from numerical simulations and pulsatile ones, and on rigid and nonrigid phantoms. Only a part of these experiments is reported here; see [11,13] for complementary details.

In Fig. 4, we show a simulated phase contrast image of constant flow obtained with JEMRIS. About 19 000 spin trajectories were calculated on a time interval of 5 s from numerical data calculated for constant flow with Feel++ and Freefem++. We used a phase contrast sequence with resolution 128, matrix 180 × 30, TE of 8 ms, TR

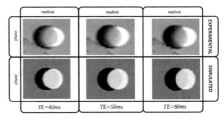

of 100 ms, Venc of 400 mm/s and Nex = 1. Computations took 15 min using 20 CPUs. We find the initial phantom geometry as expected; we can notice a lack of spins in the lower branch due to the low number of flow particles travelling along that path. The velocities measured in each branch are on par, magnitude-wise, with the initial data provided by Feel++ and Freefem++. The low resolution used for the MRI simulation leads to an averaging of the velocities in the voxel, and consequently to an underestimation of the peak velocity in each branch of the phantom (partial volume effect). It is worth mentioning that the proposed framework, although preliminary, is already efficient enough to allow for simulating subtle MRA details, and in particular to reproduce specific acquisition artifacts. This is, for instance, the case for vascular signal shift due to TE delay (first row: real data; second row: simulated data).

5   Conclusion

Beyond specific contributions to the state of the art in vessel segmentation, blood flow simulation and MRI simulation, with the purpose of providing methods both fairly validated and openly available to the whole community, the purpose of this work was to provide a full methodological framework allowing to generate virtual

MRAs from real ones, in a versatile and efficient paradigm. A software pipeline is associated to this framework, and will hopefully constitute a strong basis for facilitating research activities of the scientific community on angiographic imaging, and MRA in particular.

From a methodological point of view, we plan to further embed some solutions for generating vascular atlases [14] in this framework, thus allowing to go a step further by parameterizing the vessel geometric and topological properties. The generation of vascular atlases will however require to tackle open issues, in particular with regard to vessel registration. This will constitute our immediate further works.

References

1. Lesage, D., Angelini, E.D., Bloch, I., et al.: A review of 3D vessel lumen segmentation techniques: models, features and extraction schemes. Med. Image Anal. **13**, 819–845 (2009)
2. Cocosco, C.A., Kollokian, V., Kwan, R.K.S., et al.: BrainWeb: online interface to a 3D MRI simulated brain database. NeuroImage **5**(4 Pt 2), S425 (1997)
3. Schaap, M., Metz, C.T., van Walsum, T., et al.: Standardized evaluation methodology and reference database for evaluating coronary artery centerline extraction algorithms. Med. Image Anal. **13**, 701–714 (2009)
4. Ford, M.D., Stuhne, G.R., Nikolov, H.N., et al.: Virtual angiography for visualization and validation of computational models of aneurysm hemodynamics. IEEE Trans. Med Imaging **24**, 1586–1592 (2005)
5. Merveille, O., Miraucourt, O., Talbot, H., et al.: A variational model for thin structure segmentation based on a directional regularization. In: ICIP (2016)
6. Merveille, O., Talbot, H., Najman, et al.: Tubular structure analysis by ranking the orientation responses of path operators. Technical Report hal-01262728 (2016)
7. Thiriet, M.: Biology and Mechanics of Blood Flows, Part I: Biology of Blood Flows, Part II: Mechanics and Medical Aspects of Blood Flows. Springer, New York (2008)
8. Stoquart-Elsankari, S., Lehmann, P., Villette, A., et al.: A phase-contrast MRI study of physiologic cerebral venous flow. Cereb. Blood Flow Metab. **29**, 1208–1215 (2005)
9. Ho, H., Mithraratne, K., Hunter, P.: Numerical simulation of blood flow in an anatomically-accurate cerebral venous tree. IEEE Trans. Med Imaging **32**, 85–91 (2013)
10. Boissonnat, J.D., Chaine, R., Frey, P., et al.: From arteriographies to computational flow in saccular aneurisms: the INRIA experience. Med. Image Anal. **9**, 133–143 (2005)
11. Fortin, A., Salmon, S., Baruthio, J., et al.: High performance MRI simulation of arbitrarily complex flow: a versatile framework. Technical Report hal-01326698 (2016)
12. Staal, J.J., Abramoff, M.D., Niemeijer, M., et al.: Ridge based vessel segmentation in color images of the retina. IEEE Trans. Med. Imag **23**, 501–509 (2004)
13. Ancel, A., Fortin, A., Garnotel, S., et al.: Phantom project. Technical Report hal-01222281 (2015)
14. Passat, N., Ronse, C., Baruthio, J., et al.: Magnetic resonance angiography: from anatomical knowledge modeling to vessel segmentation. Med. Image Anal. **10**, 259–274 (2006)

Improved Diagnosis of Systemic Sclerosis Using Nailfold Capillary Flow

Michael Berks$^{(\boxtimes)}$, Graham Dinsdale, Andrea Murray, Tonia Moore,
Ariane Herrick, and Chris Taylor

University of Manchester, Manchester, UK
michael.berks@manchester.ac.uk

Abstract. Nailfold capillaroscopy (NC) allows non-invasive imaging of
systemic sclerosis (SSc) related microvascular disease. We have developed
a state-of-the-art NC system that enables fast, panoramic imaging of the
whole nailfold at high-magnification, and incorporates novel software to
make fully automated estimates of capillary structure and blood flow
velocity. We present the first results of a study in which 50 patients with
SSc, 12 with primary Raynauds phenomenon (PRP) and 50 healthy controls (HC) were imaged using the new system, and show that a combined
model of capillary measurements strongly separates SSc from HC/PRP
(ROC A_z=0.93). Including capillary flow improves model performance,
suggesting flow provides complementary information to capillary structure for diagnosing SSc.

1 Introduction

Nailfold capillaroscopy (NC) is a non-invasive optical technique for imaging
microvascular abnormalities, commonly used in the diagnosis and assessment
of systemic sclerosis (SSc) – an autoimmune connective tissue disease that is
painful, disabling and disfiguring, with high mortality. In particular, NC can
identify the characteristic structural changes in capillaries that differentiate
patients with symptoms of SSc induced Raynauds phenomenon (RP; the most
common presenting feature of SSc) from those with the more common and relatively benign primary (idiopathic) RP (PRP) [1,2].

In current clinical practice, such changes are labelled as either nor-
mal/abnormal or divided into coarse disease stages (early, active, late). However subjective labelling suffers from poor inter-observer agreement, and is not
well-suited for monitoring disease progression. With the development of drugs
with vascular remodelling potential, and increasing interest in early intervention,
there has been a move towards quantitative assessment [3,4]. Manually measuring capillary size, shape and density is labour intensive, but has been shown to
be more reproducible than qualitative assessment [3], and shows good discrim-
ination between SSc and PRP. Recent work has shown such measures can be
made automatically to the same level of accuracy as expert observers [4].

However, these *structural* changes happen on a timescale of months/years and
may not be useful for monitoring rapid changes, e.g. in a clinical trial of vasoac-
tive therapy. In contrast, capillary blood flow may respond immediately to such

© Springer International Publishing AG 2016
S. Ourselin et al. (Eds.): MICCAI 2016, Part III, LNCS 9902, pp. 344–352, 2016.
DOI: 10.1007/978-3-319-46726-9_40

interventions, whilst also providing complementary information to structural measures in routine diagnosis of SSc. Moreover, flow, as a measure of capillary *function*, can potentially provide insights into pathophysiology and markers of disease activity, both in SSc and other conditions in which the microvasculature plays a key role.

Motivated by these observations, we have developed a state-of-the-art NC system that uses a high frame rate camera to capture video sequences in which it is possible to measure red blood cell velocity in individual capillaries. The system includes software to generate high-quality static image mosaics for clinical assessment, and makes fully-automated measures of capillary structure and flow – the latter using a novel adaption of optimised optical flow [5] developed to be robust to the extremely challenging low-contrast, high noise conditions inherent in NC imaging.

While flow has been estimated previously in NC video [6,7], this was performed only at manually selected points or vessels, an approach that both introduces subjectivity and does not scale to analysing large datasets. We believe our system is the first to measure flow fully-automatically in *all* visible capillaries across the whole nailfold. Capillary blood flow has also been measured using the related technique of sidestream dark field (SDF) imaging (e.g. in [8] amongst others), however SDF requires skin contact and may be unsuitable for assessing patients with SSc.

In this paper we describe the new system, and present the first results of a trial in which it was used to image 50 healthy controls (HC), 12 patients with PRP and 50 patients with SSc. We show that automated measures of capillary structure can differentiate patients with SSc from HC/PRP providing further evidence of the validity of the technique, that a combined model provides greater predictive power than individual measures, and that including capillary blood velocity improves prediction, suggesting capillary flow can aid the diagnosis of SSc.

2 A New High Frame Rate Capillaroscopy System

The new system comprises a monochrome, high frame rate digital camera (The Imaging Source, DTK23U618, 640×480 px, 120fps) attached to a 27 mm focal length, 9 mm diameter lens, situated 152 mm from the camera sensor to produce raw video frames with a spatial resolution of 1μm per pixel. The camera is connected to a 3-D high-precision motorised stage system (Thorlabs, MTS25/M-Z8) with 25 mm of travel along each axis. This enables fast and accurate focusing and imaging mosaicking so the whole nailfold can be imaged at high-magnification. For patients unable to straighten their fingers (a common disability in SSc), the stages are mounted to a stand that can be rotated through $\sim 75°$. The system thus combines the flexibility of a hand-held capillaroscopy device with the advantages of a rigid platform for obtaining high-quality images[1].

---

[1] Videos available at http://personalpages.manchester.ac.uk/staff/Michael.Berks/ nailfolddemo.

2.1   Acquiring Images

To complement the hardware, we have developed a complete software package for acquiring image video sequences and recording associated session data. During acquisition, live video from the camera is displayed alongside a map showing the camera is current 3-D position within the $25\,mm^3$ travel permitted by the motors. The camera can be moved to any (x,y) position, either by clicking or dragging a joystick in the live display (for precision movements) or clicking in the map (for fast long range movements). Focus is controlled by moving the cameras in the z-plane using either keyboard arrows or the mouse scroll-wheel. During recording each frame is tagged with the current motor position and every 30th frame is added to a live image mosaic, registered in real-time to show the user the extent of the nailfold captured (See footnote 1).

2.2   Generating Mosaics and Capillary Videos

A complete video sequence of a nailfold typically comprises 5,000–15,000 raw frames, which are processed offline to generate high-quality static image mosaics and video sequences of each visible capillary. Consecutive frames can be separated into 3 types of segment where: (1) the motors are moving in the (x, y)-plane (*panning*); (2) the z-motor is moving (*focusing*); (3) the motors are stationary. The acquisition software limits continuous panning to guarantee that stationary segments overlap, and only these frames are used to analyse capillaries (Fig. 1a).

In the first processing step, frames within each segment are aligned and saved for later use in capillary videos (Sect. 4). The aligned frames are averaged to form a compound frame with significantly lower noise and better contrast than the

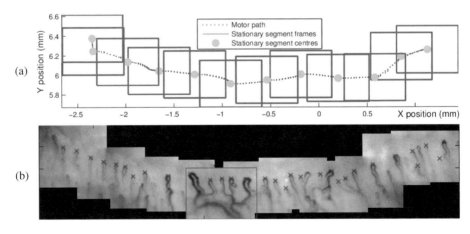

Fig. 1. Generating mosaics (a) video sequence motor positions are used to compute stationary segments and estimate the mosaic's global geometry; (b) registered mosaic, with the distal capillaries detected. The blue box marks a stationary segment from which capillary videos are extracted. (Color figure online)

raw frames [9]. To form a mosaic of the whole nailfold, the compound frames are then sequentially registered by searching for the global best match of vessel edge features, generated by non-maximally suppressing the response to a Gaussian1st derivative filter. Frames are initially aligned using their motor position (Fig. 1a). To guard against mis-registering frames with very little or no image content (a problem inherent in some nailfolds, both due to low-contrast and because disease may have destroyed capillary structure), frames that do not meet a minimum matching threshold are kept in their initial position, preventing total registration failure observed in earlier NC systems that employed mosaicking [9]. This is particularly important where capillaries are only present/visible in some regions of a nailfold, as by keeping the global geometry of the mosaic intact, we can still safely measure capillary density.

3   Measuring Capillary Structure

Having generated an image mosaic of the whole nailfold we use the method described by Berks et al. [4] to detect the distal row of capillaries (Fig. 1b). The method first predicts pixel level estimates of vesselness (V_s i.e. the probability of belonging to a vessel), vessel orientation (V_θ) and width (V_w), as outputs from random forests trained on manually labelled capillaries, with features based on a multi-scale, multi-orientation decomposition of local image structure. The pixel level maps are used to apply a second level of machine learning in which scaled and rotated image patches are extracted from candidate vessel centres and used to predict the location of nearby capillary apices. A final selection of distal row capillaries can then be made using both local image appearance and the spatial relationships between the candidate apices.

As in [4] we use the location of each distal capillary apex to compute capillary density (defined as the distance between the leftmost and rightmost distal capillaries, divided by the number of distal capillaries). In addition, using V_s we compute the set of vessel pixels connected to, and at most 100μm from the apex of each capillary, and subsequently use V_w and V_θ to compute the mean width $\bar{W}$ and orientation $\bar{\Theta}$. $\bar{W}$ is as a more robust measure of individual capillary width than a point estimate at the apex and is used to compute mean and maximum widths of all capillaries in the nailfold.

Meanwhile, $\bar{\Theta}$, is used to compute two further measures of structure: shape and derangement. Pixel orientations in V_θ are represented as angle-doubled unit vectors in the complex plane, $V_\theta(p) = \exp 2i\phi$. Thus for each capillary we can write $\bar{\Theta}$ as a complex number $S \exp 2i\bar{\phi}$ where the magnitude $S \in [0,1]$ is a measure of circular dispersion that will be higher in normal vessels (with long straight limbs and a narrow hairpin apex) than abnormally shaped capillaries. The mean of each individual capillary dispersion S in the image gives a measure of shape uniformity for the whole nailfold.

Returning to $\bar{\Theta}$, the angle $\bar{\phi}$ represents the principal direction of the capillary. Discarding S, and taking the average of the unit vectors $\hat{\Theta} = \exp 2i\bar{\phi}$ across the nailfold generates a new mean orientation, the dispersion parameter of which $\bar{D}$

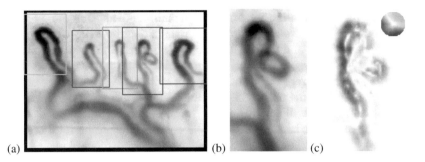

(a)   (b)   (c)

Fig. 2. Measuring capillary flow: (a) capillary bounding boxes in a stationary segment; (b) average of re-registered cropped frames from the red box (See footnote 1); (c) Estimate of vessel flow–colour denotes flow direction, intensity flow magnitude. (Color figure online)

provides a measure of the uniformity of capillary direction (derangement), again with range $[0, 1]$ and likely to be higher in nailfolds with normal structure.

The final set of structural measurements for each nailfold comprise capillary density, mean and maximum width, shape and derangement, approximately corresponding to measures made in earlier (semi-)manual quantitative analysis [3].

4   Measuring Capillary Flow

To build videos of capillary blood flow, we use the location of detected capillaries and the registered position of each compound frame in the nailfold mosaic to select the distal row capillaries visible in each stationary segment (Fig. 2a). For a given segment, we use V_s to define a bounding box around the extremities of each capillary, and use this to sample patches from the segment's frames.

The sampled patches for each capillary are re-registered using the compound frame, cropped to the capillary's bounding box, as a common target. This corrects pixel-level mis-registrations in the global frame alignment that make little difference when averaged in the static image, but significantly degrade flow estimation. Finally the registered patches are contrast normalised ready for flow estimation (Fig. 2b).

To estimate blood velocity in a capillary video, we use a multiscale version of optical flow, based on the work of Brox et al. [5]. First, we form a pyramid stack of the patches, successively smoothing and downsampling the patches at each pyramid level. We then use least-squares non-linear optimisation to compute a dense flow field in the coarsest layer. This flow field is upsampled and used to warp the patches at the next pyramid level, before recomputing spatio-temporal gradients, and optimising again to find the new flow field. The process repeats until we reach the original image resolution.

The non-linear least-squares optimisation at each level combines a data term (that the pixels should obey the standard optical flow equations and thus maintain constant brightness [10]) coupled with a smoothness term that acts to spatialy regularise the flow field (that nearby locations should have similar flow) while permitting non-linearities at object boundaries. We assume that flow is constant over time at any given location for the duration of the video, computing a single flow vector that optimally describes the observed horizontal and vertical displacements. At the finest pyramid level this effectively computes the mean flow over time at each pixel (Fig. 2c). Measuring flow in this way is considerably more robust to noise than estimating flow between pairs of frames, and is necessary to cope with the high-noise, low-contrast inherent in NC imaging. We note however that in some capillaries the assumption of constant flow over time is observably false, and thus finding the optimal compromise between robustness and measuring this temporal variability is a subject for further work.

To obtain a single measure of blood cell velocity for each capillary, we must account for the fact that a capillary may appear in multiple segments, or, particularly in the case of abnormally large capillaries, be split between segments. Rather than simply averaging flow measurements between segments, we project them back into the global geometry of the whole nailfold, and where they overlap, evaluate which segment produced a more reliable estimate.

One option is to use the residual model-fit from the top-level optimisation, although in practice we found this unreliable. Instead, we note that we do not constrain flow using V_s or V_θ and so the method will estimate non-zero flow outside of the vessel, and within the vessel may predict flow directions that do not match the predicted orientation. This provides two measures of flow reliability: firstly, using V_s we compute the ratio of mean flow magnitudes inside and outside the vessel; secondly, using V_θ we measure the mean angular difference between the flow direction and orientation at each vessel pixel.

In practice we found that selecting the segment which produced the highest vessel to background flow ratio gave best results, although work to validate measures of flow reliability are ongoing. Having projected estimations of flow from the capillary videos back to the global nailfold geometry, we take the mean flow magnitude over all distal capillaries as a single measure of blood velocity.

5   Experiments

5.1   Data

112 subjects (50 HC, 12 PRP, 50 SSc) were recruited in a tertiary referral centre for SSc and imaged using the new system. Video sequences of all 10 digits (where available) were acquired, generating 1,104 sequences. A total of 23,489 distal capillaries were detected and used to compute measures of capillary density, mean and maximum width, shape, derangement and mean flow velocity. Detecting capillaries takes ~4 mins per sequence, with processing commencing automatically in the background while live imaging continues. Flow measures are computed offline and take ~1 h per sequence, processing all capillaries sequentially. If time is a critical factor for analysis, the capillaries may be processed in parallel (e.g. on a GPU), however this was not necessary for this study.

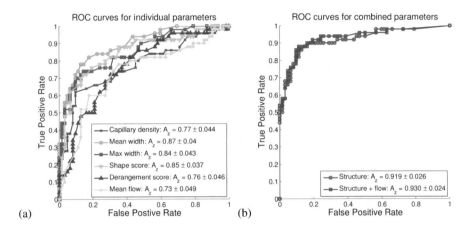

Fig. 3. ROCs for separating HC and PRP from SSc: (a) Individual measures of capillary structure and flow; (b) combined measures in a logistic regression model, with and without flow.

Table 1. Group means and standard errors and ROC A_z values for each capillary measure. ♯, †, ‡ denote significant pair-wise differences for PR vs HC, SSc vs HC, and SSc vs PR respectively.

Parameter	Subject group means ($\pm$ 2 s.e.)			ROC A_z
	HC (n=50)	PRP (n=12)	SSc (n=50)	HC,PRP v SSc
Capillary density (mm^{-1})	6.73 $\pm$ 0.34	7.28 $\pm$ 0.54	5.52 $\pm$ 0.42 †‡	0.771 $\pm$ 0.04
Mean width (μm)	11.8 $\pm$ 0.23	12.7 $\pm$ 0.74	15 $\pm$ 0.71 †‡	0.874 $\pm$ 0.04
Max width (μm)	16.5 $\pm$ 0.91	21.4 $\pm$ 2.94 $^{\sharp}$	27.4 $\pm$ 2.38 †‡	0.836 $\pm$ 0.04
Shape score ($\in [0,1]$)	0.312 $\pm$ 0.02	0.325 $\pm$ 0.03	0.249 $\pm$ 0.01 †‡	0.845 $\pm$ 0.04
Derangment score ($\in [0,1]$)	0.649 $\pm$ 0.03	0.689 $\pm$ 0.05	0.54 $\pm$ 0.03 †‡	0.761 $\pm$ 0.05
Mean flow velocity (mm s^{-1})	0.311 $\pm$ 0.05	0.383 $\pm$ 0.10	0.235 $\pm$ 0.04 †‡	0.726 $\pm$ 0.05

For each subject we computed the mean over all their gradeable digits to produce a single value for each parameter (8 subjects had one or more ungradeable digits, although all had at least 3 gradeable digits).

5.2   Results

Group means and standard errors for each structure and flow parameter are shown in Table 1. Group means for SSc are statistically significantly different to both HC and PRP for all parameters, with values matching results from earlier studies [3,4]. For each individual parameter Fig. 3a shows an ROC curve and A_z values for predicting SSc (positive) versus the combined group HC/PRP (negative)[2].

---

[2] HR/PRP are grouped both because we would not expect significant differences in their capillary measures and because detecting SSc is the most clinically relevant task.

We combined the individual parameters in a logistic regression model using HC/PRP vs SSc as a binary output variable, first using only the structural measures and then including flow. Stepwise regression was used to add/remove terms from an initial linear model fit, and in both cases max width (highly correlated with mean width) and derangement (highly correlated with shape) were discarded. In the latter model flow was retained suggesting it provides additional independent information to the structural measures. To estimate model performance we applied leave-one-out cross-validation to obtain unbiased predictions for each subject (Fig. 3b). The model of structural measures produced an A_z of 0.919, significantly greater than the best single parameter (mean width $A_z = 0.874$). Including flow further improved performance ($A_z = 0.930$), again indicating that flow contains complementary information for diagnosing SSc.

6   Conclusions

We have presented details of a new nailfold capillaroscopy system that we believe enhances the current state-of-the-art of in-vivo microvascular imaging. Carefully selected hardware components, combined with novel, bespoke software, enables fast and easy acquisition of high-quality video sequences in which both capillary structure and blood velocity are measured automatically. We have shown the results of an initial trial of the system in a case/control study in which capillary measures strongly predict patients with SSc. This should now be formally validated against current clinical practice in a prospective study. Blood flow velocity results, while preliminary, are promising and warrant further investigation, and we are currently working on validating the results, including psychovisual tests with human observers and developing a microscopic flow phantom to provide objective ground truth.

To test the sensitivity of flow measures, we are planning trials that include dynamic challenges to induce rapid changes in capillary function. Moreover the optical properties of the system may easily be adapted to assess other measures of capillary function (e.g. using multispectral imaging to assess oxygenation, or UV induced fluorescence to measure oxidative stress), providing an exciting avenue for further investigations of pathophysiology and microangiopathy.

Acknowledgements.. This work was funded by the Wellcome Trust.

References

1. Herrick, A.L.: Contemporary management of raynaud's phenomenon and digital ischaemic complications. Curr. Opin. Rheumatol. **23**, 555–561 (2011)
2. Cutolo, M., Pizzorni, C., Secchi, M.E., Sulli, A.: Capillaroscopy. Best Pract. Res. Clin. Rheumatol. **22**(6), 1093–1108 (2008)
3. Murray, A.K., Moore, T.L., Manning, J.B., Taylor, C., Griffiths, C.E.M., Herrick, A.L.: Noninvasive imaging techniques in the assessment of scleroderma spectrum disorders. Arthritis Rheum. **61**(8), 1103–1111 (2009)

4. Berks, M., Tresadern, P., Dinsdale, G., Murray, A., Moore, T., Herrick, A., Taylor, C.: An automated system for detecting and measuring nailfold capillaries. In: Golland, P., Hata, N., Barillot, C., Hornegger, J., Howe, R. (eds.) MICCAI 2014. LNCS, vol. 8673, pp. 658–665. Springer, Heidelberg (2014). doi:10.1007/978-3-319-10404-1_82

5. Brox, T., Bruhn, A., Papenberg, N., Weickert, J.: High accuracy optical flow estimation based on a theory for warping. In: Pajdla, T., Matas, J. (eds.) ECCV 2004. LNCS, vol. 3024, pp. 25–36. Springer, Heidelberg (2004). doi:10.1007/978-3-540-24673-2_3

6. Mawson, D.M., Shaw, A.C.: Comparison of CapiFlow and frame by frame analysis for the assessment of capillary red blood cell velocity. J. Med. Eng. Technol. 22(2), 53–63 (1998)

7. Shih, T.C., Zhang, G., Wu, C.C., Hsiao, H.D., Wu, T.H., Lin, K.P., Huang, T.C.: Hemodynamic analysis of capillary in finger nail-fold using computational fluid dynamics and image estimation. Microvasc. Res. 81(1), 68–72 (2011)

8. Dobbe, J.G.G., Streekstra, G.J., Atasever, B., Zijderveld, R., Ince, C.: Measurement of functional microcirculatory geometry and velocity distributions using automated image analysis. Med. Biol. Eng. Comput. 46(7), 659–670 (2008)

9. Allen, P.D., Taylor, C.J., Herrick, A.L., Moore, T.: Image analysis of nailfold capillary patterns from video sequences. In: Taylor, C., Colchester, A. (eds.) MICCAI 1999. LNCS, vol. 1679, pp. 698–705. Springer, Heidelberg (1999). doi:10.1007/10704282_76

10. Horn, B.K.P., Schunk, B.G.: Determining optical flow. Artif. Intell. 17, 185–203 (1981)

Tensor-Based Graph-Cut in Riemannian Metric Space and Its Application to Renal Artery Segmentation

Chenglong Wang[1]([⊠]), Masahiro Oda[1], Yuichiro Hayashi[2], Yasushi Yoshino[3], Tokunori Yamamoto[3], Alejandro F. Frangi[4], and Kensaku Mori[1,2]

[1] Graduate School of Information Science, Nagoya University, Nagoya, Japan
cwang@mori.m.is.nagoya-u.ac.jp
[2] Information and Communications Headquarters, Nagoya University, Nagoya, Japan
[3] Graduate School of Medicine, Nagoya University, Nagoya, Japan
[4] Electronic and Electrical Engineering Department, University of Sheffield, Sheffield, United Kingdom

Abstract. Renal artery segmentation remained a big challenging due to its low contrast. In this paper, we present a novel graph-cut method using tensor-based distance metric for blood vessel segmentation in scale-valued images. Conventional graph-cut methods only use intensity information, which may result in failing in segmentation of small blood vessels. To overcome this drawback, this paper introduces local geometric structure information represented as tensors to find a better solution than conventional graph-cut. A Riemannian metric is utilized to calculate tensors statistics. These statistics are used in a Gaussian Mixture Model to estimate the probability distribution of the foreground and background regions. The experimental results showed that the proposed graph-cut method can segment about 80 % of renal arteries with 1mm precision in diameter.

Keywords: Blood vessel segmentation · Graph-cut · Renal artery · Tensor · Hessian matrix · Riemannian manifold

1 Introduction

Blood vessel segmentation is a very basic and important problem in medical image processing. Blood vessel regions in different tissues have different features. A variety of segmentation methods were proposed to make full use of those different features. While thresholding and region-growing approaches utilize intensity-based criteria, Hessian-based methods utilize the second-order image derivatives to represent high-order local geometric information [1,2]. Other methods such as model-fitting-based methods [3] and Markov chain Monte Carlo approaches [4] have achieved excellent results in blood vessel segmentation.

Partial nephrectomy is a common treatment for kidney cancers. For surgical planning of partial nephrectomy, renal artery segmentation plays an important role. Renal arteries have lower contrast in comparison with other blood vessels

© Springer International Publishing AG 2016
S. Ourselin et al. (Eds.): MICCAI 2016, Part III, LNCS 9902, pp. 353–361, 2016.
DOI: 10.1007/978-3-319-46726-9_41

such as hepatic arteries and carotid arteries. Precise renal artery segmentation remained a big challenging. In previous work [5], we presented a two-step segmentation method, which utilized graph-cut to segment thick blood vessels and then utilized a template model to track and extract tiny blood vessels in deeper levels of the vascular tree. Although graph-cut show high robustness in segmentation tasks, it remains difficult to segment long thin tubular structures in low contrast with 1–2 voxels in diameter. This possibly stems from the fact that the optimal graph still cuts across the high-cost regions (i.e. the blood vessels) that have lower energy cost than even a cut across low-cost regions. In our previous work, a new Hessian-based dissimilarity measure was proposed to adjust the energy function to segment tiny blood vessels. The dissimilarity of two tensors is measured utilizing an Euclidean distance metric.

In this paper, we propose a tensor-based graph-cut method in a Riemannian metric space. Hessian matrix analysis is a valuable approach to represent a local geometric structure. We compute the Hessian matrix for each voxel as a "Hessian tensor". We use the Riemannian metric as a tensor measure to calculate tensors statistics. This geometric information will then be used in a Gaussian Mixture Model (GMM) to estimate the probability distribution of foreground and background regions. The main contributions of this work can be summarized as: (1) accuracy improvement of graph-cut method for small blood vessel segmentation by means of tensor analysis and (2) applying Riemannian metric to calculate the Hessian tensor statistics.

2   Method

2.1   Generation of Tensor Field

Han et al. [6] proposed a multi-scale nonlinear structure tensor (MSNST) space to extract texture features from color images. Firstly, a multi-scale structure tensor of form $\mathbf{T}_s = \alpha^{-2s} \sum_{h=1}^{H} \mathbf{T}_h$ must be constructed, where $\mathbf{T}_h$ is the structure tensor of the h-th color channel and H is the total number of color channels. s denotes the scale. Here, α is a positive constant that can be set as 2. Then, nonlinear diffusion is applied to all scales of structure tensor $\mathbf{T}_s$, and finally a MSNST space is obtained as $\Gamma = \{\hat{\mathbf{T}}_0, \hat{\mathbf{T}}_1, ..., \hat{\mathbf{T}}_{s-1}\}$.

Instead of using structure tensor, we utilize the Hessian matrix to generate a tensor representation at each voxel. This is because Hessian matrix is more appropriate to represent the blood vessel structures. Different from texture features, the most appropriate scale for each voxel to represent vessel structures can be obtained by the optimal response of Hessian-based vesselness filter [1]. The Hessian matrix is given as

$$\nabla^2 I(\mathbf{x}) = \begin{bmatrix} I_{xx}(\mathbf{x}) & I_{xy}(\mathbf{x}) & I_{xz}(\mathbf{x}) \\ I_{yx}(\mathbf{x}) & I_{yy}(\mathbf{x}) & I_{yz}(\mathbf{x}) \\ I_{zx}(\mathbf{x}) & I_{zy}(\mathbf{x}) & I_{zz}(\mathbf{x}) \end{bmatrix} \tag{1}$$

which can be regarded as a second-order tensor $\mathbf{T}_H$. Here, $I_{ij} = \dfrac{\partial^2}{\partial i \partial j} I, (i, j = \{x, y, z\})$ represents the second-order partial derivatives of the local image $I(\mathbf{x})$.

In contrast to the MSNST scheme, a multi-scale Hessian-based vesselness enhancement filter is utilized here to find the most appropriate scale for each voxel. Calculating the eigenvalues of the Hessian matrix, a vesselness measure can be obtained by determining the largest response among all scales. We use Sato's vesselness measure $\mathcal{V}$ [1] in this paper. Due to the fact that the scale with the highest response $\mathcal{V}_{max}$ is the best scale for local representation of tubular structures at each voxel, the tensor is calculated at the scale with the highest vesselness response.

Although, every voxel of image $I(\mathbf{x})$ has a scale at which it achieves its largest response of vesselness filter, most voxels actually do not belong to a vessel. Therefore, it is particularly important to reduce these "noisy tensors". In this work, we replace a *diagonal tensor* $\mathbf{T}_D$ with the tensor of the non-vessel voxels that can be expressed as

$$\mathbf{T} = \begin{cases} \mathbf{T}_H, \mathcal{V} > 0 \\ \mathbf{T}_D, \mathcal{V} \leq 0 \end{cases} \tag{2}$$

where $\mathbf{T}_D = \begin{bmatrix} \lambda_1 & 0 & 0 \\ 0 & \lambda_2 & 0 \\ 0 & 0 & \lambda_3 \end{bmatrix}$ and $\lambda_3 \gg \lambda_2 \approx \lambda_1 > 0$. $\mathbf{T}_D$ behaves as a plate-like structure in vesselness terms. An example of tensor field is shown in Fig. 1, where only tensors with $\mathcal{V} > 0$ are illustrated. The tensor visualization technique was presented by Barmpoutis et al. [7].

2.2   Tensor Metric in a Riemannian Space

Numerous studies in the diffusion tensor imaging (DTI) literature have developed methods to perform statistics over tensor space [8,9]. A key point of tensor computing is that the tensor space does not form any vector spaces, thus standard linear statistical techniques cannot be applied. The space of tensors is a type of manifold referred to as *Riemannian manifold*. The Riemannian manifold $(\mathcal{M}, g)$ consists of linear subspaces of Euclidean space, the geodesic distance on a Riemannian manifold is a continuous collection of inner products on all tangent spaces $T_x\mathcal{M}$ over the manifold $\mathcal{M}$, known as *Riemannian metric*. The Riemannian metric g makes it possible to define geometric notions on Riemannnian manifolds such as the geodesic distance, the mean tensor value, and the gradient descent.

In local coordinates, a Riemannian metric is symmetric positive definite (SPD) matrix. Therefore, as the Hessian matrix may take other forms than positive definite (not positive definite, NPD), it cannot be mapped onto a Riemannian manifold. Here, we transform the NPD Hessian matrix to a SPD matrices, meanwhile preserving the structure feature. Suppose that the tensor $\mathbf{T}^-$ is a NPD matrix. Further suppose that $\mathbf{U}$ is an invertible orthogonal matrix with columns correspond to eigenvectors. Then $\mathbf{T}^- = \mathbf{U}\mathbf{D}\mathbf{U}^{-1} = \mathbf{U}\mathbf{D}\mathbf{U}^T$ is diagonalization of the matrix $\mathbf{T}^-$. Here, $\mathbf{D} = \mathrm{diag}(d_i)$, where d_i is the i-th eigenvalue.

Taking the absolute value of $\mathbf{T}^-$, we will obtain a tensor $\mathbf{T}^+$ in space of SPD matrices Sym^+ as follows:

$$\mathbf{T}^+ = abs(\mathbf{T}^-) = \mathbf{U}\mathrm{diag}(abs(d_i))\mathbf{U}^T, \mathbf{T}^+ \in Sym^+. \tag{3}$$

Since the geometric structure is related to the ratio of absolute value of the eigenvalues, the absolute value does not alter the geometric information, i.e. it does not alter the geodesic distances. Notice that the original positive definite Hessian matrices belong to dark structures such as dark vessels ($\lambda_3 \geq \lambda_2 > \lambda_1 > 0$) and dark blob-like structures ($\lambda_3 \approx \lambda_2 \approx \lambda_1 > 0$). These matrices have already been replaced by diagonal tensors, hence the absolute value operator does not affect the segmentation result.

According to the definition in [8,9], the distance between two tensors $\mathbf{T}_1$ and $\mathbf{T}_2$ is given by

$$d(\mathbf{T}_1, \mathbf{T}_2) = \left(\sum_{i=1}^{n} \log^2 \lambda_i(\mathbf{T}_1, \mathbf{T}_2) \right)^{\frac{1}{2}}, \mathbf{T}_1, \mathbf{T}_2 \in Sym^+ \tag{4}$$

where $\lambda(\mathbf{T}_1, \mathbf{T}_2)$ returns the generalized eigenvalue of the tensors $\mathbf{T}_1$ and $\mathbf{T}_2$. and n denotes dimension which is 3 here.

The Fréchet mean is a generalization of the mean values in an arbitrary metric space that is established by minimizing the sum of squared distances: $\bar{\mathbf{T}} = \arg\min \frac{1}{N} \sum_{i=1}^{N} dist(\mathbf{T}_i, \bar{\mathbf{T}})$. The mean value in a Riemannian metric space is uniquely defined [10]. A Newton gradient descent algorithm is used to solve this minimization problem. Initially, set $\bar{\mathbf{T}}_0 = \mathbf{T}_0$. The mean tensor at step $t+1$ is given by

$$\bar{\mathbf{T}}_{t+1} = \exp_{\bar{\mathbf{T}}} \left(\frac{1}{N} \sum_{i=1}^{N} \log_{\bar{\mathbf{T}}_t}(\mathbf{T}_i) \right) = \bar{\mathbf{T}}_t^{\frac{1}{2}} \exp \left(\frac{1}{N} \sum_{i=1}^{N} \log(\bar{\mathbf{T}}_t^{-\frac{1}{2}} \mathbf{T}_i \bar{\mathbf{T}}_t^{-\frac{1}{2}}) \right) \bar{\mathbf{T}}_t^{\frac{1}{2}} \tag{5}$$

where $\exp_{\mathbf{X}}(\mathbf{\Sigma})$ is an exponential mapping that maps a point $\mathbf{X}$ on the manifold to another point on the manifold with a tangent vector $\mathbf{\Sigma}$ and its inverse mapping can also be uniquely defined as a logarithmic mapping. A simple illustration is shown in Fig. 2. See [9] for more details.

The variance σ^2 is defined as

$$\sigma^2 = \mathcal{E}[d(\bar{\mathbf{T}}, \mathbf{T})^2] = \frac{1}{N} \sum_{i=1}^{N} d(\bar{\mathbf{T}}, \mathbf{T}_i)^2 \tag{6}$$

where $\mathcal{E}[\cdot]$ denotes the expectation of a random tensor $\mathbf{T}$. The distance, mean value and variance in a Riemannian metric space are utilized in a GMM to estimate the probability distribution of each component described in Sect. 2.3.

2.3   Graph-Cut Utilizing a Tensor Riemannian Metric

Graph-cut is a powerful optimization algorithm proposed by Boykov et al. [12] in 2001. The minimal cut corresponding to a optimization solution of an energy

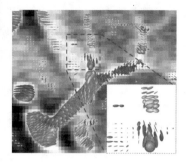

Fig. 1. A part of tensor field of CT slice. Tensors only with $\mathcal{V} > 0$ are illustrated.

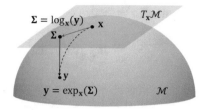

Fig. 2. Illustration of manifold mapping. $\mathbf{x}$ and $\mathbf{y}$ are two tensors (matrices) on the manifold $\mathcal{M}$ [11]. $\mathbf{\Sigma}$ is a tensor on the tangent space $T_{\mathbf{x}}\mathcal{M}$ at tensor $\mathbf{x}$. The exponential mapping $\exp(\cdot)$ projects each point at the tangent space onto the manifold

function E can be found effectively based on the max-flow/min-cut theorem. Whereas the conventional graph-cut segmentation method only utilizes low-order information such as intensity, the proposed tensor-based graph-cut method makes use of high-order information, the local geometric structure. The energy function in this work is given by

$$E(L) = \omega \underbrace{\sum_{\mathbf{x} \in \mathbb{X}} - \log \Pr(\mathbf{x}|L_{\mathbf{x}})}_{\text{intensity term}} + \underbrace{(1 - \omega) \underbrace{\sum_{\mathbf{T} \in \mathbb{T}} - \log \Pr(\mathbf{T}|L_{\mathbf{T}})}_{\text{tensor term}}}_{\text{data term}}$$

$$+ \underbrace{\varphi \sum_{\{\mathbf{x}_m, \mathbf{x}_n\} \in \mathcal{N}} V_{m,n}(\mathbf{x}_m, \mathbf{x}_n) + (1 - \varphi) \sum_{\{\mathbf{T}_m, \mathbf{T}_n\} \in \mathcal{N}'} U_{m,n}(\mathbf{T}_m, \mathbf{T}_n)}_{\text{smoothness term}} \tag{7}$$

where ω and φ are the weight parameters between the intensity-based term and the tensor-based term. $\Pr(\cdot)$ is the GMM probability that the voxel $\mathbf{x} \in \mathbb{X}$ or tensor $\mathbf{T} \in \mathbb{T}$ be assigned to the label $\{L_{\mathrm{B}}, L_{\mathrm{F}}\}$, L_{B} and L_{F} denote the background label and foreground label, respectively. Here, $\mathbf{x}_m$ and $\mathbf{x}_n$, as well as $\mathbf{T}_m$ and $\mathbf{T}_n$ are two pairs of neighboring voxels belonging to neighboring pair sets $\mathcal{N}$ and $\mathcal{N}'$. Finally, $V(\cdot, \cdot)$ and $U(\cdot, \cdot)$ represent the dissimilarity measures for neighboring voxels and neighboring tensors, respectively. Here, we focus on the tensor term. The GMM distribution can be defined as $\Pr(\mathbf{T}|\bar{\mathbf{T}}, \sigma) = \sum_k \eta_k \Pr(\mathbf{T}|\bar{\mathbf{T}}_k, \sigma_k)$, where k denotes the k-th component of GMM, and η_k is the mixture weight parameter. Therefore, the k-th Gaussian distribution of tensors can be formulated as:

$$\Pr(\mathbf{T}|\bar{\mathbf{T}}_k, \sigma_k) = \frac{1}{\sigma_k \sqrt{2\pi}} \exp\left(-\frac{d^2(\mathbf{T}, \bar{\mathbf{T}}_k)}{2\sigma_k^2}\right). \tag{8}$$

The dissimilarity measure of tensors is given by

$$U_{m,n}(\mathbf{T}_m, \mathbf{T}_n) = \frac{\exp\left(-\xi d^2(\mathbf{T}_m \mathbf{T}_n)\right)}{dist(\mathbf{T}_m, \mathbf{T}_n)} \tag{9}$$

where ξ is a contrast adaptive constant, and $dist(\cdot, \cdot)$ is the Euclidean distance.

In this work, the initial user-specified "trimap" is generated automatically. K-means clustering algorithm is applied to the vesselness enhancement result $I_\mathcal{V}$ to extract the most probable blood vessel regions as foreground regions. The procedure can then be written as:

$$\mathbf{C}' = \underset{\mathbf{C}}{\arg\min} \sum_{i=1}^{K} \sum_{\mathbf{x} \in \mathbf{c}_i} ||I_\mathcal{V}(\mathbf{x}) - \bar{I}_i||^2 \tag{10}$$

$$\mathbf{c}'_{max} = \underset{\mathbf{c}'_i}{\arg\max} \frac{1}{|\mathbf{c}'_i|} \sum_{\mathbf{x} \in \mathbf{c}'_i} |I_\mathcal{V}(\mathbf{x})| \tag{11}$$

where the set $\mathbf{C}$ consists of K initial clusters $\mathbf{c}_i$ $(i = 1, \ldots, K)$ and $\mathbf{C}'$ is the final clusters. $\bar{I}_i$ is the average intensity of set $\mathbf{c}_i$, $|\mathbf{c}'_i|$ is the number of the voxels in i-th cluster $\mathbf{c}'_i$. Voxel set $\mathbf{c}'_{max}$ is considered as most probable blood vessel regions. This scheme can effectively reduce the user's interaction complexity.

3   Experiments and Results

The proposed method was tested on seven cases of contrast-enhanced renal CT data, including six cases of renal cancer and one normal case, taken in arterial phase. All the experiments were performed on a VOI of kidney, which is a cubical data created manually containing the whole kidney region. The size, pixel spacing as well as slice spacing of the VOI data were set to $150 \times 150 \times 200$ voxels, 0.65–0.70 mm and 0.40–0.50 mm, respectively. The gold standards were created by two human experts having medical knowledge. We implemented the algorithm in C++ and evaluated it on a normal computer with an Intel Xeon CPU E5-2667 2.9 GHz 6 cores. Average computation time for one case is about 10 min. In Eq. 7, the weight parameters ω and ϕ are set to 0.8–0.9 through all experiments. Minimum and maximum detect size of Hessian vesselness filter are 1 mm and 2 mm, detect step is 1 mm.

In this study, four validation metrics, i.e. Dice Coefficient (DC), Overlapping of Centerline (OC), True Positive Ratio (TPR) and False Positive Ratio (FPR), were utilized to evaluate the proposed algorithm. OC index represents segmentation accuracy in the meaning of the branch length and the number of branches. Also, DC is the metric based on regions that is easily affected by thick branches. Both experimental results for different cases and the comparison between the previous and the new proposed graph-cut methods have been shown in Fig. 3. Quantitative evaluations of the proposed method versus the previous method have been presented in Table 1.

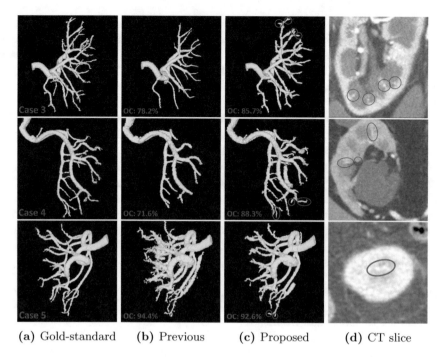

(a) Gold-standard   (b) Previous   (c) Proposed   (d) CT slice

Fig. 3. Experimental results of three cases. Each row represents one single case. (a) is gold-standard data, (b) is the result of graph-cut in previous work [5], (c) is the result of proposed graph-cut method. (d) is a part of CT images. The red circles correspond to the renal arteries marked in the (c). (Color figure online)

Table 1. Quantitative results of proposed method. For each case, boldface numerals show results of proposed method and lightface numerals show results of previous method [5]

	Data set						
	Case 1	Case 2	Case 3	Case 4	Case 5	Case 6	Case 7
OC (%)	**87.2**/79.6	**87.3**/77.9	**85.7**/82.3	**88.3**/81.8	**92.6**/94.4	**90.5**/89.3	**74.1**/70.2
DC (%)	**75.5**/73.8	**71.4**/71.3	**80.6**/82.5	**71.8**/78.7	**78.4**/69.2	**84.5**/84.5	**71.7**/88.6
FPR (%)	**0.16**/0.11	**0.14**/0.12	**0.17**/0.06	**0.13**/0.09	**0.28**/0.47	**0.05**/0.07	**0.11**/0.03
TPR (%)	**82.0**/72.3	**81.0**/77.8	**83.6**/76.0	**73.0**/78.9	**92.6**/92.6	**82.6**/86.4	**74.1**/86.0

4 Discussion and Conclusions

We have presented a tensor-based graph-cut method for blood vessel segmentation in renal CT. Firstly, a tensor field is generated by calculating the Hessian matrix. Secondly, Riemannian metric is utilized to compute statistics over tensors. Finally, these statistics are used in graph-cut framework to estimate the probability distribution of foreground and background regions. According to the

OC index, it is evident that the tensor-based graph-cut has an excellent segmentation performance at tiny blood vessels. It can extract more tiny blood vessels than previous method that is a hybrid method involving graph-cut and vessel tracking techniques. In Case 5, the previous method has a higher OC index than the proposed method, but also has a higher FPR. Serious over-segmentation is also shown in Fig. 3.

We used both intensity and tensors in the energy function of Eq. (7). This is because "tensors" only contain geometric information. However, we can only distinguish arteries from veins by the intensity difference. Thus, we solved this problem through a linear combination of intensity term and tensor term. But high weight values for tensor term may lead to over-segmentation by growing the segmentation into other tubular structures. This is the reason that the proposed method has a lower DC than previous method in several cases. For future work, we are going to find an automated method to decide the optimal weight parameters ω, φ. In addition, more experiments will be tested to assess the robustness of the proposed algorithm.

Acknowledgments. Parts of this research were supported by MEXT and JSPS KAKENHI (26108006, 26560255, 25242047), Kayamori Foundation and the JSPS Bilateral International Collaboration Grants.

References

1. Sato, Y., et al.: Three-dimensional multi-scale line filter for segmentation and visualization of curvilinear structures in medical images. Med. IA **2**(2), 143–168 (1998)
2. Frangi, A.F., Niessen, W.J., Vincken, K.L., Viergever, M.A.: Multiscale vessel enhancement filtering. In: Wells, W.M., Colchester, A., Delp, S. (eds.) MICCAI 1998. LNCS, vol. 1496, pp. 130–137. Springer, Heidelberg (1998). doi:10.1007/BFb0056195
3. Friman, O., et al.: Multiple hypothesis template tracking of small 3D vessel structures. Med. Image Anal. **14**(2), 160–171 (2010)
4. Skibbe, H., et al.: Efficient monte carlo image analysis for the location of vascular entity. IEEE Trans. Med. Imaging **34**(2), 628–643 (2015)
5. Wang, C., et al.: Precise renal artery segmentation for estimation of renal vascular dominant regions. In: SPIE Medical Imaging, pp. 97842M–97842M. International Society for Optics and Photonics (2016)
6. Han, S., Wang, X.: Texture segmentation using graph cuts in spectral decomposition based Riemannian multi-scale nonlinear structure tensor space. Int. J. Comput. Theory Eng. **7**(4), 259 (2015)
7. Barmpoutis, A., et al.: Tensor splines for interpolation and approximation of DT-MRI with applications to segmentation of isolated rat hippocampi. IEEE Trans. Med. Imaging **26**(11), 1537–1546 (2007)
8. Fletcher, P.T., Joshi, S.: Riemannian geometry for the statistical analysis of diffusion tensor data. Signal Process. **87**(2), 250–262 (2007)
9. Pennec, X., Fillard, P., Ayache, N.: A Riemannian framework for tensor computing. Int. J. Comput. Vis. **66**(1), 41–66 (2006)

10. Kendall, W.S.: Probability, convexity, and harmonic maps with small image I: uniqueness and fine existence. Proc. Lond. Math. Soc. **3**(2), 371–406 (1990)
11. Barachant, A., et al.: Classification of covariance matrices using a Riemannian-based kernel for BCI applications. Neurocomputing **112**, 172–178 (2013)
12. Boykov, Y., et al.: Fast approximate energy minimization via graph cuts. IEEE Trans. Pattern Anal. Mach. Intell. **23**(11), 1222–1239 (2001)

Automatic, Robust, and Globally Optimal Segmentation of Tubular Structures

Simon Pezold[1]([✉]), Antal Horváth[1], Ketut Fundana[1], Charidimos Tsagkas[2],
Michaela Andělová[2,3], Katrin Weier[2], Michael Amann[2],
and Philippe C. Cattin[1]

[1] Department of Biomedical Engineering, University of Basel, Basel, Switzerland
simon.pezold@unibas.ch
[2] Department of Neurology, University Hospital Basel, Basel, Switzerland
[3] Department of Internal Medicine, University Hospital Motol,
Prague, Czech Republic

Abstract. We present an automatic three-dimensional segmentation approach based on continuous max flow that targets tubular structures in medical images. Our method uses second-order derivative information provided by Frangi et al.'s vesselness feature and exploits it twofold: First, the vesselness response itself is used for localizing the tubular structure of interest. Second, the eigenvectors of the Hessian eigendecomposition guide our anisotropic total variation–regularized segmentation. In a simulation experiment, we demonstrate the superiority of anisotropic as compared to isotropic total variation–regularized segmentation in the presence of noise. In an experiment with magnetic resonance images of the human cervical spinal cord, we compare our automated segmentations to those of two human observers. Finally, a comparison with a dedicated state-of-the-art spinal cord segmentation framework shows that we achieve comparable to superior segmentation quality.

Keywords: Convex optimization · Anisotropic total variation · Vesselness

1 Introduction

Segmenting tubular structures is an important task in medical image analysis; for example, for assessing vascular diseases or tracking the progress of neurological disorders that manifest in spinal cord atrophy. Especially when used in large-scale clinical trials, largely automated segmentation is desirable to reduce the workload on clinical staff. Such automated segmentation approaches, in turn, should be robust with respect to specific choices of parameterization.

In this paper, we propose a segmentation method that fulfills both criteria: it is completely automated, and it creates segmentations of similar quality over a wide range of parameter choices. Our method adapts Yuan et al.'s continuous max flow approach [10] and combines it with an anisotropic total variation (ATV)

© Springer International Publishing AG 2016
S. Ourselin et al. (Eds.): MICCAI 2016, Part III, LNCS 9902, pp. 362–370, 2016.
DOI: 10.1007/978-3-319-46726-9_42

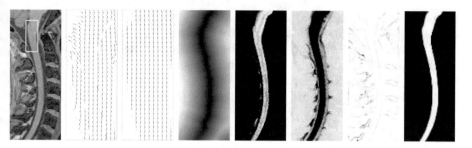

Fig. 1. *Left to right:* T1 image I of the cervical spinal cord; closeups of the vessel directions v_1 before GVF and $\tilde{v}_1$ after GVF (vectors scaled by the segmentation u^* for visualization); distance map D of the vessel ridge $\mathcal{R}$ (normalized for visualization); source capacities C_s; sink capacities C_t; nonterminal capacities C; segmentation u^*.

regularization term. ATV keeps changes of the segmentation's boundary small along the course of the tubular structure. We use Frangi et al.'s well-established vesselness feature [3] as our measure of tubularity, which we exploit twofold: both for finding the location and the orientation of the structures of interest.

The directional information of vesselness, which is usually neglected, has previously been used: Manniesing et al. [6] construct an anisotropic tensor from it for accentuating vascular structures in angiography images for image enhancement. Gooya et al. [4] use this tensor in an active contour framework for blood vessel segmentation. ATV-regularized segmentation has been generally described by Olsson et al. [7] and has been used, for example, by Reinbacher et al. [8] who segment thin structures of known volume based on first-order derivatives and a volume constraint. A review of vessel segmentation is given by Lesage et al. [5]. De Leener et al. [2] review the more specific topic of spinal cord segmentation.

Our contributions lie in incorporating Hessian-based vesselness into ATV-regularized segmentation and in integrating ATV into the continuous max flow framework [10]. To the best of our knowledge, both has not been tried, so far.

2   Methods

In Sect. 2.1, we motivate our choice of ATV regularization. In Sect. 2.2, we state the ATV-regularized segmentation problem in the continuous max flow framework and propose an algorithm for solving it. In Sect. 2.3, we describe how we incorporate the vesselness feature. In Sect. 2.4, we present our choice of flow capacities. For a good general introduction to continuous max flow, see [10].

2.1   Isotropic and Anisotropic Total Variation

Segmentation on the d-dimensional image domain $\Omega \subset \mathbb{R}^d$ can be formulated as the problem of finding a binary labeling $u : \Omega \to \{0, 1\}$ for the given image $I :$ $\Omega \to \mathcal{I}$ (e.g. with $\mathcal{I} = [0, 1]$ for a normalized single-channel image). In practice, the problem is often relaxed such that $u : \Omega \rightarrow [0,1]$, and the final labeling is determined by applying a threshold to the result of the relaxed problem [7,10].

A common regularization term in segmentation is the *total variation* TV, which minimizes the surface area of the segmented region, penalizing jumps between segmentation foreground ($u = 1$) and background ($u = 0$) and thus allowing for smooth segmentations even if I is noisy (here, $|\cdot|$ denotes the l_2 norm):

$$\text{TV}[u] = \int_\Omega |\nabla u| \, dx. \tag{1}$$

While TV is a good regularizer for many applications, it seems not optimal in the context of tubular structure segmentation. This is because TV is isotropic; that is, changes of u are penalized regardless of orientation. If we want to segment a tube, however, we would like to employ the prior knowledge that its shape ideally does not change along its course; thus we would like to penalize changes along the tube's direction more strongly than changes perpendicular to it. In other words, we would prefer an anisotropic regularization term.

In the proposed method, we thus use *anisotropic total variation* ATV [7,8]:

$$\text{ATV}[u; A] = \int_\Omega \left(\nabla u^{\mathsf{T}} A \nabla u\right)^{1/2} dx = \int_\Omega |S^{\mathsf{T}} \nabla u| \, dx \quad \text{with} \quad A = SS^{\mathsf{T}}, \tag{2}$$

where $A : \Omega \rightarrow \mathbb{R}^{d \times d}$ is strongly positive definite in the sense of Olsson et al. [7] and S is a decomposition of A. For our particular choice of A and S, see Sect. 2.3.

If we assume, as a simple three-dimensional example, that $A = \text{diag}(1, a, a)$ with $0 < a < 1$, we see that changes along the x_1 axis will be more strongly penalized than changes along x_2 and x_3. This would in fact be a meaningful choice if the tubular structure of interest was oriented along x_1. From the example we can also see that ATV is a generalization of TV, as ATV becomes TV for $a = 1$.

2.2 ATV in Continuous Max Flow

The dual formulation of the max flow problem as stated in [10], with TV replaced by ATV regularization as we propose, is given by the min cut problem

$$\min_{u \in [0,1]} \int_\Omega (1 - u) \, C_s + u \, C_t + |S^{\mathsf{T}} \nabla u| \, C \, dx, \tag{3}$$

with the source capacities C_s, sink capacities C_t, and nonterminal capacities C ($C_\cdot : \Omega \rightarrow \mathbb{R}_{\geq 0}$). Using integration by parts and the geometric definition of the scalar product, we can show for the nonterminal flow $p : \Omega \rightarrow \mathbb{R}^d$ that

$$\int_\Omega |S^{\mathsf{T}} \nabla u| \, C \, dx = \max_{|p| \leq C} \int_\Omega u \, \text{div}(Sp) \, dx. \tag{4}$$

Algorithm 1. Augmented Lagrangian–based max flow algorithm with ATV.

- Set bound $\hat{\epsilon}$, steps γ, c; calculate C, C_s, C_t, S; arbitrarily initialize p^0, p_s^0, p_t^0, u^0.
- Starting from $n = 0$, iterate until $\frac{1}{|\Omega|} \int_\Omega |\epsilon^{n+1}(x)| \, dx < \hat{\epsilon}$:

$$
\begin{cases}
\tilde{p}^{n+1} = p^n + \gamma\, S^{\mathsf{T}} \nabla \left(\mathrm{div}\,(Sp^n) - p_s^n + p_t^n - \frac{u^n}{c} \right) \\
p^{n+1} = \frac{\tilde{p}^{n+1}}{|\tilde{p}^{n+1}|} \min\left\{ |\tilde{p}^{n+1}|, C \right\} \quad \text{if } \tilde{p}^{n+1} \neq 0 \quad \text{else} \quad 0 \\
p_s^{n+1} = \min\left\{ \left(\frac{1-u^n}{c} + \mathrm{div}\,(Sp^{n+1}) + p_t^n \right), C_s \right\} \\
p_t^{n+1} = \min\left\{ \left(\frac{u^n}{c} - \mathrm{div}\,(Sp^{n+1}) + p_s^{n+1} \right), C_t \right\} \\
\epsilon^{n+1} = c \left(\mathrm{div}\,(Sp^{n+1}) - p_s^{n+1} + p_t^{n+1} \right) \\
u^{n+1} = u^n - \epsilon^{n+1}.
\end{cases}
$$

Together with the respective equalities for C_s, C_t and the source and sink flows $p_s, p_t : \Omega \to \mathbb{R}$ (see Eqs. (18) and (19) in [10]), we derive the primal–dual formulation as $\max_{p_s, p_t, p} \min_{u \in [0,1]} E\,[p_s, p_t, p, u]$ with

$$
E = \int_\Omega (1 - u)\, p_s + u\, p_t + u\, \mathrm{div}\,(Sp) \, dx = \int_\Omega p_s + u\, (\mathrm{div}\,(Sp) - p_s + p_t) \, dx, \quad (5)
$$

subject to the flow capacity constraints $p_s \leq C_s$, $p_t \leq C_t$, and $|p| \leq C$.

Making use of the anisotropic coarea formula in [7], it can be shown that any u^ℓ for a threshold $\ell \in (0, 1)$, given by

$$
u^\ell(x) = \begin{cases} 1, & u^*(x) > \ell \\ 0, & u^*(x) \leq \ell \end{cases} \quad \text{with} \quad u^* = \arg\min_{u \in [0,1]} E, \quad (6)
$$

is a globally optimal solution for the binary problem corresponding to Eq. (3). Following [10], we add an augmented Lagrangian term to Eq. (5), gaining

$$
\max_{p_s, p_t, p} \min_{u \in [0,1]} \int_\Omega p_s + u\, (\mathrm{div}\,(Sp) - p_s + p_t) - \frac{c}{2} \left(\mathrm{div}\,(Sp) - p_s + p_t \right)^2 dx \quad (7)
$$

as the final problem, which we propose to solve with Algorithm 1.

2.3   ATV Regularization with Vesselness

Frangi et al. [3] examine the Hessian matrices; that is, the second-order derivatives, in the scale space of the volumetric image I to calculate what they call vesselness. The idea is to determine from the ratios of the Hessians' eigenvalues how closely the local structure in I resembles a tube.

In particular, let $\mathcal{S}$ be a predefined set of scales that roughly match the expected tube radii. For each scale $s \in \mathcal{S}$, let $H_s(x)$ denote its Hessian approximation in x, calculated by convolving I with Gaussian derivatives of standard deviation s. Let $\lambda_{i,s}(x)$ $(i = 1, 2, 3)$ denote the sorted eigenvalues

$(|\lambda_{1,s}| \leq |\lambda_{2,s}| \leq |\lambda_{3,s}|)$ and $v_{i,s}(x)$ corresponding eigenvectors of H_s, such that

$$H_s = V_s \Lambda_s V_s^\mathsf{T} \quad \text{with} \quad V_s = [v_{1,s}|v_{2,s}|v_{3,s}], \quad \Lambda_s = \mathrm{diag}\,(\lambda_{1,s}, \lambda_{2,s}, \lambda_{3,s}). \quad (8)$$

Note that $V_s^\mathsf{T} = V_s^{-1}$, as H_s is symmetric. Assuming bright tubular structures on dark background, the vesselness response is $\nu(x) = \max_{s \in \mathcal{S}} \nu_s(x)$, where

$$\nu_s = \begin{cases} 0, & \lambda_{2,s} \geq 0 \text{ or } \lambda_{3,s} \geq 0 \\ \left(1 - \exp(\frac{-1}{2w_1^2}\frac{\lambda_{2,s}^2}{\lambda_{3,s}^2})\right) \exp(\frac{-1}{2w_2^2}\frac{\lambda_{1,s}^2}{\lambda_{2,s}\lambda_{3,s}}) \left(1 - \exp(\frac{-\sum_i \lambda_{i,s}^2}{2w_3^2})\right), & \text{else,} \end{cases}$$
$$(9)$$

with the weighting factors $w_i \in \mathbb{R}_{>0}$. The eigenvectors for ν are $V = [v_1|v_2|v_3]$, with $v_i = v_{i,s^*}$ and $s^* = \arg\max_{s \in \mathcal{S}} \nu_s$. In the original description of [3], no use of V is made. In our approach, we use the eigenvectors to steer the ATV regularizer. We observe that in points where ν is high, v_1 points along the local vessel orientation [6]. Recall that we want to regularize strongly along the direction of the vessel. Unfortunately, we cannot use v_1 directly for this purpose, as it reliably gives the vessel's direction in the vessel center only, where ν is the highest. Therefore, we use the concept of gradient vector flow (GVF) [9] to first propagate the directions from places where ν is high to regions where ν is low, creating a smoothly varying vector field. The necessary steps are as follows.

Let $\mathcal{R}$ be the set of vesselness ridge points; that is, the local maxima of ν, down to a noise threshold. As both $-v_1$ and v_1 are valid eigenvectors, we have to make sure that the vectors of neighboring points approximately point in the same rather than the opposite direction, so that they don't cancel each other out when diffusing them via GVF. Thus, we fix their signs beforehand, gaining $\bar{v}_1$: We calculate the minimum spanning tree over the ridge points $\mathcal{R}$, select a root point, keep its sign, and traverse the tree. For each child point, we choose $\bar{v}_1$ as either $-v_1$ or v_1, depending on which one maximizes the dot product (i.e. minimizes the angle) with its parent's $\bar{v}_1$. After traversal, the signs of the v_1 for all remaining domain points $x \in \Omega \backslash \mathcal{R}$ are fixed w.r.t. their closest point in $\mathcal{R}$, following the same rule. We scale all $\bar{v}_1$ with ν, apply GVF, and scale the resulting vectors back to unit length, gaining $\tilde{v}_1$. A comparison of the vector field before and after sign adjustment and GVF is shown in Fig. 1.

Finally, we recomplete $\tilde{v}_1$ to an orthonormal basis $\tilde{V} = [\tilde{v}_1|\tilde{v}_2|\tilde{v}_3]$. The particular choice of $\tilde{v}_2, \tilde{v}_3$ does not matter, as we will treat all directions perpendicular to $\tilde{v}_1$ the same when regularizing. From $\tilde{V}$, we construct A, S for Eq. (2) as

$$A = \tilde{V}\tilde{A}\tilde{V}^\mathsf{T} \quad \text{and} \quad S = \tilde{V}\tilde{A}^{1/2} \quad \text{with} \quad \tilde{A} = \mathrm{diag}\,(1, a, a) \quad \text{and} \quad 0 < a \leq 1.$$
$$(10)$$

Notice the similarity to A in the example at the end of Sect. 2.1: The idea of regularizing one direction stronger than the others remains the same; however, as we now scale with $\tilde{A} = \mathrm{diag}\,(1, a, a)$ in the new basis $\tilde{V}$, we target the actual local vessel direction $\tilde{v}_1$ rather than a fixed axis.

2.4 Flow Capacities

For the source and sink capacities C_s, C_t of Eqs. (3) and (5), we use a combination of the normalized image intensities and the distances to the vessel ridge points $\mathcal{R}$. Intuitively, using the intensities enables the distinction of foreground (i.e. the vessel) and background (i.e. everything else), while the distances w.r.t. $\mathcal{R}$ isolate the vessel surrounding. This helps avoiding oversegmentations in case other structures have intensities similar to those of the vessel of interest. More formally, let $D : \Omega \rightarrow \mathcal{D} = \mathbb{R}_{\geq 0}$ be a Euclidean distance map of $\mathcal{R}$, and let $I : \Omega \rightarrow \mathcal{I} = [0, 1]$ be the normalized image. Let p_b^D, p_f^D, p_b^I, p_f^I be predefined estimates of the background and foreground probability densities for $\mathcal{D}$ and $\mathcal{I}$, with $p^D : \mathcal{D} \rightarrow \mathbb{R}_{\geq 0}$ and $p^I : \mathcal{I} \rightarrow \mathbb{R}_{\geq 0}$. We calculate C_s, C_t as

$$C_s (x) = \frac{1}{q} \max \{r(x), 0\}, \quad \text{with} \quad r(x) = \ln \left(\frac{p_f^D (D(x)) \cdot p_f^I (I(x)) + \varepsilon}{p_b^D (D(x)) \cdot p_b^I (I(x)) + \varepsilon} \right),$$
(11)

$$C_t (x) = \frac{1}{q} \max \{-r(x), 0\}, \quad q = \ln \left(\frac{\max\{\hat{p}_b^D \cdot \hat{p}_b^I, \ \hat{p}_f^D \cdot \hat{p}_f^I\} + \varepsilon}{\varepsilon} \right),$$
(12)

where $\hat{p} = \max p$. The small positive constant ε avoids zero logarithms and zero divisions in r. Normalization with q ensures that $C_s, C_t \in [0, 1]$, which eases their balancing with the nonterminal capacities C of Eqs. (3) and (5).

Using C, we try to move the segmentation boundary to image edges by making C small where the intensity gradient magnitude is high and vice versa:

$$C(x) = w \exp \left(-1/\varsigma^2 \ |\nabla I(x)|^2 \right) \quad \text{with} \quad w, \varsigma \in \mathbb{R}_{>0},$$
(13)

where ς controls C's sensitivity regarding the size of $|\nabla I|$ and w balances C and C_s, C_t. For an example of the capacities, see Fig. 1.

3 Experiments and Results

Implementation: Most of the method's steps can be described as *embarrassingly parallel*, which means they can be calculated independently for different voxels. This is true, for example, for the vesselness ν, GVF, the capacities C_s, C_t, C, and large parts of Algorithm 1. For this reason, we ported code to the GPU wherever possible. To reduce memory consumption, which is still a limiting factor for GPU programming, we represent the pointwise basis matrices $\tilde{V}$ in Eq. (10) as equivalent unit quaternions. Derivatives are approximated using forward (∇, Algorithm 1), backward (div, Algorithm 1), and central (∇, Eq. 13) differences. *Parameterization:* For all experiments, the following parameters were chosen. Algorithm 1: $\hat{\epsilon} = 10^{-6}$, $\gamma = 0.11 \Delta x^2$, $c = 0.2 \Delta x^2$ (Δx: minimum voxel edge length in mm); GVF: 316 iterations with a regularization parameter of $\mu = 3.16$ and step size determined as defined and described in [9]; Eq. (6): $\ell = 0.5$; Eq. (9): $w_1 = w_2 = 0.5$ as suggested in [3], w_3 determined following [3]; Eq. (12): $\varepsilon = 10^{-9}$.

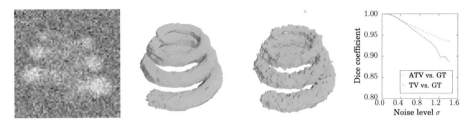

Fig. 2. Phantom experiment. *Left to right:* Mean intensity projection at $\sigma = 1.5$; segmentation with ATV; segmentation with TV; Dice coefficients w.r.t. ground truth (GT) for all noise levels σ.

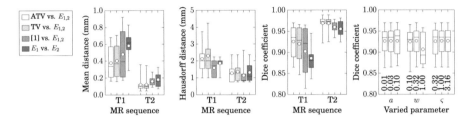

Fig. 3. Spinal cord experiment. *Left to right:* Mean surface distances for ATV/TV/ *PropSeg* [1] vs. E_1 and E_2; corresponding Hausdorff distances; corresponding Dice coefficients; T1 Dice coefficients for ATV vs. E_1 and E_2 with varying parameter values (central bar: median, circle: mean, box limits: 25/75th percentile, whiskers: extrema).

Helical Phantom. In this simulation experiment, we rendered images of a synthetic helical phantom with values in $[0, 1]$ to which we added Gaussian noise of standard deviation σ (Fig. 2). The phantom's tube radius varied between 3 mm and 6 mm, so we set $\mathcal{S} = [2.5\,\text{mm}, 7.2\,\text{mm}]$ (16 scales) in Eq. (9). We segmented the images with TV and ATV regularization, setting $a = 1$ and $a = 0.03$ in Eq. (10), respectively. We modeled $p^I_\cdot$ as normal distributions, using the true background, foreground, and noise level values. For the sake of simplicity, we set $p^D_\cdot = 1$ always. For w and ς in Eq. (13), we made grid searches for each noise level, using the Dice coefficients w.r.t. the ground truth as optimization criterion.

Figure 2 shows the Dice coefficients for the best w, ς combinations. The advantage of ATV becomes apparent as soon as the noise level increases.

Spinal Cord. In this experiment with real data, two clinical experts (E_1, E_2) manually segmented 10 MR scans (5 T1, 5 T2) of the healthy human cervical spinal cord over the C1–C3 region. For each image, we then used the remaining four images of the same sequence (T1/T2) to estimate $p_\cdot$ and to find an optimal parameter combination for a, w, ς. The distributions $p_\cdot$ were estimated from the manual labelings of the remaining four images, modeling p_b as mixtures of four Gaussians and p_f as normal distributions. We set $\mathcal{S} = [2\,\text{mm}, 4\,\text{mm}]$ (16 scales) in Eq. (9). The parameters a, w, ς were optimized via grid search, using the mean

Dice coefficients of the remaining four images w.r.t. their manual segmentations as optimization criterion. These distributions and the determined optimum parameterization were then used to segment the left-out image for evaluation of the method. For comparison with the state of the art, we also segmented all images with *PropSeg* [1].

Figure 3 shows the averaged mean surface distances, Hausdorff distances, and Dice coefficients w.r.t. their manual segmentations. Especially the T1 images profit from ATV, as they have both a lower resolution (T1: $1 \times 1 \times 1 \text{ mm}^3$, T2: $0.75 \times 0.38 \times 0.38 \text{ mm}^3$) and a lower contrast-to-noise ratio (about one eighth) than the T2 images. On the right, Fig. 3 shows the Dice coefficients for applying a wide range of parameter values to the T1 images, demonstrating the robustness of our method w.r.t. parameterization. For each varied parameter, the others were kept constant ($a = 0.03$, $w = 0.32$, $\varsigma = 1.00$).

4   Discussion and Conclusion

We presented a fully automated method for the segmentation of tubular structures. For a single image of 256^3 voxels, the complete process of calculating the vesselness, GVF, capacities, and segmentation takes about 1 to 1.5 min (GPU: Nvidia GeForce GTX 770). Although image segmentation in general and tubular structure segmentation in particular have often been addressed, the results of comparison with a state-of-the-art approach lead us to believe that our method may be of value to the scientific community. Future experiments will have to show in more detail how strong is the dependence of the segmentation quality on the outcome of the Frangi vesselness response and what is the influence of a particular GVF parameterization in this context. Furthermore, the use of alternative vesselness indicators will have to be considered. We provide our reference implementation at https://github.com/spezold/miccai2016.

References

1. De Leener, B., Kadoury, S., Cohen-Adad, J.: Robust, accurate and fast automatic segmentation of the spinal cord. NeuroImage **98**, 528–536 (2014)
2. De Leener, B., Taso, M., Cohen-Adad, J., Callot, V.: Segmentation of the human spinal cord. Magn. Reson. Mater. Phys., Biol. Med. **29**(2), 125–153 (2016)
3. Frangi, A.F., Niessen, W.J., Vincken, K.L., Viergever, M.A.: Multiscale vessel enhancement filtering. In: Wells, W.M., Colchester, A.C.F., Delp, S.L. (eds.) MICCAI 1998. LNCS, vol. 1496, pp. 130–137. Springer, Heidelberg (1998)
4. Gooya, A., Liao, H., Sakuma, I.: Generalization of geometrical flux maximizing flow on Riemannian manifolds for improved volumetric blood vessel segmentation. Comput. Med. Imaging Graph. **36**(6), 474–483 (2012)
5. Lesage, D., Angelini, E.D., Bloch, I., Funka-Lea, G.: A review of 3D vessel lumen segmentation techniques: models, features and extraction schemes. Med. Image Anal. **13**(6), 819–845 (2009)
6. Manniesing, R., Viergever, M.A., Niessen, W.J.: Vessel enhancing diffusion: a scale space representation of vessel structures. Med. Image Anal. **10**(6), 815–825 (2006)

7. Olsson, C., Byrod, M., Overgaard, N., Kahl, F.: Extending continuous cuts: anisotropic metrics and expansion moves. In: 2009 IEEE 12th International Conference on Computer Vision, pp. 405–412 (2009)
8. Reinbacher, C., Pock, T., Bauer, C., Bischof, H.: Variational segmentation of elongated volumetric structures. In: 2010 IEEE Conference on Computer Vision and Pattern Recognition (CVPR), pp. 3177–3184 (2010)
9. Xu, C., Prince, J.L.: Snakes, shapes, and gradient vector flow. IEEE Trans. Image Process. **7**(3), 359–369 (1998)
10. Yuan, J., Bae, E., Tai, X.C.: A study on continuous max-flow and min-cut approaches. In: 2010 IEEE Conference on Computer Vision and Pattern Recognition (CVPR), pp. 2217–2224 (2010)

Dense Volume-to-Volume Vascular Boundary Detection

Jameson Merkow[1]([✉]), Alison Marsden[2], David Kriegman[1], and Zhuowen Tu[1]

[1] University of California, San Diego, USA
jmerkow@eng.ucsd.edu
[2] Stanford University, Stanford, USA

Abstract. In this work, we tackle the important problem of dense 3D volume labeling in medical imaging. We start by introducing HED-3D, a 3D extension of the state-of-the-art 2D edge detector (HED). Next, we develop a novel 3D-Convolutional Neural Network (CNN) architecture, I2I-3D, that predicts boundary location in volumetric data. Our fine-to-fine, deeply supervised framework addresses three critical issues to 3D boundary detection: (1) efficient, holistic, end-to-end volumetric label training and prediction (2) precise voxel-level prediction to capture fine scale structures prevalent in medical data and (3) directed multi-scale, multi-level feature learning. We evaluate our approaches on a dataset consisting of 93 medical image volumes with a wide variety of anatomical regions and vascular structures. We show that our deep learning approaches out-perform the current state-of-the-art in 3D vascular boundary detection (structured forests 3D), by a large margin, as well as HED applied to slices. Prediction takes about one minute on a typical $512 \times 512 \times 512$ volume, when using GPU.

1 Introduction

The past decade has witnessed major progress in computer vision, graphics, and machine learning, due in large part to the success of technologies built around the concept of "image patches". Many patch-centric approaches fall into the category of "sliding-window" methods [3,9,11] that consider dense, overlapping windows. Patch-centric approaches limit us in terms of computational complexity and long-range modeling capabilities. Fully convolutional neural networks (FCN) [7] achieved simultaneous performance and full image labeling. Holistically-Nested Edge Detector (HED) [13] applied this approach to image-to-image object boundary detection. HED significantly improved the state-of-the-art in edge detection, and did so at a fraction of the computational cost of previous CNN-based edge/boundary detection algorithms. Another member of the FCN family, UNet [10], adapted this architecture for neuronal segmentation.

Volume-to-volume learning has yet to garner the same attention as image-to-image labeling. One approach applies 2D prediction schemes on images generated by traversing the volume on an anatomical plane then recombining predictions into a volume. However, volumetric features exist across three spatial dimensions, therefore it is crucial to process this data where those features exist.

© Springer International Publishing AG 2016
S. Ourselin et al. (Eds.): MICCAI 2016, Part III, LNCS 9902, pp. 371–379, 2016.
DOI: 10.1007/978-3-319-46726-9_43

The current state-of-the-art in vessel wall detection uses a 3D patch-to-patch approach along with domain features, *a-priori* information, and a structured forest classifier [9]. In that work, the authors mitigate computational cost of patch-centric classifiers by using a sampling scheme and limiting their dataset to certain types of vascular structures. This method side-steps patch-centric inefficiency by limiting accurate prediction to a subset of structures and anatomical regions. Volumetric labeling using a CNN approach has been attempted [14], but the high computational cost of these frameworks preclude them from accurate end-to-end volumetric prediction.

A secondary challenge lies in detecting small structures prevalent in medical volume data. In contrast to objects in natural images, anatomical structures are often small, and resolution may be limited by acquisition. In fact, small anomalies are often of greater importance than the larger structures. These factors manifest a unique challenge for dense labeling of medical volumes.

In this work, we first extend HED (2D-CNN) to HED-3D for direct dense volume labeling; we then propose a novel 3D-CNN architecture, I2I-3D, for precise volume-to-volume labeling. Our approach tackles three key issues in dense medical volume label prediction: (1) efficient volumetric labeling of medial data using 3D, volume-to-volume CNN architectures, (2) precise fine-to-fine and volume-to-volume labeling, (3) nested multi-scale learning. We extend the typical fine-to-coarse architecture by adding an efficient means to process high resolution features late in the network, enabling precise voxel-level prediction that benefit from coarse level guidance and nested multi-scale representations. We evaluate our approach against the state-of-the-art in vessel wall detection.

2   Dense Volume-to-Volume Prediction

2.1   Pixel Level Prediction in 2D Images

Fully convolutional neural networks [7] were among the first methods to adapt the fine-to-coarse structure to dense pixel-level prediction. The FCN architecture added element-wise summations to VGGNet [2] that link coarse resolution predictions to layers with finer strides. However, it has been shown that pulling features directly from bottom layers to top layers is sub-optimal as the fine-level features have no coarse-level guidance [4]. HED [13] produced top accuracy on the BSDS500 dataset [8] with an alternative adaptation of VGGNet which fused several boundary responses at different resolutions with weighted aggregation. However, HED's fine-to-coarse framework leaves fundamental limitations to precise prediction and a close look at the edge responses produced by HED reveals many thick orphan edges. HED only achieves top accuracy after boundary refinement via non-maximum suppression (NMS) and morphological thinning. This approach is often sufficient for 2D tasks, however, it is less reliable in volumetric data. Furthermore, NMS fails when the prediction resolution is lower than the object separation resolution.

In these architectures, the most powerful outputs (in terms of predictive power) lack the capability to produce fine resolution predictions. Not only is this problematic for making high resolution predictions, but coarse representations inform finer resolution predictions and finer resolution distinctions often require complex predictive power. UNet [10] addressed some of these issues by adding more convolutional layers, and using a loss function that penalizes poor localization of adjacent structures. However, UNet does not directly learn nested multi-level interactions and the large number of dense layers hinder efficiency in 3D tasks.

2.2 Precise Multi-Scale Voxel Level Prediction

Our framework addresses these crucial issues to volume-to-volume labeling and applies them to vascular boundary detection in medical volumes. Our proposed network, I2I-3D, consists of two paths: a fine-to-coarse path and a multi-scale coarse-to-fine path. The fine-to-coarse network structure follows popular network architecture and generates features with increasing feature abstraction and greater spatial extent. By adding side outputs and a fusion layer, we obtain an efficient 3D-CNN: HED-3D. As expected, HED-3D struggles to localize small vascular structures, and requires a secondary path to increases prediction resolution. I2I-3D uses a secondary path to learn complex multi-scale interactions in a coarse-to-fine fashion creating a fine-to-fine architecture.

Each stage of the coarse-to-fine path incorporates abstract representations with higher resolution features to produce fine resolution responses that benefit from multi-scale influences and coarse level guidance. Special 'mixing' layers and two convolution layers combine these two inputs to minimize a multi-scale, deeply supervised loss function. Here, deep supervision [6], plays an important role through multiple loss functions that reward multi-scale integration at each stage. Cascading this process results in features with large projective fields at high resolution. Later layers benefit from abstract features, coarse level guidance, and multi-scale integration; this culminates in a top most layer with the best predictive power and highest resolution. Figure 1 depicts the layer-wise connected 3D convolutional neural network architectures of I2I-3D and HED-3D.

2.3 Formulation

We denote our input training set of N volumes by $S = \{(X_n, Y_n), n = 1, \ldots, N\}$, where sample $X_n = \{x_j^{(n)}, j = 1, \ldots, |X_n|\}$ denotes the raw input volume and $Y_n = \{y_j^{(n)}, j = 1, \ldots, |X_n|\}, y_j^{(n)} \in \{1, .., K\}$ denotes the corresponding ground truth label map. For our task, $K = 2$, here we define the generic loss formulation. We drop n for simplicity, as we consider volumes independently. Our goal is to learn network parameters, $\mathbf{W}$, that enable boundary detection at multiple resolutions. Our approach produces M multi-scale outputs with $\frac{1}{2^{M-1}}$ input resolution. Each output has an associated classifier whose weights are denoted $\mathbf{w} = (\mathbf{w}^{(1)}, \ldots, \mathbf{w}^{(M)})$. Loss for each of these outputs is defined as:

$$\mathcal{L}_{\text{out}}(\mathbf{W}, \mathbf{w}) = \sum_{m=1}^{M} \ell_{\text{out}}^{(m)}(\mathbf{W}, \mathbf{w}^{(m)}), \tag{1}$$

where ℓ_{out} denotes the volume-level loss function. Loss is computed over all voxels in a training volume X and label map Y. Specifically, we define the following cross-entropy loss function used in Eq. (1):

$$\ell_{\text{out}}^{(m)}(\mathbf{W}, \mathbf{w}^{(m)}) = -\sum_k \sum_{j \in Y_k} \log \Pr(y_j = k | X; \mathbf{W}, \mathbf{w}^{(m)}) \tag{2}$$

where Y_k denotes the voxel truth label sets for the kth class. $\Pr(y_j = k | X; \mathbf{W}, \mathbf{w}^{(m)}) = \sigma(a_j^{(m)}) \in [0, 1]$ is computed using sigmoid function $\sigma(.)$ on the activation value at voxel j. We obtain label map predictions $\hat{Y}_{\text{out}}^{(m)} = \sigma(\hat{A}_{\text{out}}^{(m)})$, where $\hat{A}_{\text{out}}^{(m)} \equiv \{a_j^{(m)}, \ j = 1, \ldots, |Y|\}$ are activations of the output of layer m. Putting everything together, we minimize the following objective function via standard stochastic gradient descent:

$$(\mathbf{W}, \mathbf{w}) = \operatorname{argmin}(\mathcal{L}_{\text{out}}(\mathbf{W}, \mathbf{w})) \tag{3}$$

During testing, given image X we obtain label map predictions from the output layers: $\hat{Y}_{\text{top}} = \text{I2I}(X, (\mathbf{W}, \mathbf{w}))$, where $\text{I2I}(\cdot)$ denotes the label maps produced by our network.

3   Network Architecture and Training

The coarse-to-fine path of I2I-3D, we mimic VGGNet's [2] design with domain specific modifications. First, we truncate at the fourth pooling layer resulting in a network with 10 convolutional layers at four resolutions. Second, we decrease the filter count of the first two convolution layers to 32. Lastly, we replace max pooling with average pooling. For our HED-3D framework, we place deep supervision at side-outputs at each convolution layer just prior to pooling, as in [13]. These side-outputs are fused via weighted aggregation.

I2I-3D adds a pathway to HED-3D's architectures to combines multi-scale responses into higher resolution representations. The second structure follows an inverted pattern of the fine-to-coarse path; it begins at the lowest resolution and upsamples in place of pooling. Each stage of the coarse-to-fine path contains a mixing layer and two convolutional layers. Mixing layers take two inputs: one from the corresponding resolution in fine-to-coarse path and a second from the output of the previous (coarser) stage in the coarse-to-fine path. Mixing layers concatenate inputs and do a specialized $1 \times 1 \times 1$ convolution operation to mix multi-resolution input features. Mixing layers are similar to reduction layers in GoogLeNet [12] but differ in usage and initialization. Mixing layers directly hybridize low resolution and fine-to-coarse features, while maintaining network efficiency. Mixing layer output is pass through two convolutional layers to spatially mix the two streams. Each coarse-to-fine stage is deeply supervised after the final convolution layer, just prior to upsampling. These side outputs push each stage to produce higher quality predictions by incorporating information from the lower resolution, more abstract representations These outputs are

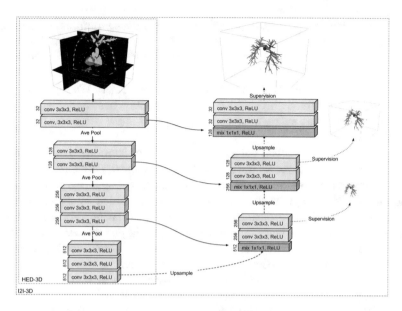

Fig. 1. The proposed network architecture I2I-3D. Our architecture couples fine-to-coarse and coarse-to-fine convolutional structures and multi-scale loss to produce dense voxel-level labels at input resolution. The number of channels is denoted on the left of each convolution layer, arrows denote network connections and operations.

only used to promote multi-scale integration at each stage, and are phased out, leaving single output at the top-most layer.

We begin by describing the training procedure for HED-3D. We, first, load pre-trained weights (details in Sect. 4) and place deep supervision at each of the four multi-scale outputs and at the fusion output. We iteratively train starting with a learning rate of $1e^{-7}$ and decimate every $30k$ iterations. Weight updates occur after every iteration till convergence.

For I2I-3D, we attach a coarse-to-fine path and move deep supervision to new multi-scale outputs. Each stage is initialize to produce the identity mapping of the fine-to-coarse input. We decrease all learning rates in the fine-to-coarse path to $\frac{1}{100}$ and train until loss plateaus. These hyper-parameters force the network to learn multi-scale features at each stage in order to minimize loss at each resolution. Finally, we return learning rate multipliers to 1, remove all supervision on all outputs except the highest resolution, and train until convergence.

4   Experimentation and Results

In [9], the authors use direct voxel overlap for evaluation, however, this metric fails to account for any localization error in boundary prediction and over-penalizes usable boundaries that do not perfectly overlap with ground truth boundaries. The metrics used here a 3D extension of the BSDS benchmark metrics [1] which are standard protocols for evaluating boundary contours in natural images.

These metrics find match correspondences between ground truth and predicted contour boundaries. Matched voxels contribute to true positive counts, and unmatched voxels contribute to fall-out and miss rates. We report three performance measures: fixed threshold F measure (ODS), best per-image threshold F measure (OIS), and average precision (AP) and show precision-recall curves for each classifier.

Our dataset includes all 38 volumes used in [9] but introduces an 55 additional volumes to form an expanded dataset with 93 volumes. This dataset includes a variety of anatomical regions, including: abdominal, thoracic, cerebral, vertebral, and lower extremity regions. All volumes are accompanied by 3D models which were expertly built for computational blood flow simulation. Volumes were captured from individual patients for clinically indicated purposes via magnetic resonance (MR) or computed tomography (CT) imaging. Volumes include normal physiologies as well as a variety of pathologies including: aneurysms, stenoses, peripheral artery disease, congenital heart disease, and dissection. The dataset contains various arterial vessel types, but only one structure is annotated per volume. All volumes were obtained from http://www.vascularmodel.com.

We split volumes into training, validation, and test sets, each set contains 67, 7 and 19 volumes respectively and consist of both CT and MR data. Since volumes contain incomplete annotation, only voxels inside annotated vessels and those within 20 voxels of the vessel wall are considered during evaluation.

We pre-process each volume by whitening voxel intensities and cropping them into overlapping, $96 \times 96 \times 48$, segments. A single segment takes about one second to process on a NVidia K40 GPU and a typical volume ($512 \times 512 \times 512$) takes less than a minute. As a result of inconsistent annotation, we only train on volumes that contain over 0.25% labeled vessel voxels (approx. 1000 of $442,368$ voxels).

Our networks are implemented in the popular *Caffe* library [5] where methods were extended for 3D when necessary. Fine-to-coarse weights were generated by pre-training a randomly initialized network on entire vessel label prediction for a fixed number of iterations (50k) with a high learning rate. These labels produce less overall loss, preventing unstable gradients from developing during back-propagation.

We compare I2I-3D to the current state-of-the-art [9], a 2D-CNN baseline (HED) [13] and our HED-3D architecture. HED (in 2D) was trained without modification on individual slices from each volume. We also compare against the widely used 3D-Canny edge detector.

Figures 2 and 3 show the results of our experimentation. Figure 3 indicates that our method out-performs all other methods, including the current state-of-the-art. We also notice that 3D-CNN approaches considerably improves average precision over 2D-CNN when comparing results from HED and HED-3D. The precision-recall curves reveal that I2I-3D consistently boosts precision over HED-3D indicating that our fine-to-fine multi-scale architecture improves localization.

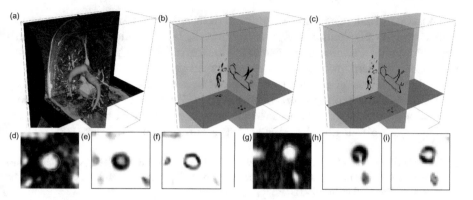

Fig. 2. Results of our HED-3D and I2I-3D vessel boundary classifiers. (a) Input volume and ground truth (in blue). (b) HED-3D result. (c) I2I-3D result. (d), (g) vessel cross section and ground truth (in blue). (e), (h) HED-3D cross section result. (f), (i) I2I-3D cross section result. (Color figure online)

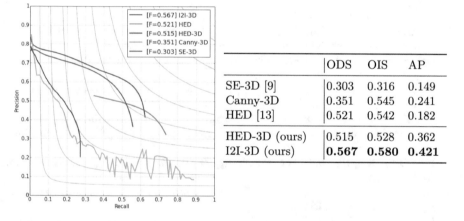

	ODS	OIS	AP
SE-3D [9]	0.303	0.316	0.149
Canny-3D	0.351	0.545	0.241
HED [13]	0.521	0.542	0.182
HED-3D (ours)	0.515	0.528	0.362
I2I-3D (ours)	**0.567**	**0.580**	**0.421**

Fig. 3. (left) Precision recall curves comparing our approach with state-of-the-art, our baseline methods. (right) Performance metrics of our approach and baselines.

In Fig. 2, we see the results of I2I-3D characterized by stronger and more localized responses when compared to HED-3D, showing the benefit of our fine-to-fine, multi-scale learning approach. The fine-to-coarse architecture of HED and HED-3D generate low resolution responses resulting in poor localization of tiny structures and a weaker edge response. This indicates that I2I-3D's multi-scale representation enable precise localization.

5   Conclusion

We have proposed two network structures, HED-3D and I2I-3D, that address major issues in efficient volume-to-volume labeling. Our HED-3D framework demonstrates that processing volumetric data natively in 3D, improves performance over its 2D counterpart; our framework, I2I-3D, efficiently learns multiscale hierarchal features and generates precise voxel-level predictions at input resolution. We demonstrate through experimentation, that our approach is capable of fine localization and achieves state-of-the-art performance vessel boundary detection without explicit *a-priori* information. We provide our source code and pre-trained models to ensure that our approach can be applied to variety of medical applications and domains at: https://github.com/jmerkow/I2I.

Acknowledgments. Z.T. is supported by NSF IIS-1360566, NSF IIS-1360568, and a Northrop Grumman Contextual Robotics grant. We are grateful for the generous donation of the GPUs by NVIDIA.

References

1. Arbelaez, P., Maire, M., Fowlkes, C., Malik, J.: Contour detection and hierarchical image segmentation. PAMI **33**(5), 898–916 (2011)
2. Chatfield, K., Simonyan, K., Vedaldi, A., Zisserman, A.: Return of the devil in the details: delving deep into convolutional nets. In: BMVC (2014)
3. Dollár, P., Zitnick, C.L.: Fast edge detection using structured forests. In: PAMI (2015)
4. Hariharan, B., Arbeláez, P., Girshick, R., Malik, J.: Hypercolumns for object segmentation and fine-grained localization. In: CVPR (2014)
5. Jia, Y., Shelhamer, E., Donahue, J., Karayev, S., Long, J., Girshick, R., Guadarrama, S., Darrell, T.: Caffe: convolutional architecture for fast feature embedding. preprint arXiv:1408.5093 (2014)
6. Lee, C.Y., Xie, S., Gallagher, P., Zhang, Z., Tu, Z.: Deeply-supervised nets. In: AISTATS (2015)
7. Long, J., Shelhamer, E., Darrell, T.: Fully convolutional networks for semantic segmentation. In: CVPR (2014)
8. Martin, D.R., Fowlkes, C.C., Malik, J.: Learning to detect natural image boundaries using local brightness, color, and texture cues. PAMI **26**(5), 530–549 (2004)
9. Merkow, J., Tu, Z., Kriegman, D., Marsden, A.: Structural edge detection for cardiovascular modeling. In: Navab, N., Hornegger, J., Wells, W.M., Frangi, A.F. (eds.) MICCAI 2015. LNCS, vol. 9351, pp. 735–742. Springer, Heidelberg (2015). doi:10.1007/978-3-319-24574-4_88
10. Ronneberger, O., Fischer, P., Brox, T.: U-Net: convolutional networks for biomedical image segmentation. In: Navab, N., Hornegger, J., Wells, W.M., Frangi, A.F. (eds.) MICCAI 2015. LNCS, vol. 9351, pp. 234–241. Springer, Heidelberg (2015). doi:10.1007/978-3-319-24574-4_28
11. Roth, H.R., Lu, L., Farag, A., Shin, H.-C., Liu, J., Turkbey, E.B., Summers, R.M.: DeepOrgan: multi-level deep convolutional networks for automated pancreas segmentation. In: Navab, N., Hornegger, J., Wells, W.M., Frangi, A.F. (eds.) MICCAI 2015. LNCS, vol. 9349, pp. 556–564. Springer, Heidelberg (2015). doi:10.1007/978-3-319-24553-9_68

12. Szegedy, C., Liu, W., Jia, Y., Sermanet, P., Reed, S., Anguelov, D., Erhan, D., Vanhoucke, V., Rabinovich, A.: Going deeper with convolutions. In: CVPR (2015)
13. Xie, S., Tu, Z.: Holistically-nested edge detection. In: ICCV (2015)
14. Zheng, Y., Liu, D., Georgescu, B., Nguyen, H., Comaniciu, D.: 3D deep learning for efficient and robust landmark detection in volumetric data. In: Navab, N., Hornegger, J., Wells, W.M., Frangi, A.F. (eds.) MICCAI 2015. LNCS, vol. 9349, pp. 565–572. Springer, Heidelberg (2015). doi:10.1007/978-3-319-24553-9_69

HALE: Healthy Area of Lumen Estimation for Vessel Stenosis Quantification

Sethuraman Sankaran[1(✉)], Michiel Schaap[1], Stanley C. Hunley[1],
James K. Min[2], Charles A. Taylor[1], and Leo Grady[1]

[1] HeartFlow Inc., Redwood City, CA, USA
ssankaran@heartflow.com
[2] Department of Radiology, Weill-Cornell Medical College, New York, NY, USA

Abstract. One of the most widely used non-invasive clinical metric for
diagnosing patients with symptoms of coronary artery disease is %steno-
sis derived from cCTA. Estimation of %stenosis involves two steps -
the measurement of local diameter and the measurement of a reference
healthy diameter. The estimation of a reference healthy diameter is challenging, especially in diffuse, ostial and bifurcation lesions. We develop a
machine learning algorithm using random forest regressors for the estimation of healthy diameter using downstream and upstream properties of
coronary tree vasculature as features. We use a population-based estimation, in contrast to single patient estimation that is used in the majority
of the literature. We demonstrate that this method is able to predict the
diameter of healthy sections with a correlation coefficient of 0.95. We then
estimate %stenosis based on the ratio of the local vessel diameter to the
estimated healthy diameter. Compared to a reference anisotropic kernel
regression method, the proposed method, HALE (Healthy Area of Lumen
Estimation), has a superior area under curve (0.90 vs 0.83) and operating
point sensitivity/specificity (90 %/85 % vs 82 %/76 %) for the detection
of stenoses. We also demonstrate superior performance of HALE against
invasive quantitative coronary angiography (QCA), compared to the reference method (mean absolute error: 14 % vs 31 %, p < 0.001).

Keywords: Healthy lumen diameter · Stenosis detection · Coronary
artery disease

1 Introduction

Coronary artery disease (CAD) is one of the leading causes of death and
may result in acute events such as plaque rupture which demands immediate
care or gradual events such as accumulation of plaque which leads to progres-
sive anatomic narrowing resulting in ischemia. Coronary computed tomography
angiography (cCTA) provides information on the degree of anatomical narrowing
(stenosis) in different regions of the coronary artery tree. The degree of stenosis,
called %stenosis, is a widely used clinical measure to decide between performing invasive angiography and pressure measurements or deferment of invasive
measurements. The estimation of %stenosis is usually performed categorically

© Springer International Publishing AG 2016
S. Ourselin et al. (Eds.): MICCAI 2016, Part III, LNCS 9902, pp. 380–387, 2016.
DOI: 10.1007/978-3-319-46726-9_44

(e.g. 0 %, 1–30%, 31–49%, 50–69%, 70–100%) in the clinic, or, less frequently, sent to a core lab with expert readers for analysis. Quantitative computed tomography (QCT) and QCA are methods where %stenosis is estimated as a number between 0 % (healthy vessel) and 100 % (complete obstruction). QCA is invasive, while QCT, evaluated on cCTA, is time consuming and generally performed in a core lab. The method we present enables automatic measurement of %stenosis given a lumen segmentation. The main novelty is that we estimate the healthy diameter with respect to a database of healthy sections from other patients, in contrast to regressing from individual patient data.

Different methods for stenosis detection and quantification were compared on a set of cCTAs in the 2012 MICCAI stenosis challenge [1]. The goal was to quantify results in a set of patients who were evaluated by expert readers and QCA, and to report diagnostic performance and differences in stenosis grade. For most of the algorithms, this process had, built into it, (i) a centerline detection algorithm, (ii) a lumen segmentation algorithm and (iii) a stenosis detection step. We believe that (iii) by itself has scope for improvement based on the best performing methods in literature, as shown later. Therefore, we use the same lumen segmentation to analyze the performance of all stenosis detection algorithms. Towards this, a lumen segmentation is read by expert readers and stenosed sections are annotated, which are then compared to the proposed method to quantify performance. We use the acronym HALE for the proposed method (Healthy Area of Lumen Estimation). HALE is designed to predict healthy lumen diameter, and thereby also enables the prediction of healthy lumen area and evaluation of %stenosis. We believe that HALE, when used with a state-of-the-art lumen segmentation algorithm, can be used as an accurate and efficient QCT tool. Kirisli et al. [1] conclude the MICCAI stenosis challenge by stating that "Given a similar accurate lumen segmentation, robust kernel regression outperforms the other approaches and is a good approach to quantify lesions from accurate lumen segmentation". The quoted method [2] uses a robust kernel regression approach with a radial basis function applied on the segmented lumen radius profile. Later, it was suggested that natural discontinuities in lumen radii at bifurcations can be accounted for by using an anisotropic kernel [3].

While focal coronary disease is captured well by many methods in literature, diffuse and ostial coronary artery disease are difficult to diagnose due to the absence of a clear reference lumen diameter. Huo et al. [4] suggested that epicardial volume, length and lumen area are related by a power-law and that the coefficient of power-law separates subjects with and without diffuse disease, indicating only the presence or absence of diffuse lumen narrowing without specifying where the disease is present. In this work, we present a general framework that can identify regions of lumen narrowing in (coronary) arteries, including focal, diffuse, ostial and bifurcation disease. The (coronary) arteries are split into sections or stems, and each stem is associated with features corresponding to its crown (downstream vasculature), root (upstream vasculature) and sibling (the other child vessel of its parent, if available). We predict the healthy diameter of the stem using a machine learning method trained on these features on a database of 6000 stems (from 200 patients) and tested on 4697 stems (150 patients). We demonstrate that HALE performs better than state-of-the-art techniques over different lesion characteristics including the challenging cases of diffuse and ostial disease.

2 Methods

The first step in our process is the extraction of a coronary centerline tree and lumen segmentation. Following this, trained CT readers evaluate the lumen segmentation and make corrections, as necessary. Since manual annotation of diseased sections is performed on the lumen segmentation rather than the cCTA, performance does not depend on the algorithm used for centerline detection and lumen segmentation and many available methods may be used [5,6]. In the section below, we first describe the process of manual annotation of sections of disease. Then, we describe the proposed method, HALE, including definition of features and estimation of healthy lumen diameter. We then discuss how we evaluate %stenosis and the metrics used for validation.

2.1 Manual Annotation

Trained readers of cCTA assess lumen segmentation on a cohort of patients and identify locations of lumen narrowing (i.e. %stenosis $\geq 50\%$). This process mimics the process of reading %stenosis from CT scans in the clinic, i.e. estimated visually rather than assessing a reference diameter and evaluating the ratio of minimum lumen diameter to the reference diameter. To provide confidence in the readings, each patient is assessed by three readers and only sections that have a consensus read are used for training and testing. For convenience, the coronary trees are split into sections, where each section is marked either as diseased or healthy. Sections are split using locations of bifurcations as separators. The rationale for using bifurcation as separators is that flow rate in a given section being constant, a healthy vessel maintains its radius within a section to preserve a homeostatic state of wall shear stress.

2.2 Data-Driven Estimation of Healthy Radius

The approach we outline here aims to estimate healthy vessel diameter. Regions of disease are evaluated by dividing the difference between the estimated healthy diameter and local diameter with the estimated healthy diameter, and comparing it to a diagnostic threshold of 50 %. Our approach maps metrics derived from the epicardial vasculature to a healthy diameter using a machine learning approach, which is trained on a database of sections annotated as healthy.

In contrast to previously published methods, we do not solely rely on the patient's vasculature to determine the healthy diameter at a given location. We use a machine-learning approach relying on a population of 6000 healthy stems from 200 patients. This enables a better identification of non-focal stenosis morphologies such as long diffuse lesions, ostial lesions, or lesions which are present along an entire section. To determine features of the machine learning algorithm, we first evaluate local diameter using maximum inscribed spheres. An alternative approach is to derive average diameter from the area of lumen along the normal to centerlines. This approach was not used as it provides inaccurate values near bifurcations. To assess the healthy lumen diameter, we first split the lumen segmentation into stem-crown-root units. A stem is the section for which we are evaluating healthy diameter. A crown refers to its downstream vasculature and a root refers to its upstream vasculature. We also identify a sibling vessel which is the other child of the parent vessel. By definition, all the features are not available for all stems (e.g. ostial sections do not have a root unit and terminal sections do not have a crown unit) and are given a default special value of -1. The crown, root and sibling units for a stem are shown in Fig. 1.

Our approach omits one stem at a time and uses features from the rest of the vascular tree to infer the healthy lumen diameter of the stem under consideration. For each stem in a given coronary vasculature, the following features, hypothesized to be relevant, are extracted for the corresponding crown, root and sibling vessels (when available) - average, maximum and minimum lumen area (A), volume (V), length (L), V/A, and V/L. We also use a feature (d_m) derived from Murray's law [7], which is a physiologic model of how the diameters of parent (d_p) and daughter vessels are related. This feature is calculated as $d_m = (d_p^3 - d_s^3)^{1/3}$, where d_s is the diameter of its sibling vessel.

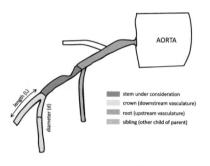

Fig. 1. A schematic of the method used is shown. The coronary tree is split into many stem-crown-root units. Stems are defined based on branch points as separators with the corresponding crown and root being the downstream and upstream vasculatures respectively. Features are derived from epicardial volume, length and lumen diameter.

We use random forest regression [8] to predict the healthy lumen diameter. Random forests are known to be effective and powerful for high dimensional and heterogeneous features. Random forests employ an ensemble of decision trees, each of which is composed of a random subset of features and training data. The values from the decision trees are pooled together and averaged to compute the final predictor of healthy lumen diameter (d_p). Percent stenosis is evaluated from the ratio of the local lumen diameter (d_l) to the predicted healthy lumen diameter as $\alpha = \max\left(0\,\%, \left(1 - \frac{d_l}{d_p}\right) \times 100\,\%\right)$. We use 50 trees with an average of 5 features per tree (chosen based on a 5-fold cross validation).

Results of the random forest regressor on a test set of 4697 stems (from 150 patients) are evaluated by assessing sensitivity, specificity and area under the receiver-operator characteristic (ROC) curve. Sections annotated by readers as

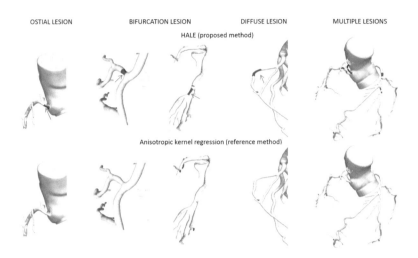

Fig. 2. Comparison of the machine learning method (top) with an anisotropic kernel method [3] (bottom) on patients with (from left) ostial, bifurcation, diffuse and multiple lesions. Anisotropic kernels can minimize the effect of steep changes in healthy lumen area across bifurcations [3] but is unable to detect lesions in the examples shown above in contrast to HALE. Regions with $\alpha \geq 50\%$ are shown in red. (Color figure online)

diseased are considered positive, which are further classified as "true positive" if the random forest predicts %stenosis $\geq o\%$ or "false negative" otherwise, where the operating point o can be different for each method. Similarly, sections which are annotated as healthy are classified as "true negative" if the random forest predicts %stenosis $< 50\%$ and "false positive" otherwise. Sensitivity (Se) and specificity(Sp) are defined as

$$Se = \frac{TP}{TP + FN}, \ Sp = \frac{TN}{TN + FP}$$

An ROC curve is plotted by evaluating the sensitivity and specificity for different value of cutoffs used to define sections of disease, (i.e.) $\alpha \leq x \ \ \forall x \in [0\%, 100\%]$.

3   Results

We implemented the robust kernel regression [2] and anisotropic kernel regression methods [3] to serve as a baseline. We refer to anisotropic kernel regression as the "reference" method since it outperformed the robust kernel regression method in our dataset (shown later). First, we use HALE and evaluate healthy lumen diameter and subsequently %stenosis on five patients with either ostial lesions, bifurcation lesions, diffuse lesions or a combination thereof. Figure 2 shows a map of regions identified as diseased using HALE and the reference anisotropic kernel regression method, suggesting that the latter fails to capture non-focal lesions.

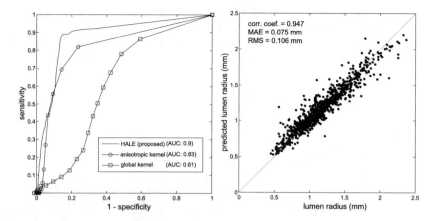

Fig. 3. The figure on the left demonstrates superior performance of HALE (area under the curve (AUC) : 0.90) compared to anisotropic kernel (AUC: 0.83) and global kernel methods (AUC:0.61). The figure on the right shows a comparison of the predicted and measured lumen radius in vessel sections marked healthy by human evaluation.

To quantify the overall performance of the algorithm, we predict healthy diameter and assess presence of stenosis on 150 patients (4697 sections) distinct from those used for training. A scatterplot of average radius of sections annotated as healthy compared to their estimated healthy radius is shown in Fig. 3. The correlation coefficient between the predicted and the measured healthy lumen diameter is 0.947, with a mean absolute error of 0.150 mm and a root mean squared error of 0.212 mm. The operating point sensitivity and specificity for detecting %stenosis using HALE is 90 %/85 % (operating point, o is 48 %), compared to 77 %/52 % using a global kernel regression method and 82 %/76 % using the reference anisotropic kernel regression method (operating point, o is 32 %). The receiver operator characteristic (ROC) curves for the three methods are compared in Fig. 3 with the area under curve being 0.90 (HALE), 0.83 (anisotropic kernel regression) and 0.61 (global kernel regression).

Next, we apply the method on patients who underwent a coronary angiography and the corresponding diseased locations were identified and quantified using QCA by an independent expert at a core laboratory. Coronary QCA data from a subset of the DeFACTO clinical trial [9] (Clinicaltrials.gov # NCT01233518) is used as the reference ground truth data. Performance of HALE and the reference method against QCA data on 69 measured vessel segments is tabulated in Table 1. There is a significant improvement in mean absolute error (MAE) and an insignificant difference in correlation coefficient, evaluated on the same lumen segmentation. Figure 4 compares locations of disease identified by HALE, the reference method, CTA and QCA evaluated by a core-lab for a severely diseased patient with multiple locations of lumen narrowing. The results show that HALE is able to identify four lesions out of five identified by CTA (only four of these are identified by QCA due to distal loss of contrast).

Table 1. The mean absolute error (MAE) of HALE is significantly better (p < 0.001, for both healthy diameter and %stenosis) and correlation coefficient (R) is slightly better but not significant (p = 0.47 for healthy diameter and p = 0.36 for %stenosis) compared to the reference method, both using QCA data as the ground truth.

Method	Metric	Bias	MAE	R	Slope	Intercept
Reference (anisotropic kernel)	healthy dia. (mm)	−0.52	0.58	0.76	0.51	0.90
HALE (machine learning)	healthy dia. (mm)	0.29	0.50	0.77	0.61	1.42
Reference (anisotropic kernel)	%stenosis	−31 %	31 %	0.54	0.98	−0.30
HALE (machine learning)	%stenosis	−13 %	14 %	0.58	0.85	−0.04

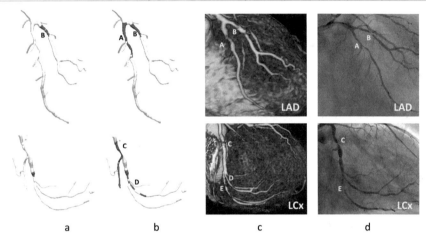

a   b   c   d

Fig. 4. Comparison of (a) HALE and (b) anisotropic kernel method on a severely diseased coronary artery with (c) five identified regions of lumen narrowing in CTA and (d) four stenosed regions identified by QCA, showing that HALE is able to identify four of the lesions while only one was identified by the anisotropic kernel regression method. Regions with $\alpha \geq 50\%$ are shown in red in panels (a) and (b). (Color figure online)

In comparison, the reference method is able to identify only a single lesion. This example demonstrates that with an accurate lumen segmentation algorithm, we are able to evaluate lesions with complex morphologies.

4   Discussion

We proposed a method that quantifies stenoses by first training a machine learning method on healthy vessel sections. We hypothesized that a set of features derived from the geometry of the downstream vasculature, upstream vasculature, and sibling vessel can be used to estimate the healthy vessel dimensions of a given section. To test this, we partitioned the geometry into various "stem-crown-root" units and used metrics such as epicardial vascular volume, lumen area, centerline lengths and other metrics derived from these. We also used a feature motivated from Murray's law that relates lumen diameter of parent sections to its daughter sections, though the impact of the feature itself was modest. We extracted patient-specific metrics, omitting one section at a time, and using a database of these metrics, mapped them to a healthy lumen diameter. We obtained a correlation coefficient of 0.947 with a mean absolute error of 0.15 mm for predicting lumen diameter of healthy sections. HALE had an operating point sensitivity/specificity of 90 %/85 % for detecting stenoses. The mean absolute error in quantifying the degree of stenosis reduced from 31 % using the reference method to 14 % using HALE, with QCA being the ground truth.

The kernel-regression based methods are able to capture regions of focal narrowing but not the other disease morphologies, likely because they rely heavily on local patient-specific data without accounting for population data. The method for detection of diffuse lesions by Huo et al. [4], on the other hand, uses a population-based cutoff tailored to, solely, the presence or absence of diffuse lesions. We posit that the higher mean absolute error and lower bias in quantifying degree of stenosis by the reference method is because regressing on a single patient lumen area results in underestimation of healthy lumen radius.

The proposed method, HALE, can be used with any lumen segmentation algorithm, and is fully reproducible and takes only a few seconds. Depending on the application, HALE can be used with an automated lumen segmentation algorithm for on site evaluation of %stenosis, or be used with a semi-automated method offline or in a core-lab setting. It is our belief that an accurate QCT assessment tool would involve the coupling of an accurate lumen segmentation algorithm with an accurate algorithm for evaluation of %stenosis.

References

1. Kirisli, H.A., et al.: Standardized evaluation framework for evaluating coronary artery stenosis detection, stenosis quantification and lumen segmentation algorithms in computed tomography angiography. Med. Image Anal. **17**(8), 859–876 (2012)
2. Shahzad, R., et al.: Automatic segmentation, detection and quantification of coronary artery stenoses on CTA. Int. J. Cardiovasc. Imaging **29**(8), 1847–1859 (2013)
3. Sankaran, S., Grady, L., Taylor, C.A.: Fast computation of hemodynamic sensitivity to lumen segmentation uncertainty. IEEE TMI **34**(12), 2562–2571 (2015)
4. Huo, Y., et al.: CT-based diagnosis of diffuse coronary artery disease on the basis of scaling power laws. Radiology **268**(3), 694–701 (2013)
5. Lesage, D., et al.: A review of 3D vessel lumen segmentation techniques: models, features and extraction schemes. Med. Image Anal. **13**(6), 819–845 (2009)
6. Schaap, M., et al.: Standardized evaluation methodology and reference database for evaluating coronary artery centerline extraction algorithms. Med. Image Anal. **13**(5), 701–714 (2009)
7. Sherman, T.F.: On connecting large vessels to small. The meaning of Murray's law. J. Gen. Physiol. **78**(4), 431–453 (1981)
8. Breiman, L.: Random forests. Mach. Learn. **45**(1), 5–32 (2001)
9. Min, J.K., et al.: Diagnostic accuracy of fractional flow reserve from anatomic CT angiography. JAMA **308**(12), 1237–1245 (2012)

3D Near Infrared and Ultrasound Imaging of Peripheral Blood Vessels for Real-Time Localization and Needle Guidance

Alvin I. Chen$^{(\boxtimes)}$, Max L. Balter, Timothy J. Maguire, and Martin L. Yarmush

Rutgers University, Piscataway, NJ 08854, USA
alvin.chen@rutgers.edu

Abstract. This paper presents a portable imaging device designed to detect peripheral blood vessels for cannula insertion that are otherwise difficult to visualize beneath the skin. The device combines near infrared stereo vision, ultrasound, and real-time image analysis to map the 3D structure of subcutaneous vessels. We show that the device can identify adult forearm vessels and be used to guide manual insertions in tissue phantoms with increased first-stick accuracy compared to unassisted cannulation. We also demonstrate that the system may be coupled with a robotic manipulator to perform automated, image-guided venipuncture.

1 Introduction

Peripheral vascular access is one of the most commonly performed clinical procedures in the world and is a pivotal step in the diagnosis and treatment of many medical conditions. Oftentimes, however, it can be difficult to identify suitable blood vessels, particularly in patients with small vessels, dark skin, or a high body mass [1]. It may also be difficult to estimate the depth of the vessel or accurately insert the needle due to the lack of visibility through the skin.

A number of imaging tools have been introduced in recent years to assist clinicians in performing vascular access. Optical imaging systems most commonly utilize near infrared (NIR) light, as the decreased scattering of NIR light through tissue may allow otherwise occluded vessels up to 3 mm below the skin to be detected. Meanwhile, to visualize vessels beyond a few millimeters in depth, ultrasound (US) imaging is generally preferred. Unfortunately, when either imaging modality is used alone, trade-offs must be made between image resolution, penetration depth, and field-of-view (FOV). Furthermore, for the imaging tools to provide clinical benefit, improvements in vessel visualization must be translated into an increase in needle insertion accuracy.

To address these challenges, we have developed a portable device for peripheral vessel imaging (Fig. 1a) that uses NIR light to detect vessels over the FOV of an adult forearm; US to provide local high-resolution scans of a selected vessel target; and image analysis routines to segment and track the vessels in 3D at video rates. This paper describes the hardware and software design of the NIR+US imaging device and provides evidence of the device's clinical potential - both as a standalone tool and as a means for image-guided robotic cannulation.

© Springer International Publishing AG 2016
S. Ourselin et al. (Eds.): MICCAI 2016, Part III, LNCS 9902, pp. 388–396, 2016.
DOI: 10.1007/978-3-319-46726-9_45

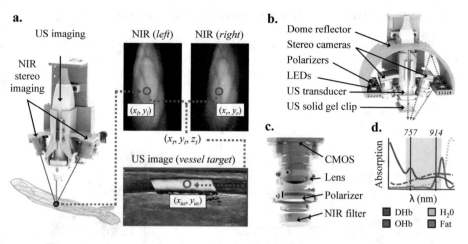

Fig. 1. Bimodal NIR+US vessel imaging. **(a)** The two imaging modalities are combined to provide 3D position information for needle guidance. **(b)** Main imaging hardware components. Red lines show the light path when using the inverted reflection imaging configuration. **(c)** Miniaturized optical components in each NIR camera subsystem. **(d)** 757 and 914 nm LEDs are used to maximize absorption from deoxyhemoglobin (DHb) and oxyhemoglobin (OHb) while minimizing absorption due to water and fat. (Color figure online)

2 Methods

2.1 Bimodal NIR+US Vessel Imaging

Near Infrared Stereo Imaging: The main components of the NIR imaging subsystem are shown in Figs. 1b and c. The light source consists of six arrays of light emitting diodes (LEDs) with wavelengths of 757 and 914 nm. The wavelengths were selected to maximize absorption due to blood while minimizing absorption due to water and fat [2] (Fig. 1d). A cylindrical reflector is used to redirect the upward emitted light back toward the skin in a diffuse manner (Fig. 1b). Two miniature CMOS cameras (VRmUsb12, VRMagic UAB, DEU) form a stereo vision system that acquires 752×480 images at 40 frames per second (fps). Each camera is coupled with a wide-angle (120°) lens, a 750 nm long-pass filter, and a NIR polarizing filter oriented orthogonal to a second set of polarizers above the LED arrays. The camera parameters are computed based on geometric calibration using circular control points [3].

Ultrasound Imaging: US transducers may be easily interchanged within the system depending on resolution requirements. In this study we used a high-frequency (18 MHz) linear array transducer with 100 μm element pitch (L18-10L30H-4, Telemed UAB, LTU) (Fig. 1a and b). The transducer provides B-mode and Color Doppler images at up to 40 fps and with sufficient resolution to delineate vessels 1 mm in diameter or greater. Solid polyacrylamide hydrogel is used in place of liquid ultrasound gel to improve device usability.

2.2 Segmentation, 3D Reconstruction, and Motion Tracking

The image analysis routines (Fig. 2) are executed on a laptop computer equipped with a CUDA-enabled GPU. During the procedure, the clinician selects a target vessel (x_t, y_t, z_t) for cannulation using the graphical user interface (GUI).

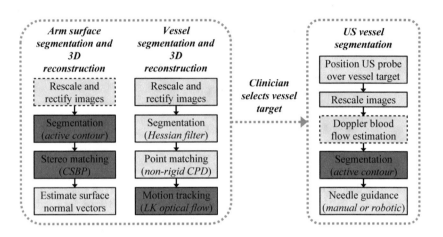

Fig. 2. Overview of the NIR and US image analysis framework. Gray boxes indicate routines performed on the CPU. Red boxes indicate GPU-enabled computations. (Color figure online)

Arm Segmentation Based on Active Contours: Gradient vector flow (GVF) based active contour segmentation [4] is then performed to extract the 2D region-of-interest (ROI) of the arm in each image (Fig. 3a). We used GVF active contours for its insensitivity to initialization and ability to move into concavities. The computation is accelerated with a CUDA-optimized OpenCL implementation of GVF [5]. In the first frame, the contour is initialized by threshold and morphological operations. In all subsequent frames, the contours are initialized using the segmentation result from the preceeding frame.

Vessel Segmentation Using Curvilinear Filters: The vessels are segmented based on the assumption that they have a curvilinear line- or tube-like structure. Specifically, a Difference of Gaussians filter is first used to enhance line structures in the image (Fig. 3b). A Hessian-based filtering method [6] is then performed to enhance tubular structures (Fig. 3c).

Stereo Reconstruction: The 3D positions (x_i, y_i, z_i) along each vessel are computed by extracting feature points i and performing point registration between the left and right stereo images. We use the local intensity maxima of the distance map of the vessel segmentation images as feature points (Fig. 3d). The points lie along the vessel centerlines (Fig. 3e), and the intensity of each point represents the vessel diameter about i. Non-rigid point registration [7] is constrained to

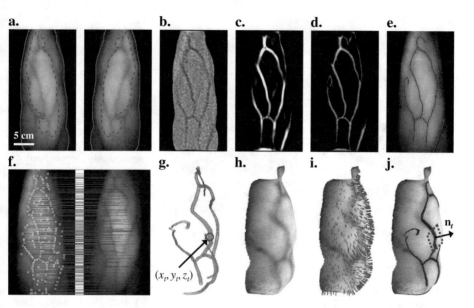

Fig. 3. Image analysis of NIR images. (a) Segmentation of left and right forearm images, including GVF initialization (blue) and final result (red). (b–e) Edge enhancement, Hessian vessel enhancement, distance transform, and skeleton. (f) Point registration (white squares) along epipolar lines (red stripes). (g) 3D reconstruction of vessels (red) and vessel target (blue circle). (h) 3D arm surface and (i) surface normals (blue arrows). (j) Normal vector $\mathbf{n_t}$ and tangent plane (blue square) about vessel target. (Color figure online)

occur only along the epipolar lines between the stereo cameras (Fig. 3f). The resulting 3D vessel geometry is shown in Fig. 3g.

In addition to vessel reconstruction, the 3D arm surface is also extracted when the full 6-DOF pose information $(x_i, y_i, z_i, \alpha_i, \beta_i, \gamma_i)$ about each feature point i can be utilized, i.e. for robotic guidance. Here, we use a CUDA-optimized belief propagation algorithm [8] for real-time dense stereo correspondence. Figure 3h shows the resulting 3D point cloud of the arm. The surface normal vectors about each 3D point (Fig. 3i) define the pose of the vessels below (Fig. 3j).

Vessel Motion Tracking: Pairwise vessel feature points are tracked between every frame using OpenCV CUDA-optimized Lucase-Kanade pyramidal optical flow [9]. Pairs are discarded if either point deviates from the epipolar line beyond a minimum tolerance. At every fifth frame, newly registered feature points are used to update the vessel target based on proximity to the optical flow position.

Vessel Segmentation from US Images: To isolate the target vessel in the US image after the transducer is lowered over the skin, we again apply the GVF active contour model for segmentation at every second frame. As with the forearm segmentation from NIR images, the contour is initialized in the first US frame by threshold and morphological operations. The US system may also be

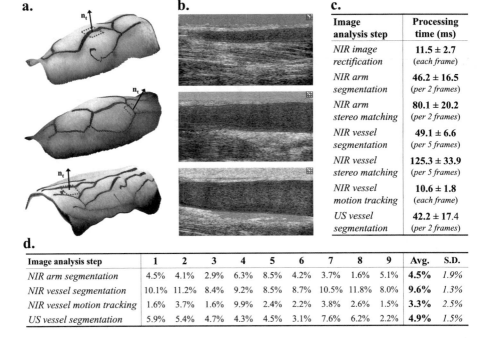

a.

b.

c.

Image analysis step	Processing time (ms)
NIR image rectification	**11.5 ± 2.7** (each frame)
NIR arm segmentation	**46.2 ± 16.5** (per 2 frames)
NIR arm stereo matching	**80.1 ± 20.2** (per 2 frames)
NIR vessel segmentation	**49.1 ± 6.6** (per 5 frames)
NIR vessel stereo matching	**125.3 ± 33.9** (per 5 frames)
NIR vessel motion tracking	**10.6 ± 1.8** (each frame)
US vessel segmentation	**42.2 ± 17.4** (per 2 frames)

d.

Image analysis step	1	2	3	4	5	6	7	8	9	Avg.	S.D.
NIR arm segmentation	4.5%	4.1%	2.9%	6.3%	8.5%	4.2%	3.7%	1.6%	5.1%	**4.5%**	*1.9%*
NIR vessel segmentation	10.1%	11.2%	8.4%	9.2%	8.5%	8.7%	10.5%	11.8%	8.0%	**9.6%**	*1.3%*
NIR vessel motion tracking	1.6%	3.7%	1.6%	9.9%	2.4%	2.2%	3.8%	2.6%	1.5%	**3.3%**	*2.5%*
US vessel segmentation	5.9%	5.4%	4.7%	4.3%	4.5%	3.1%	7.6%	6.2%	2.2%	**4.9%**	*1.5%*

Fig. 4. Imaging assessment on 9 adult subjects. (**a**) Representative NIR segmentation and 3D reconstruction results. (**b**) Representative US segmentation results, with initialization shown in blue and final contours in red. (**c**) Average per-frame processing times. (**d**) Root mean squared errors relative to manual segmentation and tracking. (Color figure online)

used to confirm blood flow by displaying Color Doppler images onto the GUI during the procedure. Finally, US is useful to visualize the needle within the tissue; vessels may also roll or deflect during insertion, and this may only be detected with US. Ongoing work is focused on implementing needle segmentation and tracking approaches as an added means of safety and image feedback.

3   Results and Discussion

3.1   Assessment of NIR+US Vessel Imaging in 9 Adult Subjects

The speed and accuracy of each image analysis step were investigated on 9 adult subjects (Fig. 4). Representative NIR segmentation, 3D reconstruction, and US segmentation results are shown in Figs. 4a and b. Figure 4c lists the average processing times for each step. Unsurprisingly, the stereo matching routines were the most demanding (80 and 125 ms). The remaining steps each required less than 50 ms. The overall frame rate was maintained at 10.8 fps by executing independent steps in parallel and carrying out demanding computations over multiple frames.

Figure 4d shows root mean squared errors (RMSE) for the arm segmentation, NIR vessel segmentation, vessel tracking, and US vessel segmentation steps over 30 s relative to manual segmentation and tracking. Errors are expressed as a % of the average per-frame segmentation area or motion displacement. The greatest error (9.6 %) was observed in the NIR vessel segmentation step, largely due to the removal of small disconnected segments during post-processing. However, removal of these segments is not expected to affect insertion accuracy, as clinicians preferentially target long, continuous vessels when performing venipuncture.

Average RMSE's for the NIR arm segmentation and US vessel segmentation steps were 4.5 % and 4.9 %, respectively. The errors were mostly due to inaccuracies in the initialization of the active contours. While the GVF algorithm is relatively more stable to initialization, the accuracy was nevertheless affected in a small number of cases. Currently we are investigating more robust approaches to initialize the GVF contour, including implementing region growing techniques or utilizing the US speckle statistics or Doppler image information.

The NIR vessel motion tracking step resulted in an average RMSE of 3.3 %. The largest tracking error occurred on Subject 4 due to a rapid arm motion that caused the vessel target to be lost. In such circumstances, the vessel target must be reselected. As an alternative to Lucas-Kanade optical flow tracking, dense optical flow algorithms [10] could potentially be implemented to enforce spatial smoothness constraints on the optical flow fields. It may also be possible to adapt the non-rigid point registration approach used here for stereo registration to perform motion tracking. However, the increased robustness of these alternative techniques will need to be weighed against their added computational costs.

NIR stereo reconstruction errors were not assessed in these studies, since such errors are more readily evaluated in conjunction with robotic cannulation. A focus of future studies will be to evaluate the reliability of the stereo correspondence approach under noise by comparing reconstruction errors in human subjects to previous results by our group on patterned tracking targets.

3.2   Comparison of Unassisted Manual, NIR+US Guided Manual, and NIR+US Guided Robotic Cannulations in Phantoms

In addition to using NIR+US imaging to assist in manual cannulations, it is also possible to couple the imaging system with a robotic needle insertion mechanism. The main advantage of robotic guidance is the ability to precisely update the position and orientation of the needle in real-time based on image feedback. Compared to manual cannulation, a robotic system may minimize errors due to misalignments between the needle and vessel, vessel rolling and deformation during insertion, and random arm motions. Previously, we described the mechanical design of a robotic venipuncture device [11, 12] (Fig. 5a) and demonstrated early results in multilayered gelatin-based phantoms simulating the mechanical, optical, and ultrasonic properties of human skin, vessels, and blood [13]. However, the full algorithmic framework had not been implemented, and the performance of the robot was not compared to manual techniques.

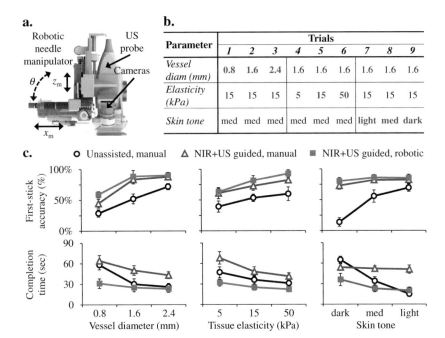

Fig. 5. Cannulation testing in tissue phantoms. (a) NIR+US imaging system coupled with robotic needle manipulator. (b) Phantom conditions used to assess cannulation performance. (c) First-stick accuracy and completion times of unassisted, image-guided, and robotic cannulation. Error bars indicate deviations for 12 trials.

Here, we evaluated the effects of vessel diameter, tissue elasticity, and skin tone on the first-stick accuracy and completion time of unassisted manual cannulation, NIR+US guided manual cannulation, and NIR+US guided robotic cannulation. Cannulations were performed on phantoms containing vessels with diameters of 0.8, 1.6, and 2.4 mm, tissue elasticities of 5, 15, and 50 kPa, and skin pigmentation matching that of light, medium, and dark toned patients (Fig. 5b). For each condition, 12 trials were conducted, and all manual trials were carried out by an expert clinician. Cannulation success was defined as the collection of at least 1 mL of blood mimicking fluid perfused through the phantom vessels.

The use of NIR+US guidance was observed to increase first-stick accuracy compared to unassisted cannulation, most notably in difficult conditions, i.e. small vessels, low elasticity, and dark skin tone (Fig. 5c). However, completion time was also seen to increase. Meanwhile, robotic cannulation increased accuracy and decreased completion time compared to manual techniques. These findings suggest a potential for improvement in venipuncture accuracy using image-guidance and for increased efficiency using robotic insertion. Additional measures of success, including the distance of the needle tip from the vessel center, the extent of random needle motion within the tissue, and the average blood volume collected, will be assessed in future studies. The effects of insertion parameters, such needle gauge, insertion speed, and insertion angle, will also be investigated. Finally, collaborative features between the imaging system, the robot, and the operator will be further developed to facilitate clinical translation.

4   Conclusion

In this paper, a device for 3D vessel imaging using NIR and US was introduced. Methods to segment and track the vessels, and to estimate 3D structure, were described and evaluated in human imaging trials. As demonstrated through cannulation experiments in tissue phantoms, the device may be used as an assistive tool or coupled with a robotic system for automated venipuncture. Further clinical development will entail a comprehensive investigation into the robustness of the imaging and image guidance approach, as well as the safety and usability of the robotic platform, in patients with difficult veins.

Acknowledgments. This work was supported by a National Institutes of Health (NIH) Research Grant (R01 EB020036), an NIH NIGMS Biotechnology Training Grant (T32 GM008339), an NIH Graduate Fellowship (F31 EB018191), and a National Science Foundation Graduate Fellowship (DGE 0937373).

References

1. Walsh, G.: Difficult peripheral venous access: recognizing and managing the patient at risk. J. Assoc. Vasc. Access **13**(4), 198–203 (2014)
2. Bashkatov, A.N., Genina, E.A., Kochubey, V.I., Tuchin, V.V.: Optical properties of human skin, subcutaneous and mucous tissues in the wavelength range from 400 to 2000 nm. J. Phys. D. Appl. Phys. **38**(15), 2543–2555 (2005)
3. Heikkila, J.: Geometric camera calibration using circular control points. IEEE Trans. Pattern. Anal. Mach. Intell. **22**(10), 1066–1077 (2000)
4. Xu, C., Prince, J.L.: Snakes, shapes, and gradient vector flow. IEEE Trans. Image Process. **7**(3), 359–369 (1998)
5. Smistad, E., Elster, A.C., Lindseth, F.: Real-time gradient vector flow on GPUs using openCL. J. Real Time Image Process **10**(1), 67–74 (2015)
6. Frangi, A.F., Niessen, W.J., Vincken, K.L., Viergever, M.A.: Multiscale vessel enhancement filtering. In: Wells, W.M., Colchester, A.C.F., Delp, S.L. (eds.) MICCAI 1998. LNCS, vol. 1496, p. 130. Springer, Heidelberg (1998)
7. Myronenko, A., Song, X.: Point set registration: coherent point drift. IEEE Trans. Pattern. Anal. Mach. Intell. **32**(12), 2262–2275 (2010)
8. Yang, Q., Wang, L., Yang, R., Stewénius, H., Nistér, D.: Stereo matching with color-weighted correlation, hierarchical belief propagation, and occlusion handling. IEEE Trans. Pattern. Anal. Mach. Intell. **31**(3), 492–504 (2010)
9. Lucas, B.D., Kanade, T.: An iterative image registration technique with an application to stereo vision. In: Proceedings of the 7th International Joint Conference on Artificial Intelligence, IJCAI 1981, vol. 2, pp. 674–679 (1981)
10. Brox, T., Bruhn, A., Papenberg, N., Weickert, J.: High accuracy optical flow estimation based on a theory for warping. In: Pajdla, T., Matas, J.G. (eds.) ECCV 2004. LNCS, vol. 3024, pp. 25–36. Springer, Heidelberg (2004)

11. Chen, A.I., Balter, M.L., Maguire, T.J., Yarmush, M.L.: Real-time needle steering in response to rolling vein deformation by an image-guided autonomous venipuncture robot. In: 2015 IEEE/RSJ International Conference on Intelligent Robots and Systems (IROS), pp. 2633–2638 (2015)
12. Balter, M.L., Chen, A.I., Maguire, T.J., Yarmush, M.L.: Adaptive kinematic control of a 9-DOF robotic venipuncture device based on stereo vision, ultrasound, and force guidance. IEEE Trans. Ind. Electron. (in press)
13. Chen, A.I., Balter, M.L., Chen, M.I., Gross, D., Alam, S.K., Maguire, T.J., Yarmush, M.L.: Multilayered tissue mimicking skin and vessel phantoms with tunable mechanical, optical, and acoustic properties. Med. Phys. **43**(6), 3117 (2016)

The Minimum Cost Connected Subgraph Problem in Medical Image Analysis

Markus Rempfler[1(✉)], Bjoern Andres[2], and Bjoern H. Menze[1]

[1] Department of Informatics and Institute for Advanced Study,
Technical University of Munich, Munich, Germany
markus.rempfler@tum.de

[2] Max Planck Institute for Informatics, Saarbrücken, Germany

Abstract. Several important tasks in medical image analysis can be stated in the form of an optimization problem whose feasible solutions are connected subgraphs. Examples include the reconstruction of neural or vascular structures under connectedness constraints.

We discuss the minimum cost connected subgraph (MCCS) problem and its approximations from the perspective of medical applications. We propose (a) objective-dependent constraints and (b) novel constraint generation schemes to solve this optimization problem exactly by means of a branch-and-cut algorithm. These are shown to improve scalability and allow us to solve instances of two medical benchmark datasets to optimality for the first time. This enables us to perform a quantitative comparison between exact and approximative algorithms, where we identify the geodesic tree algorithm as an excellent alternative to exact inference on the examined datasets.

1 Introduction

The *minimum cost connected subgraph* (MCCS) optimization problem arises in several medical image analysis tasks, most prominently for segmenting neural structures [1] or reconstructing vascular networks [2], where the maximum a posteriori (MAP) subgraph under connectedness constraints is inferred. Variations of this optimization problem have been proposed for anatomical labelling of vasculature [3] or artery-vein separation [4]. Imposing connectedness serves as regularizer, suppressing spurious detections and complementing incomplete observations, and it is often a requirement for further processing steps, e.g. if the reconstructed vasculature shall be used for biophysical simulations.

While [1–4] successfully solve an MCCS problem on heavily preprocessed, application-specific, sparse graphs, it would also be interesting to enforce connectedness on both very dense or large grid-graphs, for example in low-level segmentation tasks (Fig. 1, left), for 3D/4D reconstruction problems (Fig. 1, middle and right) or when it is not possible to reliably reduce the candidate graphs size.

Electronic supplementary material The online version of this chapter (doi:10.1007/978-3-319-46726-9_46) contains supplementary material, which is available to authorized users.

© Springer International Publishing AG 2016
S. Ourselin et al. (Eds.): MICCAI 2016, Part III, LNCS 9902, pp. 397–405, 2016.
DOI: 10.1007/978-3-319-46726-9_46

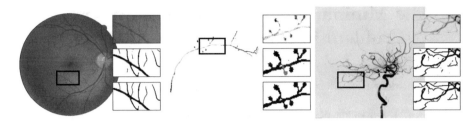

Fig. 1. *Examples for the MCCS on grid graphs.* **Left:** Segmentation of vasculature in retinal images. **Middle:** Reconstruction of a neuron from a 3D stack. Excessive disconnected components are shown in red for better visibility. **Right:** Delineation of vessels in a digital subtraction angiography (DSA) time series. The detail views show: raw image (**top**), without connectedness (**middle**) and with connectedness (**bottom**). Imposing connectedness constraints, i.e. requiring an MCCS, helps to reconnect disconnected terminals and remove spurious detections without penalizing thin tubular structures. (Color figure online)

In these cases, however, the computational complexity becomes challenging. In fact, it was shown to be NP-hard in [5]. Nowozin and Lampert [6] propose an exact algorithm that tightens an outer polyhedral relaxation of the connected subgraph polytope by cutting planes. However, without guarantee to terminate in polynomial time, it was found to be too slow to solve typical instances of medical benchmark datasets to optimality. To this end, two heuristical algorithms were proposed by Chen et al. [7] and Stühmer et al. [8]. They either use an approximative formulation of the connected subgraph polytope by means of a precomputed geodesic shortest path tree [8] or iteratively solve a surrogate problem that is based on altered weights of the original problem [7]. Both approaches are fast enough for medical applications and were reported to yield qualitatively promising results. A quantitative comparison, however, has been prevented by the prohibitively expensive computation of exact solutions to the MCCS problem.

In this paper, we revisit the MCCS in an integer linear programming (ILP) framework for MAP estimation under connectedness constraints. First, we contribute to the exact optimization by proposing (a) *objective-dependent constraints* that reduce the size of the polytope and hence, reduce the number of potential solutions to explore, and (b) *constraint generation strategies* beyond the standard *nearest* and *minimal* separator strategy, which we show to have a strong impact on the runtime of the ILP. Both propositions together enable us to compute the MCCS on several instances of two medical benchmark datasets – addressing vessel segmentation and neural fiber reconstruction – to optimality. Our second contribution is a first quantitative comparison of the exact algorithm and the two heuristics in terms of runtime, objective function and semantic error metrics.

2   Background

We are interested in the most likely binary labeling $\mathbf{x} \in \{0,1\}^{|V|}$ of the nodes V in the graph $G = (V, E)$. A node i is active if $x_i = 1$. By imposing connectedness constraints, i.e. $\mathbf{x} \in \Omega$, the MAP estimate becomes a MCCS problem:

$$\mathbf{x}^* = \underset{\mathbf{x} \in \{0,1\}^{|V|}}{\arg\max} P\left(\mathbf{X} = \mathbf{x} | I, \Omega\right) = \underset{\mathbf{x} \in \Omega}{\arg\max} P\left(\mathbf{X} = \mathbf{x} | I\right), \qquad (1)$$

where I is the image evidence and Ω denotes the set of $\mathbf{x}$ that are connected subgraphs of G. In this section, we discuss two formulations of Ω, the exact formulation that follows [6] and the geodesic tree formulation of [8].

2.1 Exact Connectedness

Following [6], we can describe Ω with the following set of linear inequality constraints

$$\forall i, j \in V, (i,j) \notin E : \forall \mathcal{S} \in S(i,j) \quad x_i + x_j - 1 \le \sum_{k \in \mathcal{S}} x_k, \qquad (2)$$

where $\mathcal{S}$ is a set of vertices that separate i and j, while $S(i,j)$ is the collection of all vertex separator sets for i and j. In other words, if two nodes i and j are active, then they are not allowed to be separable by any set of inactive nodes. Thus, a path of active nodes has to exist. In practice, this set of constraints is too large to be generated in advance. However, given a labelling $\mathbf{x}$ we can identify at least a subset of the violated connectedness constraints in polynomial time, add them to the ILP and search for a new feasible solution. This approach is known as *lazy constraint generation*. In Sect. 3.2, we detail on identifying and adding these constraints.

Rooted case. In many medical segmentation problems, it is reasonable to assume that a root node can be identified aforehand with an application-specific detector, manually or by a heuristic, such as picking the strongest node in the largest component. If a known root r exists, it suffices to check connectedness to the root node instead of all pairs of active nodes. The constraints in (2) then become

$$\forall i \in V \setminus \{r\}, (r,i) \notin E : \forall \mathcal{S} \in S(i,r) \quad x_i \le \sum_{k \in \mathcal{S}} x_k. \qquad (3)$$

2.2 Geodesic Tree Connectedness

Alternative to the exact description of all connected subgraphs that we discussed in the previous section, we can formulate a connectedness prior as in [8] on a *geodesic shortest path tree* $T(G) = (V, A \subseteq E)$ rooted in r. Here, $T(G)$ is precomputed based on the unary potentials, i.e. with edge weights defined as $f(i,j) = \frac{1}{2}\left(\max(w_i, 0) + \max(w_j, 0)\right)$. The set of feasible solutions is then given by the inequalities:

$$\forall i \in V \setminus \{r\}, (p,i) \in T(G) \quad x_i \le x_p, \qquad (4)$$

where p is the parent of i in the geodesic tree $T(G)$. With this set of constraints, a node i can only be active if his parent p in the geodesic tree is also active, thus connecting all active nodes to the root r along the branches of $T(G)$. Advantages of this approach are that only $|V| - 1$ constraints are necessary to describe the set of feasible solutions and that the relaxation is tight. On the other hand, the inequalities of (4) describe a strict subset of (3), unless $T(G) = G$. Hence it might discard an optimal solution that is feasible in (3).

3 Methods

Given the probabilistic model $P(\mathbf{X} = \mathbf{x}|I)$ of (1) is a random field over $G = (V, E)$, we can write its MAP estimator $\mathbf{x}^* = \arg\max_{\mathbf{x} \in \{0,1\}} P(\mathbf{X} = \mathbf{x}|I, \Omega)$ as an ILP. We will assume for the remaining part that $P(\mathbf{X} = \mathbf{x}|I) = \prod_{i \in V} P(x_i|I)$, leading to the ILP:

$$\text{minimize} \quad \sum_{i \in V} w_i x_i, \tag{5}$$

$$\text{s.t.} \quad \mathbf{x} \in \Omega, \tag{6}$$

$$\mathbf{x} \in \{0, 1\}^{|V|}, \tag{7}$$

where (6) are the connectedness constraints, i.e. either (3) or (4), (7) enforces integrality, and w_i are the weights that can be derived as $w_i = -\log \frac{P(x_i=1|I)}{1-P(x_i=1|I)}$. Higher order terms of the random field can be incorporated by introducing auxiliary binary variables and according constraints as done in [2]. Note, however, that [7] reported problem instances with weak or no pairwise potentials – as we are addressing them here – to be amongst the most difficult.

3.1 Objective-Dependent Constraints

Given the problem with unary terms, we observe that, for any connected component $\mathcal{U} \subset V$ composed of *unfavourable* nodes only, i.e. $\forall i \in \mathcal{U}, w_i > 0$, it can only be active in the optimal solution if there are at least two active nodes in its neighbourhood:

$$\forall i \in \mathcal{U} \quad 2x_i \leq \sum_{j \in \cup_{k \in \mathcal{U}} \delta(k) \setminus \mathcal{U}} x_j, \tag{8}$$

where $\delta(k)$ is the set of neighbouring nodes to k. In other words, unfavourable nodes can not form a leaf in the optimal solution (otherwise, removing the unfavourable nodes would give us a better solution without loosing connectedness). In the special case of $|\mathcal{U}| = 1$, we can add the constraint from the beginning. This removes feasible solutions from Ω that are a priori known to be suboptimal, hence reducing the search space in the optimization and making it unnecessary to add a large set of separator inequalities.

Higher-order weights. Even though we only define (8) for unary weights, it is possible to adapt the constraint to higher-order models by changing the condition to $w_i + \min_{j \in \delta(i)} w_{ij} > 0$, provided the pairwise weights w_{ij} are only introduced for neighbouring nodes i, j such that $(i, j) \in E$.

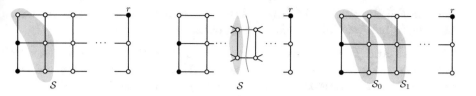

Fig. 2. *Constraint generation strategies.* Illustration of the nearest separator (left), minimal separator (middle) and *k*-nearest (right) strategies. Active nodes are shown in black, inactive nodes are white and the identified separator sets S are marked in blue. S is subsequently used to generate the corresponding constraint in (2) or (3). (Color figure online)

3.2   Constraint Generation Strategies

The extensive number of inequalities needed for (3) makes it necessary to identify violated constraints during the optimization and add them to the problem. We note that it suffices to treat individual connected components as one entitity, since establishing a connection automatically connects all pairs of nodes between them. Identifying violated constraints boils down to finding a vertex separator set S between two disconnected, active components in the current solution. The constraints corresponding to S are then generated according to (2) or (3) for all nodes in the given connected component.

At the heart of this technique is the observation that only a subset of inequalities is active at the optimum of a given problem instance. However, depending on the choice of the inequalities that we add in each step, we may explore (and therefore construct) different parts of the polytope Ω, most likely requiring a different number of iterations.

In the following, we first review the two standard strategies, namely the *nearest* and *minimal* separator, and then propose several novel, alternative strategies.

Nearest separator. In this standard approach, the vertex separator set in the immediate neighbourhood of the active component is picked for generating the new constraint. This strategy has been used, for example, in [2]. It is motivated by its simplicity and the fact that it often coincides with the minimal separator strategy for small components.

Minimal separator. A minimal (in terms of $|S|$) separator set is obtained by solving a max-flow problem between any two disjoint active components at hand and selecting the smaller vertex set on either side of the resulting min-cut. For the max-flow, we set the flow capacity c in edge (i, j) as $c(i, j) = \max(1 - x_i, 1 - x_j)$. The strategy was applied in [6].

Equidistant separator. Alternatively, we can identify the separator set S that is equidistant to the current active component and all other components by running a BFS from either side. Similar to the max-flow of the minimal separator, the distance measure is only accounting for non-active nodes. This strategy originates in the observation that the weakest evidence between two components is often found half-way into the connecting path.

k-Nearest and k-Interleave. We run a BFS from the active component C and collect the k (disjoint) separator sets $\{\mathcal{S}_n\}_{n=0}^{k-1}$ composed of all nodes with identical distance. The search terminates if k equals the number of nodes in C or if another active node is reached. For the k-interleave, only separators with even distance are chosen. The intuition behind these strategies is that a wider range of neighbours (and their neighbours) has to be considered for the next solution.

4   Experiments and Results

Datasets and Preprocessing. We conduct experiments on two medical datasets: First, on the DRIVE database of retinal images [9], each being 565×584 px. We use the probability estimates $P(x_i = 1|I)$ for a pixel i being vasculature from the recent state-of-the-art approach of [10] for our unaries. Second, we run experiments on the olfactory projection fibers (OPF) dataset [11], composed of 8 3D confocal microscopy image stacks. We use the stacks prepared in [1], where we estimate $P(x_i = 1|I)$ of voxel i being part of the fiber by a logistic regression on the image intensities. We segment the nerve fiber under the requirement of connectedness on the 3D grid graph of $256 \times 256 \times n$ nodes with $n \in \{30, \ldots, 51\}$ depending on the case. The probability $P(x_i = 1|I)$ of voxel i being part of the fiber is estimated by a logistic regression on the image intensities. Both datasets are illustrated in Fig. 1.

Optimization. We solve the ILP (5) by the branch-and-cut algorithm of the solver Gurobi [12] with a default relative gap of 10^{-4}. Objective-dependent constraints for single nodes (Sect. 3.1) are added from the beginning. For the exact connectedness (Sect. 2.1), the strategies described in Sect. 3.2 are implemented as a callback: Whenever the solver arrives at an integral solution $\mathbf{x}'$, violated constraints are identified and added to the model. If no such violation is found, i.e. $\mathbf{x}'$ is already connected, then it is accepted as new current solution $\mathbf{x}^*$. For the geodesic tree connectedness (Sect. 2.2), all constraints are added at once. In order to arrive at a fair comparison, we define the root node for both approaches.

Experiment: Objective-dependent constraints. To examine the impact of the objective-dependent constraints, we subsample 25 subimages of 64×64 px from the DRIVE instances and run the ILP once with and once without the additional first order constrains of (8). As shown in Fig. 3, we find that all strategies benefit from the additional constraints.

Experiment: Comparing exact and approximative algorithms. We compare exact and geodesic tree MCCS on both datasets. On 2D images, we additionally compare to the method by [7] called Topocut. As a baseline, we compute the maximum connected component in the non-constrained solution (Max-comp). The results are presented in Fig. 4 and Table 1 (additional information *per instance* is provided in the supplement). We observe that 6/8 and 12/20 instances

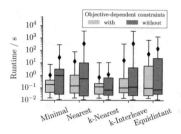

Fig. 3. Runtime with and without the proposed objective-dependent constraints on 64×64 instances. Mean values are depicted by ♦, whiskers span $[\min, \max]$ values. Unsolved instances are excluded for readability. We find that all strategies benefit from the additional constraints. Additional *per-instance* information can be found in the supplement.

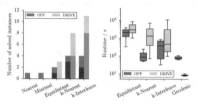

Fig. 4. Left: Number of solved instances per strategy. The darker bar indicates how often a strategy was the *fastest* to solve an instance. **Right:** Runtime on solved instances. Strategies with too few solved instances are not included. k-Nearest and k-Interleave are found to be the most successful exact strategies

Table 1. Segmentation scores in terms of **F1**-score, (**P**recision, **R**ecall) in % on the solved instances. All approaches outperform the baseline (MaxComp), while no significant difference can be found between them

	OPF		DRIVE	
	F1	(P, R)	F1	(P, R)
Maxcomp	68.5	(67.7, 71.9)	78.7	(87.2, 72.1)
Geodesic	76.2	(69.1, 85.4)	80.1	(86.2, 75.2)
Topocut	-	-	80.1	(86.4, 74.9)
Exact	76.2	(69.1, 85.4)	80.1	(86.2, 75.2)

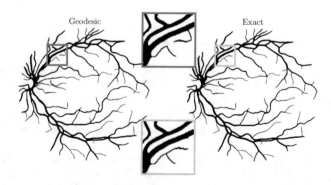

Fig. 5. Comparison of exact and approximative connectedness: Major differences as the one indicated are encountered mainly if solutions are competing under the model $P(\mathbf{X} = \mathbf{x}|I)$ and thus almost equivalent w.r.t. objective value.

were solved to optimality with our propositions, while standard strategies solved ≤ 1. k-Nearest and k-interleave are the two most successful exact strategies in terms of solved instances and speed. In terms of segmentation scores, the two heuristics are on par with the exact algorithm, while all of them outperform the baseline. We find the geodesic approach to match the exact solution with respect to objective values in all instances (within a relative difference of 10^{-4}), whereas Topocut often obtains slightly lower objective values than the geodesic approach. A qualitative comparison between an exact and geodesic solution is presented in Fig. 5.

5   Conclusions

We have shown that exact optimization of the MCCS, as it is typical for neural and vascular structure reconstruction tasks, strongly benefits from the proposed objective-dependent constraints and the constraint generation strategies. In a first quantitative comparison between exact and approximative approaches on two datasets, we found that the geodesic tree formulation is a fast, yet highly competitive alternative to exact optimization.

While we focussed on large grid-graphs that are most important for low-level segmentation and reconstruction, we expect that our findings transfer to MCCS problems and related ILP-based formulations on sparse graphs, e.g. those discussed in [1–4], and thus consider this a promising direction for future work. Besides, it will be interesting to investigate the effect of our propositions in the presence of higher-order terms.

Acknowledgments. With the support of the Technische Universität München – Institute for Advanced Study, funded by the German Excellence Initiative (and the European Union Seventh Framework Programme under grant agreement n 291763).

References

1. Türetken, E., Benmansour, F., Andres, B., et al.: Reconstructing curvilinear networks using path classifiers and integer programming. IEEE TPAMI, preprint (2016)
2. Rempfler, M., Schneider, M., Ielacqua, G.D., et al.: Reconstructing cerebrovascular networks under local physiological constraints by integer programming. Med. Image Anal. **25**(1), 86–94 (2015)
3. Robben, D., Türetken, E., Sunaert, S., et al.: Simultaneous segmentation and anatomical labeling of the cerebral vasculature. Med. Image Anal. **32**, 201–215 (2016)
4. Payer, C., et al.: Automated integer programming based separation of arteries and veins from thoracic CT images. Med. Image Anal. preprint (2016)
5. Vicente, S., Kolmogorov, V., Rother, C.: Graph cut based image segmentation with connectivity priors. In: Proceedings of CVPR, pp. 1–8 (2008)
6. Nowozin, S., Lampert, C.H.: Global connectivity potentials for random field models. In: Proceedings of CVPR, pp. 818–825 (2009)

7. Chen, C., Freedman, D., Lampert, C.H.: Enforcing topological constraints in random field image segmentation. In: Proceedings of CVPR, pp. 2089–2096 (2011)
8. Stühmer, J., Schroder, P., Cremers, D.: Tree shape priors with connectivity constraints using convex relaxation on general graphs. In: Proceedings of ICCV, pp. 2336–2343 (2013)
9. Staal, J.J., Abramoff, M.D., Niemeijer, M., et al.: Ridge based vessel segmentation in color images of the retina. IEEE TMI **23**(4), 501–509 (2004)
10. Ganin, Y., Lempitsky, V.: N^4-fields: neural network nearest neighbor fields for image transforms. In: Cremers, D., Reid, I., Saito, H., Yang, M.-H. (eds.) ACCV 2014. LNCS, vol. 9004, pp. 536–551. Springer, Heidelberg (2015). doi:10.1007/978-3-319-16808-1_36
11. Brown, K.M., Barrionuevo, G., Canty, A.J., et al.: The DIADEM data sets. Neuroinformatics **9**(2), 143–157 (2011)
12. Gurobi Optimization, I.: Gurobi Optimizer Reference Manual (2015)

ASL-incorporated Pharmacokinetic Modelling of PET Data With Reduced Acquisition Time: Application to Amyloid Imaging

Catherine J. Scott[1]([✉]), Jieqing Jiao[1], Andrew Melbourne[1],
Jonathan M. Schott[2], Brian F. Hutton[3,4], and Sébastien Ourselin[1,2]

[1] Translational Imaging Group, CMIC, University College London, London, UK
catherine.scott.14@ucl.ac.uk
[2] Dementia Research Centre, Institute of Neurology,
University College London, London, UK
[3] Institute of Nuclear Medicine, University College London, London, UK
[4] Centre for Medical Radiation Physics, University of Wollongong,
Wollongong, NSW, Australia

Abstract. Pharmacokinetic analysis of Positron Emission Tomography (PET) data typically requires at least one hour of image acquisition, which poses a great disadvantage in clinical practice. In this work, we propose a novel approach for pharmacokinetic modelling with significantly reduced PET acquisition time, by incorporating the blood flow information from simultaneously acquired arterial spin labelling (ASL) magnetic resonance imaging (MRI). A relationship is established between blood flow, measured by ASL, and the transfer rate constant from plasma to tissue of the PET tracer, leading to modified PET kinetic models with ASL-derived flow information. Evaluation on clinical amyloid imaging data from an Alzheimer's disease (AD) study shows that the proposed approach with the simplified reference tissue model can achieve amyloid burden estimation from 30 min [18F]florbetapir PET data and 5 min simultaneous ASL MR data, which is comparable with the estimation from 60 min PET data (mean error = −0.03). Conversely, standardised uptake value ratio (SUVR), the alternative measure from the data showed a positive bias in areas of higher amyloid burden (mean error = 0.07).

1 Introduction

Position Emission Tomography (PET) is currently the most sensitive *in vivo* molecular imaging technique to provide a non-invasive assay of the human body. Dynamic PET image data acquired following the injection of a radioactive tracer allows the use of pharmacokinetic modelling techniques to quantify a range of biological, physiological and biochemical parameters. However, a typical dynamic PET scan requires at least 1 h to sufficiently cover the underlying processes. The long scan duration is prohibitive for routine clinical use, where time is limited, and data integrity is risked by the increased chance of subject motion.

© Springer International Publishing AG 2016
S. Ourselin et al. (Eds.): MICCAI 2016, Part III, LNCS 9902, pp. 406–413, 2016.
DOI: 10.1007/978-3-319-46726-9_47

Currently clinical imaging in PET is often performed using single time point estimates (static imaging) of tracer uptake, such as the standardised uptake value ratio (SUVR). SUVR, a semi-quantitative measure of uptake, is the ratio of the activity concentration within a region relative to the concentration in a tissue which is free from the imaging target, called the reference region. It usually requires 10 min of PET data, which are acquired once non-specifically bound tracer reaches equilibrium between a region and the reference tissue, approximately 50 min or more post injection. This measure is expected to correlate with fully quantitative estimates derived from the full dynamic PET data. However, changes in blood flow affect the delivery of the tracer to tissue and consequently alter the tracer concentration in the tissue when a static image is acquired. Without the blood flow information contained in the early dynamic data, there is no way to account for the influence of the changes in blood flow, thus SUVR values can be biased. This has been highlighted in longitudinal studies, where pathophysiological changes in blood flow have caused spurious changes in SUVR values which do not reflect imaging target abundance [1]. The estimates derived by kinetic modelling are not biased in this way, as the full dynamic curve contains blood flow information, which is parametrised within the model.

In neuroimaging, cerebral blood flow can be measured using arterial spin labelled (ASL) MRI, where magnetically tagged blood is used as an endogenous contrast agent. With the advent of PET-MRI scanners, this information can be acquired concurrently with PET data. Therefore the blood flow information from the ASL can be used in pharmacokinetic analysis when the early part of a dynamic PET scan, which involves blood flow, is not collected. This will lead to the reduction of PET acquisition time needed to perform pharmacokinetic modelling.

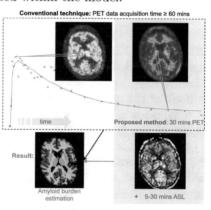

Fig. 1. Dynamic PET acquisition for amyloid burden quantification and time reduction for the proposed method.

In this work, we propose a novel approach for combining PET and ASL information to derive the parameters of interest with a greatly reduced scanning time, Fig. 1. To our knowledge, this is the first time that ASL blood flow estimates have been used to perform PET kinetic analysis to reduce image acquisition time. We evaluated the proposed approach in an AD study using [18F]florbetapir, a PET radiotracer that binds to amyloid-β, which is considered to be an important target in the AD brain.

2   Methods

2.1   CBF Estimation with ASL MRI

The cerebral blood flow (CBF) map is estimated from pseudo continuous arterial spin labelling (PCASL) data using the relationship established in [2]. The parameter values used in this work were $0.9\,\mathrm{ml/g}$ for the plasma/tissue partition coefficient, a blood $T1$ value of $1650\,\mathrm{ms}$, and a labelling efficiency of 0.85.

2.2   Amyloid-β Burden Estimation with SRTM

In this work, the simplified reference tissue model (SRTM) [3] was used to quantify the PET data. SRTM describes the tracer-target interaction using a single tissue compartment model. Using the tracer time activity curve in the reference region $C_R(t)$ as an input function, the operational equation between the tracer time activity curve in the target tissue $C_T(t)$ and $C_R(t)$ is formulated as:

$$C_T(t) = R_1 C_R(t) + \left(k_2 - R_1 \frac{k_2}{1 + BP_{ND}}\right) C_R(t) \otimes e^{-\frac{k_2}{1 + BP_{ND}}t}, \qquad (1)$$

where t denotes time and $t = 0$ at tracer injection, R_1 is the local rate of delivery in the target tissue relative to reference tissue, k_2 is the rate constant from target tissue to blood, BP_{ND} is the binding potential that is proportional to the density of amyloid-β, and $\otimes$ denotes the convolution operator. Cerebellar grey matter is used as the reference region to derive $C_R(t)$ as it is considered to be devoid of amyloid-β in this study [4]. BP_{ND}, as the outcome measure of interest to represent the amyloid-β burden, can then be estimated together with R_1 and k_2 by performing curve-fitting using (1) with $C_T(t)$ and $C_R(t)$ extracted from PET data acquired from tracer injection over a sufficient duration. We used a linearised version of SRTM [5] to calculate BP_{ND}, R_1 and k_2 from dynamic PET data of 0:60 min as the gold standard.

2.3   SRTM with Incomplete PET Scan and CBF

Population-Based Extrapolation of Reference Input $C_{R(t)}$. To estimate BP_{ND} using the PET data where the early part from the tracer injection is absent ($t \in [t_s, t_e]$, $t_s > 0$), firstly extrapolation is required to have the reference input $C_R(t)$ for $t \in [0, t_s]$ so that the convolution term in (1) can be calculated. In this work the whole reference input $C_R(t)$ for $t \in [0, t_e]$ was generated using a single tissue compartment model $C_R(t) = K_1' e^{-k_2' t} \otimes \alpha AIF(t)$. If we assume $AIF(t)$, $t \in [0, t_e]$ is a population arterial input function with α being an individual scaling factor, k_2' a population rate constant from reference tissue to blood, and K_1' an individual rate constant from blood to reference tissue, then $K_1' \alpha$ can be estimated by scaling a measured population-based reference input curve $C_R^p(t)$, $t \in [0, t_e]$ to match the individual $C_R(t)$, $t \in [t_s, t_e]$ to generate $C_R(t)$, $t \in [0, t_e]$.

R_1 Estimation with CBF. ASL is used to measure the CBF, flow denoted by F, which is converted into a pseudo R_1 estimate to use in SRTM. R_1 is defined as $R_1 = K_1/K_1'$ where K_1 is the rate constant from blood to target tissue and K_1' is the rate constant from blood to reference tissue.

Based on the Renkin-Crone model, the relationship between K_1 and F can be described as

$$K_1 = EF = \left(1 - e^{-\frac{PS}{F}}\right) F, \qquad (2)$$

where E denotes the net extraction, P is the vessel permeability and S the surface area. Under common physiological conditions of flow, where PS is high ($> 3\,\mathrm{ml}$ $\cdot 100\,\mathrm{g}^{-1} \cdot \mathrm{min}^{-1}$), the relationship between K_1 and flow F is linear. In the absence of knowledge on PS across the brain, we assume that it is sufficiently high such that the relationship between K_1 and F, and in turn the relationship between R_1 and F, can be approximated as a linear function. Linear regression between R_1 and F was performed on a group of subjects, and the linear relationship was then applied to a different group of subjects to convert CBF to a pseudo R_1 value for estimating BP_{ND} with incomplete PET data.

SRTM with CBF-derived R_1 and Extrapolated $C_{R(t)}$. Rewrite (1) as $C_T'(t) = \phi C_R(t) \otimes e^{-\theta t}$, where $C_T'(t) = C_T(t) - R_1 C_R(t)$ is calculated from the $C_T(t)$ and $C_R(t)$ extracted from the measured PET data for $t \in [t_s, t_e]$, and R_1 is derived from the CBF. Here, $\phi = k_2 - R_1 k_2/(1 + BP_{ND})$ and $\theta = k_2/(1 + BP_{ND})$ are unknown. To solve ϕ and θ, we used the basis functions defined in [5] to precalculate the convolution term using the extrapolated $C_R(t)$, $t \in [0, t_e]$ with a range of biologically plausible values for θ. BP_{ND} and k_2 are then derived from ϕ, θ and the CBF-derived R_1.

3   Experiments and Results

Data. We evaluated the proposed method on data from 11 cognitively normal subjects participating in Insight 46, a neuroimaging sub-study of the MRC National Survey of Health and Development, who underwent amyloid PET and multi-modal MR imaging on a Siemens Biograph mMR PET/MR scanner. List mode PET data were acquired for 60 min following intravenous injection of [18F]florbetapir, a radiotracer that binds to amyloid-β. For PET image reconstruction, simultaneously acquired structural MR was used to synthesise CT data and calculate the μ-map [6]. Dynamic PET data were binned into 15 s × 4, 30 s × 8, 60 s × 9, 180 s × 2, 300 s × 8 time frames, and reconstructed using the manufacturer's software with corrections for dead-time, attenuation, scatter (based on the synthesised CT), randoms and normalisation. PCASL data were acquired using a 3D GRASE readout with voxels of 1.88 × 1.88× 4 mm. 10 control-label pairs were acquired with a pulse duration and post labelling delay of 1800 ms.

Data Processing Framework. T1-weighted images were parcellated [7] into amygdala, pons, brainstem, cerebellum (white and grey separately), hippocampus, cerebral white matter, putamen, thalamus and 6 cortical grey matter

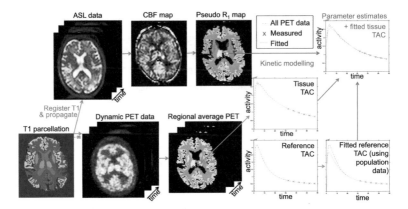

Fig. 2. Overview- parcellation is registered to PET and ASL to calculate regional average values. ASL data is converted into CBF-derived R_1 values using the linear regression relationship. A population reference tissue time activity curve of 0:60 min combined with the measured reference tissue data (30:60 min) is used with the CBF-derived R_1 and the measured PET tissue data (30:60 min), to apply the modified simplified reference tissue model to estimate BP_{ND}.

regions, with left and right hemispheres combined. The T1-weighted image was rigidly registered to both ASL and PET space, and the transformation was propagated to the parcellation. Regional average CBF values were calculated, and the PET time activity curves were averaged across the region prior to kinetic modelling. PET data acquired during 30:60 min were used to evaluate the proposed method. To estimate the reference region activity in the missing time frames, a population averaged reference input was extracted from 14 age matched subjects with 60 min [18F]florbetapir PET data. To establish the relationship between the CBF and R_1 values, linear regression was performed on data from 5 subjects and the proposed approach was tested on the remaining 6 subjects. A summary of the data processing framework is shown in Fig. 2.

3.1   Comparison of Proposed Method with Gold Standard

Figure 3a shows BP_{ND}, the measure of the amyloid burden, estimated using the proposed method with 30:60 min data plotted against the gold standard using the full 60 min dynamic data. Linear regression of all subjects and regions shows that the proposed method offers a good approximation of the gold standard as it closely follows the line of identity (blue dashed line), which is within the 95 % confidence interval (CI) of the regression (shaded area). Furthermore, subject specific Pearson correlation coefficients, ρ, show a high linear correlation.

The alternative measure used in clinical practice, $SUVR - 1$, was calculated from PET data over 50:60 min for comparison, Fig. 3b. Whilst ρ is still high for each subject, a clear bias is shown as $SUVR - 1$ overestimates the binding potential at higher values. The mean error quantifies the bias between the estimates and the gold standard which is 0.0740 for $SUVR - 1$, indicative of the

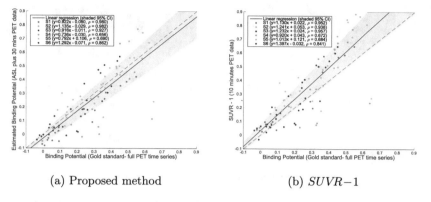

(a) Proposed method   (b) $SUVR-1$

Fig. 3. Estimated amyloid burden against the gold standard value calculated using full PET time series. (Color figure online)

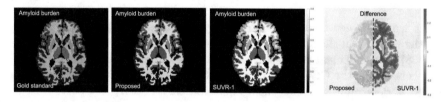

Fig. 4. Regional average binding potential maps for (left to right) gold standard, proposed method, $SUVR - 1$, difference maps compared to gold standard.

systematic overestimation, compared to -0.0311 for the proposed method. The proposed method also has a lower mean square error (0.0151 compared to 0.0247 for $SUVR-1$), and variance (0.0142 compared to 0.0194 for $SUVR-1$). Figure 4 shows BP_{ND} maps for a subject, comparing the gold standard with the proposed method and $SUVR - 1$ regionally. The proposed method shows good agreement with the gold standard, with slight overestimation of the cortical white matter. For the $SUVR - 1$ estimation, amyloid burden is greatly overestimated within both grey and white matter structures. The difference map shows that the errors in the proposed method are far lower than for $SUVR - 1$.

3.2 Influence of R_1 Estimation on Amyloid Quantification

Whilst Fig. 3a demonstrates a high similarity between binding potential estimation using the gold standard and the proposed method, there is a noise component which introduces variation around the line of identity. This is due to noise in the PET data, noise in the CBF-derived R_1 estimate from the ASL data, and inaccuracies in the estimation of the reference tissue input.

To demonstrate the influence of the CBF-derived R_1 estimate using ASL data, the proposed method was applied using the R_1 estimated using the gold standard technique instead of the CBF-derived R_1. The population input function and 30:60 min PET data were used as before. This represents the optimal

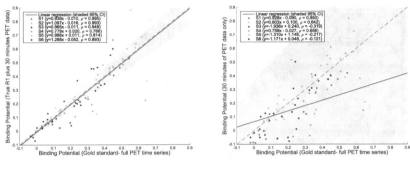

(a) 30:60 mins PET + gold standard R_1 (b) 30:60 mins PET data only

Fig. 5. Estimated binding potential plotted against the gold standard value calculated using full PET time series

case in which R_1 can be determined exactly from the ASL data. Figure 5a shows that the variance in the binding potential estimate has been reduced (from 0.0142 to 0.008), and the linear regression line lies along identity with a narrow CI. This is expected since the CBF map from the ASL is noisy, and linear regression performed to determine the relationship between CBF and R_1 was performed with only 5 subjects, and therefore may not be generalisable. However, for the data used in this study the estimation of R_1 from CBF is sufficiently accurate that the BP_{ND} estimates between the proposed method using CBF-derived R_1 and gold standard R_1 are comparable and there is a reduced bias in the estimates.

Figure 5b compares BP_{ND} estimation using 30:60 min PET data only to the gold standard to demonstrate the need of a CBF-derived R_1. Due to the lack of data to support the kinetic modelling, the results are noisy and extreme parameter estimates occurred for some regions. These points are beyond the display range in Fig. 5b and have skewed the linear regression such that it no longer follows the identity line, and the 95 % CI extends beyond that shown.

4 Discussion and Conclusion

This work demonstrates that the proposed method produces estimates of amyloid burden which are comparable to full pharmacokinetic modelling of 0:60 min [18F]florbetapir PET data, using just 30:60 min of PET data together with blood flow information from ASL. The proposed method is more accurate than the simplified estimate of amyloid burden, $SUVR - 1$, which showed a positive bias especially at higher binding potential values. The results of the proposed technique depend on the CBF-derived R_1 estimate from the ASL data. The ASL data used here were acquired for only 5 min without motion correction, and thus susceptible to artefacts and noise. Linear regression between CBF and R_1 using just 5 subjects could produce errors which may propagate to the binding potential estimation. To reduce the influence of errors in the CBF maps on the parameter estimation, a more complex kinetic model will be explored in future work to penalise the deviation of R_1 estimation from the CBF-derived R_1 value. The relationship between CBF from ASL and PET R_1 will be further explored to tune this regularisation scheme. The application of this technique to PET tracers which bind to other biological targets of interest will also be explored.

Acknowledgments. This work was supported by the EPSRC UCL Centre for Doctoral Training in Medical Imaging (EP/L016478/1), UCL Leonard Wolfson Experimental Neurology Centre (PR/ylr/18575), EPSRC (EP/H046410/1, EP/J020990/1, EP/K005278), MRC (MR/J01107X/1), NIHR UCLH Biomedical Research Centre (inc. High Impact Initiative, BW.mn.BRC10269). Insight 1946 receives funding from Alzheimer's Research UK (ARUK-PG2014-1946), MRC Dementia Platform UK (CSUB19166) and The Wolfson Foundation, and support from Avid Radiopharmaceuticals, a wholly owned subsidiary of Eli Lilly. We are grateful to the Insight 46 participants for their involvement in this study.

References

1. Cselényi, Z., Farde, L.: Quantification of blood flow-dependent component in estimates of beta-amyloid load obtained using quasi-steady-state standardized uptake value ratio. J. Cereb. Blood Flow Metab. **35**, 1–9 (2015)
2. Melbourne, A., Toussaint, N., Owen, D., Simpson, I., Anthopoulos, T., De Vita, E., Atkinson, D., Ourselin, S.: Niftyfit: a software package for multi-parametric model-fitting of 4D magnetic resonance imaging data. Neuroinformatics **14**(3), 319–337 (2016)
3. Lammertsma, A., Hume, S.: Simplified reference tissue model for PET receptor studies. Neuroimage **158**(4), 153–158 (1996)
4. Klunk, W.E., Engler, H., Nordberg, A., Wang, Y., Blomqvist, G., Holt, D.P., Bergström, M., Savitcheva, I., Huang, G.F., Estrada, S., Ausén, B., Debnath, M.L., Barletta, J., Price, J.C., Sandell, J., Lopresti, B.J., Wall, A., Koivisto, P., Antoni, G., Mathis, C., Långström, B.: Imaging brain Amyloid in Alzheimer's disease with pittsburgh compound-B. Ann. Neurol. **55**(3), 306–319 (2004)
5. Gunn, R.N., Lammertsma, A.A., Hume, S.P., Cunningham, V.J.: Parametric imaging of ligand-receptor binding in PET using a simplified reference region model. NeuroImage **6**(4), 279–287 (1997)
6. Burgos, N., Cardoso, M.J., Thielemans, K., Modat, M., Dickson, J., Schott, J.M., Atkinson, D., Arridge, S.R., Hutton, B.F., Ourselin, S.: Multi-contrast attenuation map synthesis for PET/MR scanners: assessment on FDG and florbetapir PET tracers. Eur. J. Nucl. Med. Mol. Imaging **42**(9), 1447–1458 (2015)
7. Cardoso, M.J., Modat, M., Wolz, R., Melbourne, A., Cash, D., Rueckert, D., Ourselin, S.: Geodesic information flows: spatially-variant graphs and their application to segmentation and fusion. IEEE TMI **99**, 1976–1988 (2015)

Probe-Based Rapid Hybrid Hyperspectral and Tissue Surface Imaging Aided by Fully Convolutional Networks

Jianyu Lin[1,2(✉)], Neil T. Clancy[1,3], Xueqing Sun[1,3], Ji Qi[1,3], Mirek Janatka[4,5], Danail Stoyanov[4,5], and Daniel S. Elson[1,3]

[1] Hamlyn Centre for Robotic Surgery, Imperial College London, London, UK
[2] Department of Computing, Imperial College London, London, UK
[3] Department of Surgery and Cancer, Imperial College London, London, UK
[4] Centre for Medical Image Computing, University College London, London, UK
[5] Department of Computer Science, University College London, London, UK

Abstract. Tissue surface shape and reflectance spectra provide rich intra-operative information useful in surgical guidance. We propose a hybrid system which displays an endoscopic image with a fast joint inspection of tissue surface shape using structured light (SL) and hyperspectral imaging (HSI). For SL a miniature fibre probe is used to project a coloured spot pattern onto the tissue surface. In HSI mode standard endoscopic illumination is used, with the fibre probe collecting reflected light and encoding the spatial information into a linear format that can be imaged onto the slit of a spectrograph. Correspondence between the arrangement of fibres at the distal and proximal ends of the bundle was found using spectral encoding. Then during pattern decoding, a fully convolutional network (FCN) was used for spot detection, followed by a matching propagation algorithm for spot identification. This method enabled fast reconstruction (12 frames per second) using a GPU. The hyperspectral image was combined with the white light image and the reconstructed surface, showing the spectral information of different areas. Validation of this system using phantom and *ex vivo* experiments has been demonstrated.

Keywords: Structured light · Hyperspectral imaging · Endoscopy · Deep learning

1 Introduction

Tissue surface shape measurement is a tool for both surgical navigation and pathology detection. For example, morphological appearance could assist in colonic polyp detection [1]. In addition intra-operative tissue surface shape can be combined with pre-operative imaging modalities like CT or MRI, aiding surgical navigation [2]. SL is an active stereo technique used for surface reconstruction, provides similar reconstruction accuracy to passive stereo, and outperforms methods like shape-from-shading and time-of-flight. Due to its non-reliance on object surface texture, SL has shown potential in textureless tissue surface reconstruction in surgical environments [2]. A typical SL

© Springer International Publishing AG 2016
S. Ourselin et al. (Eds.): MICCAI 2016, Part III, LNCS 9902, pp. 414–422, 2016.
DOI: 10.1007/978-3-319-46726-9_48

system consists of a projector and camera. A pattern decoding step finds the correspondences between the camera and/or projector image planes, and enables surface reconstruction by triangulation for a specific camera-projector position.

Spectral imaging techniques including HSI and multispectral (MSI) implementations, measure the reflectance spectra at particular locations in an image, and have useful clinical applications in discriminating tissues which are indistinguishable under white light [3]. MSI has been used to monitor perfusion and tissue oxygen saturation intra-operatively in the bowel [4], during transplant surgery, and vascular procedures [5]. The high resolution of HSI, compared to multispectral imaging (MSI), can also enable more quantitative analysis allowing extraction of structural information or identification of disease markers in tissue using machine learning algorithms [6]. Previously combination of spectral and 3D information using MSI systems has been attempted [7, 8], but acquisition time has limited the spectral resolution to tens of wavelengths or less. To the best of our knowledge, this is the first time HSI (hundreds of wavelengths) has been combined with 3D reconstruction techniques based on SL and we believe that this solution to the compromise of spectral versus spatial resolu-tion can allow highly accurate rapid distinction between different pathologies.

Computational image analysis involves the development of a robust near real-time algorithm to decode the projected pattern for 3D tissue surface reconstruction, based on deep learning and a pattern-specific feature matching method. Recently, advances in hardware have made solving large-scale problems using Convolutional Neural Networks (CNN) possible in a reasonable amount of time. Long et al. proposed to use Fully Convolutional Networks (FCN) for pixelwise semantic segmentation, exceeding the state-of-the-art segmentation [9]. FCN has the benefits of non-dependency on the manually extracted features, combining both global and local information, and fast execution time. In the field of microscopic imaging, FCN has been used to detect and segment cells successfully [10]. So in this work FCN is applied for pattern decoding to detect projected spots. We also show that even with a limited amount of training images (n = 17) by data augmentation FCN still performs robustly and accurately.

2   Materials and Methods

2.1   Hybrid Structured Light and Hyperspectral Imager (SLHSI)

The system is built around a custom optical fibre assembly (Fibertech Optica, Inc., Canada) similar to that in our previous work [11, 12]. It is a 2.5 m long incoherent bundle of 171 50 μm core fibres arranged in a linear array at one end and a circular bundle at the other (Fig. 1). A 20 mm working distance GRIN lens (GRINtech GmbH, Germany) is attached distally. The probe's outer diameter is 2.8 mm.

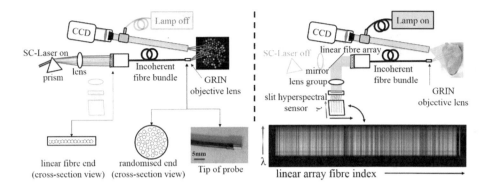

Fig. 1. Left: setup in SL mode, and the physical appearance of the miniaturised probe (lower left). Right: setup in HSI mode and the captured spectrograph image (lower right)

SL. A 4 W supercontinuum laser, dispersed by a prism, is coupled into the probe's linear array (Fig. 1). The GRIN lens projects an image of the bundle's end face which, due to the incoherent fibres, is a mixture of multi-coloured spots. The pattern is reflected by the object, collected by a laparoscope (Karl Storz GmbH, Germany) and imaged onto a CCD (Prosilica GX1050C; Allied Vision Technologies, Inc., USA).

HSI. With the laser switched off a white light source (Xenon 300; Karl Storz GmbH, Germany) is activated. Reflected light is collected by the probe and directed, via a 45° mirror on a motorised flipper mount (MFF101; Thorlabs Ltd., UK), towards a 250/50 mm focal length lens combination to form a demagnified image of the fibre array on the slit of a HSI camera (Nano-Hyperspec; Headwall Photonics, Inc., USA) (Fig. 1).

Correspondences between SL and HSI. The incoherent bundling of fibres in the probe meant that the mapping between an individual fibre's HSI spectral line and its position in the object plane had to be determined. This was done by projecting the SL pattern onto a white screen and imaging it with a separate hyperspectral camera [4] to determine each spot's mean wavelength. These could then be linked to the corresponding HSI sensor locations by sorting their wavelengths from shortest to longest.

Spectral processing. For each fibre in the HSI image its corresponding pixel columns were averaged to reduce signal noise. The linear wavelength-pixel row relationship was calibrated by illuminating the probe with laser light of known wavelengths and recording the positions of the intensity maxima. Each fibre's spectrum was divided by the corresponding signal from a white reference target (Spectralon; Labsphere, Inc., USA) to correct for wavelength-dependent transmission characteristics of the system. Further processing to generate absorbance spectra and determine relative haemoglobin concentration in tissue was performed as described previously [4].

2.2 3D Tissue Surface Reconstruction

SL system calibration. During calibration the projector can be regarded as an inverse camera. The calibration method has been described previously [13]. Besides, a virtual projector image (reference image) is generated from an SL pattern on a white plane using the probe intrinsic parameter and the homography [14]. It functions like the image from the second camera in passive stereo, facilitating pattern decoding.

Pattern decoding – spot detection. In this system projected spots with different colour are considered as features. In surgical environments spot detection is the key challenging step for accurate pattern decoding. An algorithm based on FCN has been employed to detect the spots in endoscopic images robustly in near real-time despite confounding factors such as blood, smoke or non-uniform illumination.

Our FCN model (Fig. 2 (a)) consists of two parts: the contractive and the expansive phases. The former halves image size and doubles the feature dimension at each step. At the end of this phase, each neuron has an effective receptive field of 16 × 16 pixels, and the feature dimension of its output volume is 512. The expansive phase also contains four steps, where each step upsamples image, fuses the upsampled output and the convoluted output from the counterpart in the contractive phase, and then convolutes to decrease the feature dimension. This expansive phase thus combines the coarse "what" and fine "where" information, resulting in a pixel-wise prediction of the whole image. The output of this model is a 2-channel image with the same size as the input image. Each channel indicates the "probabilities" of being foreground (spots) or background. The loss function is evaluated using the softmax function.

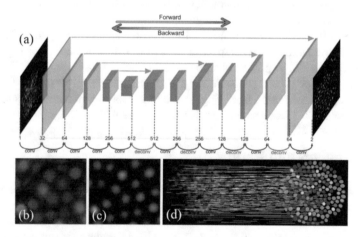

Fig. 2. (a) The deployed FCN model; (b) Cropped SL image; (c) Density map of the cropped SL image; (d) Feature matching between the captured (left) and the reference SL image (right)

For training 17 captured images have been used and image argumentation including resizing, flipping, and rotation, was applied to increase the training set. Input image size was halved to increase speed. During training the manual segmentations of the SL images were used as the desired label images. The training included a coarse training and a fine tuning, each with momentum 0.9 and weight decay 0.0005. The former had a learning rate of 0.0000005 until 80000 iterations, while the latter had 0.0000001 until 150000 iterations. In prediction the subtraction between the foreground and background channels was used as the "density map" of spot detection (Fig. 2 (c)). Both training and prediction were applied using Caffe [15]. In prediction the spot centres were detected at the local maxima locations of the density map.

Pattern decoding- spot matching. Like feature matching in passive stereo, detected spots should be matched to counterparts in the reference image for 3D reconstruction. On the reference image the spots were manually segmented offline.

The spot matching algorithm is based on colour and neighbourhood information detected using Delaunay triangulation. Neighbourhood areas of spots were defined according to distances between neighbours. Then a customised feature descriptor was defined for each spot. Taking the spot as the area centre, its feature descriptor was a 32×3 matrix, each row of which represented the colour in one direction on the area boundary. Only one feature descriptor was generated per spot in the captured SL image, while 32 descriptors starting from different directions were generated per spot in the reference image, taking rotation into consideration.

Epipolar lines were used to constrain the matching search space. The smallest distance between a spot descriptor on the captured image and all 32 descriptors of a spot on the reference image was used to describe the distance between them. The match with closest distance smaller than a threshold was chosen. This was followed by a pruning procedure based on neighbourhood information. An iterative method was then applied: matching was propagated to other neighbouring unmatched spots, followed by pruning, until the number of matches stops changing.

Combination of SL and HSI. With calibration and spot matching the 3D tissue surface could be triangulated. Hyperspectral data from different fibres, corresponding to individual spots, could be projected onto the reconstructed surfaces, providing a hybrid view of both the spectral and shape information relating to the target tissue. The computation time for reconstruction from single SL image was ~ 80 ms on a PC (OS: Ubuntu 14.04; processor: i7-3770; graphics card: NVIDIA GTX TITAN X).

3   Experiments and Results

Phantom and *ex vivo* tissue experiments have been carried out to validate the SL reconstruction and demonstrate hybrid hyperspectral and surface shape imaging.

SL Reconstruction. In SL mode the angle between the probe and the camera is ~10–15°, baseline ~3 cm, working distance 5–9 cm, with the endoscope optical axis roughly perpendicular to the tissue surface. Previous work has shown that the projected spot patterns are robust to changes in background albedo, due to their narrow bandwidth [11]. It was also found that, given an accurate calibration and perfect feature matching, reconstruction error can reach 0.7 mm at a working distance of ~10 cm [13]. Thus, the reconstruction accuracy mainly depends on the pattern decoding results. Here we provide the validation of feature matching from a silicone heart phantom, and *ex vivo* experiments on ovine heart and liver. Each group of validation data contains 10 images chosen randomly from recorded videos. Automatic feature matching results were compared with those from manual annotation. The true positive, annotated matches, together with the matching sensitivity and precision are listed in Table 1.

Table 1. Validation of feature matching. Manual annotation is used as the ground truth.

Object	Annotated matches	True positive	Sensitivity	Precision
Silicone heart phantom	170 ± 1	154 ± 17	0.907 ± 0.101	0.997 ± 0.004
Ovine heart	134 ± 8	113 ± 10	0.844 ± 0.038	0.997 ± 0.006
Ovine liver	128 ± 11	110 ± 13	0.861 ± 0.052	0.994 ± 0.005

Table 1 shows that the pattern decoding algorithm functions robustly with both the phantom and even some challenging *ex vivo* data, with feature matching sensitivity higher than 0.8, and precision 0.99. Compared with previous work [13], this shows a much higher sensitivity for feature matching due to the high spot detection accuracy achievable with FCN. Meanwhile, the near real-time performance of FCN guarantees its real-world practicality. The specified feature descriptor which accounts for pattern rotation, not only functions robustly but also simplifies the matching procedure.

HSI validation. Reflectance spectra from spot regions on a Macbeth colour chart, indicated by the SL pattern in Fig. 3(a), are plotted in Fig. 3(b) alongside those measured by a spectrometer (USB4000HR; Ocean Optics, Inc., USA). In each panel the SLHSI system's mapping procedure returns the correct reflectance spectrum for each location, with a mean spectral error of 10 % between the SLHSI and the gold standard.

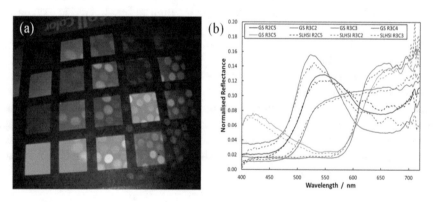

Fig. 3. (a) Macbeth colour chart illuminated with SL. (b) Reflectance spectra from selected colour panels of the chart, with *R* and *C* indicating the row and column, respectively. Data from the hybrid system (SLHSI) are plotted alongside the high resolution spectrometer results (GS).

To demonstrate combined shape and spectral information acquisition a cylindrical three-coloured target was imaged (Fig. 4). Mean reflectance curves for each region show peaks in the red, green and blue, and convolution with a colour CCD's spectral sensitivity allows RGB data recovery, shown in the surface mesh overlay (Fig. 4 (c)).

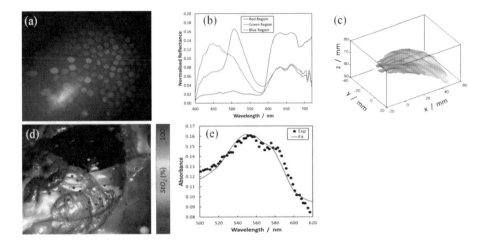

Fig. 4. (a) Three-coloured cylindrical target with SL. (b) Mean reflectance spectra for each of the target's regions. (c) 3D reconstruction coloured by RGB values generated from spectra in (b). (d) Murine abdomen with StO_2 overlay. (e) Tissue absorbance spectrum and model fit.

Reflectance spectra from a murine abdomen, imaged *post mortem*, were used to calculate the absorbance spectrum for each spot location and extract tissue oxygen saturation (StO2) using a method described previously [4]. StO2 at various spot locations is shown in Fig. 4 (d), along with an absorbance spectrum from one region (Fig. 4 (e)). Spectra that did not match the model well (r2 < 0.8) were rejected. Mean StO2 in the abdomen is low (14 ± 10 %), as expected for an *ex vivo* experiment.

According to the colour chart validation, this system can measure sample reflectance spectra accurately. This conclusion should apply to other objects including *in vivo* tissue. The main differences to be expected *in vivo* are higher StO2 values and breathing/peristalsis-related movement. The difference in StO2 will only affect the measured spectral shape. Tissue motion will not introduce much spectral artefact as each fibre's signal is acquired in a single snapshot (100 ms).

4   Discussion and Conclusion

We have developed a flexible rapid hybrid system capable of 3D sensing and HSI, using a motorised flipper mirror to switch between modes. The probe's size and flexibility means that it is compatible with standard clinical endoscopic tools for assessing the gastrointestinal tract and abdomen, while its imaging capabilities can enable clinical studies based on previous work in measurement of oxygenation dynamics [4], tissue classification [3] and augmentation of the clinician's view with pre-operative data [2].

SL mode enabled surface reconstruction of up to 171 data points, using a random-coloured spot pattern; while HSI measured the reflectance spectra of the same regions in one exposure. In addition, an accurate and fast 3D reconstruction algorithm was proposed, using FCN with specific feature descriptors, resulting in near real-time measurement of tissue surface even with low quality images. Future work will focus on system reliability and practicality enhancements, including compatibility with existing clinical instruments and sterilisability. Pilot studies on freshly excised tissue from human surgical procedures are planned and will allow testing of the system against histology, while further preclinical work will enable evaluation and optimisation of performance *in vivo*.

Acknowledgements. This work is funded by ERC 242991 and an Imperial College Confidence in Concept award. Jianyu Lin is supported by IGHI scholarship. Neil Clancy is supported by Imperial College Junior Research Fellowship. Danail Stoyanov is funded by EPSRC (EP/N013220/1, EP/N022750/1, EP/N027078/1, NS/A000027/1) and the EU-Horizon2020 (H2020-ICT-2015-688592).

References

1. Schwartz, J.J., Lichtenstein, G.R.: Magnification endoscopy, chromoendoscopy and other novel techniques in evaluation of patients with IBD. Tech. Gastrointest. Endosc. **6**, 182–188 (2004)
2. Maier-Hein, L., Mountney, P., Bartoli, A., Elhawary, H., Elson, D., Groch, A., Kolb, A., Rodrigues, M., Sorger, J., Speidel, S., Stoyanov, D.: Optical techniques for 3D surface reconstruction in computer-assisted laparoscopic surgery. Med. Image Anal. **17**, 974–996 (2013)
3. Lu, G., Fei, B.: Medical hyperspectral imaging: a Rev. J. Biomed. Opt. **19**, 010901 (2014)
4. Clancy, N.T., Arya, S., Stoyanov, D., Singh, M., Hanna, G.B., Elson, D.S.: Intraoperative measurement of bowel oxygen saturation using a multispectral imaging laparoscope. Biomed. Opt. Express **6**, 4179–4190 (2015)
5. Clancy, N.T., Arya, S., Corbett, R., Singh, M., Stoyanov, D., Crane, J.S., Duncan, N., Ebner, M., Caro, C.G., Hanna, G., Elson, D.S.: Optical measurement of anastomotic oxygenation dynamics. In: Biomedical Optics 2014, BS3A.23. Optical Society of America (2014)
6. Akbari, H., Halig, L.V., Schuster, D.M., Osunkoya, A., Master, V., Nieh, P.T., Chen, G.Z., Fei, B.: Hyperspectral imaging and quantitative analysis for prostate cancer detection. J. Biomed. Opt. **17**, 0760051–07600510 (2012)
7. Clancy, N.T., Lin, J., Arya, S., Hanna, G.B., Elson, D.S.: Dual multispectral and 3D structured light laparoscope. In: Proceedings of SPIE, Multimodal Biomedical Imaging X, vol. 9316, p. 93160C (2015)
8. Clancy, N.T., Stoyanov, D., James, D.R.C., Di Marco, A., Sauvage, V., Clark, J., Yang, G.-Z., Elson, D.S.: Multispectral image alignment using a three channel endoscope *in vivo* during minimally invasive surgery. Biomed. Opt. Express **3**, 2567–2578 (2012)
9. Long, J., Shelhamer, E., Darrell, T.: Fully convolutional networks for semantic segmentation. In: The IEEE Conference on Computer Vision and Pattern Recognition (CVPR) (2015)
10. Ronneberger, O., Fischer, P., Brox, T.: U-Net: convolutional networks for biomedical image segmentation. In: Navab, N., Hornegger, J., Wells, W.M., Frangi, A.F. (eds.) MICCAI 2015, Part III. LNCS, vol. 9351, pp. 234–241. Springer, Heidelberg (2015). doi: 10.1007/978-3-319-24574-4_28
11. Clancy, N.T., Stoyanov, D., Maier-Hein, L., Groch, A., Yang, G.-Z., Elson, D.S.: Spectrally encoded fiber-based structured lighting probe for intraoperative 3D imaging. Biomedical Optics Express **2**, 3119–3128 (2011)

12. Maier-Hein, L., Groch, A., Bartoli, A., Bodenstedt, S., Boissonnat, G., Chang, P.L., Clancy, N.T., Elson, D.S., Haase, S., Heim, E., Hornegger, J., Jannin, P., Kenngott, H., Kilgus, T., Muller-Stich, B., Oladokun, D., Rohl, S., dos Santos, T.R., Schlemmer, H.P., Seitel, A., Speidel, S., Wagner, M., Stoyanov, D.: Comparative validation of single-shot optical techniques for laparoscopic 3-D surface reconstruction. IEEE Trans. Med. Imaging **33**, 1913–1930 (2014)

13. Lin, J., Clancy, N.T., Elson, D.S.: An endoscopic structured light system using multispectral detection. Int. J. CARS **10**, 1941–1950 (2015)

14. Lin, J., T.Clancy, N., Stoyanov, D., Elson, D.S.: Tissue surface reconstruction aided by local normal information using a self-calibrated endoscopic structured light system. In: Navab, N., Hornegger, J., Wells, W.M., Frangi, A.F. (eds.) MICCAI 2015, Part I. LNCS, vol. 9349, pp. 405–412. Springer, Heidelberg (2015). doi:10.1007/978-3-319-24553-9_50

15. Jia, Y., Shelhamer, E., Donahue, J., Karayev, S., Long, J., Girshick, R., Guadarrama, S., Darrell, T.: Caffe: convolutional architecture for fast feature embedding. In: Proceedings of the 22nd ACM International Conference on Multimedia, pp. 675–678. ACM, Orlando (2014)

Efficient Low-Dose CT Denoising by Locally-Consistent Non-Local Means (LC-NLM)

Michael Green[1], Edith M. Marom[2], Nahum Kiryati[1],
Eli Konen[2], and Arnaldo Mayer[2(✉)]

[1] Department of Electrical Engineering, Tel-Aviv University, Tel-Aviv, Israel
green1@mail.tau.ac.il, nk@eng.tau.ac.il
[2] Diagnostic Imaging, Sheba Medical Center, Affiliated to the Sackler School of Medicine,
Tel-Aviv University, Tel-Aviv, Israel
{edith.marom,eli.konen,arnaldo.mayer}@sheba.health.gov.il

Abstract. The never-ending quest for lower radiation exposure is a major challenge to the image quality of advanced CT scans. Post-processing algorithms have been recently proposed to improve low-dose CT denoising after image reconstruction. In this work, a novel algorithm, termed the locally-consistent non-local means (LC-NLM), is proposed for this challenging task. By using a database of high-SNR CT patches to filter noisy pixels while locally enforcing spatial consistency, the proposed algorithm achieves both powerful denoising and preservation of fine image details. The LC-NLM is compared both quantitatively and qualitatively, for synthetic and real noise, to state-of-the-art published algorithms. The highest structural similarity index (SSIM) were achieved by LC-NLM in 8 out of 10 denoised chest CT volumes. Also, the visual appearance of the denoised images was clearly better for the proposed algorithm. The favorable comparison results, together with the computational efficiency of LC-NLM makes it a promising tool for low-dose CT denoising.

1 Introduction

In the last decade, low dose CT scan techniques have been successful at reducing radiation exposure of the patient by tens of percent, narrowing the gap with X-ray radiographs [1]. However, generating diagnostic grade images from very low SNR projections is too demanding for the classical filtered back-projection algorithm [2]. Iterative-reconstruction algorithms [3] have been successful at the task and were implemented by most commercial CT scan developers. These methods, however, are computationally very demanding, generally requiring significantly longer reconstruction times [1] and expensive computing power.

In recent years, post-processing algorithms have been proposed to denoise low-dose CT after the back-projection step [1, 4–8]. In [6], a previous high quality CT scan is registered to the low dose scan and a (non-linearly) filtered difference is computed. Eventually, a denoised scan is obtained by adding the filtered difference to the co-registered high quality scan. The method assumes the availability of an earlier scan and depends on registration accuracy.

© Springer International Publishing AG 2016
S. Ourselin et al. (Eds.): MICCAI 2016, Part III, LNCS 9902, pp. 423–431, 2016.
DOI: 10.1007/978-3-319-46726-9_49

In [1], a modified formulation of the block matching and 3-D filtering (BM3D) algorithm [9] is combined with a noise confidence region evaluation (NCRE) method that controls the update of the regularization parameters. Results are shown for a few phantom and human CT slices.

Non-local mean (NLM) filters [10] have also been proposed for low-dose CT denoising [4, 5, 7]. In [5], the weights of the NLM filters are computed between pixels in the noisy scan and an earlier, co-registered, high quality scan. Artificial streak noise is added to the high quality scan to improve weights accuracy. In [4], a dataset of 2-D patches (7×7) is extracted from high quality CT slices belonging to several patients. At each position in the noisy scan, the 40 Euclidean nearest-neighbors patches (hereafter denoted *filtering patches*) of the local 7×7 patch (hereafter denoted *query* patch) are found by exhaustive search in the patch dataset. The denoised value at each position is computed by NLM filtering of these 40 nearest-neighbor patches. While the method does not need previous co-registered scans, it requires the extraction of 40 nearest-neighbor patches for every pixel, at high computational cost. The method shows initial promising results, although it was validated on a very small set of 2-D images. It suggests that small CT patches originating from different scans for the same body area (chest in that case) contain similar patterns.

We further observe that in [4], local consistency in the filtered image is not explicitly enforced: the *filtering patches* are just required to be similar to the query patch, but not to neighboring patches which still have a significant overlap with the query patch. As a result, fine details may be filtered out in the denoised image.

In this work, we propose a computationally efficient algorithm for the denoising of low-dose CT scans after image reconstruction. By using a database of high-SNR patches to filter the pixels while locally enforcing spatial consistency, the proposed algorithm achieves both powerful denoising and preservation of fine image details and structures. The remainder of this paper is organized as follows: The LC-NLM algorithm is detailed in Sect. 2 and validated on synthetic and real noisy data in Sect. 3. A discussion concludes the paper in Sect. 4.

2 Methods

The main steps of the proposed method, shown in Fig. 1 (left), are divided in two major parts: The creation of the patch dataset, which is performed only once, and the denoising of input low-dose (*LD*) scans. Both steps will be described in detail in the following subsections.

2.1 Patch Dataset Creation

The idea is to create a dataset of high SNR patches to approximate visually similar noisy patches in the *LD* scans. It is therefore necessary for the dataset to represent as much as possible the variability of the patches in order to increase the chance to find a good match. However, due to memory and performance limitations, the size of the patch dataset must be limited. Randomly sampling the full dataset is not a good option as most

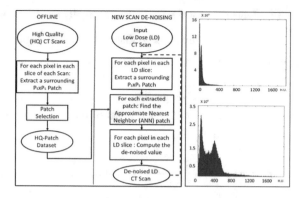

Fig. 1. (left) The main steps of the proposed method; (right) Patch variance histogram for the patch dataset: (top) for random sampling; (bottom) for roulettte wheel selection.

of the patches have fairly constant values as can be seen from the patch standard deviation (SD) histogram (Fig. 1, top-right). We propose a patch selection step in which patches containing more signal variation have a higher probability of being included in the dataset. For this purpose, a roulette wheel (RW) selection scheme [11] is implemented. RW samples uniformly a virtual disk along which patch indices are represented by variable length segments. The higher the patch SD, the longer the segment and accordingly the probability to select it. The resulting SD histogram for the selected patches (Fig. 1, bottom-right) is clearly more balanced than for the random selection case.

2.2 Denoising of Low Dose (*LD*) Scans

Given an input *LD* CT scan, a $P_s \times P_s$ patch centered at each pixel position is extracted in every slice. The approximate nearest neighbor (ANN) is then found for each patch using the state-of-the-art randomized kd-trees algorithm [12] implemented in the Fast

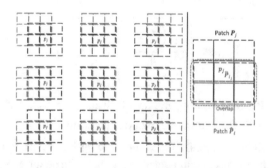

Fig. 2. (left) Pixel p_j can be viewed as the intersection of P_s^2 partially overlapping $P_s \times P_s$ patches (red). In the example $P_s = 3$; (right) patch $\hat{P}_i$ contributes to the denoised value $\hat{p}_j$ via its pixel $\hat{P}_{i_j}$, which the way noisy pixel p_j is perceived by high-SNR patch $\hat{P}_i$. (Color figure online)

Library for ANN (FLANN) [13] for the Euclidean norm. These patches will be designated as *high-SNR* patches. Any given pixel p_j, distant by at least $\dfrac{P_s}{2}$ pixels from the slice borders, can be viewed as the intersection of P_s^2 overlapping $P_s \times P_s$ patches. An example is shown in Fig. 2 (left) for $P_s = 3$.

Let NN_{p_j} be the set of P_s^2 high-SNR patches returned as nearest-neighbor of the P_s^2 overlapping patches. We propose to compute the denoised value $\hat{p}_j$ at pixel p_j as a function of the patches belonging to N_{p_j} (Eq. 1):

$$\hat{p}_j = F\left(\hat{P}_1, \dots, \hat{P}_{P_s^2}\right) \; for \; \hat{P}_i \in \left(NN_{p_j}\right) \tag{1}$$

where $F\left(\underline{X}\right) : \mathcal{R}^{P_s^2} \to \mathcal{R}$ and $i = 1 \dots P_s^2$. A simple choice of F may be the average of all the pixels from the same location as p_j, leading to (Eq. 2):

$$\hat{p}_j = \frac{1}{P_s^2} \sum_{i=1}^{P_s^2} \hat{P}_{i_j} \; for \; \hat{P}_i \in \left(NN_{p_j}\right) \tag{2}$$

where $\hat{P}_{i_j}$ stands for pixel value in patch $\hat{P}_i$ at the location overlapping with pixel p_j. In this approach, each overlapping patch $\hat{P}_i$, (Fig. 2, right, in red) contributes to the denoised value $\hat{p}_j$ via its pixel $\hat{P}_{i_j}$, which is the way noisy pixel p_j is perceived by high-SNR patch $\hat{P}_i$.

A more powerful choice for F, inspired by the non-local means (NLM) filters [10], is to weight the contributions $\hat{P}_{i_j}, i = 1 \dots P_s^2$ by a similarity measure between $\hat{P}_i$ and the original noisy patch centered in p_j, formalized by (Eq. 3):

$$\hat{p}_j = \frac{\sum_{i=1}^{P_s^2} \exp\left(-\dfrac{D\left(P_j, \hat{P}_i\right)}{h^2}\right) \hat{P}_{i_j}}{\sum_{i=1}^{P_s^2} \exp\left(-\dfrac{D\left(P_j, \hat{P}_i\right)}{h^2}\right)}, \hat{P}_i \in \left(NN_{p_j}\right) \tag{3}$$

where $h = P_s \cdot \gamma > 0$ is the filtering parameter [10] and γ a constant, P_j is the noisy patch centered in p_j and $D(P_j, \hat{P}_i)$ is the average L_1 distance between the overlapping pixels of P_j and $\hat{P}_i$ (Fig. 2, right, in green). Thus, surrounding high-SNR $\hat{P}_i$ patches with high similarity to P_j at their overlap will contribute more to the denoised value of p_j. Consequently, the proposed method explicitly promotes local-consistency in the denoised image, resulting in a locally-consistent non-local means (LC-NLM) algorithm. Eventually, to further boost the denoising effect, the LC-NLM can be applied iteratively several times (Fig. 1, left, dashed line) as will be shown in the experiments.

3   Experiments

Quantitative validation on real data requires the availability of high-SNR and *LD* CT scans pairs acquired with exactly the same body position and voxel size for each subject. As these conditions are difficult to meet in practice, we have adopted the pragmatic approach proposed in [4]: *LD* scans were generated by adding artificial noise to real high-SNR CT scans. Zero-mean additive Gaussian noise ($\sigma = 2000$) was added to the sinogram re-computed from the high-SNR slices before returning to the image space.

A dataset was built from 10 high-SNR real full chest scans (voxel size $= 1 \times 1 \times 2.5$ mm^3) and the 10 corresponding synthetic *LD* scans. The patch size, P_s, and the γ constant, were set to 5 and 18, respectively, for all the experiments. A leave-one-out cross validation methodology was implemented: 10 training-test sets were generated, keeping each time another single *LD* scan for testing and using the remaining 9 high-SNR scans to build the high-SNR patch dataset (training set). The training set was generated using the roulette wheel methodology (see Sect. 2) to sample 2 % of the total number of patches in the 9 training scans while preserving inter-patch variability. The structural similarity index (SSIM) [14] was used to quantify the similarity between the denoised *LD* scan and the corresponding high-SNR scan used as ground truth. For a pair of *LD* and high-SNR patches, denoted P_1 and P_2, respectively, the SSIM is given by (Eq. 4):

$$SSIM\left(P_1, P_2\right) = \frac{(2\mu_1\mu_2 + c_1)(2\sigma_{12} + c_2)}{(\mu_1^2 + \mu_2^2 + c_1)(\sigma_1^2 + \sigma_2^2 + c_2)} \tag{4}$$

where, μ_1, μ_2 and σ_1, σ_2 are the mean and standard deviation, respectively, for P_1 *and* P_2, and σ_{12} their covariance. We set the constants $c_1 = 6.5$, $c_2 = 58.5$ and quantized the pixels to [0 255], as suggested in [4]. The LC-NLM was compared to three state-of-the-art denoising algorithms: (1) The original NLM [10] as implemented in [1] with default parameters, except for *max_dist*, that was set to 3. (2) Our implementation of the patch-database-NLM (PDB-NLM) [4] with parameters taken from [4]. (3) BM3D [9] with code and parameters from [1, 15], respectively.

In Table 1, the average *SSIM* is given for the LC-NLM (1-4 iterations), NLM and BM3D algorithms for the 10 scans datasets. Due to its very high running time, the PDB-NLM algorithm is compared to LC-NLM for a single representative slice per scan in separate Table 2. In this case, leave-one-out is performed on a total dataset of 10 slice pairs *(LD* and high-SNR), instead of 10 full scans. In 8 out of 10 cases, the best *SSIM* score (bold in Tables 1 and 2) is obtained for the proposed LC-NLM algorithm. In two cases alone (#2 & #8), BM3D reached a higher score than LC-NLM. For LC-NLM, the *SSIM* generally improved for 3–4 iterations before decreasing.

Table 1. Average *SSIM* for 10 full scans: LC-NLM vs. other methods (best score in bold)

case #	LC-NLM, it#1	LC-NLM, it#2	LC-NLM, it#3	LC-NLM, it#4	NLM [10]	BM3D [9]
1	0.614	**0.633**	0.629	0.620	0.463	0.623
2	0.549	0.600	0.619	0.624	0.513	**0.639**
3	0.563	0.601	**0.614**	0.608	0.478	0.610
4	0.571	0.610	**0.627**	0.620	0.490	0.625
5	0.595	**0.605**	0.595	0.581	0.419	0.584
6	0.609	0.62	**0.625**	0.615	0.447	0.618
7	0.589	**0.611**	0.607	0.598	0.453	0.606
8	0.608	0.636	0.639	0.634	0.494	**0.643**
9	0.600	**0.618**	0.614	0.605	0.454	0.607
10	0.589	**0.594**	0.581	0.567	0.410	0.579

Table 2. LC-NLM vs PDB-NLM (PDB-NLM) [4] for the 10 slices dataset (best score in bold)

slice #	LC-NLM it#1	LC-NLM it#2	LC-NLM it#3	LC-NLM it#4	PDB-NLM [4]
1	0.571	0.616	0.631	**0.635**	0.620
2	0.616	0.646	**0.650**	0.64	0.638
3	0.565	0.614	0.631	**0.636**	0.620
4	0.587	0.632	0.648	**0.653**	0.637
5	0.639	0.670	**0.677**	0.675	0.667
6	0.639	0.667	**0.669**	0.66	0.661
7	0.591	**0.611**	0.609	0.601	0.600
8	0.587	0.634	0.649	**0.652**	0.638
9	0.527	0.624	**0.657**	0.648	0.645
10	0.572	0.621	0.637	**0.641**	0.628

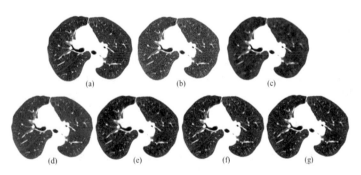

Fig. 3. A sample slice for case #2: (a) Original image; (b) synthetic low-dose image; (c) NLM [10]; (d) BM3D [9]; (e) PDB-NLM [4]; (f) iter.2 of LC-NLM; (g) iter.3 of LC-NLM.

A sample slice for case #2 is shown in Fig. 3. The original high-SNR slice (a) is shown alongside the corresponding synthetic *LD* image (b), the NLM, BM3D, PDB-NLM results (c–e), and the LC-NLM results for 2 and 3 iterations (f–g). BM3D performed significantly better than NLM, but over-smoothed the fine lung texture while PDB-NLM and LC-NLM better preserved fine details and resulted in more realistic and contrasted images (Table 3).

Table 3. Average running time for the denoising of a CT slice by the compared algorithms.

LC-NLM (1 iter.)	NLM [10]	BM3D [9]	PDB-NLM [4]
~4 s	~7 s	~16 s	~1800 s

In Fig. 4, a pathological free-breathing porcine slice (1 mm thick), acquired at both (a) normal (120 kVp–250 mAs) and (b) low-dose (80 kVp–50 mAs) is shown after denoising the low-dose acquisition by: (c) NLM [10], (d) BM3D [9], (e) PDB-NLM [4], (f) LC-NLM-2iterations, and (g) LC-NLM-3iterations. In the highlighted area (red), a 3 mm part-solid nodule (yellow box, a–g) was further magnified (g). The solid part of the nodule is clearly visible (thick arrows) only in the normal-dose slice (a) and the LC-NLM outputs (f–g). Conversely, a barely distinguishable smeared spot is observed (thin arrow) for BM3D [9] (d), while the nodule has completely disappeared with NLM [10] (c) and PDB-NLM[4] (e), and is undistinguishable from noise in the low-dose slice (b). The dose length product (DLP) was 670.2 and 37.7 mGy·cm for normal and low-dose porcine scans, respectively, reflecting a dose reduction of about 94 % between them.

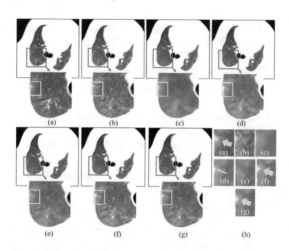

Fig. 4. Porcine CT scan slice acquired at (a) 120 kVp and 250 mAs, and (b) 80 kVp and 50 mAs. Low dose slice denoised by: (c) NLM [10]; (d) BM3D [9]; (e) PDB-NLM [4]; (f) LC-NLM-2iter; (g) LC-NLM-3iter. The highlighted lung area (red) is zoomed-in. (h) Zoomed view of a 3 mm part-solid nodule (yellow boxes) for images a–g. The solid part of the nodule is only clearly visible (thick arrows) in the normal-dose slice (a) and the LC-NLM outputs (f–g). A barely distinguishable smeared spot is observed (thin arrow) for BM3D [9] (d), while it has completely disappeared with NLM [10] (c) and PDB-NLM [4] (e), and is undistinguishable from noise in the low-dose slice (b). (Color figure online)

4 Conclusions

We have presented a computationally efficient algorithm for the denoising of *low dose* (LD) CT scans. The LC-NLM algorithm uses a database of high-SNR *filtering* patches to denoise low-dose scans. By explicitly enforcing similarity between the *filtering* patches and the spatial neighbors of the *query* patch, the LC-NLM better preserves fine structures in the denoised image. The algorithm compared favorably to previous state-of-the-art methods both qualitatively and quantitatively. While PDB-NLM produced better visual results than the other published algorithms (NLM and BM3D), it required prohibitive running times and, also in contrast to LC-NLM, was unable to preserve fine pathological details such as a tiny 3 mm nodule. Moreover, PDB-NLM [4] performs exhaustive search of 40-nearest neighbors. An efficient approximate-NN (ANN) implementation of [4] would strongly affect quality as patch similarity degrades rapidly with the ANN's neighbor order. This problem is avoided with LC-NLM which uses only 1st order ANNs, thus a much better approximation than the 40th. The encouraging results and the computational efficiency of LC-NLM make it a promising tool for significant dose reduction in lung cancer screening of populations at risk without compromising sensitivity. In future research, the patch dataset will be extended to include pathological cases and the method will be further validated on large datasets of real LD-scans in the framework of prospective studies.

References

1. Hashemi, S., Paul, N.S., Beheshti, S., Cobbold, R.S.: Adaptively tuned iterative low dose ct image denoising. Comput. Math. Methods Med. **2015** (2015)
2. Pontana, F., Duhamel, A., Pagniez, J., Flohr, T., Faivre, J.-B., Hachulla, A.-L., Remy, J., Remy-Jardin, M.: Chest computed tomography using iterative reconstruction vs filtered back projection (Part 2): image quality of low-dose CT examinations in 80 patients. Eur. Radiol. **21**(3), 636–643 (2011)
3. Beister, M., Kolditz, D., Kalender, W.A.: Iterative reconstruction methods in X-ray CT. Physica Med. **28**(2), 94–108 (2012)
4. Ha, S., Mueller, K.: Low dose CT image restoration using a database of image patches. Phys. Med. Biol. **60**(2), 869 (2015)
5. Xu, W., Mueller, K.: Efficient low-dose CT artifact mitigation using an artifact-matched prior scan. Med. Phys. **39**(8), 4748–4760 (2012)
6. Yu, H., Zhao, S., Hoffman, E.A., Wang, G.: Ultra-low dose lung CT perfusion regularized by a previous scan. Acad. Radiol. **16**(3), 363–373 (2009)
7. Zhang, H., Ma, J., Wang, J., Liu, Y., Lu, H., Liang, Z.: Statistical image reconstruction for low-dose CT using nonlocal means-based regularization. Comput. Med. Imaging Graph. **38**(6), 423–435 (2014)
8. Ai, D., Yang, J., Fan, J., Cong, W., Wang, Y.: Adaptive tensor-based principal component analysis for low-dose CT image denoising (2015)
9. Dabov, K., Foi, A., Katkovnik, V., Egiazarian, K.: Image denoising by sparse 3-D transform-domain collaborative filtering. IEEE Trans. Image Process. **16**(8), 2080–2095 (2007)

10. Buades, A., Coll, B., Morel, J.M.: A non-local algorithm for image denoising. In: IEEE Computer Society Conference on Computer Vision and Pattern Recognition, CVPR 2005. IEEE (2005)
11. Goldberg, D.E.: Genetic Algorithms in Search Optimization and Machine Learning, vol. 412. Addison-wesley, Reading Menlo Park (1989)
12. Silpa-Anan, C., Hartley, R.: Optimised KD-trees for fast image descriptor matching.In: IEEE Conference on Computer Vision and Pattern Recognition, CVPR 2008. IEEE (2008)
13. Muja,M., Lowe, D.G.: Fast approximate nearest neighbors with automatic algorithm configuration. In: VISAPP, no. 1 (2009)
14. Wang, Z., Bovik, A.C., Sheikh, H.R., Simoncelli, E.P.: Image quality assessment: from error visibility to structural similarity. IEEE Trans. Image Process. **13**(4), 600–612 (2004)
15. Lebrun, M.: An analysis and implementation of the BM3D image denoising method. Image Process. Line **2**, 175–213 (2012)

Deep Learning Computed Tomography

Tobias Würfl$^{(\boxtimes)}$, Florin C. Ghesu, Vincent Christlein, and Andreas Maier

Pattern Recognition Laboratory, Friedrich-Alexander-University
Erlangen-Nuremberg, Erlangen, Germany
wuerflts@outlook.com

Abstract. In this paper, we demonstrate that image reconstruction can be expressed in terms of neural networks. We show that filtered back-projection can be mapped identically onto a deep neural network architecture. As for the case of iterative reconstruction, the straight forward realization as matrix multiplication is not feasible. Thus, we propose to compute the back-projection layer efficiently as fixed function and its gradient as projection operation. This allows a data-driven approach for joint optimization of correction steps in projection domain and image domain. As a proof of concept, we demonstrate that we are able to learn weightings and additional filter layers that consistently reduce the reconstruction error of a limited angle reconstruction by a factor of two while keeping the same computational complexity as filtered back-projection. We believe that this kind of learning approach can be extended to any common CT artifact compensation heuristic and will outperform hand-crafted artifact correction methods in the future.

1 Introduction

X-ray computed tomography scanning has become a standard procedure in diagnosis of certain diseases or trauma. In virtually every scanning system heuristic steps exist to compensate for artifacts from scatter, beam-hardening, or other sources of artifacts. A simple heuristic approach for compensation of limited angle artifacts is shown in the work of Riess et al. [9]. The method introduces heuristic compensation weights for the filtered back-projection (FBP) algorithm that reduce the loss in mass from the reduced number of views. While demonstrating significant improvements in image quality, the approach lacks any theoretical guarantees for the weighting procedure. The approach is one amongst many "hand-crafted" artifact reduction methods.

Neural networks have been employed for reconstruction. Argyrou et al. [1] already show an approach of learning 2-D reconstruction with a zero hidden layer neural network. The main disadvantage of their approach is the large number of synapses required. Thus, this method methods requires an impractical amount of memory and training examples and an extension to 3-D seems impossible.

Recent developments in deep learning also suggest that deeper architectures should be explored and regularization is necessary for training such networks. A method presented by Cierniak [2] uses a back-projection then filtering approach and employs a Hopfield neural network to solve the image deblurring problem.

© Springer International Publishing AG 2016
S. Ourselin et al. (Eds.): MICCAI 2016, Part III, LNCS 9902, pp. 432–440, 2016.
DOI: 10.1007/978-3-319-46726-9_50

This approach bypasses the problem of too many parameters by fixing them in the back-projection step and degenerates the reconstruction problem to an image-based filtering approach.

A different approach by de Medeiros et al. [6] exploits the sparsity of the back-projection matrix to fit it into memory. However, this approach is not able to involve any training since the sparse structure would be undone in the training step.

In MRI-reconstruction Hammernik et al. [5] have shown an approach of learning sparsifying transforms and potential functions.

In this paper, we propose a fully differentiable back-projection layer for parallel-beam and fan-beam projection as well as a weighting layer. This enables various neural network architectures for reconstruction to be trained end-to-end. The distinctive advantage of our approach is that we are also able to learn heuristics that are applied in the projection domain *before* back-projection. This way we can replace heuristic correction methods with learned optimal solutions. Also we can jointly optimize different correction methods to improve their results when applied simultaneously. We present an example where we jointly optimize compensation weights, the reconstruction filter and a non-linear image filtering algorithm. In addition we propose a method for regularizing the optimization by pre-training. We evaluate our method using realistic data.

2   Methodology

We first describe the mapping of a filtered back-projection algorithm to a basic neural network architecture for reconstruction in Sect. 2.1. For this architecture we derive the forward and backward computation of our novel back-projection layer, cf. Sect. 2.2). In Sect. 2.3 we extend the architecture to fan-beam reconstruction by deriving a novel weighting layer that implements the special topology of this operation. and a fan-beam layer (Sect. 2.3). Eventually, we evaluate these architectures in Sect. 2.5).

2.1   Mapping FBP to Neural Networks

The input-vector x to the neural network corresponds to the whole sinogram, while the output-vector y corresponds to the whole reconstruction. As loss function every regression loss function is applicable, e. g., the l_2 norm: $\|x - y\|_2$. The filtering is a convolution with a high pass filter and can directly be mapped to a convolutional layer. Typically, convolutional layers in neural networks use comparably small filter kernels which are calculated in spatial domain. In comparison, a convolution in the Fourier domain is advantageous for reconstruction because (i) the high pass filters have infinite support, thus, they are as large as the number of detector pixels, and (ii) reduce computational complexity. Rectified linear units (ReLU) as non-linear activation functions can enforce the constraint of non-negativity of the reconstruction. As last step back-projection has to be mapped to a layer in a neural network. We begin with the discrete formulation of FBP:

$$f(u,v) \approx \frac{\pi}{N} \sum_{n=1}^{N} q(u\cos(\theta_n) + v\sin(\theta_n), \theta_n), \tag{1}$$

where $f(u,v)$ denotes the function to be reconstructed, s is a position on the detector, N denotes the number of projections and $q(s, \theta_n)$ denotes the filtered projections. Since we sample the function $q(s, \theta_n)$ only at discrete positions of s (denoted as $q_{m,n}$), a one-dimensional interpolation has to be performed, i.e.,:

$$f(u,v) \approx \frac{\pi}{N} \sum_{n=1}^{N} \sum_{m=1}^{M} w_m(u, v, \theta_n) \cdot q_{\left\lceil u\cos(\theta_n) + v\sin(\theta_n) - \frac{M+2}{2} + m \right\rceil, n}, \tag{2}$$

where $w_m(u, v, \theta_n)$ are the interpolation weights and M is an even integer denoting the number of interpolation coefficients.

A well known activation model of a neuron is [3]:

$$f(y_i) = f\left(\sum_{j=1}^{N} w_{ij} x_j + w_{j0} \right). \tag{3}$$

When we set our activation function to be the identity $f(x) = x$ and all bias weights w_{j0} to zero it follows $f(y_i) = \sum_{j=1}^{N} w_{ij} x_j$. Let us change the indexation of $f(y_i)$ to $f(x_i, y_j)$ which denotes a pixel of a reconstruction of Size $I \times J$. Similarly we change the indexation of x to that of the filtered sinogram $q_{m,n}$:

$$f(x_i, y_j) = \sum_{n=1}^{N} \sum_{m=1}^{M} w_{i+(j-1)\cdot I, m+(n-1)\cdot M} \cdot q_{m,n}. \tag{4}$$

We can compute Eq. (2) only at some discrete u, v positions and choose, without loss of generality, the interpolation size big enough to cover the length of the detector by zero-padding the signal as needed.

$$f(u_i, v_j) \approx \frac{\pi}{N} \sum_{n=1}^{N} \sum_{m=1}^{M} w_m(u_i, v_j, \theta_n) \cdot q_{m,n} \tag{5}$$

Equation (5) is equivalent to Eq. (4) if we choose:

$$w_{i+j\cdot I, m+(n-1)\cdot M} = \frac{\pi}{N} w_m(u_i, v_j, \theta_n). \tag{6}$$

This general result holds for arbitrary interpolation techniques. The most important case being the linear interpolation which will yield only up to two non-zero coefficients for every M interpolation coefficients resulting in an extremely sparse matrix.

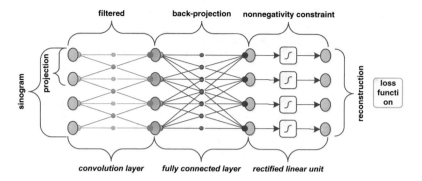

Fig. 1. Parallel-beam neural network architecture

Plugging in our convolution layer, the output for our neural network architecture is finally calculated as:

$$f(x_i, y_j) = \max\left[0, \sum_{n=1}^{N}\sum_{m=1}^{M}\frac{\pi}{N}w_m(u_i, v_j, \theta_n)\cdot\left(\sum_{k=-M/2}^{M/2} w_k \cdot p_{m-k,n}\right)\right]. \quad (7)$$

This shows that our neural network architecture implements a filtered back-projection algorithm. Note that the network's weights for initialization are known from the original derivation of the filtered back-projection. Figure 1 shows this basic architecture for parallel-beam reconstruction. We mapped each step of the FBP algorithm into a corresponding layer.

2.2 Parallel-Beam Back-Projection Layer

To solve the problem of fitting the parameters of the FCL, which represents the back-projection operator, into memory we propose a novel back-projection layer. This layer has no adjustable parameters. During the forward-pass of the network the coefficients $w_{i,j}$ of the matrix $\mathbf{W}_l$ are computed, where l denotes the index of this layer. This is calculated incrementally using the update rule

$$\mathbf{y}_l = \mathbf{W}_l\mathbf{y}_{l-1} \quad (8)$$

similar to the traditional back-projector in FBP. Since this layer has no adjustable weights in its backward pass only the gradient with respect to the lower layers has to be calculated. For FCLs this corresponds to calculating:

$$\mathbf{E}_{l-1} = \mathbf{W}_l^T\mathbf{E}_l, \quad (9)$$

where $\mathbf{E}_{l-1}$ represents the error of the next lower layer of the network. Since the back-projection operator is the transpose of the projection operator [11], one algorithm for the backward-pass is readily available. An alternative way is to recalculate the weights as in the forward-pass and apply them to the error.

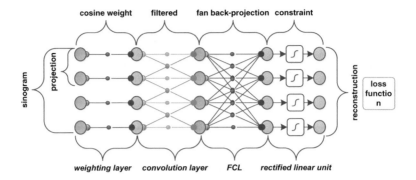

Fig. 2. Fan-beam neural network architecture

2.3   Extension to Fan-Beam Reconstruction

The extension of the well known FBP algorithm to the fan-beam projection model consists of a cosine weighting of the projections and weighted back-projection. Figure 2 shows this extended architecture for fan-beam reconstruction.

Weighting Layer. A layer that performs only weighing has the very sparse structure of a diagonal matrix. This can be exploited to construct a special weighting layer that enforces sparsity. This layer has exactly N training parameters, where N is the dimensionality of the input and output vectors. The forward-pass can be calculated using Eq. (8) which corresponds to an element-wise multiplication of the input with the weights. For the backward-pass we employ Eq. (9). Since $\mathbf{W}^T = \mathbf{W}$ holds for diagonal matrices, the backward-pass of this layer is an element-wise multiplication of the weights with the error of the next higher layer. The gradient with respect to the weights of a FCL is calculated by $\mathbf{G}_l = \mathbf{E}_l \mathbf{y}_{l-1}$.

Fan-Beam Back-Projection Layer. The derivation of the forward and backward pass of a fan-beam layer is identical to the parallel-beam layer. The weights are calculated differently and a distance weighting is applied to every element of the sum [11]. But the backward pass can also be implemented as fan-beam projection.

2.4   Convergence and Overfitting

The advances in deep learning have shown that regularization is crucial to the performance of neural networks. Because of the high dimensionality of our reconstruction networks, regularization is important to achieve convergence and to prevent overfitting. Popular methods are weight-decay, dropout [10] and pre-training. Weight-decay is not effective for this learning problem because the scaling of the data is crucial when using the l_2 norm as a loss function. Dropout is normally very effective for fully connected layers because it can prevent co-adaptation of features. However for this large scale regression problem, co-adaptation is required and all weights depend upon each other. Pre-training can be applied directly using knowledge of existing FBP algorithms. Discretized solutions are known for all layers: the convolutional layer uses the ramp filter, and the weighting layer accounts for cosine-weighting or redundancy weighting. These initializations can be used for a very effective pre-training.

2.5   Experiments

We present two applications of our proposed neural network architecture. For both we use slices of reconstructions of real patient data of size 512×512. These slices are downsized by a factor of 0.7 and embedded into a zero image of the original size to prevent truncation artifacts. We perform a ten-fold cross validation on 2378 slices of ten different patients.

The presented layers have been implemented with GPU-acceleration using the Caffe Framework. We also implemented the weight initializations used as pre-training as so called weight-fillers in the framework. The implementation will be released upon publication of the paper.

Limited Angle Parallel-Beam Reconstruction. In our first experiment, we explore improvements of parallel-beam architectures for limited angle reconstruction with five degree of missing data. We use 175 projections with an angular increment of one degree. The training target is the original image, which was used to simulate the projections. Our neural network architecture is the presented basic architecture for parallel beam reconstruction, with an additional weighting layer between the filtering and the back-projection operation. Since the data is incomplete, this problem can only be solved approximately without any regularizing assumptions. Thus, we place a *maxout* [4] filtering cascade on top of the network to introduce a non-linear filtering. We change the reconstruction filter to a 2D filter with a kernel size of 5. The values of the reconstruction kernel outside the third column are initialized to zero. The weighting layer is initialized with every value set to one, while the reconstruction filter is set to the well known Ramachandran-Lakshminarayan filter [8] discretization. The maxout network is initialized with Gaussian distributed random values.

Limited Angle Fan-Beam Reconstruction. In the second experiment, we learn compensation weights for a limited-angle problem with 180 projections up to 180 degree. We use our basic architecture for fan-beam reconstruction. The weights of the weighting layer are initialized with the well known Parker weights [7] multiplied with cosine weights. The reconstruction filter is set to the Ramachandran-Lakshminarayan filter discretization. As training target we employ a reconstruction with 360 projections of full scan data. During the training, only the weights receive a non-zero learning rate.

3   Evaluation

We found experimentally that the different layers require individual learning rates. The reconstruction filter was found to be extremely sensitive. The weighting-layer before the back-projection layer generally tolerates large learning rates.

For the parallel-beam problem we found Caffe's "RMSPROP" solver with the decay of 0.02 effective. The global learning rate was set to 10^{-6} while the reconstruction filter's learning rate had to be set to 10^{-15} to prevent divergence. For this problem online training turned out to be more effective than mini-batch or batch learning. The relative root-mean-square error, averaged over the test sets, drops from 6.78e−03 % for the classical FBP to only 3.54e−3 %. Hereby, our method outperforms the conventional FBP with enforcing the non-negativity constraint for every case by a factor of nearly two.

For the fan-beam experiment, we used Caffe's "ADAGRAD" solver and online training. We could set our learning rate for the weighting layer to $2 \cdot 10^2$ without divergent behaviour. The relative root-mean-square error averaged over the test sets dropped from 5.31e−03 % for FBP to 3.92e−03 % for our method.

Ground Truth   FBP   NN

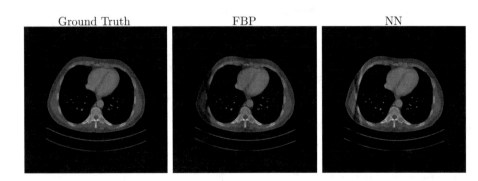

Fig. 3. Reconstruction results using 360°, 180° FBP, and 180° NN.

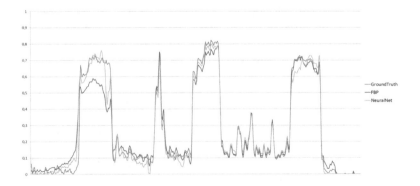

Fig. 4. Cross sections through the images of Fig. 3

Figures 3 and 4 show that the loss of mass could be corrected well, despite the architecture being equivalent to FBP.

4   Conclusion

We propose to use deep learning techniques to replace heuristic compensation steps in CT reconstruction. This enables various new architectures which can account for many artifact types. Evaluations of the reconstruction results show improved image quality compared to FBP while still retaining the same computational demands. We could successfully learn compensation layers for limited-angle tomography. Presumably, most artifact compensation methods in CT can be mapped to convolutional neural networks which will also enable to learn scatter compensation and beam-hardening.

Acknowledgments. The authors would like to thank Dr. Cynthia McCollough, the Mayo Clinic, the American Association of Physicists in Medicine funded by grants EB017095 and EB017185 from the National Institute of Biomedical Imaging and Bioengineering for providing the used data.

References

1. Argyrou, M., Maintas, D., Tsoumpas, C., Stiliaris, E.S.: Tomographic image reconstruction based on artificial neural network (ANN) techniques. In: Proceedings of 2012 IEEE Nuclear Science Symposium and Medical Imaging Conference Record (NSS/MIC), pp. 3324–3327. IEEE (2012)
2. Cierniak, R.: A new approach to image reconstruction from projections using a recurrent neural network. Int. J. Appl. Math. Comput. Sci. **18**, 147–157 (2008). AMCS
3. Duda, R.O., Hart, P.E., Stork, D.G. (eds.): Pattern Classification. Wiley, New York (2000)
4. Goodfellow, I.J., Warde-farley, D., Mirza, M., Courville, A., Bengio, Y.: Maxout networks. In: Proceedings of The 30th International Conference on Machine Learning, vol. 28, pp. 1319–1327 (2013)
5. Hammernik, K., Knoll, F., Sodickson, D., Pock, T.: Learning a variational model for compressed sensing mri reconstruction. In: Proceedings of the International Society of Magnetic Resonance in Medicine (ISMRM) (2016)
6. de Medeiros, L.F., da Silva, H.P., Ribeiro, E.P.: Tomographic image reconstruction of fan-beam projections with equidistant detectors using partially connected neural networks. In: Learning and Nonlinear Models - Revista da Sociedade Brasileira de Redes Neurais, vol. 1, pp. 122–130. Sociedade Brasileira de Redes Neurais (2003)
7. Parker, D.L.: Optimal short scan convolution reconstruction for fan beam CT. Med. Phys. **9**(2), 254–257 (1982)
8. Ramachandran, G.N., Lakshminarayanan, A.V.: Three-dimensional reconstruction from radiographs and electron micrographs: application of convolutions instead of fourier transforms. Proc. Nat. Acad. Sci. **68**(9), 2236–2240 (1971)

9. Riess, C., Berger, M., Wu, H., Manhart, M., Fahrig, R., Maier, A.: TV or not TV? that is the question. In: Leahy, R.M., Qi, J. (eds.) Fully Three-Dimensional Image Reconstruction in Radiology and Nuclear Medicine, pp. 341–344, June 2013

10. Srivastava, N., Hinton, G., Krizhevsky, A., Sutskever, I., Salakhutdinov, R.: Dropout: a simple way to prevent neural networks from overfitting. J. Mach. Learn. Res. **15**, 1929–1958 (2014)

11. Zeng, G.L. (ed.): Medical Image Reconstruction. Springer, New York (2009)

Axial Alignment for Anterior Segment Swept Source Optical Coherence Tomography via Robust Low-Rank Tensor Recovery

Yanwu Xu[1(✉)], Lixin Duan[2], Huazhu Fu[1], Xiaoqin Zhang[3],
Damon Wing Kee Wong[1], Baskaran Mani[4], Tin Aung[4], and Jiang Liu[1,5]

[1] Institute for Infocomm Research, Agency for Science,
Technology and Research, Singapore, Singapore
yaxu@i2r.a-star.edu.sg
[2] Amazon, Seattle, USA
[3] Wenzhou University, Wenzhou, China
[4] Singapore Eye Research Institute, Singapore, Singapore
[5] Cixi Institute of Biomedical Engineering,
Ningbo Institute of Materials Technology and Engineering,
Chinese Academy of Sciences, Ningbo, China

Abstract. We present a one-step approach based on low-rank tensor recovery for axial alignment in 360-degree anterior chamber optical coherence tomography. Achieving translational alignment and rotation correction of cross-sections simultaneously, this technique obtains a better anterior segment topographical representation and improves quantitative measurement accuracy and reproducibility of disease related parameters. Through its use of global information, the proposed method is more robust compared to using only individual or paired slices, and less sensitive to noise and motion artifacts. In angle closure analysis on 30 patient eyes, the preliminary results indicate that the proposed axial alignment method can not only facilitate manual qualitative analysis with more distinct landmark representation and much less human labor, but also can improve the accuracy of automatic quantitative assessment by 2.9%, which demonstrates that the proposed approach is promising for a wide range of clinical applications.

1 Introduction

The optical system resides in the anterior segment of the human eye, which consists of the cornea, iris and crystalline lens, as shown in Fig. 1A and C. Pathological changes in this area can drastically degrade vision and even result in blindness [1–3]. Quantitative assessments of the anterior segment are thus essential to a wide range of clinical applications [2–5].

Nowadays swept source optical coherence tomography (SS-OCT) is the most advanced technology for eye imaging, which has significantly improved imaging

This work is funded by A*STAR BEP Grant (152 148 0034) and NSFC Grant (61511130084).

S. Ourselin et al. (Eds.): MICCAI 2016, Part III, LNCS 9902, pp. 441–449, 2016.
DOI: 10.1007/978-3-319-46726-9_51

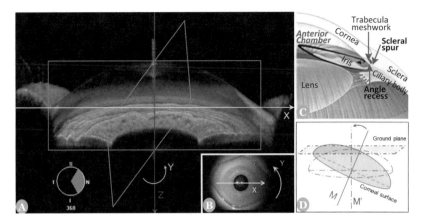

Fig. 1. A: swept source optical coherence tomography of anterior segment, where each *A-scan* is captured along the Z axis, each *B-scan* is captured along the X axis, and a 360-degree circular scan is performed along the Y axis. **B:** top view of the 360-degree anterior segment imaging process. **C:** anatomical structure of anterior segment around the angle. **D:** illustration of axial alignment of corneal surface reconstructed from aligned B-scans.

speed and detection sensitivity in comparison to traditional OCT technologies. Most recently, anterior segment SS-OCT (AS-SS-OCT) [1,6,7] has been developed for 3D imaging of the anterior segment of the human eye. Nevertheless, it is still hard to use SS-OCT to capture well-aligned B-scans along the X axis, due to involuntary eye motions and the relatively low density of raster scans.

As a fundamental problem for all SS-OCT based imaging technologies, *translational misalignment* reduction has been studied for SS-OCT retinal scans [8,9]. However, in the context of the anterior segment, we additionally need to correct the tilt of B-scans, due to the *rotational misalignment* caused by the positioning of an eye [10] and the fixation lag of the instrument [1] (which ignores eye movement during the imaging process [8,9]). As shown in Fig. 1D, the task is to tilt the axis M of the corneal surface to the ideal axis M' which is perpendicular to the ground plane. This is crucial to conduct accurate and reproducible quantitative measurements [1] of the anterior segment for various parameters that depend only on the actual geometry of the anterior chamber structure, e.g., cornea thickness map [1], central anterior chamber depth [2,3] and iris-trabecular contact (ITC) index [5].

To our knowledge, no such work has been done, although its importance has been highlighted in AS-SS-OCT instrument design works [1,6]. We formally refer to this problem as the *axial alignment* problem, which will be studied in this work. Currently, axial alignment and clinical parameter measurement rely on manual marking of landmarks (e.g., scleral spur [4,5]). And no fully automated approach has ever been reported. In this work, we propose a **one-step** method to simultaneously solve the alignment and rotation issues by using robust low-rank tensor recovery, based on the symmetry characteristic of the anterior segment structure. Our proposed method effectively utilizes the global information from the entire volume to reduce the sensitivity to noise and blur, and generates more reliable and smooth results. Moreover, our method is able to solve other general alignment problems when the input data is represented by a tensor. To verify the effectiveness of the proposed axial alignment algorithm, we perform extensive experiments on anterior chamber angle (ACA) analysis to qualitatively and quantitatively examine the improvements from performing axial alignment.

2   Proposed Method

2.1   Problem Formulation

An AS-SS-OCT volume, consisting of n_3 cross-sectional slices, can be viewed as a 3D tensor (see the *left* of Fig. 2), denoted as $\mathcal{D} \in \mathbb{R}^{n_1 \times n_2 \times n_3}$, where n_i is a positive integer. An ideal 360-degree AS-SS-OCT scan does not contain any noise or artifacts and its cross-sectional slices are all well aligned with each other. And thus, the tensor representation of an AS-SS-OCT volume should exhibit a *low-rank* structure, which is denoted as $\mathcal{A}$. However, artifacts from the AS-SS-OCT machine and small disturbances of the eyes (e.g., the involuntary axial movement) during the scan process may break the low-rank structure. In this work, we propose an axial alignment method by recovering the ideal low-rank structure $\mathcal{A}$ from a real OCT volume tensor $\mathcal{D}$, by taking into account the imaging difference $\mathcal{E}$ as well as by introducing a set of transformations $\mathrm{T} = \{\tau_1, \ldots, \tau_{n_3}\}$ to correct the misalignment and rotation. With the above, mathematically we have:

$$\mathcal{D} \circ \mathrm{T} = \mathcal{A} + \mathcal{E}, \tag{1}$$

where $\mathcal{D} \circ \mathrm{T}$ means applying every transformation τ_k to the corresponding OCT image $\mathcal{A}[:,:,k], k = 1, \ldots, n_3$. Additionally in this work, we assume that only a small fraction of the image pixels are corrupted by imaging artifacts, and hence $\mathcal{E}$ becomes a sparse error term. Therefore, with $\mathcal{A}$ being low-rank and $\mathcal{E}$ being sparse, we formally present the axial alignment problem as follows:

$$\min_{\mathcal{A},\mathcal{E},\mathrm{T}} \quad \mathrm{rank}(\mathcal{A}) + \lambda\|\mathcal{E}\|_0, \quad \text{s.t.} \quad \mathcal{D} \circ \mathrm{T} = \mathcal{A} + \mathcal{E}. \tag{2}$$

2.2   Solution

Note that it is not a trivial task to directly solve (2). Instead, we propose to decompose the rank of $\mathcal{A}$ by using the tensor rank definition [13] based on the Tucker decomposition [14]. Specifically, under the Tucker decomposition, $\mathcal{A}$ can be viewed as a rank-(r_1, r_2, r_3) tensor, where r_i is the rank of the unfolding matrix $\mathcal{A}_{(i)}$. And then $\mathrm{rank}(\mathcal{A})$ becomes a linear combination of $\mathrm{rank}(\mathcal{A}_{(i)})$'s, i.e., $\mathrm{rank}(\mathcal{A}) = \sum_{i=1}^{3} \omega_i \cdot \mathrm{rank}(\mathcal{A}_{(i)})$, where $\omega_i \in [0,1]$ is the predefined weight

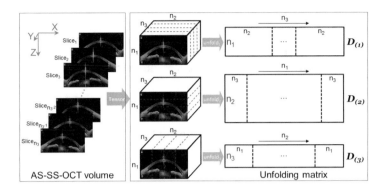

Fig. 2. *Left:* An AS-SS-OCT volume comprised of n_3 B-scans. *Right:* Tensor unfolding along each order

for the corresponding unfolding matrix $\mathcal{A}_{(i)}$, and $\sum_{i=1}^{3} \omega_i = 1$ is assumed to make the definition consistent with the form of the matrix. This decomposition step is essentially equivalent to first naturally unfolding the original tensor $\mathcal{A}$ to the unfolding matrices $\mathcal{A}_{(i)}$'s and then directly working on the combination of the ranks of $\mathcal{A}_{(i)}$'s. It is worth mentioning that minimizing the ranks of $\mathcal{A}_{(i)}$'s is intuitively meaningful in our studied problem. Specifically, enforcing the low rank of $\mathcal{A}_{(2)}$ and $\mathcal{A}_{(3)}$ will achieve good image alignment among the corresponding B-scans along the X and Z axes respectively, while keeping the low rank of $\mathcal{A}_{(1)}$ will correct the rotation of B-scans along the Z axis[1] [15]. So together, we can achieve both good image alignment and rotational correction in our axial alignment task for an input AS-SS-OCT volume.

Since it is still not easy to directly minimize $\sum_{i=1}^{3} \omega_i \cdot \mathrm{rank}(\mathcal{A}_{(i)})$ (due to the nonconvexity and discontinuity of the rank operation), we propose to replace each rank operation by using the corresponding nuclear norm which is a convex approximation. As a result, we approximate $\mathrm{rank}(\mathcal{A})$ by using:

$$\mathrm{rank}(\mathcal{A}) = \sum_{i=1}^{3} \omega_i \cdot \mathrm{rank}(\mathcal{A}_{(i)}) \approx \sum_{i=1}^{3} \omega_i \|\mathcal{A}_{(i)}\|_*. \tag{3}$$

Moreover, following [16], we replace the ℓ_0-norm in (2) with its convex surrogate ℓ_1-norm. In addition, since the constraint $\mathcal{D} \circ \mathrm{T} = \mathcal{A} + \mathcal{E}$ in (2) is non-linear, similar to [16], we approximate the constraint by linearizing it based on the first-order Taylor expansion (assuming the change in τ_k is small). And together with (3), we approximate our original problem by using the following one:

$$\min_{\mathcal{A},\mathcal{E},\mathrm{T}} \sum_{i=1}^{3} \omega_i \|\mathcal{A}_{(i)}\|_* + \lambda \|\mathcal{E}\|_1, \quad \text{s.t.} \quad \mathcal{D} \circ \mathrm{T} + \Delta\hat{\mathrm{T}} = \mathcal{A} + \mathcal{E}, \tag{4}$$

---

[1] As illustrated in Fig. 2, $\mathcal{A}_{(1)}$, $\mathcal{A}_{(2)}$ and $\mathcal{A}_{(3)}$ are obtained by unfolding $\mathcal{A}$ along the Z, X and Y axes, respectively.

where $\Delta\hat{T} = \text{fold}_3\left(\left(\sum_{k=1}^{n_3} J_k \Delta T \epsilon_k \epsilon_k^\top\right)^\top\right)$, $\text{fold}_3(\cdot)$ is the inverse operation of the mode-3 unfolding[2], J_k represents the Jacobian of $\mathcal{A}[:,:,k]$ w.r.t. the k-th transformation τ_k, and ϵ_k denotes the standard basis.

To solve (4), we first introduce a matrix B_i to replace $\mathcal{A}_{(i)}$ for each i, which decouples the interdependencies among the $\mathcal{A}_{(i)}$'s and relaxes (4), and then we arrive at the following optimization problem:

$$\min_{\mathcal{A},\mathcal{E},\mathrm{T},B_i} \sum_{i=1}^{3} \omega_i \|B_i\|_* + \lambda\|\mathcal{E}\|_1, \text{ s.t. } B_i = \mathcal{A}_{(i)}, \mathcal{D} \circ \mathrm{T} + \Delta\hat{\mathrm{T}} = \mathcal{A}+\mathcal{E}. \quad (5)$$

The optimization problem in (5) can be solved by employing the augmented Lagrange multiplier (ALM) method [17]. After solving (5) to obtain the optimal T^*, we can effectively correct both the alignment and rotation of all the OCT images from a test OCT imaging volume $\mathcal{D}$, by performing $\mathcal{D} \circ \mathrm{T}^*$, which is also the final result of axial alignment for $\mathcal{D}$.

2.3   Discussion

The proposed method is a relatively generalized approach which can be extended to different use cases. For instance, single images can be rectified by setting $\omega_3 = 0$ or get aligned without the need of rotation correction by setting $\omega_1 = 0$. Also, since the tensor representation can be extended to a higher order, we may be able to align multiple volumes from different or the same eyes along the axial direction to facilitate comparison, and our method may have potential to become a platform for pathology discovery in a series of images from different time instances. Moreover, the obtained error term $\mathcal{E}^*$, after solving (2), can be used to (1) capture pixel-wise differences for image denoising, deblurring and corruption recovery; and (2) detect outliers caused by artifacts or lesions. We will consider the above mentioned use cases as our future work.

3   Experiments

Since anterior chamber angle (ACA) analysis is the major application of anterior segment imaging (which has attracted much attention from clinicians [2,3,5] and computer-aided-diagnosis researchers [11,12]), we employ it for performance measurement on axial alignment. Specifically, based on ACA analysis, we investigate different manual/semi-automatic and fully automatic methods, by performing both visual comparison and qualitative evaluation.

3.1   Dataset and Experimental Setup

A total of 30 AS-SS-OCT volumes of 30 patients' eyes are used for the experiment. Each volume contains 128 slices, and each slice captures two angles at a

---

[2] To give an example, the inverse operation of the mode-i unfolding on an unfolding matrix $\mathcal{A}_{(i)}$ restores the original tensor $\mathcal{A}$, i.e., $\mathcal{A} = \text{fold}_i(\mathcal{A}_{(i)})$.

resolution of 1680×900. Among the 30 AS-SS-OCT volumes, 16 of them have primary angle closure (PAC) and the other 14 have open angle controls (OAC) [5,11,12]. For our method, we empirically set $\omega_1 = 0.5, \omega_2 = 0.25, \omega_3 = 0.25$ and $\lambda = 0.8$. On average, it takes about 20 mins to process each volume on a 3.2 GHz CPU with 24 GB RAM using MATLAB code. Optimizations for speed are certainly possible [17].

3.2   Qualitative Evaluation

The qualitative evaluation is based on each single volume. The corresponding 128 slices of a volume are averaged before and after axial alignment in order to visually compare whether it can help identify PAC and OAC. In current clinical practice, this task totally relies on manual assessment, i.e., for each 360-degree scan, the ophthalmologists manually mark the landmarks (seen in Fig. 1C) such as scleral spur (SS) and angle recess (AR) on four or more slices, to calculate parameters such as ITC index [5] (which needs axial adjustment), angle opening distance (AOD) [3], etc., or directly classify each angle as open or closed. As reported in [5], at least 16 labeled slices (32 angles) are required to guarantee a relatively reliable angle closure grading, which is very time consuming and subjective, and may be inaccurate due to a low sampling ratio.

As illustrated in Fig. 3, it is clear that in general the averaged slices after axial alignment are visually much better than the ones before axial alignment, which provides a clearer *summarization* of each AS-SS-OCT volume to facilitate qualitative assessment of angle closure, with much less human labor involved, compared to conventional practice (1 vs 16+). Note that among the six averaged aligned slices, Fig. 3C$_2$ still has a bit of blurring at the iris regions. This is due to the considerable scale change caused by bad eye positioning (i.e., imaging does not focus on or aim at the geometrical corneal center), which unfortunately cannot be recovered without introducing distortion.

In addition, as reported in [4], previously the SS points could not even be manually located in 30 % or more of angles, which greatly hampers quantitative analysis of a large number of ACA parameters related to SS [3,4]. However, as demonstrated in Fig. 3, the SS points are more distinct in well-aligned averaged cross-sectional slices. This not only can facilitate manual or semi-automatic quantitative analysis, but may also be used to develop a new fully automatic quantitative measurement tool for angle closure assessment, which will be investigated in our future work.

3.3   Quantitative Evaluation

The quantitative experiments are based on classifying each individual angle to open or closed, and the ground truth of the 7680 angles is labeled by a group of ophthalmologists from a hospital. The ITC in each ACA is located using the algorithm proposed in [12], and then a linear SVM classifier is used to classify each angle as open or closed, using HOG or HEP features as proposed in [11, 12], respectively. We compare the classification accuracy before and after axial

Average of unaligned slices (**D**)   Average of axial aligned slices (**DoT***)

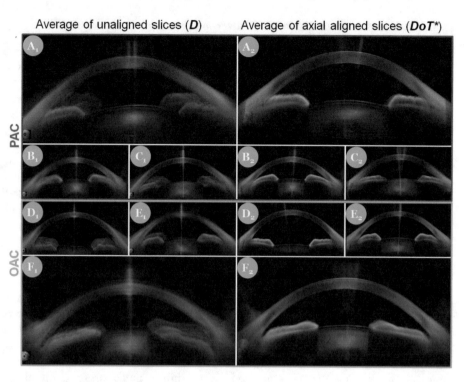

Fig. 3. Illustration of averaged cross-sectional slices before (*left column*) and after (*right column*) axial alignment.

alignment to investigate how the proposed axial alignment facilitates automatic ACA classification.

We performed ten repeated 2-fold cross-validation experiments, *i.e.*, for each testing round, half of all the volumes with PAC and OAC are randomly selected to train a classifier, and the other half are used for testing; then the training and testing data are swapped to perform the test again. We assess the performance using balanced accuracy ($\bar{P}$) with a fixed 85 % specificity (P_-) and area under ROC curve (AUC) which evaluates the overall performance. The optimal parameters of each method are chosen following [11,12]. For more details, readers may refer to [11,12].

Table 1. Performance comparisons for ACA classification before and after axial alignment (denoted as $AL+$ in the table) (P-value < 0.01)

Method	HOG [11]	AL+HOG	HEP [12]	AL+HEP
AUC	0.840±0.060	0.864±0.071	0.856 ±0.078	**0.871 ±0.057**
$\bar{P}(\%)$	73.5±8.5	76.9±8.9	76.9 ±8.8	**78.0 ±8.6**

The results shown in Table 1 indicate the following:

1. Comparing the classification accuracy of each individual method before and after axial alignment, we can see that both methods gain a certain improvement, which demonstrates that the proposed axial alignment has the ability to improve angle closure detection accuracy. Specifically, the HOG based method improves 2.9 % and HEP improves 1.8 % in terms of AUC, which might be explained as HOG being relatively more sensitive to rotation compared to HEP.

2. Comparing the two methods under the same axial alignment condition (with/without), HEP features outperform HOG features, which was also observed in [12]. This might be because HEP is extracted from down-sampled images with very low resolution, and thus has larger tolerance to rotational and translational misalignment.

4   Conclusion

In this work, we proposed a one-step method based on robust low-rank tensor recovery to solve the new yet fundamental axial alignment problem for AS-SS-OCT imaging. The preliminary experiments on angle closure analysis demonstrate that our proposed method not only can facilitate manual qualitative assessments, but also can significantly improve the accuracy of automatic quantitative assessments. This method thus exhibits much promise for other clinical applications besides anterior segment analysis.

References

1. Gora, M., Karnowski, K., Szkulmowski, M., Kaluzny, B.J., Huber, R., Kowalczyk, A., Wojtkowski, M.: Ultra high-speed swept source OCT imaging of the anterior segment of human eye at 200 kHz with adjustable imaging range. Opt. Express **17**(17), 14880–14894 (2009)
2. Lim, S.H.: Clinical applications of anterior segment optical coherence tomography. J. Ophthalmol. Article ID 605729, 12 (2015)
3. Maslin, J.S., Barkana, Y., Dorairaj, S.K.: Anterior segment imaging in glaucoma: an updated review. Indian J. Ophthalmol. **63**(8), 630–640 (2015)
4. Sakata, L.M., Lavanya, R., Friedman, D.S., Aung, H.T., Seah, S.K., Foster, P.J., Aung, T.: Assessment of the scleral spur in anterior segment optical coherence tomography images. Arch Ophthalmol. **126**(2), 181–185 (2008)
5. Mishima, K., Tomidokoro, A., Suramethakul, P., Mataki, N., Kurita, N., Mayama, C., Araie, M.: Iridotrabecular contact observed using anterior segment three-dimensional OCT in eyes with a shallow peripheral anterior chamber. Invest. Ophthalmol. Vis. Sci. **54**(7), 4628–4635 (2013)
6. Li, P., Johnstone, M., Wang, R.K.: Full anterior segment biometry with extended imaging range spectral domain optical coherence tomography at 1340 nm. J. Biomed. Opt. **19**(4), 046013 (2014)
7. The cornea/anterior segment OCT SS-1000 'CASIA'. http://www.tomey.com/Products/OCT/SS-1000CASIA.html

8. Xu, J., Ishikawa, H., Wollstein, G., Kagemann, L., Schuman, J.S.: Alignment of 3-D optical coherence tomography scans to correct eye movement using a particle filtering. IEEE Trans. Med. Image **31**(7), 1337–1345 (2012)
9. Montuoro, A., Wu, J., Waldstein, S., Gerendas, B., Langs, G., Simader, C., Schmidt-Erfurth, U.: Motion artefact correction in retinal optical coherence tomography using local symmetry. In: Golland, P., Hata, N., Barillot, C., Hornegger, J., Howe, R. (eds.) MICCAI 2014, Part II. LNCS, vol. 8674, pp. 130–137. Springer, Heidelberg (2014)
10. Navarro, R., González, L., Hernández, L.: Optics of the average normal cornea from general and canonical representations of its surface topography. J. Opt. Soc. Am. A. Opt. Image Sci. Vis. **23**(2), 219–232 (2006)
11. Xu, Y., Liu, J., Tan, N.M., Lee, B.H., Wong, D.W.K., Baskaran, M., Perera, S., Aung, T.: Anterior chamber angle classification using multiscale histograms of oriented gradients for glaucoma subtype identification. In: IEEE Engineering in Medicine and Biology Society, pp. 3167–3170 (2012)
12. Xu, Y., Liu, J., Cheng, J., Lee, B.H., Wong, D.W.K., Baskaran, M., Perera, S., Aung, T.: Automated anterior chamber angle localization and glaucoma type classification in OCT images. In: IEEE Engineering in Medicine and Biology Society, pp. 7380–7383 (2013)
13. Liu, J., Musialski, P., Wonka, P., Ye, J.: Tensor completion for estimating missing values in visual data. IEEE Trans. Pattern Anal. Mach. Intell. **35**(1), 208–220 (2013)
14. Kolda, T., Bader, B.: Tensor decompositions and applications. SIAM Rev. **51**(3), 455–500 (2009)
15. Xu, Y., Liu, J., Wong, D.W.K., Baskaran, M., Perera, S., Aung, T.: Similarity-weighted linear reconstruction of anterior chamber angles for glaucoma classification. In: IEEE International Symposium on Biomedical Imaging, pp. 693–697 (2016)
16. Peng, Y., Ganesh, A., Wright, J., Ma, Y.: RASL: robust alignment by sparse and low-rank decomposition for linearly correlated images. In: CVPR, pp. 2233–2246 (2013)
17. Lin, Z., Chen, M., Wu, L., Ma, Y.: The augmented lagrange multiplier method for exact recovery of corrupted low-rank matrices. UIUC Technical report UILU-ENG-09-2215 (2009)
18. Yang, J., Yuan, X.: Linearized augmented lagrangian and alternating direction methods for nuclear norm minimization. Math. Comput. **82**(281), 301–329 (2013)

3D Imaging from Video and Planar Radiography

Julien Pansiot[(✉)] and Edmond Boyer

LJK, Inria Grenoble, Grenoble, France
{julien.pansiot,edmond.boyer}@inria.fr

Abstract. In this paper we consider dense volumetric modeling of moving samples such as body parts. Most dense modeling methods consider samples observed with a moving X-ray device and cannot easily handle moving samples. We propose a novel method that uses a surface motion capture system associated to a single low-cost/low-dose planar X-ray imaging device for dense in-depth attenuation information. Our key contribution is to rely on Bayesian inference to solve for a dense attenuation volume given planar radioscopic images of a moving sample. The approach enables multiple sources of noise to be considered and takes advantage of limited prior information to solve an otherwise ill-posed problem. Results show that the proposed strategy is able to reconstruct dense volumetric attenuation models from a very limited number of radiographic views over time on simulated and in-vivo data.

1 Introduction

The ability to capture intrinsic body structure in motion is of interest in a number of fields related to medical imaging such as computer-assisted surgery, biomechanics, and sports science. Many applications consider video or depth cameras and infer skeletal motion from surface observations using prior models. However, this strategy does not provide real measures on the internal structure and the estimated skeleton does not match the actual bone structure due to multiple factors such as inaccurate skeletal model and complex elastic tissue motion. With the aim to provide better measures to observe intrinsic structures in motion, and validation purposes, we investigate in this paper a new strategy that recovers dense 3D volumetric models of moving samples.

To this purpose, we combine a video-based surface motion capture system that provides motion cues, with a single static planar X-ray imaging device that captures the inner structure. We present the first step towards three-dimensional volumetric motion capture by investigating first rigidly moving samples, assuming limited prior knowledge on the captured samples. A key concept of our approach compared to traditional tomography is that it does not consider motion as low-amplitude noise to be corrected, but at the contrary as a source of information, ensuring the capture of X-ray images from multiple viewpoints.

As a result, the proposed configuration can consider moving samples as well as several sensors (*eg.* two X-ray devices). Yet less accurate than a CT-scanner, it yields a less expensive low-dose solution, taking benefit of equipment widely available in clinical environments.

© Springer International Publishing AG 2016
S. Ourselin et al. (Eds.): MICCAI 2016, Part III, LNCS 9902, pp. 450–457, 2016.
DOI: 10.1007/978-3-319-46726-9_52

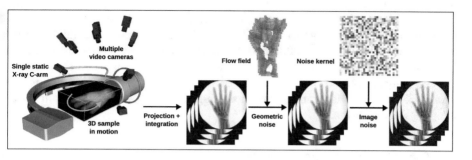

Fig. 1. X-ray image formation model for a moving sample observed by a single static planar X-ray device. Video cameras are used to recover the sample motion.

Our volumetric reconstruction method builds on super-resolution techniques [6] to optimally exploit X-ray samples and infer 3D attenuation. It relies on an X-ray image formation model (see Fig. 1) accounting for 2D sensor noise as well as 3D geometric errors. This model is associated with a volumetric L_1 smoothness prior to constrain the reconstruction, allowing for a limited number of input views. All these elements are integrated within a Bayesian framework for backward inference.

To summarize, the key contribution introduced in this paper is a Bayesian approach to 3D imaging of a moving sample which accounts for both sensor and calibration inaccuracies using a generative model.

2   Related Work

Currently, the two well-established classes of methods to recover attenuation models are planar radiography and Computed Tomography (CT). The former can capture motion at competitive frame rates with a low dose, but is limited to integrated two-dimensional information. The latter, in the form of Multi-Detector CT (MDCT) and Electron Beam CT (EBCT), can capture accurate dense 3D volumetric attenuation models at up to 30 fps, yet exposing patients to higher ionising radiations, present much higher costs, and limited versatility.

For these reasons, few-views cone-beam computed tomography (CBCT) techniques [4] have gained interest. Several methods have been devised to reconstruct relatively accurate 3D attenuation models from a limited number of cone-beam images [1,10]. Nevertheless these methods are limited to static samples.

The combination of motion capture and emission tomography has also been investigated but either requires markers [7], or is designed for low-amplitude motion correction [5]. Similarly, motion correction in tomography has been largely covered in traditional CT/PET [3] as well as CBCT [11]. Again, our strategy differs since we consider motion as a mean to vary viewpoints which helps capturing moving samples.

A method to reconstruct 3D attenuation from a limited number of arbitrary X-ray views was proposed in [9], but assumes reasonably good calibration.

The general approach by [8] reconstructs volumetric attenuation from a limited number of X-ray views of a moving object which motion is estimated using videos. While building on a similar concept, we take however a different and more formal generative strategy inspired by image super resolution [6]. In this domain, Bayesian inference methods have demonstrated their ability to optimally exploit noisy observations with uncertainty modelling and we extend them to our X-ray imaging configuration.

3   Generative Image Model

As mentioned, our generative model builds on existing image formation model [6] to explain the X-ray images given the 3D model. Our method takes as input a set of X-ray images of a rigidly moving sample. The images are first registered in a common framework using the motion estimated by a multi-view motion capture system. A dense attenuation model of the moving sample, represented as a voxel grid, is then reconstructed using the entire X-ray image sequence.

We detail below the main components of this model. In order to account for the multiple sources of noise present in the acquisition process, we introduce a generative image formation model, as illustrated in Fig. 1. This model is associated with a sparse prior, $ie.$ a TV-norm.

3.1   Image Formation

We discretise the continuous absorbance problem in 3D as a weighted sum over the voxels v_j along the given ray ω, d_j being the distance covered within the voxel v_j and μ_j the attenuation assumed uniform within v_j, defining the absorbance $I(\omega)$ in function of the emitted and transmitted intensities L_0 and $L(\omega)$:

$$I(\omega) = \log \frac{L(\omega)}{L_0} = -\sum_{j \in \omega} d_j \mu_j. \tag{1}$$

In real scenarii however, several sources of noise affect the image formation, and therefore a more comprehensive image formation model must be devised as illustrated in Fig. 1. We consider a sequence of images $I = \{I_i\}$ acquired from a volume discretised as a voxel grid with attenuations $V = \{\mu_j\}$. For each image I_i we have:

1. A known projection and integration matrix P_i composed of the coefficients d_j obtained from motion capture. In the ideal case, we would have $P_i V = I_i$. We denote the projection matrix concatenation for all images $P = \{P_i\}$.
2. A 2D image noise variance θ_i accounting for the light source, the amplifier, and the imaging sensor.
3. Geometric noise, $ie.$ the errors in the projection P_i. This includes the inaccuracy in the motion and projection estimation as well as the deviation from purely rigid motion. It is modeled by a warping matrix F_i.

3.2   Bayesian Model

Our aim is to recover the 3D attenuation V given the absorbance image sequence I, $ie.$ to invert the model described previously. For this purpose we rely on a MAP estimation to find the optimal solution in terms of attenuation and noise:

$$\{V^*, \{F_i\}^*, \{\theta_i\}^*\} = \underset{V, \{F_i\}, \{\theta_i\}}{\operatorname{argmax}} \; p(V, \{F_i\}, \{\theta_i\})|\{I_i\}), \tag{2}$$

where, assuming statistical conditional independence between images given the attenuation model:

$$p(V, \{F_i\}, \{\theta_i\})|\{I_i\}) \propto p(V) \prod_i p(F_i) \prod_i p(\theta_i) \prod_i p(I_i|V, F_i, \theta_i). \tag{3}$$

3.3   Priors and Image Likelihood

Geometric noise appears as a result of calibration inaccuracies and non exactly rigid object motions. We modeled it by a warping function F_i, estimated using the optical flow w_i [2] between the observed image I_i and the generated one P_iV.

As the inverse problem (3) is ill-posed and noise-ridden, we introduce noise and model priors. Given the nature of the data typically observed, the sparsity of the derivative responses is used as a prior for the 3D attenuation volume as in [6]:

$$p(V) = \eta^{dim(V)} e^{-\eta \|\nabla V\|}, \tag{4}$$

where η is the gradient weight. The minimisation of the L_1 norm of the gradient, or Total Variation TVL_1, favours continuous volumes separated by potentially high, albeit localised gradients.

The likelihood distribution is modeled as an exponential distribution:

$$p(I_i|V, F_i, \theta_i) = \theta_i^{dim(I_i)} e^{-\theta_i \|I_i - F_iP_iV\|}. \tag{5}$$

where the 2D image noise variance θ_i follows a Gamma distribution [6].

4   Model Estimation

In order to solve for the parameters in the MAP estimation (2), we use a coordinate descent scheme [6], that iteratively cycles through the independent estimation of each parameter: the original volume V using expressions (4) and (5), image noise variance θ_i, and the motion noise warp F_i as detailed in Sect. 3.3.

Attenuation Volume. Given the current estimates for the warping function F_i and noise θ_i, we estimate the volume based on the image set $\{I_i\}$ and the gradient prior η with Iteratively Reweighted Least Squares (IRLS) to minimise:

$$V^* = \underset{V}{\operatorname{argmin}} \sum_i \theta_i \|F_iP_iV - I_i\| + \eta \|\nabla V\|. \tag{6}$$

Image/Sensor Noise. Given the current volume V of N voxels and flow field F_i we estimate the image noise variance θ_i based on the residual error following a gamma distribution:

$$\theta_i^* = \frac{\alpha + N - 1}{\beta + \overline{x}} \text{ with } \overline{x} = \sum_{q=1}^{N} |(I_i - F_i P_i V)(q)|, \tag{7}$$

Geometric Correction. The residual motion is estimated using the optical flow $\dot{w}_i$ [2] between the observed image I_i and the projected volume $P_i V$. Given the current volume V and the noise variance θ_i, we estimate the flow w_i associated to the warp matrix F_i. We then reformulate the data term in (6) as:

$$\sum_i \theta_i \| P_i V - F_i^{-1} I_i \|. \tag{8}$$

5   Experiments

Three sets of experiment were carried out to validate the proposed framework. First the CT scan of a phantom model was used to simulate image observations. Secondly, the phantom model was placed into our hardware platform. And third, an in-vivo hand was captured and reconstructed using the proposed framework.

5.1   Simulated Radiographic and Video Data from CT

A forearm phantom, consisting of a real human forearm skeleton cast in resin was first scanned with a regular CT device. A complete capture pipeline was then simulated from the phantom scan which was rendered by 10 virtual video cameras and one virtual planar X-ray image[1]. The phantom scan model was then moved artificially, following roughly a 180 degrees rotation. The phantom motion was estimated using video and Iterative Closest Point for comparison with [8]. The proposed approach was then applied to the simulated data.

The performance of individual components of the algorithm were analysed independently, as illustrated in Fig. 2. We note that on simulated data, our approach exhibits slightly better contrast than ART (higher Mutual Information (MI) score). We also evaluate the sensitivity of our method with respect to the number of input frames, as illustrated in Fig. 3. These experiments show that for the given dataset, main skeletal structures can be recovered with as little as 16 frames. However, finer features such as bone cavities require at least 32 frames.

Furthermore we reduce the motion range from 180 to 90 degrees, which clearly impacts the volumetric estimation quality, as illustrated in Fig. 4. Raycasting rendering of the volume yields sharper results for poses within the original motion range, due to increased sampling density, as illustrated in Fig. 5.

---

[1] Input data and more results for simulated and in-vivo experiments are available here: http://morpheo.inrialpes.fr/people/pansiot/sup/2016_Pansiot_MICCAI.mp4.

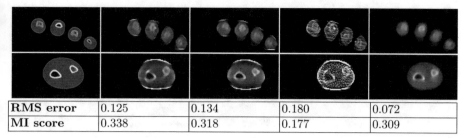

| RMS error | 0.125 | 0.134 | 0.180 | 0.072 |
| MI score | 0.338 | 0.318 | 0.177 | 0.309 |

Fig. 2. Results on simulated data (2 selected slices, RMS, and Mutual Information (MI) score). Left-to-right: ground-truth CT scan, proposed method, without optical flow, without TVL_1 prior, ART [8]. Without TVL_1 prior, the algorithm does not converge. The contrast is better with the proposed approach (better MI as compared to ART) even though artefacts appear on the edges as a result of aliasing during the data simulation process (higher RMS as compared to ART). ART performs relatively well in part due to the fact that simulated data are close to the noiseless theoretical model.

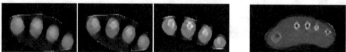
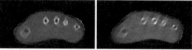

Fig. 3. Results on simulated data (selected slice) based on varying numbers of input frames. Left-to-right: 8, 16, and 32 frames. Skeletal structures are visible with 16 frames when detailed features require 32 frames.

Fig. 4. Results on simulated data (selected slice) based on varying input angular range. Left: 32 frames roughly distributed over 180 degrees; right: over 90 degrees.

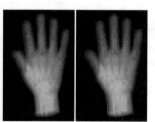

Fig. 5. Results on the simulated data (raycasting rendering) based on varying input angular range. Left: 32 frames roughly distributed over 180 degrees; right: over 90 degrees. The rendered viewpoint falls within the range of the original 90 degrees motion, but not on an original viewpoint, leading to sharper rendering due to locally denser sampling.

5.2 In-Situ Forearm Phantom

The proposed platform is composed of ten colour video cameras and a single X-ray C-arm. The forearm phantom presented here above was placed into the capture platform and moved manually to follow roughly a 180 degree rotation. The volumetric results were compared to the original CT model. Unlike the simulated experiment, the CT model and the model reconstructed with the C-arm images are in different poses since they correspond to 2 different acquisitions

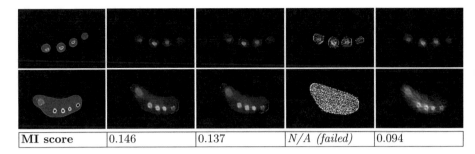

| MI score | 0.146 | 0.137 | *N/A (failed)* | 0.094 |

Fig. 6. Results on the forearm phantom (2 selected slices and Mutual Information (MI) score). Left-to-right: ground-truth CT scan, proposed method, without optical flow, without TVL_1 prior, ART [8]. Without optical flow, artefacts are visible, for example in the bone cavities. The ART method produces much noisier results.

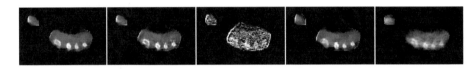

Fig. 7. Results on the in-vivo hand with different priors (selected slice). Left-to-right: TVL_1 weight $\eta = 2$; $\eta = 1$; $\eta = 0$ (no TVL_1 prior); no optical flow prior; ART [8]. The first three reconstructions demonstrate the favourable impact of the TVL_1 prior. Comparing the first and fourth reconstruction (no optical flow), we observe less artefacts with flow and the bones are better resolved, in particular the index. ART exhibits a lot of under-sampling artefacts that cannot be recovered without priors.

of the phantom, as illustrated in Fig. 6. Furthermore, the energy spectrum of the CT scanner and that of the low-dose X-ray C-arm are different. Hence, the two models are first registered using multi-resolution Mutual Information (MI). The MI score is provided for quantitative comparison, being invariant to attenuation spectrum. Unlike the simulated case, this experiment shows that the proposed method performs significantly better than ART. In particular, the use of optical flow for motion noise compensation allows to retain a fair level of detail, whilst the TVL_1 norm prior constrains the ill-posed problem without excessive blurring.

5.3   In-Vivo Human Hand

Finally, an actual in-vivo human hand was moved in the field, again following roughly a rotation movement over 20 frames. The results presented in Fig. 7 demonstrate the benefit of our approach which improves the results in some specific areas which we attribute to local (*ie.* non-rigid) motion. This demonstrates the interest of the generative model with the optical flow correction and the TV L1 regularization over more traditional approaches for few-view CBCT.

6   Conclusions and Future Work

In this paper we have presented a novel generative model to estimate a dense volumetric attenuation model of a rigidly moving object using motion tracking and a single planar X-ray device. Our framework contributes with an approach that takes benefit of object motion to accumulate evidence on the object inner structure. To this aim, we have introduced a Bayesian approach that optimally exploits X-ray information while enabling for acquisition noise. Our experiments show that the TVL_1 prior on the attenuation volume fundamentally contributed to convergence without excessive blurring, and that geometric noise can be effectively corrected using optical flow. This work considers rigid motion and we are currently investigating non-rigid motion.

Acknowledgments. This research was partly funded by the KINOVIS project (ANR-11-EQPX-0024).

References

1. Bang, T.Q., Jeon, I.: CT reconstruction from a limited number of X-ray projections. World Acad. Sci. Eng. Technol. **5**(10), 488–490 (2011)
2. Bruhn, A., Weickert, J., Schnörr, C.: Lucas/Kanade meets Horn/Schunck: Combining local and global optic flow methods. Int. J. Comput. Vis. **61**(3), 211–231 (2005)
3. Dawood, M., Lang, N., Jiang, X., Schafers, K.: Lung motion correction on respiratory gated 3-D PET/CT images. TMI **25**(4), 476–485 (2006)
4. Feldkamp, L.A., Davis, L.C., Kress, J.W.: Practical cone-beam algorithm. J. Opt. Soc. Am. (JOSA) A **1**(6), 612–619 (1984)
5. Hutton, B.F., Kyme, A.Z., Lau, Y.H., Skerrett, D.W., Fulton, R.R.: A hybrid 3-D reconstruction/registration algorithm for correction of head motion in emission tomography. IEEE Trans. Nucl. Sci. **49**(1), 188–194 (2002)
6. Liu, C., Sun, D.: On Bayesian adaptive video super resolution. TPAMI **36**(2), 346–360 (2014)
7. McNamara, J.E., Pretorius, P.H., Johnson, K., Mukherjee, J.M., Dey, J., Gennert, M.A., King, M.A.: A flexible multicamera visual-tracking system for detecting and correcting motion-induced artifacts in cardiac SPECT slices. Med. Phys. **36**(5), 1913–1923 (2009)
8. Pansiot, J., Reveret, L., Boyer, E.: Combined visible and X-ray 3D imaging. In: MIUA, London, pp. 13–18, July 2014
9. Sidky, E.Y., Kao, C.M., Pan, X.: Accurate image reconstruction from few-views and limited-angle data in divergent-beam CT. J. X-Ray Sci. Technol. **14**(2), 119–139 (2006)
10. Yang, G., Hipwell, J.H., Hawkes, D.J., Arridge, S.R.: A nonlinear least squares method for solving the joint reconstruction and registration problem in digital breast tomosynthesis. In: MIUA, pp. 87–92 (2012)
11. Zhang, Q., Hu, Y.C., Liu, F., Goodman, K., Rosenzweig, K.E., Goodman, K., Mageras, G.S.: Correction of motion artifacts in cone-beam CT using a patient-specific respiratory motion model. Med. Phys. **37**(6), 2901–2909 (2010)

Semantic Reconstruction-Based Nuclear Cataract Grading from Slit-Lamp Lens Images

Yanwu Xu[1(✉)], Lixin Duan[2], Damon Wing Kee Wong[1],
Tien Yin Wong[3], and Jiang Liu[1,4]

[1] Institute for Infocomm Research, Agency for Science,
Technology and Research, Singapore, Singapore
yaxu@i2r.a-star.edu.sg
[2] Amazon, Seattle, USA
[3] Singapore Eye Research Institute, Singapore, Singapore
[4] Cixi Institute of Biomedical Engineering,
Ningbo Institute of Materials Technology and Engineering,
Chinese Academy of Sciences, Beijing, China

Abstract. Cataracts are the leading cause of visual impairment and blindness worldwide. Cataract grading, i.e. assessing the presence and severity of cataracts, is essential for diagnosis and progression monitoring. We present in this work an automatic method for predicting cataract grades from slit-lamp lens images. Different from existing techniques which normally formulate cataract grading as a regression problem, we solve it through reconstruction-based classification, which has been shown to yield higher performance when the available training data is densely distributed within the feature space. To heighten the effectiveness of this reconstruction-based approach, we introduce a new semantic feature representation that facilitates alignment of test and reference images, and include locality constraints on the linear reconstruction to reduce the influence of less relevant reference samples. In experiments on the large ACHIKO-NC database comprised of 5378 images, our system outperforms the state-of-the-art regression methods over a range of evaluation metrics.

1 Introduction

Cataracts are a clouding of the lens that reduces transmission of light to the retina. They may be caused by a variety of factors, including age, ultraviolet radiation, and genetics. This obstruction of light can seriously impair vision and may even progress into blindness [1]. Due to its prevalence particularly among the elderly, there is a need to screen for them in an efficient and cost-effective manner.

Most commonly, cataracts develop in the nucleus, which is the central layer of the lens. The opacification and coloration caused by nuclear cataracts is visible in cross-sectional views of the lens in slit-lamp images. Currently, nuclear cataracts are diagnosed by ophthalmologists directly using a slit-lamp microscope, or graded by clinicians who assess the presence and severity of a cataract

© Springer International Publishing AG 2016
S. Ourselin et al. (Eds.): MICCAI 2016, Part III, LNCS 9902, pp. 458–466, 2016.
DOI: 10.1007/978-3-319-46726-9_53

by comparing slit-lamp images against a set of protocol photographs [2–4] such as that shown in Fig. 1. However, manual assessments can be both subjective and time-consuming [4].

The need for objectivity and efficiency in nuclear cataract grading has led to the development of several computer-aided systems [5–10]. These systems generally operate with three main steps: lens structure detection, feature extraction, and severity prediction. Most prior art formulate the severity prediction as a regression problem on certain visual features. In the state-of-the-art method of [5], bag-of-features (BOF) descriptors are extracted from RGB and HSV color channels of different lens sections, and group sparsity regression (GSR) is used to jointly select the features, parameters and models for grading. In [6], 21 pre-defined features are extracted from different sections of the lens, and then are fed into a pre-learned RBF kernel-based Support Vector Regressor (SVR) to estimate the cataract grade.

While regression-based methods have achieved higher accuracy than other previous techniques, we observe that the dense sampling of cataract grades in the available training data allows for a more direct grading prediction. When training samples are densely distributed in the feature space, higher accuracy can be achieved through reconstruction from the samples, where class membership of an input is estimated based on reconstruction accuracy from similar instances within each class. Compared to regression, a reconstruction-based approach is less reliant on discriminative feature quality and more robust to small inter-class margins, such as those that exist for the continuous space of cataract grades. These advantages of reconstruction-based classification have been exploited for human gait recognition [11], where a large number of training samples are densely distributed in a feature space that is compact due to the relatively narrow range of gait differences.

For nuclear cataract grading, however, the reconstruction-based approach is ineffective when employed in a straightforward manner. In our preliminary tests, linear reconstruction of lens images after alignment and size normalization of lens sections led to grading performance much lower than the state-of-the-art *BOF+GSR* method [5]. This is mainly due to inadequate lens alignment. Since lenses vary in both size and shape, a non-rigid structural alignment of lenses is needed for accurate reconstruction, but is challenging to accomplish. To address this problem, we propose to model the test and reference images with a new semantic representation of lens structure that is less sensitive to slight misalignments, instead of processing in the original raw image space. In addition, we improve the accuracy of reconstruction-based cataract grade prediction by accounting for the degree of similarity between the test image and reference images. By ignoring reference images that are not well-aligned to the test image as done in the similarity ranking-based CBMIR approach [8], the alignment issue is further diminished.

Our proposed method essentially follows the manual grading protocol, as it directly compares with reference images through the alignment and reconstruction procedure, and it compares intensity/color and contrast patterns via the

Nuclear
Cataract
Grade

Standard
Lens
Photograph

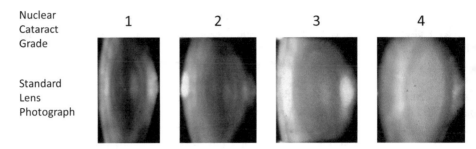

Fig. 1. Standard photographs of the Wisconsin nuclear cataract grading system. From left to right, the severity of the nuclear cataracts increases, with greater brightness and lower contrast between anatomical landmarks. In addition, the color of the nucleus and posterior cortex exhibits more of a yellow tint due to brunescence.

semantic feature representation. With this approach, our system attains higher overall performance than the state-of-the-art, and has the potential to be applied to other ocular diseases such as angle closure glaucoma detection and optical cup localization.

2   Nuclear Cataract Grading Through Semantic Reconstruction

We formulate nuclear cataract grading as a linear reconstruction problem with a similarity-weighted constraint. For a given slit-lamp test image, our algorithm follows the steps of lens structure detection, semantic feature extraction, and linear reconstruction with reference images.

2.1   Lens Structure Detection

Detection of lens structures in slit-lamp images is a well-studied problem with effective solutions [5–10]. For this purpose, we employ techniques similar to those used in [5,6]. As illustrated in Fig. 2, the lens structure detection proceeds with the following steps:

1. Using the active shape model based lens structure detection proposed in [6], each lens image is separated into three sections: anterior cortex, nucleus, and posterior cortex. The visual axis is located as well.
2. A lens cross-section is extracted around the visual axis, using a bounding box with a height of h pixels ($h = 128$ in our implementation) to obtain the central parts of the nucleus, anterior cortex and posterior cortex.
3. Features are extracted from only the nucleus and posterior cortex sections, since the anterior cortex contains no discriminant information for nuclear cataract grading [5]. This practice is also supported by clinical protocol [4], where nuclear cataracts are graded based on the intensity and visibility of nuclear landmarks and the color of the nucleus and posterior cortex.

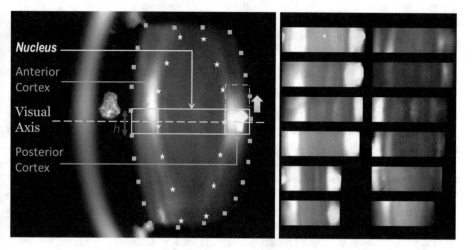

Fig. 2. Left: illustration of lens structure detection, with the initially detected lens structure (solid yellow boxes) and final detected posterior cortex (dashed yellow box). Right: examples of detected lens cross-sections. On the left are initially detected cross-sections with sharp reflections in the posterior cortex. On the right are cross-sections that were detected without the posterior cortex reflections. Since the anterior cortex will be discarded, reflections there need not be avoided. (Color figure online)

4. As illustrated on the right side of Fig. 2, bright spots may appear in the extracted posterior cortex section, due to reflections of the photographic flash. The presence of these sharp reflections may greatly reduce grading accuracy, so we avoid them by simply shifting the bounding box of the posterior cortex vertically with a step size of $h/2$ until it has a mean scaled value lower than a threshold value θ_p, where $\theta_p = 192$ in our implementation.

2.2 Semantic Feature Representation

After detection, the posterior cortex is divided into $s \times s$ ($s = 3$ in our implementation) half-overlapping grid cells, and the nucleus is partitioned into $s \times 2s$ half-overlapping grid cells. For each of the RGB and HSV color channels[1], a grid cell is represented by its mean intensity $\hat{t}$ and entropy e, defined as $e = -\sum_{l=0}^{255} p_l \log p_l$ where p_l is the probability of intensity l in the grid for a given color channel. With this data, each image is represented by a feature vector with $3 \times s \times s \times 6 \times 2 = 36s^2$ dimensions.

With the downsampling and half-overlapping grid cells, this representation becomes less sensitive to slight misalignments caused by differences in lens shape. We note that the feature vectors used in previous works such as [6], though containing features such as intensity ratios and edge strength that are useful

---

[1] HSV values are linearly scaled to the range $[0, 255]$ for consistency with the RGB channels.

for discriminative classification, are less suitable for dealing with the alignment problem, which is critical to the success of reconstruction-based techniques.

2.3 Similarity Weighted Linear Reconstruction (SWLR)

Suppose we have a dictionary that consists of n reference images, denoted by $\mathbf{D} = \{\mathbf{d_1}, \mathbf{d_2}, \cdots, \mathbf{d_n}\} \in \mathbb{R}^{f \times n}$ where each column d_i denotes a reference image expressed by its semantic feature vector. For a given test image expressed as $\mathbf{y} \in \mathbb{R}^{f \times 1}$, we compute the optimal linear reconstruction coefficients $\mathbf{w} \in \mathbb{R}^{n \times 1}$, $\sum_{i=1}^{n} w_i = 1$, $w_i \geq 0$, that minimize the reconstruction error $||\mathbf{y} - \mathbf{Dw}||^2$. Our objective function also includes a cost term that penalizes the use of references that are less similar to the test image. Let us denote the costs for the reference images in $\mathbf{D}$ as the vector $\mathbf{c} = \{c_1, c_2, \cdots, c_n\}^\top \in \mathbb{R}^{n \times 1}$, where c_i is the cost of using $\mathbf{d_i}$ for reconstruction. The overall cost term can then be expressed as $||\mathbf{c} \odot \mathbf{w}||^2$ where $\odot$ denotes the Hadamard product. Combining this cost term with the reconstruction error gives the following objective function:

$$\min_{\mathbf{w}} ||\mathbf{y} - \mathbf{Dw}||^2 + \lambda||\mathbf{c} \odot \mathbf{w}||^2, \quad s.t. \sum_{i=1}^{n} w_i = 1, w_i \geq 0, \tag{1}$$

where $\lambda > 0$ is a regularization parameter. This objective can be minimized in closed form using the Lagrange multiplier method:

$$\mathbf{w} = \frac{1}{\mathbf{1}^\top (\hat{\mathbf{D}}^\top \hat{\mathbf{D}} + \lambda \mathbf{C}^\top \mathbf{C})\mathbf{1}} (\hat{\mathbf{D}}^\top \hat{\mathbf{D}} + \lambda \mathbf{C}^\top \mathbf{C})^{-1} \mathbf{1},$$
$$\hat{\mathbf{D}} = (\mathbf{1} \otimes \mathbf{y} - \mathbf{D}), \tag{2}$$

where $\mathbf{C} = \text{diag}(\mathbf{c})$ and $\otimes$ denotes the Kronecker product. The cost c_i is defined as the χ^2-distance between the test image $\mathbf{y}$ and the i-th reference image $\mathbf{d_i}$, i.e.,

$$c_i = \sum_{j=1}^{f} \frac{(y_j - d_{i,j})^2}{2(y_j + d_{i,j})}, \tag{3}$$

where $d_{i,j}$ denotes the j-th entry of reference image $\mathbf{d_i}$. We note that the inclusion of entropy in the semantic feature helps to exclude misaligned references in the SWLR algorithm, since high entropy indicates the presence of structural variations, and differences in entropy caused by misalignment are penalized by this cost function.

Finally, the test image is graded as $\mathbf{w}^\top \mathbf{g}$, where $\mathbf{g}$ denotes the corresponding cataract grades of reference images in dictionary $\mathbf{D}$.

3   Experiments

To evaluate our method, we first compare it to the state-of-the-art nuclear cataract grading methods [5,6]. We then validate its major components by comparing to versions of our technique with certain components replaced.

3.1 Experimental Setting

Dataset. All the experiments are performed on the large ACHIKO-NC dataset used in [5,6], which is comprised of 5378 images with decimal grading scores that range from 0.3 to 5.0. The scores are determined by professional graders based on the Wisconsin protocol [4]. The protocol takes the ceiling of each decimal grading score as the integral grading score, *i.e.*, a cataract with a decimal grading score of 2.4 has an integral grading score of 3. ACHIKO-NC consists of 94 images of integral grade 1, 1874 images of integral grade 2, 2476 images of integral grade 3, 897 images of integral grade 4, and 37 images of integral grade 5. All left eye images are flipped horizontally so that they can be processed in the same way as right eye images.

Evaluation Criteria. For a fair comparison to prior art, we measure grading accuracy using the same four evaluation criteria as in [5,6], namely the exact integral agreement ratio (R_0), the percentage of decimal grading errors ≤ 0.5 ($R_{e0.5}$), the percentage of decimal grading errors ≤ 1.0 ($R_{e1.0}$), and the mean absolute error (ε), which are defined as

$$
R_0 = \frac{|\lceil G_{gt} \rceil = \lceil G_{pr} \rceil|_0}{N}, \qquad R_{e0.5} = \frac{||G_{gt} - G_{pr}| \leq 0.5|_0}{N},
$$
$$
R_{e1.0} = \frac{||G_{gt} - G_{pr}| \leq 1.0|_0}{N}, \qquad \varepsilon = \frac{\sum |G_{gt} - G_{pr}|}{N},
\tag{4}
$$

where G_{gt} denotes the ground-truth clinical grade, G_{pr} denotes the predicted grade, $\lceil \cdot \rceil$ is the ceiling function, $|\cdot|$ denotes the absolute value, $|\cdot|_0$ is a function that counts the number of non-zero values, and N is the number of testing images ($N = |G_{gt}|_0 = |G_{pr}|_0$). $R_{e0.5}$ has the most narrow tolerance among the four evaluation criteria, which makes it more significant in evaluating the accuracy of grading.

Testing Method. To examine generalization ability, we follow the repeated test settings in [5], *i.e.*, in each round, 100 training samples are randomly selected from all the 5378 images, with 20 images for each grade, and the remaining 5278 images are used for testing. In training, optimal parameters are selected for each method by cross-validation, where half of the images (50 images with 10 per grade) are used as the dictionary, the other half used for testing, and the set of parameters with the smallest average ε is chosen. The result of each round is obtained by testing the remaining 5278 images using all the 100 images as the dictionary together with the determined optimal parameters.

3.2 Comparison to State-of-the-art Regression Methods

We first compare our method to the state-of-the-art techniques, namely **BOF+GSR** [5] and **RBF ϵ-SVR** [6], using the same dataset, experimental

Table 1. Cataract grading performance vs. state-of-the-art regression based methods

Method	R_0	$R_{e0.5}$	$R_{e1.0}$	ε
Proposed SF+SWLR	**0.696±0.008**	**0.871±0.007**	**0.991±0.001**	**0.332±0.006**
BOF+GSR [5]	0.682±0.004	0.834±0.005	0.985±0.001	0.351±0.004
RBF ϵ-SVR [6]	0.658±0.014	0.824±0.016	0.981±0.004	0.354±0.014
SF+RBF ϵ-SVR	0.645±0.018	0.826±0.020	0.875±0.010	0.449±0.018
Our improvement over [5]	2.05 %	4.44 %	0.61 %	5.41 %

setting and reporting methods. The results are listed in Table 1, where **SF** refers to the proposed semantic feature and **SWLR** refers to the proposed similarity weighted linear reconstruction method. According to the results, our method is shown to surpass [5,6] in all four evaluation criteria.

In Table 1, our method is also compared to the application of **RBF ϵ-SVR** on the proposed semantic feature. The results show that the proposed feature has less discriminative power than the features used in [5,6]. This is not unexpected, since our semantic feature is designed for more robust alignment rather than discriminative power. In addition, our method has an extra advantage over [6] in that a more detailed segmentation of the lens is not needed for extracting discriminative features.

In summary, reconstruction and regression are two significantly different approaches to solve the cataract grading problem. The proposed **SWLR** selects more relevant sample *images* for *each individual testing image* to perform grading, while **GSR** selects more discriminative *feature vector entries* over *all training images* and assumes that good prediction can be obtained with these features on all the test images.

3.3   Comparison to Alternative Versions of Our Method

To validate the components of our technique, we compare it to alternative versions without the similarity based regularizer (referred to as **LR**), and by applying **SWLR** on different feature sets. The results are given in Table 2, and the following observations can be made:

- Comparing **SWLR** to **LR** shows that the similarity constraint is helpful for selecting more relevant/representative reference images for each individual test image. With better reconstruction, the performance is improved. We note that applying **LR** on only the k-nearest neighbours (k-NN) also does not yield performance as high as **SWLR**, since k cannot be fixed to a value that is suitable for all test images. By contrast, **SWLR** can adaptively determine a set of proper reference images to reconstruct each individual test image.
- Comparing **SWLR** using different feature sets shows that though some features may have greater discriminative power, they are less suitable in the context of reconstruction-based classification.

Table 2. Cataract grading performance using different reconstruction techniques and features

Method	Feature	R_0	$R_{e0.5}$	$R_{e1.0}$	ε
Proposed SWLR	*Proposed SF*	**0.696±0.008**	**0.871±0.007**	**0.991±0.001**	**0.332±0.006**
LR	*Proposed SF*	0.685±0.009	0.846±0.010	0.986±0.002	0.348±0.009
Proposed SWLR	*BOF* [5]	0.586±0.035	0.758±0.031	0.815±0.018	0.484±0.019
Proposed SWLR	[6]	0.655±0.021	0.773±0.027	0.801±0.014	0.406±0.017

3.4 Discussion

Similarity Metric. We compared our **SWLR** method using different similarity metrics, namely χ^2 distance and Gaussian distance, defined as $\exp(\|\mathbf{y} - \mathbf{d_i}\|^2/\sigma^2)$ where σ is a parameter that accounts for imaging noise. It was observed that χ^2 distance is more effective than Gaussian distance for the proposed feature representation, with metrics of (R_0, $R_{e0.5}$, $R_{e1.0}$, ε) for χ^2 distance being (0.696±0.008, 0.871±0.007, 0.991±0.001, 0.332±0.006) and for Gaussian distance being (0.688±0.009, 0.868±0.007, 0.990±0.001, 0.337±0.007).

Processing Speed. On a four-core 2.4 GHz PC with 16 GB RAM, our method takes 17.73 s on average to process an image, with 1.36 s for feature extraction and only 0.001 s for prediction because of the small dictionary size. This processing speed slightly exceeds the 20.45 s per image of [5], which takes 4.23 s for feature extraction and 0.00001 s for prediction. It is also faster than the 25.00 s per image of [6], which spends 8.76 s for feature extraction and 0.02 s for prediction.

4 Conclusion

For grading the severity of nuclear cataracts from slit-lamp lens images, we proposed a reconstruction-based approach with a new semantic feature representation and a similarity weighted regularizer. In tests on the *ACHIKO-NC* dataset comprised of 5378 images, our approach achieves significant improvements over the state-of-the-art regression based methods [5,6]. In future work, we plan to elevate performance by introducing a feature selection mechanism and investigating other similarity metrics.

References

1. Kanski, J.J.: Clinical Ophthalmology – A systematic Approach. Elsevier Butterworth-Heinemann, Edinburgh (2007)
2. Thylefors, B., Chylack Jr., L.T., Konyama, K., Sasaki, K., Sperduto, R., Taylor, H.R., West, S.: A simplified cataract grading system. Ophthalmic Epidemiol. **9**(2), 83–95 (2002)
3. Chylack, L., Wolfe, J., Singer, D., Leske, M.C., Bullimore, M.A., Bailey, I.L., Friend, J., McCarthy, D., Wu, S.Y.: The lens opacities classificatin system III. Arch Ophthalmol. **111**(6), 831–836 (1993)

4. Klein, B., Klein, R., Linton, K., Magli, Y., Neider, M.: Assessment of cataracts from photographs in the beaver dam eye study. Ophthalmology **97**, 1428–1433 (1990)
5. Xu, Y., Gao, X., Lin, S., Wong, D.W.K., Liu, J., Xu, D., Cheng, C.Y., Cheung, C.Y., Wong, T.Y.: Automatic grading of nuclear cataracts from slit-lamp lens images using group sparsity regression. In: Mori, K., Sakuma, I., Sato, Y., Barillot, C., Navab, N. (eds.) MICCAI 2013, Part II. LNCS, vol. 8150, pp. 468–475. Springer, Heidelberg (2013)
6. Li, H., Lim, J.H., Liu, J., Mitchell, P., Tan, A., Wang, J., Wong, T.: A computer-aided diagnosis system of nuclear cataract. IEEE Trans. Biomed. Eng. **57**, 1690–1698 (2010)
7. Fan, S., Dyer, C.R., Hubbard, L., Klein, B.: An automatic system for classification of nuclear sclerosis from slit-lamp photographs. In: Ellis, R.E., Peters, T.M. (eds.) MICCAI 2003. LNCS, vol. 2878, pp. 592–601. Springer, Heidelberg (2003)
8. Huang, W., Li, H., Chan, K.L., Lim, J.H., Liu, J., Wong, T.Y.: A computer-aided diagnosis system of nuclear cataract via ranking. In: Yang, G.-Z., Hawkes, D., Rueckert, D., Noble, A., Taylor, C. (eds.) MICCAI 2009, Part II. LNCS, vol. 5762, pp. 803–810. Springer, Heidelberg (2009)
9. Duncan, D.D., Shukla, O.B., West, S.K., Schein, O.D.: New objective classification system for nuclear opacification. J. Opt. Soc. Am. **14**, 1197–1204 (1997)
10. Khu, P.M., Kashiwagi, T.: Quantitating nuclear opacification in color scheimpflug photographs. Invest. Ophthalmol. Vis. Sci. **34**, 130–136 (1993)
11. Xu, D., Huang, Y., Zeng, Z., Xu, X.: Human gait recognition using patch distribution feature and locality-constrained group sparse representation. IEEE Trans. Image Process. **21**(1), 316–326 (2012)

Vessel Orientation Constrained Quantitative Susceptibility Mapping (QSM) Reconstruction

Suheyla Cetin[1(✉)], Berkin Bilgic[2], Audrey Fan[3], Samantha Holdsworth[3], and Gozde Unal[4]

[1] Faculty of Engineering and Natural Sciences, Sabanci University, Istanbul, Turkey
suheylacetin@sabanciuniv.edu
[2] Athinoula A. Martinos Center for Biomedical Imaging, Charlestown, USA
berkin@nmr.mgh.harvard.edu
[3] Department of Radiology, Stanford University, Stanford, USA
{auddie,sjhold}@stanford.edu
[4] Department of Computer Engineering, Istanbul Technical University, Istanbul, Turkey
gozde.unal@itu.edu.tr

Abstract. QSM is used to estimate the underlying tissue magnetic susceptibility and oxygen saturation in veins. This paper presents vessel orientation as a new regularization term to improve the accuracy of l_1 regularized QSM reconstruction in cerebral veins. For that purpose, the vessel tree is first extracted from an initial QSM reconstruction. In a second step, the vascular geometric prior is incorporated through an orthogonality constraint into the QSM reconstruction. Using a multi-orientation QSM acquisition as gold standard, we show that the QSM reconstruction obtained with the vessel anatomy prior provides up to 40 % RMSE reduction relative to the baseline l_1 regularizer approach. We also demonstrate in vivo OEF maps along venous veins based on segmentations from QSM. The utility of the proposed method is further supported by inclusion of a separate MRI venography scan to introduce more detailed vessel orientation information into the reconstruction, which provides significant improvement in vessel conspicuity.

Keywords: QSM · Susceptibility MRI · QSM reconstruction · Vessel orientation constraint

1 Introduction

Susceptibility MRI provides exquisite contrast of the venous vasculature due to the presence of paramagnetic deoxyhemoglobin molecules in cerebral veins. Although susceptibility-weighted imaging has gained popularity due to its ability to depict the veins in clinical applications such as stroke and traumatic brain injury [1], this method suffers from non-local and orientation-dependent effects that may preclude accurate identification of brain vessels.

© Springer International Publishing AG 2016
S. Ourselin et al. (Eds.): MICCAI 2016, Part III, LNCS 9902, pp. 467–474, 2016.
DOI: 10.1007/978-3-319-46726-9_54

As an alternative, vessel segmentation can be performed directly on QSM derived from MRI phase images [2]. Because dipolar field patterns have been deconvolved during QSM reconstruction, segmentation of vasculature on QSM images is expected to outperform magnitude- or phase- based approaches. Automated vessel detection may also provide anatomical priors to improve quantification of brain physiology from QSM, including oxygen extraction fraction (OEF) in cerebral veins. Baseline OEF is an important physiological parameter for tissue health in normal brain function and many cerebrovascular diseases [3]. Reliable estimation of OEF depends on robust and accurate QSM reconstruction within venous structures.

In this study, we present a new regularization constraint to the existing l_1-norm regularized QSM reconstruction [4,5]. The new regularization constraint incorporates prior information about the vessel anatomy and the orientation. The vessel orientation prior is estimated by extracting the vessel tree. This process uses high order vessel tractography on the QSM data itself or on separate angiography images [2].

2   Method

2.1   Segmentation

To extract a brain vessel tree from a given QSM or angiographic image volume, we utilized a recent framework based on a higher order tensor vessel tractography by [2,6]. The method in [2] involves a unified mathematical formulation which models the n-furcations, i.e. bifurcations or higher order junctions in vessel trees, jointly with tubular sections. A general Cartesian tensor is embedded into a 4-dimensional space so that antipodal asymmetries in Y-junction-like situations, which are abundant in vascular trees, can be accurately modeled. Starting from a few seed points (e.g. 5–6), an entire cerebral vein tree can be captured from the QSM by this technique, which provides the vessel orientation, its centerline (central lumen line), its thickness (vessel lumen diameter), locations of branching points, and lengths of branches. The extracted knowledge of centerlines permits OEF computation [7] along the vasculature. The only interaction to the method is providing seed points which lends itself to a simple practical vessel extraction process. The computation time for segmentation of the whole vessel tree is on the order of minutes (<10 min).

2.2 l_1-regularized QSM Reconstruction

To quantify oxygenation along brain vessels requires recovery of the underlying tissue susceptibility distribution from MRI observations of magnetic field perturbations. Tissue susceptibility χ is related to the measured field map ϕ via the formulation $\mathbf{DF}\chi = \mathbf{F}\phi$, where $\mathbf{F}$ is the Fourier transform operator and $\mathbf{D}$ $= 1/3 - k_z^2/k^2$ is the susceptibility kernel in k-space. Due to the presence of zeros on the conical surface along the magic angle in this kernel, the solution of this system necessitates additional regularization.

Most popular types of existing QSM reconstruction techniques can be formulated by penalizing l_1-norm of gradients in three dimensions [5], and can be expressed as an unconstrained convex optimization problem, minimizing

$$\underset{\chi}{argmin} \ \frac{1}{2} \left\| \mathbf{F}^{-1}\mathbf{DF}\chi - \phi \right\|_2^2 + \alpha \cdot \left\| \mathbf{G}\chi \right\|_1 \tag{1}$$

where α is the regularization parameter and $\mathbf{G} = [\mathbf{G}_x; \mathbf{G}_y; \mathbf{G}_z]$ is the gradient operator in three spatial directions.

2.3 l_1-regularized QSM Reconstruction with Vessel Orientation (VO) Constraint

We propose a new regularization term to be added to Eq. 1. As a regularizer, we use the dot product between the $\mathbf{G}\chi$ and the orientation vector $\mathbf{V} = [\mathbf{V}_x; \mathbf{V}_y; \mathbf{V}_z] \in \mathbb{R}^3$. The new regularization term incorporates prior information about the vessel anatomy and the orientation. We expect OEF (and thus susceptibility) along the vessel direction to be relatively smooth. Thus, the $\mathbf{G}\chi$ inside a vessel should be orthogonal to the $\mathbf{V}$, and the dot product between $\mathbf{G}\chi$ and $\mathbf{V}$ should be small. The final constraint is weighted by a dilated vessel mask $\mathbf{M}$: $\left\| \mathbf{M}(\mathbf{G} \cdot \mathbf{V})\chi \right\|_1$, where the structuring element in the dilation is a cylinder and the size of its radius is the half of the vessel radius. Over each cross section of the vessel along the centerline, $\mathbf{V}$ is defined at each voxel as the difference between two consecutive centerline points. Then, $\mathbf{V}$ is weighted by a smooth surface which enhances it along the edges and suppresses along the centerline of the vessel and outside of $\mathbf{M}$.

Hence, the l_1-regularized and vessel orientation constrained reconstruction problem reads as:

$$\underset{\chi}{argmin} \ \frac{1}{2} \left\| \mathbf{F}^{-1}\mathbf{DF}\chi - \phi \right\|^2 + \alpha \cdot \left\| \mathbf{G}\chi \right\|_1 + \lambda \left\| \mathbf{M}(\mathbf{G} \cdot \mathbf{V})\chi \right\|_1 \tag{2}$$

where α and λ are the regularization parameters. We perform the optimization by non-linear conjugate gradient with backtracking line-search using 200 iterations [8].

3 Experimental Results

In this section, we will show the results of the l_1-regularized QSM reconstruction with vessel orientation (VO) constraint on: (Sect. 3.1) a ground truth in vivo validation data; (Sect. 3.2) in vivo QSM volumes acquired on ten healthy volunteers; (Sect. 3.3) a single in vivo QSM volume registered with a contrast-enhanced Fast Spin Echo MRI (MFAST) data. The regularization parameters (α, λ) were determined by parameter sweeping based on the validation data. The values $(\alpha = 8.3 \cdot 10^{-4}, \lambda = 3.5 \cdot 10^{-2})$ that minimized the normalized root mean square error (RMSE) relative to the true χ were selected to be the optimal setting, and applied in all experiments.

3.1   Validation Data

A ground truth in vivo QSM dataset is obtained using 3D-Gradient Echo (GRE) acquisition at 12 different head orientations relative to the main magnetic field. Since the dipole kernel $\mathbf{D}$ varies as a function of the angle between the subject's head and the main field, an overdetermined system can be formed using data from multiple orientations to mitigate the ill-conditioning of dipole inversion. This technique is termed Calculation Of Susceptibility through Multiple Orientation Sampling (COSMOS), and obviates the need for additional regularization [9] to provide ground-truth quality susceptibility maps. For this acquisition, a healthy volunteer (female, age 30) was scanned with a 32-channel head coil on a Siemens 3T Trio system using TR/TE $= 35/25$ ms at 1 mm isotropic resolution with BW $= 100$ Hz/pixel upon 15-fold acceleration with the Wave-CAIPI sequence [10]. Raw phase images were processed using Laplacian unwrapping [11] and SHARP background removal [12] to yield tissue phase images from each orientation, which were jointly inverted to provide the COSMOS χ solution. Using the COSMOS reconstruction as the ground truth χ map (Fig. 1(a)), the field map ϕ was simulated using the forward dipole model $\phi = \mathbf{F}^{-1}\mathbf{DF}$, and Gaussian noise ($\sigma = 0.01$) was added.

Starting from the noisy field map (Fig. 1(b)), l_1-reconstruction results in 8.37 % RMSE which is calculated in the whole volume (Fig. 1(c)). We segmented the vessel tree from the χ map using the higher order tensor based vessel extraction method described in Sect. 2.1. Figure 1(d) depicts the extracted vessel tree, where 7 seed points are selected for the segmentation. l_1 regularized reconstruction with VO constraint has RMSE error of 5.13 % for the overall data (Fig. 1(e)). The results show that the improvement in the accuracy of the reconstruction with our vessel orientation constraint over the existing l_1 reconstruction is 40 % along the whole data. Qualitatively, it can be observed that smaller vessels are more visible in the reconstructions regularized with the additional VO constraint (Fig. 1(e)).

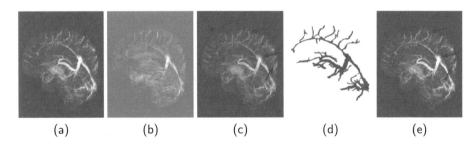

(a)   (b)   (c)   (d)   (e)

Fig. 1. Simulations result from ground truth susceptibility phantom. (a) Original χ field; (b) noisy normalized field map (input to QSM reconstruction); (c) l_1 regularized reconstructed χ field (8.37 % RMSE); (d) the extracted vessel tree (7 seed points are selected); (e) l_1 regularized reconstructed with VO constraint χ field (5.13 % RMSE). Arrows point out the reconstruction comparisons on the sample veins.

3.2   3D-GRE Volunteer Data

Ten young, healthy volunteers were scanned with a 32-channel coil on a Siemens 3T Trio system. 3D-GRE in vivo images for susceptibility mapping were acquired with full flow-compensation along each axis at all echoes. Axial magnitude and phase images were collected with TR = 23 ms; TE = 7.2/17.7 ms; resolution = 0.875 × 0.875 × 1 mm³, matrix = 226 × 256 × 144; and BW = 260 Hz/pixel. Phase images were combined offline and processed with Laplacian unwrapping [11]. Background field was removed with SHARP filtering [12] and QSM reconstruction was performed with a l_1 regularized reconstruction technique [4].

Figure 2 depicts the QSM map, centerlines and surfaces of the vessel trees on two healthy volumes. We compute the OEF values [7] after the l_1 regularized reconstruction with VO constraint on the same subjects. Mean OEF across all veins are $33.3 \pm 4\%$, $35.7 \pm 7\%$, $31.7 \pm 3\%$, $38.6 \pm 5\%$, $37.4 \pm 6\%$, $33.8 \pm 3\%$, $33.7 \pm 2\%$, $35.7 \pm 5\%$, $31.9 \pm 4\%$, and $34.3 \pm 9\%$ respectively, for each of ten subjects. Estimated OEF for straight sinus, sagittal sinus, pial vessels are $46.3 \pm 6\%$, $36.4 \pm 4\%$, $31.8 \pm 3\%$, respectively, in average of ten subjects. Furthermore, we display the OEF values on the vessel surfaces of the sample two subjects, where the VO constraint is shown to improve conspicuity of smaller vessels (Fig. 3).

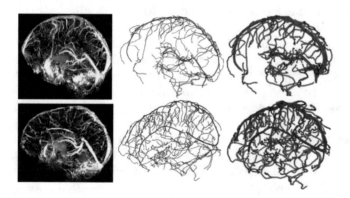

Fig. 2. (Left) original QSM map; (Middle) extracted centerlines of the vessels; (Right) surface renderings for the vessels are shown for two healthy subjects.

3.3   QSM + MFAST Data

The approach in Sect. 3.2 first uses standard QSM reconstruction (generic prior) and segments the vessels from this initial estimate of susceptibility. Here we test the hypothesis that vessel tree extraction from a separate angiographic volume offers improved vascular priors for OEF quantification from QSM maps.

With IRB approval, patients were scanned on a 3T GE scanner (MR750, GE Healthcare Systems, Waukesha, WI) with an 8-channel head-coil. A flow compensated 3D parallel-imaging-accelerated multi-echo (ME)-GRE sequence

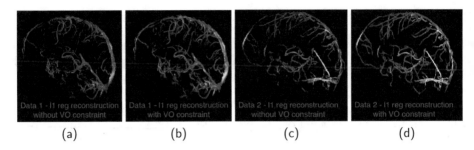

Fig. 3. OEF visualization on two sample subjects from ten data volume (shown in hot colors); l_1 regularized QSM reconstruction without (a, c) and with (b, d) VO constraint for the two subjects respectively.

was used with the following parameters: Axial plane, FOV $= 22$ cm, matrix size $= 384 \times 256$, number of partitions $= 66$, resolution $= 0.6 \times 0.9 \times 2\,\text{mm}^3$, acceleration factor $= 2$, flip angle $= 15°$, TR $= 36$ ms, seven echoes ranging from TE $= 4$ ms-33 ms (4.8 ms increments), scan time $= 5.44$ min. On completion of the scan, the raw data from the scanner were automatically reconstructed using compiled threaded MATLAB (MathWorks Inc., Natick, MA, USA) code.

A ferumoxytol-enhanced MRA using 3D SPGR was designed with short repetition time (TR) $= 4$ ms and echo time (TE) $= 1$ ms. The sequence was fat suppressed with FOV $= 26$ cm, matrix size $= 416 \times 416$, resolution $= 0.625 \times 0.625\,\text{mm}^2$ and 180 slices with 1 mm thickness. The excitation was done with a flip angle of 15 degrees, and receiver bandwidth of 62.5 kHz. The scan time was reduced by not acquiring the corners of ky-kz space, producing an acquisition time of 5.46 min.

We first extracted the brain using FSL [13] from MFAST data, then registered MFAST and QSM data with a rigid registration using the MedInria software [14]. Using the QSM reconstruction as the reference χ map, the field map ϕ was simulated using the forward dipole model, and Gaussian noise was added ($\sigma = 0.02$). Then, we segmented the vessel tree from QSM data and MFAST data separately. Figure 4 (Top) shows the vessel tree segmentation from QSM and MFAST data, respectively. We use morphological operators to separate veins from arteries for the MFAST data. Figure 4 (Bottom) visualizes the results of: (Left) QSM reconstruction without the vessel orientation prior; (Middle) QSM reconstruction with the vessel orientation prior where the vessel tree is segmented from the QSM data; (Right) QSM reconstruction with the vessel orientation prior where the vessel tree is segmented from the MFAST data. The results show the enhancements along the veins using our VO prior in the reconstructions. The amount of detail captured in the vessel tree extracted from the MFAST data volume, which is then incorporated into the QSM reconstruction through the VO regularizer clearly reveals the benefits of the new regularizer term.

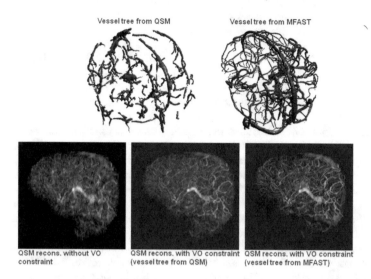

Fig. 4. Top: Left-vessel tree extraction from QSM data (Extr. 1), Right-vessel tree extraction from MFAST data (Extr. 2); Bottom: (Left) QSM reconstruction without VO, (Middle) l_1-reg QSM data reconstructed with VO constraint (Extr. 1), (Right) l_1-reg QSM data reconstructed with VO constraint (Extr. 2).

4   Conclusion

We developed a method that improves the accuracy of l_1 regularized QSM reconstruction [4,5] with a new regularization constraint, vessel orientation. Quantitative performance of our method was demonstrated on a ground truth phantom data. Furthermore, we performed the experiments on ten QSM images reconstructed from MRI phase and presented the mean OEF results for all veins in each volume and major vessel segments. On two sample subjects, we showed that the OEF maps along the vessel direction are relatively smooth. Finally, we compared the QSM reconstructions on a QSM volume acquired with an additional contrast, the MFAST. We showed the results for QSM reconstructions with and without vessel orientations where the vessel trees were segmented from QSM and MFAST data respectively. This experiment implied that when the segmentation becomes more detailed and accurate, the quality of the reconstruction increases. Use of the vessel orientation constraint increased OEF values (Fig. 3), such that our results are more in line with physiological OEF values reported by O-15 PET imaging [15]. This observation suggests that the use of anatomical prior helps mitigate partial volume effects and over-smoothing associated with traditional regularized QSM reconstruction. The new OEF values may also reflect less underestimation due to vessel orientation because of the vascular prior. In future work we will pursue the idea of extracting the vessel prior from the enhanced QSM image and iterating the whole procedure a few times which can lead to an improvement. We will also monitor both the number of vessel branches and OEF values over iteration number.

References

1. Hammond, K.E., Lupo, J.M., Xu, D., Veeraraghavan, S., Lee, H., Kincaid, A., Vigneron, D.B., Manley, G.T., Nelson, S.J., Mukherjee, P.: Microbleed detection in traumatic brain injury at 3T and 7T: comparing 2D and 3D gradient-recalled echo (GRE) imaging with susceptibility-weighted imaging (SWI). In: ISMRM, p. 248 (2009)
2. Cetin, S., Unal, G.: A higher-order tensor vessel tractography for segmentation of vascular structures. IEEE TMI **34**(10), 2172–2185 (2015)
3. Christen, T., Bolar, D.S., Zaharchuk, G.: Imaging brain oxygenation with mri using blood oxygenation approaches: methods, validation, and clinical applications. Am. J. Neuroradiol. **34**, 1113–1123 (2012)
4. Bilgic, B., Fan, A.P., Polimeni, J.R., Cauley, S.F., Bianciardi, M., Adalsteinsson, E., Wald, L.L., Setsompop, K.: Fast quantitative susceptibility mapping with l1-regularization and automatic parameter selection. MRM **72**(5), 1444–1459 (2014)
5. de Rochefort, L., Liu, T., Kressler, B., Liu, J., Spincemaille, P., Lebon, V., Wu, J., Wang, Y.: Quantitative susceptibility map reconstruction from MR phase data using bayesian regularization: validation and application to brain imaging. MRM **63**(1), 194–206 (2010)
6. Cetin, S., Demir, A., Yezzi, A.J., Degertekin, M., Unal, G.: Vessel tractography using an intensity based tensor model with branch detection. IEEE TMI **32**(2), 348–363 (2013)
7. Fan, A.P., Bilgic, B., Gagnon, L., Witzel, T., Bhat, H., Rosen, B.R., Adalsteinsson, E.: Quantitative oxygenation venography from MRI phase. MRM **72**(1), 149–159 (2014)
8. Lustig, M., Donoho, D., Pauly, J.M.: Sparse MRI: the application of compressed sensing for rapid MR imaging. MRM **58**(6), 1182–1195 (2007)
9. Liu, T., Spincemaille, P., de Rochefort, L., Kressler, B., Wang, Y.: Calculation of susceptibility through multiple orientation sampling (cosmos): a method for conditioning the inverse problem from measured magnetic field map to susceptibility source image in MRI. MRM **61**(1), 196–204 (2009)
10. Bilgic, B., Xie, L., Dibb, R., Langkammer, C., Mutluay, A., Ye, H., Polimeni, J.R., Augustinack, J., Liu, C., Wald, L.L., Setsompop, K.: Rapid multi-orientation quantitative susceptibility mapping. NeuroImage **125**, 1131–1141 (2016)
11. Li, W., Wu, B., Liu, C.: Quantitative susceptibility mapping of human brain reflects spatial variation in tissue composition. NeuroImage **55**(4), 1645–1656 (2011)
12. Schweser, F., Deistung, A., Lehr, B.W., Reichenbach, J.R.: Quantitative imaging of intrinsic magnetic tissue properties using MRI signal phase: an approach to in vivo brain iron metabolism. NeuroImage **54**(4), 2789–2807 (2011)
13. Smith, S.M.: Fast robust automated brain extraction. Hum. Brain Mapp. **17**(3), 143–155 (2002)
14. Toussaint, N., christophe Souplet, J., Fillard, P.: Medinria: medical image navigation and research tool by INRIA. In: Proceedings of MICCAI Workshop (2007)
15. Bremmer, J.P., Berckel, B.N.M., Persoon, S., Kappelle, L.J., Lammertsma, A.A., Kloet, R., Luurtsema, G., Rijbroek, A., Klijn, C.J.M., Boellaard, R.: Day-to-day test-retest variability of CBF, CMRO2, and OEF measurements using dynamic 15O pet studies. Mol. Imag. Biol. **13**(4), 759–768 (2010)

Spatial-Angular Sparse Coding for HARDI

Evan Schwab$^{(\boxtimes)}$, René Vidal, and Nicolas Charon

Center for Imaging Science, Johns Hopkins University, Baltimore, USA
eschwab3@jhu.edu

Abstract. High angular resolution diffusion imaging (HARDI) can produce better estimates of fiber orientation and richer sets of features for disease classification than diffusion tensor imaging. However, existing HARDI reconstruction algorithms require a large number of gradient directions, making the acquisition time too long to be clinically viable. State-of-the-art compressed sensing methods can reduce the number of measurements needed for accurate reconstruction by exploiting angular sparsity at each voxel, but the global sparsity level is therefore bounded below by the number of voxels. In this work, we aim to find a significantly sparser representation of HARDI by exploiting redundancies in both the spatial and angular domains jointly with a global HARDI basis. However, this leads to a massive global optimization problem over the whole brain which cannot be solved using existing sparse coding methods. We present a novel Kronecker extension to ADMM that exploits the separable spatial-angular structure of HARDI data to efficiently find a globally sparse reconstruction. We validate our method on phantom and real HARDI brain data by showing that we can achieve accurate reconstructions with a global sparsity level corresponding to less then one atom per voxel, surpassing the absolute limit of the state-of-the-art.

1 Introduction

Diffusion magnetic resonance imaging (dMRI) is a 6D neuroimaging modality that produces 3D q-space signals at every voxel of a 3D brain MRI volume and can be used to estimate the orientation and integrity of neuronal fiber bundles *in vivo*. Diffusion tensor imaging (DTI), which models the probability of water diffusion in each voxel with a 3D Gaussian distribution, requires a relatively low number of q-space signal measurements. While this makes DTI well-suited for clinical research, the diffusion tensor cannot model multiple fiber orientations crossing in a single voxel.

High angular resolution diffusion imaging (HARDI) can provide more accurate estimations of anatomical fiber networks than DTI by estimating a higher-order probability distribution function. However, HARDI reconstruction algorithms require a larger number of q-space directions, which leads to a significantly longer patient scan time in comparison to DTI. As a consequence, HARDI has not been broadly accepted as a clinically viable dMRI protocol. Therefore, reducing HARDI scan times to the rate of DTI while maintaining accurate orientation estimation is an important open question in HARDI research.

© Springer International Publishing AG 2016
S. Ourselin et al. (Eds.): MICCAI 2016, Part III, LNCS 9902, pp. 475–483, 2016.
DOI: 10.1007/978-3-319-46726-9_55

Compressed sensing (CS) is a very useful tool to solve problems of this type and hinges on finding a sparse representation of a signal with respect to some basis. If such a sparse representation exists, CS can recover nearly perfect signals with sub-Nyquist sampling, allowing the potential to reduce signal acquisition time. Many approaches [9] have applied CS to dMRI protocols like multi-shell/single-shell HARDI and DSI to sparsely reconstruct signals, estimate orientation distribution functions (ODFs), fiber orientation distribution functions (FODs) [4], and ensemble average propagators (EAPs) [7], using dictionary learning or fixed sparsifying bases such as spherical ridgelets/wavelets [15], spherical polar Fourier bases, spherical Fourier-Bessel bases, directional radial bases, higher order tensors, and many more. These approaches reduce the number of q-space measurements needed from hundreds to tens by representing a q-space signal with as few q-space basis atoms as possible. However, since these methods compute one sparse representation for each and every voxel, the sparsest representation they can possibly achieve is with a single atom per voxel. Since spatial correlations between atoms are not exploited, these methods are still likely to represent a brain volume with millions of possibly redundant parameters.

In practice, measurements from neighboring voxels share much of the same information, hence there may exist further redundancies in the spatial domain when signals are modeled sparsely over the angular domain alone. Therefore, to reduce the number of measurements further, recent work [3,8,10,11] aims to apply CS to DSI/HARDI in the joint (k,q)-space. These methods apply joint (k,q) undersampling but still only apply sparse coding in the angular domain. Some works add sparse spatial regularization such as total-variation, yet with disjoint spatial and angular terms, global sparsity is still limited by the size of the data and (k,q)-CS may not be fully utilized.

In this paper, we propose to model HARDI signals using a global spatial-angular basis. However, because of the large size and complexity of HARDI data, optimizing over an entire HARDI volume is a computationally challenging problem. Our main contribution is an efficient joint spatial-angular sparse coding algorithm that exploits a separable model of the spatial and angular domains of HARDI data. With this proposed framework we aim to efficiently find a significantly sparser HARDI representation than state-of-the-art voxel-based methods can theoretically allow. In future work, joint spatial-angular sparse coding will allow us to more naturally apply (k,q)-CS with joint undersampling [8,11] to further reduce the total number of HARDI measurements.

2   HARDI Data Representation

Angular (Voxel-Based) HARDI Representation. For each voxel v in a HARDI brain volume $\Omega \subset \mathbb{R}^3$, q-space measurements are acquired at gradient directions $\vec{g} \in \mathbb{S}^2$ and are modeled by an angular (spherical) basis, $\{\gamma_i(\vec{g})\}_{i=1}^{N_\Gamma}$, with N_Γ atoms such that $s_v(\vec{g}) = \sum_{i=1}^{N_\Gamma} a_i \gamma_i(\vec{g})$ where $s_v(\vec{g})$ denotes the HARDI signal at voxel v measured at gradient direction $\vec{g}$. Classical HARDI reconstruction methods model the q-space signals from each voxel separately and add a regularization term $\mathcal{R}$ to enforce desirable properties such as spatial coherence, ODF non-negativity, or sparsity. Some recent methods [1,5,12,13] have considered simultaneous voxel-based reconstruction over an entire volume by solving

$$A^* = \arg\min_{A} ||S - \Gamma A||_F^2 + \lambda\mathcal{R}(A), \tag{1}$$

where $S = [s_1 \ldots s_V] \in \mathbb{R}^{G \times V}$ is the concatenation of signals $s_v \in \mathbb{R}^G$ sampled at G gradient directions over V voxels, $A = [a_1 \ldots a_V] \in \mathbb{R}^{N_\Gamma \times V}$ is the concatenation of coefficients and $\Gamma \in \mathbb{R}^{G \times N_\Gamma}$ is the discretization of the basis γ. While these methods attempt to reduce redundancies by adding spatial regularization, signal reconstruction still only operates on angular basis Γ at every voxel.

Spatial-Angular HARDI Representation. In this work, we propose to model the HARDI signal $\mathcal{S}(v, \vec{g})$ based on a single global basis, say $\varphi(v, \vec{g})$, to explicitly reduce redundancies in both the spatial and angular domains. However, typical HARDI contains on the order of $V \approx 100^3$ voxels each with $G \approx 100$ q-space measurements for a total of $100^4 \approx 100$ million signal measurements. Since many sparse coding applications often use bases that are over-redundant, this leads to a massive matrix Φ of size greater than $100^4 \times 100^4$. Therefore efficiently optimizing over a global basis is a very difficult problem. To overcome this challenge, we introduce additional structure on the dictionary atoms by considering separable functions over Ω and $\mathbb{S}^2$, namely a set of atoms of the form $\varphi(v, \vec{g})_{i,j} = (\psi_j(v)\gamma_i(\vec{g}))$, where $\psi(v)$ is a spatial basis for Ω with N_Ψ atoms. The HARDI signal may then be decomposed as:

$$\mathcal{S}(v, \vec{g}) = \sum_{i=1}^{N_\gamma} \sum_{j=1}^{N_\psi} c_{i,j}\psi_j(v)\gamma_i(\vec{g}) = \sum_{k=1}^{N_\psi N_\gamma} c_k \varphi_k(v, \vec{g}), \tag{2}$$

where $c = [c_k] \in \mathbb{R}^{N_\psi N_\Gamma}$ is the vectorization of $C = [c_{i,j}] \in \mathbb{R}^{N_\Gamma \times N_\Psi}$. In discretized form, our global basis φ is the separable Kronecker product matrix $\Phi \triangleq \Psi \otimes \Gamma \in \mathbb{R}^{VG \times N_\Psi N_\Gamma}$ with $\Psi \in \mathbb{R}^{V \times N_\Psi}$ and $\Gamma \in \mathbb{R}^{G \times N_\Gamma}$ such that

$$s = \begin{pmatrix} s_1 \\ s_2 \\ \vdots \\ s_V \end{pmatrix} = \begin{pmatrix} \Psi_{1,1}\Gamma & \Psi_{1,2}\Gamma & \cdots & \Psi_{1,N_\Psi}\Gamma \\ \Psi_{2,1}\Gamma & \Psi_{2,2}\Gamma & \cdots & \Psi_{2,N_\Psi}\Gamma \\ \vdots & \vdots & \ddots & \vdots \\ \Psi_{V,1}\Gamma & \Psi_{V,2}\Gamma & \cdots & \Psi_{V,N_\Psi}\Gamma \end{pmatrix} \begin{pmatrix} c_1 \\ c_2 \\ \vdots \\ c_{N_\Psi N_\Gamma} \end{pmatrix} = \Phi c. \tag{3}$$

Alternatively, in matrix form, (3) can be written compactly as $S = \Gamma C \Psi^\top$. In the special case of $\Psi = I_V$, the identity, we can see this leads to the state-of-the-art voxel-based formulation (1) with $C \equiv A$.

For HARDI, ODFs, p, can be estimated globally for all voxels with a single equation $p(v, \vec{x}; c) = \frac{1}{4\pi} + \tilde{\Phi}(v, \vec{x})c$, where $\tilde{\Phi}(v, \vec{x}) \triangleq \Psi(v) \otimes \tilde{\Gamma}(\vec{x})$ and $\tilde{\Gamma}(\vec{x})$ is the transformed angular basis into the space of ODFs for $\vec{x} \in \mathbb{S}^2$. This novel global formulation could provide a nice framework for HARDI applications like enforcing global non-negativity, extracting global features or global fiber segmentation. Though this current spatial-angular formulation may be specific to HARDI, our framework is generalizable to any dMRI protocol such as DSI, or multi-shell methods, by choosing an appropriate Γ which represents these data in q-space.

3   Efficient Globally Sparse HARDI Reconstruction

With our proposed spatial-angular basis representation of HARDI, the goal of this paper is to accurately reconstruct an entire HARDI volume with fewer atoms than the state-of-the-art voxel-based methods can theoretically allow. To find a globally sparse representation c, we aim to solve the l_1 minimization problem:

$$c^* = \arg\min_c \frac{1}{2}||s - \Phi c||_2^2 + \lambda||c||_1, \tag{4}$$

where $\lambda > 0$ is the sparsity trade-off parameter. The Alternating Direction Method of Multipliers (ADMM) [2] is a popular method for solving (4), however, its application in the case of a large dictionary Φ remains prohibitive. To reduce computation, we first note that when using over-redundant dictionaries (i.e., $V < N_\Psi, G < N_\Gamma$), it is more efficient to apply ADMM to the dual of (4) so that we can switch from calculating $\Phi^\top \Phi$ of size $N_\Psi N_\Gamma \times N_\Psi N_\Gamma$ to $\Phi\Phi^\top$ of size $VG \times VG$. The dual of (4) is:

$$\max_\alpha -\frac{1}{2}||\alpha||_2^2 + \alpha^\top s \text{ s.t. } ||\Phi^\top \alpha||_\infty \leq \lambda, \tag{5}$$

and update equations of the Dual ADMM (DADMM) [6] are given by:

$$\alpha_{k+1} = (I + \eta\Phi\Phi^\top)^{-1}(s - \Phi(c_k - \eta\nu_k)) \tag{6}$$

$$\nu_{k+1} = P_\lambda^\infty(\frac{c_k}{\eta} + \Phi^\top \alpha_{k+1}) \tag{7}$$

$$c_{k+1} = \text{shrink}_{\lambda\eta}(c_k + \eta\Phi^\top \alpha_{k+1}), \tag{8}$$

where $P_\lambda^\infty(x)$ is an element-wise projection to $[-\lambda, \lambda]$, $\text{shrink}_\rho(x)$ is the soft-threshold operator and $\eta > 0$ is an optimization parameter. The globally sparse output vector c^* minimizes the primal problem (4). DADMM reduces inner product computations to matrices of smaller size $G \times V$ instead of $N_\Gamma \times N_\Psi$ and is therefore not dependent on the size of basis but only on the size of the data. Furthermore, soft-thresholding is now done directly on c, which reduces the number of iterations for reaching a sparsity level by building up from 0 atoms instead of descending down from the total $N_\Psi N_\Gamma$ atoms. However, this naïve formulation with large Φ still has complexity $O(GVN_\Gamma N_\Psi)$ per iteration. Even submitting Φ into memory may be an issue, as well as the expensive cost of an inverse. We address this issue by exploiting the separability of Φ to perform computations with the much smaller Ψ and Γ. Our proposed method, called Kronecker DADMM, exploits the Kronecker product in two ways:

1. Kronecker SVD. Computing $(I + \eta\Phi\Phi^\top)^{-1}$ for large Φ is challenging and even taking an SVD to reduce the inverse to a diagonal of singular values is $O((GV)^2 N_\Gamma N_\Psi)$. Instead, we can exploit the Kronecker product and compute separate SVDs of the smaller $\Psi\Psi^\top$ and $\Gamma\Gamma^\top$. Let $\Psi\Psi^\top = U_\Psi \Sigma_\Psi U_\Psi^\top$ and $\Gamma\Gamma^\top = U_\Gamma \Sigma_\Gamma U_\Gamma^\top$, then we have $(I + \eta\Phi\Phi^\top)^{-1} = (U_\Psi \otimes U_\Gamma)(I + \eta(\Sigma_\Psi \otimes \Sigma_\Gamma))^{-1}(U_\Psi \otimes U_\Gamma)^\top$, where the inverse is now simply taken over a diagonal matrix. Computing these two SVDs is now of complexity $O(V^2 N_\Psi + G^2 N_\Gamma)$. In the case of tight frames, such as Wavelets, where $\Psi\Psi^\top = I$, we can significantly reduce computations to only involve Γ. We then simplify computations for (6) by pre-multiplication, setting $\alpha' \triangleq (U_\Psi \otimes U_\Gamma)^\top \alpha$, $s' \triangleq (U_\Psi \otimes U_\Gamma)^\top s$ and $\Phi' \triangleq (U_\Psi \otimes U_\Gamma)^\top \Phi = (U_\Psi \otimes U_\Gamma)^\top (\Psi \otimes \Gamma) = (U_\Psi^\top \Psi) \otimes (U_\Gamma^\top \Gamma) \triangleq (\Psi' \otimes \Gamma')$. [6] proves that we can now replace our original variables with α', s', and Φ' and our primal and dual optimization problems do not change.

2. Kronecker Matrix Formulation. We can further reduce the size of our problem and avoid any computations with Φ' by using the Kronecker product matrix formulation of (3) to write $\Phi'(c_k - \eta\nu_k) = \Gamma'(C_k - \eta\mathcal{V}_k)\Psi'^\top$, where C and $\mathcal{V}$ are the $N_\Gamma \times N_\Psi$ matrix forms of c and ν. Likewise, $\Phi'^\top \alpha' = \Gamma'^\top A'\Psi'$, where A' is the $G \times V$ matrix form of α' and we can pre-compute $S' = U_\Gamma^\top S U_\Psi$ where S is the $G \times V$ matrix form of s. To fit the $G \times V$ matrix dimensions, we simplify diagonal $(I + \eta(\Sigma_\Psi \otimes \Sigma_\Gamma))^{-1}$ to $\Sigma_\eta^{-1} \triangleq 1/(1 + \eta\Sigma)$ where $\Sigma \triangleq d_\Gamma d_\Psi^\top$ and d_Ψ and d_Γ are the diagonals of Σ_Ψ and Σ_Γ. This Kronecker matrix formulation has a significantly reduced complexity of $O(GV N_\Psi)$ per iteration compared with $O(GV N_\Gamma N_\Psi)$ for the naïve approach. Furthermore, in the case where Ψ is a tight frame transformation, such as Wavelets, for which $\Psi' = \Psi$, fast decomposition and reconstruction algorithms can be used to replace multiplication by Ψ and $\Psi^\top$ reducing complexity to $O(GV \log_2(N_\Psi))$.

Algorithm 1. (Kron-DADMM)

Precompute: $S', \Gamma', \Psi', \Sigma$.
Initialize: $k = 0, C_0 = 0, \mathcal{V}_0 = 0$. Choose: $\eta_0, \lambda, \epsilon$.
while Duality Gap $> \epsilon$ **do**
   1: $A'_{k+1} = \Sigma_{\eta_k}^{-1} \circ (S' - \Gamma'(C_k - \eta_k\mathcal{V}_k)\Psi'^\top)$;
   2: $\mathcal{V}_{k+1} = P_\lambda^\infty(\frac{1}{\eta_k}C_k + \Gamma'^\top A'_{k+1}\Psi')$;
   3: $C_{k+1} = \text{shrink}_{\lambda\eta_k}(C_k + \eta_k\Gamma'^\top A'_{k+1}\Psi')$;
   4: $\eta_{k+1} = \min(\frac{||S' - \Gamma'C_{k+1}\Psi'^\top||_F^2 ||C_{k+1}||_F^2}{2\lambda||\Gamma'C_{k+1}\Psi'^\top||_F^2}, \frac{||S||_1}{\lambda GV})$
   5: $\Sigma_{\eta_{k+1}}^{-1} = 1/(1 + \eta_{k+1}\Sigma)$
   6: $k = k + 1$;
end while
Return: globally sparse representation C^*

Our proposed algorithm for globally sparse HARDI reconstruction (Kron-DADMM) is presented in Algorithm 1. The symbol "$\circ$" in Step 1 denotes element-wise matrix multiplication. We follow [6] to update penalty parameter η and stop when the duality gap is sufficiently small.

4   Experiments

Data Sets. We provide experiments on the ISBI 2013 HARDI Reconstruction Challenge Phantom dataset, a $50 \times 50 \times 50$ volume consisting of 20 phantom fibers crossing intricately within an inscribed sphere, measured with $G = 64$ gradient directions (SNR = 30). Figures 1 and 2 show quantitative signal error vs. sparsity and qualitative ODF estimations at specific sparsity levels, respectively. We also experimented on a real $128 \times 128 \times 26$ HARDI brain volume with $G = 384$ from the Hippocampal Connectivity Project (FOV: 192, resolution: 1.5 mm isotropic, b-value: 1400 s/mm^2, TR/TE: 3500/86). Figure 3 shows sparse reconstruction using Kron-DADMM with Haar-SR compared to full voxel-based SH reconstruction. We can achieve a good reconstruction with $\sim$2 atoms per voxel in about 2.5 h.

Choice of Spatial and Angular Bases. *Spatial* (Ψ): A popular choice of sparsifying basis for MRI is a wavelet basis. For our experiments we compared Haar and Daubechies wavelets to get an indication of which can more sparsely represent the spatial organization of HARDI. Importantly, we also compared to state-of-the-art voxel-wise methods by simply choosing the identity I as the spatial basis. We compare these basis choices in terms of sparsity and reconstruction error in Fig. 1 (left). *Angular* (Γ): The over-complete spherical ridgelet/wavelet (SR/SW) basis pair [15] has been shown to sparsely model HARDI signals/ODFs. We also compare this to the popular SH basis, though for order L the SH is a low-pass truncation and does not exude sparse signals. With order $L = 4$, SH and SR have $N_\Gamma = 15$ and $N_\Gamma = 1169$ atoms, respectively. We compare these angular choices in Fig. 1 (right). As a note, these basis choices are preliminary and future work will involve exploring more advanced basis options to increase sparsity.

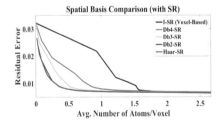 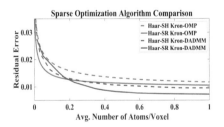

Fig. 1. Phantom Data. Left: Comparison of various spatial basis choices using Kron-DADMM paired with the SR angular basis. Haar-SR achieves the lowest residual ($\sim$0.074) with the sparsest number of coefficients ($\sim$0.5). The black line is voxel-based angular reconstruction where the identity I is the chosen spatial basis. Voxel-based is unable to achieve sparsity below 1 atom/voxel without forcing some voxels to 0 atoms. Right: Comparison between Kron-OMP and Kron-DADMM. Kron-OMP takes 40 h to reach 1 atom/voxel, while Kron-DADMM takes 40 min and provides better accuracy. SR outperforms SH basis as expected.

Voxel-Based Full Reconstruction SH 15 Atoms/Voxel (Non-Sparse)	Global Sparse Reconstruction, SR-Haar 0.728 Avg Atoms/Voxel, 0.0074 Residual	Voxel-Based Sparse Reconstruction, SR 1.57 Avg Atoms/Voxel, 0.0075 Residual

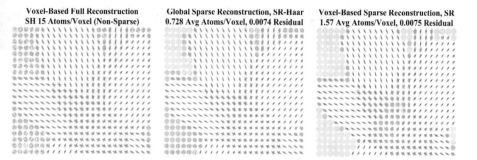

Fig. 2. Phantom Data. Comparison of Kron-DADMM with Haar-SR (middle) and voxel-based I-SR (right) against a full voxel-based least squares reconstruction with SH (left). The global reconstruction provides a more accurate signal with less than 1 atom per voxel while the voxel-based sparse reconstruction has difficulty estimating crossing fibers at this sparsity level and is forced to model isotropic ODFs with 0 atoms.

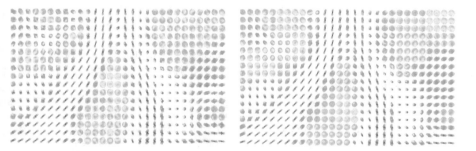

Fig. 3. Real Data. Global sparse reconstruction via Kron-DADMM with Haar-SR basis (right) compared to full voxel-based least squares reconstruction with SH basis (left). We can achieve an accurate reconstruction with only 2.23 atoms/voxel.

Comparison with a Baseline Algorithm. Orthogonal Matching Pursuit (OMP) is a widely used algorithm to approximate a solution to the l_0 problem by greedily selecting and orthogonalizing the K basis atoms that are most correlated with signal s. The Kronecker OMP (Kron-OMP) proposed in [14] exploits bases with separable structure but the method still needs to orthogonalize a $K \times K$ matrix where the sparsity level K empirically approaches the number of voxels $V \approx 100^4$. Because of this, our implementation takes on the order of 40 h to optimize over the phantom dataset compared to 40 min for Kron-DADMM. The results are presented in Fig. 1 (right).

5 Conclusion

We have presented a new efficient algorithm for globally sparse reconstruction of HARDI using a global basis representation which exploits spatial-angular separability to significantly reduce computational complexity. Our experiments show that greater sparsity for the representations may be achieved using spatial-angular bases instead of voxel-based approaches. So far, these were conducted as a proof-of-concept with dictionaries involving very simple spatial wavelet bases such as Haar, but the versatility of the algorithm enables the use of possibly more adequate directional Wavelets (e.g. shearlets, curvelets) or dictionary learning strategies, which are both important directions for future work. Our next step is to develop spatial-angular sensing matrices to jointly subsample (k,q)-space using a form of Kronecker CS. Finally, a globally sparse representation can be utilized in many other areas of HARDI applications including fiber segmentation, global tractography, global feature extraction, and sparse disease classification.

Acknowledgements. This work funded by JHU startup funds.

References

1. Auría, A., Daducci, A., Thiran, J.-P., Wiaux, Y.: Structured sparsity for spatially coherent fibre orientation estimation in diffusion MRI. NeuroImage **115**, 245–255 (2015)
2. Boyd, S., Parikh, N., Chu, E., Peleato, B., Eckstein, J.: Distributed optimization and statistical learning via the alternating direction method of multipliers. Found. Trends Mach. Learn. **3**(1), 1–122 (2010)
3. Cheng, J., Shen, D., Basser, P.J., Yap, P.-T.: Joint 6D k-q space compressed sensing for accelerated high angular resolution diffusion MRI. In: Ourselin, S., Alexander, D.C., Westin, C.-F., Cardoso, M.J. (eds.) IPMI 2015. LNCS, vol. 9123, pp. 782–793. Springer, Heidelberg (2015). doi:10.1007/978-3-319-19992-4_62
4. Feng, Y., Wu, Y., Rathi, Y., Westin, C.-F.: Sparse deconvolution of higher order tensor for fiber orientation distribution estimation. Artif. Intell. Med. **65**(3), 229–238 (2015)
5. Goh, A., Lenglet, C., Thompson, P.M., Vidal, R.: Estimating orientation distribution functions with probability density constraints and spatial regularity. In: Yang, G.-Z., Hawkes, D., Rueckert, D., Noble, A., Taylor, C. (eds.) MICCAI 2009, Part I. LNCS, vol. 5761, pp. 877–885. Springer, Heidelberg (2009)
6. Goncalves, H.R.: Accelerated sparse coding with overcomplete dictionaries for image processing applications. Ph.D. thesis (2015)
7. Gramfort, A., Poupon, C., Descoteaux, M.: Denoising and fast diffusion imaging with physically constrained sparse dictionary learning. Med. Image Anal. **18**(1), 36–49 (2014)
8. Mani, M., Jacob, M., Guidon, A., Magnotta, V., Zhong, J.: Acceleration of high angular and spatial resolution diffusion imaging using compressed sensing with multichannel spiral data. Magn. Reson. Med. **73**(1), 126–138 (2015)
9. Ning, L., et al.: Sparse reconstruction challenge for diffusion MRI: validation on a physical phantom to determine which acquisition scheme and analysis method to use? Med. Image Anal. **26**(1), 316–331 (2015)
10. Ning, L., Setsompop, K., Michailovich, O.V., Makris, N., Shenton, M.E., Westin, C.-F., Rathi, Y.: A joint compressed-sensing and super-resolution approach for very high-resolution diffusion imaging. NeuroImage **125**, 386–400 (2016)

11. Sun, J., Sakhaee, E., Entezari, A., Vemuri, B.C.: Leveraging EAP-sparsity for compressed sensing of MS-HARDI in $(\mathbf{k}, \mathbf{q})$-space. In: Ourselin, S., Alexander, D.C., Westin, C.-F., Cardoso, M.J. (eds.) IPMI 2015. LNCS, vol. 9123, pp. 375–386. Springer, Heidelberg (2015). doi:10.1007/978-3-319-19992-4_29
12. Ouyang, Y., Chen, Y., Wu, Y.: Vectorial total variation regularisation of orientation distribution functions in diffusion weighted MRI. Int. J. Bioinform. Res. Appl. **10**(1), 110–127 (2014)
13. Ouyang, Y., Chen, Y., Wu, Y., Zhou, H.M.: Total variation and wavelet regularization of orientation distribution functions in diffusion MRI. Inverse Prob. Imaging **7**(2), 565–583 (2013)
14. Rivenson, Y., Adrian, S.: Compressed imaging with a separable sensing operator. IEEE Signal Process. Lett. **16**(6), 449–452 (2009)
15. Tristán-Vega, A., Westin, C.-F.: Probabilistic ODF estimation from reduced HARDI data with sparse regularization. In: Fichtinger, G., Martel, A., Peters, T. (eds.) MICCAI 2011. LNCS, vol. 6892, pp. 182–190. Springer, Heidelberg (2011). doi:10.1007/978-3-642-23629-7_23

Compressed Sensing Dynamic MRI Reconstruction Using GPU-accelerated 3D Convolutional Sparse Coding

Tran Minh Quan and Won-Ki Jeong[(✉)]

Ulsan National Institute of Science and Technology (UNIST), Ulsan, South Korea
{quantm,wkjeong}@unist.ac.kr

Abstract. In this paper, we introduce a fast alternating method for reconstructing highly undersampled dynamic MRI data using 3D convolutional sparse coding. The proposed solution leverages Fourier Convolution Theorem to accelerate the process of learning a set of 3D filters and iteratively refine the MRI reconstruction based on the sparse codes found subsequently. In contrast to conventional CS methods which exploit the sparsity by applying universal transforms such as wavelet and total variation, our approach extracts and adapts the temporal information directly from the MRI data using compact shift-invariant 3D filters. We provide a highly parallel algorithm with GPU support for efficient computation, and therefore, the reconstruction outperforms CPU implementation of the state-of-the art dictionary learning-based approaches by up to two orders of magnitude.

1 Introduction

Dynamic cardiac MRI is considered as the gold standard among several imaging modalities in heart function diagnosis. However, due to its long acquisition time, its clinical application has been limited to non-time-critical ones. Recent research advances in Compressed Sensing (CS) have been successfully applied to MRI [8] to reduce acquisition time. Nevertheless, CS-MRI poses a new challenge – the reconstruction time also increases because it needs to solve an in-painting inverse problem in the frequency domain (i.e., k-space). Therefore, accelerating the reconstruction process is a top priority to adopt CS framework to fast MRI diagnosis.

Conventional CS-MRI reconstruction methods have exploited the sparsity of signal by applying universal sparsifying transforms such as Fourier (e.g., discrete Fourier transform (DFT) or discrete cosine transform (DCT)), Total Variation (TV), and Wavelets (e.g., Haar, Daubechies, etc.). This research direction has focused on accelerating the sparsity-based energy minimization problem, with [10] or without hardware supports [7]. Some strategies were designed to accelerate the minimization process such as using TV plus nuclear norm [14] or proposed the solver in other sparsity domain such as low-rank technique [9,12]. More recently, the other approaches leveraging the state-of-the-art data-driven

S. Ourselin et al. (Eds.): MICCAI 2016, Part III, LNCS 9902, pp. 484–492, 2016.
DOI: 10.1007/978-3-319-46726-9_56

method, i.e., dictionary learning [2] (DL), have been proposed to further enhance the reconstruction quality [3,5,6,11]. However, the existing learning-based methods suffer from the drawback of patch-based dictionary (i.e., redundant atoms and longer running times).

Convolutional sparse coding (CSC) is a new learning-based sparse representation that approximates the input signal with a superposition of sparse feature maps convolved with a collection of filters. This advanced technique replaces the patch-based dictionary learning process with an energy minimization process using a convolution operator on the image domain, which leads to an element-wise multiplication in frequency domain, derived within Alternating Direction Method of Multiplier (ADMM) framework [4], and later its direct inverse problem is introduced by Wohlberg [13]. CSC can generate much compact dictionaries due to its *shift-invariant* nature of filters, and the pixel-wise computation in Fourier domain maps well to parallel architecture. However, such advanced machine learning approaches have not been fully exploited in CS-MRI literature yet. Therefore, in this paper, we propose a novel CS dynamic MRI reconstruction that exploits the compactness and efficiency of 3D CSC. The proposed 3D CSC directly encodes both spatial and temporal features from dynamic cardiac 2D MRI using a compact set of 3D atoms (i.e., filters) without regularizers enforcing temporal coherence (e.g., total variation along the time axis). We also show that the proposed method maps well to data-parallel architecture, such as GPUs, for further accelerating its running time significantly, up to two orders of magnitude faster compared to the state-of-the-art CPU implementation of CS-MRI using patch-based dictionary learning. To the best of our knowledge, this is the first CS-MRI reconstruction method based on GPU-accelerated 3D CSC.

2   Method

Figure 1 is a pictorial description of the proposed method. If the inverse Fourier transform is directly applied to undersampled MRI k-space data (Fig. 1a ×4 undersampling), the reconstructed images will suffer from artifacts (Fig. 1b). The zero-filling reconstruction will serve as an initial guess for our iterative reconstruction process with randomly initialized filters, e.g., a collection of 16 atoms of size 9×9×9 as shown in Fig. 1d. Then the image and filters are iteratively updated until they converge as shown in Fig. 1c, e and f.

The proposed CS-MRI reconstruction algorithm is a process of finding s (i.e., a stack of 2D MR images for a given time duration) in the energy minimization problem defined as follows:

$$\min_{d,x,s} \frac{\alpha}{2} \left\| s - \sum_k d_k * x_k \right\|_2^2 + \lambda \sum_k \|x_k\|_1$$
$$s.t. : \|R\mathcal{F}_2 s - m\|_2^2 < \varepsilon^2, \|d_k\|_2^2 \leqslant 1 \tag{1}$$

where d_k is the k-th filter (or atom in the dictionary) and x_k, is its corresponding sparse code for s. In Eq. (1), the first term measures the difference between s

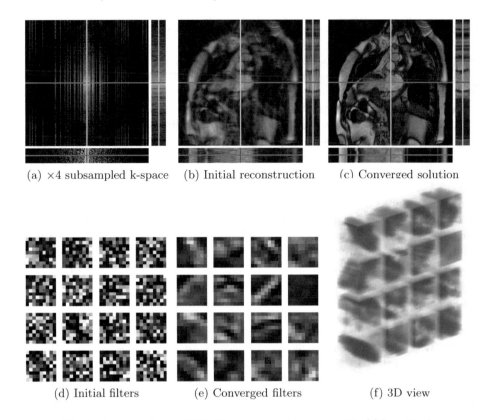

(a) ×4 subsampled k-space   (b) Initial reconstruction   (c) Converged solution

(d) Initial filters   (e) Converged filters   (f) 3D view

Fig. 1. An overview of CS-MRI reconstruction using 3D CSC method.

and its sparse approximation $s - \sum_k d_k * x_k$, weighted by α. The second term is the sparsity regularization of x_k using an $\ell 1$ norm with a weight λ instead of an $\ell 0$ norm as used in [2,5,6]. The rest of the equation is the collection of constraints - the first constraint enforces the consistency between undersampled measurement m and the undersampled reconstructed image using the mask R and the Fourier operator $\mathcal{F}$, and the second constraint restricts the Frobenius norm of each atom d_k within a unit length. In the following discussion, we will use a simplified notation without indices k and replace the result of Fourier transform of a given variable by using the subscript f (for example, d_f is the simplified notation for $\mathcal{F}d$ in 3D domain and s_{f_2} is the simplified notation for $\mathcal{F}_2 s$ in 2D spatial domain) to derive the solution of Eq. (1). Therefore, problem 1 can be rewritten using auxiliary variables y and g for x and d as follows:

$$\min_{d,x,g,y,s} \quad \frac{\alpha}{2} \left\| s - \sum d * x \right\|_2^2 + \lambda \left\| y \right\|_1$$
$$s.t. : x - y = 0, \|R\mathcal{F}_2 s - m\|_2^2 < \varepsilon^2, g = \mathcal{P}roj(d), \|g\|_2^2 \leqslant 1 \qquad (2)$$

where g and d are related by a projection operator as a combination of a truncated matrix followed by a padding-zero matrix in order to make the dimension of g same as that of x. Since we will leverage Fourier transform to solve this problem, g should be zero-padded to make its size same as g_f and x_f. The above constrained problem can be rebuilt in an unconstrained form with dual variables u, h, and further regulates the measurement consistency and the dual differences with γ, ρ, and σ, respectively:

$$\min_{d,x,g,y,s} \frac{\alpha}{2} \left\| s - \sum d * x \right\|_2^2 + \lambda \|y\|_1 + \frac{\gamma}{2} \|R\mathcal{F}_2 s - m\|_2^2$$
$$+ \frac{\rho}{2} \|x - y + u\|_2^2 + \frac{\sigma}{2} \|d - g + h\|_2^2 \ s.t. : g = \mathcal{P}roj(d), \ \|g\|_2^2 \leqslant 1 \quad (3)$$

Then we can solve problem (3) by iteratively finding the solution of independent smaller problems, as described below:

Solve for x:

$$\min_x \frac{\alpha}{2} \left\| \sum d * x - s \right\|_2^2 + \frac{\rho}{2} \|x - y + u\|_2^2 \quad (4)$$

If we apply the Fourier transform to the (4), it becomes:

$$\min_{x_f} \frac{\alpha}{2} \left\| \sum d_f x_f - s_f \right\|_2^2 + \frac{\rho}{2} \|x_f - y_f + u_f\|_2^2 \quad (5)$$

Then the minimum solution of (5) can be found by taking the derivative of (5) with respect to x_f and setting it to zero as follows:

$$\left(\alpha D_f^H D_f + \rho I \right) x_f = D_f^H s_f + \rho \left(y_f - u_f \right) \quad (6)$$

Note that the notation D_f stands for the concatenated matrix of all diagonalized matrices d_{fk} as follows: $D_f = [diag(d_{f1}), ..., diag(d_{fk})]$ and D_f^H is the complex conjugated transpose of D_f.

Solve for y:

$$\min_y \lambda \|y\|_1 + \frac{\rho}{2} \|x - y + u\|_2^2 \quad (7)$$

y for $\ell 1$ minimization problem can be found by using a shrinkage operation:

$$y = \mathcal{S}_{\lambda/\rho} \left(x + u \right) \quad (8)$$

Update for u: The update rule for u can be defined as a fixed- point iteration with the difference between x and y (u converges when x and y converge each other) as follows:

$$u = u + x - y \quad (9)$$

Solve for d:

$$\min_d \frac{\alpha}{2} \left\| \sum d * x - s \right\|_2^2 + \frac{\sigma}{2} \|d - g + h\|_2^2 \quad (10)$$

Similar to x, d can be solved in the Fourier domain:

$$\min_{d_f} \quad \frac{\alpha}{2} \left\| \sum d_f x_f - s_f \right\|_2^2 + \frac{\sigma}{2} \|d_f - g_f + h_f\|_2^2 \tag{11}$$

$$\left(\alpha X_f^H X_f + \sigma I \right) d_f = X_f^H s_f + \sigma \left(g_f - g_f \right) \tag{12}$$

where X_f stands for the concatenated matrix of all diagonalized matrices x_{fk} as follows: $X_f = [diag(x_{f1}), ..., diag(x_{fk})]$ and X_f^H is the complex conjugated transpose of X_f.

Solve for g:

$$\min_g \quad \frac{\sigma}{2} \|d - g + h\|_2^2 \qquad s.t. : \qquad g = \mathcal{P}roj(d), \|g\|_2^2 \leqslant 1 \tag{13}$$

g can be found by taking the inverse Fourier transform of d_f. This projection should be constrained by suppressing the elements which are outside the filter size d_k, and followed by normalizing its $\ell 2$-norm to a unit length.

Update for h: Similar to u, the update rule for h can be defined as follows:

$$h = h + d - g \tag{14}$$

Solve for s:

$$\min_s \quad \frac{\alpha}{2} \left\| s - \sum d * x \right\|_2^2 + \frac{\gamma}{2} \|R \mathcal{F}_2 s - m\|_2^2 \tag{15}$$

The objective function of (15) can be transformed into 2D Fourier domain:

$$\min_{s_{f_2}} \quad \frac{\alpha}{2} \left\| s_{f_2} - \mathcal{F}_t^H \sum d_f x_f \right\|_2^2 + \frac{\gamma}{2} \|R s_{f_2} - m\|_2^2 \tag{16}$$

Since d_f and x_f obtained previously in 3D Fourier domain, we need to bring it onto the same space by applying an inverse Fourier transform along time-axis $\mathcal{F}_t^H$. Then s_{f_2} can be found by solving the following linear system:

$$\left(\gamma R^H R + \alpha I \right) s_{f_2} = \gamma R^H m + \alpha \mathcal{F}_t^H \sum d_f x_f \tag{17}$$

Note that the efficient solutions of (6), (12) and (17) can be determined via the Sherman-Morrison formula for independent linear systems as shown in [13]. To this end, after the iteration process, s will be the results of applying a 2D inverse Fourier transform $\mathcal{F}_2^H$ on s_{f_2}.

Implementation Details: Since the above derivation consists only Fourier transform and element-wise operations, it maps well to data-parallel architecture, such as GPUs. We used MATLAB to implement the proposed method using the GPU. We set $\alpha = 1$, $\gamma = 1$, $\lambda = 0.1$, $\rho = 10$, $\sigma = 10$ and keep refining the filter banks as well as the reconstruction iteratively until they converge.

3   Result

In order to assess the performance of the proposed method, we compared our algorithm with the stage-of-the-art dictionary learning-based CS reconstruction from Caballero et. al. [5], and the conventional CS reconstruction using wavelet and total variation energy from Quan et. al. [10]. We used three cardiac MRI datasets from The Data Science Bowl [1] – 2 chamber view (2ch), 4 chamber view (4ch), and short axis view (sax). Each dataset consists of 30 frames of a 256×256 image across the cardiac cycle of a heart. In the experiment, we used 3D atoms of size $9 \times 9 \times 9$ and CS-undersampling factor was set to $\times 4$.

Running Time Evaluation: In order to make this direct performance comparison of learning-based methods between the proposed one and Caballero et al. [5], we measured wall clock running time of both methods on a PC equipped with an Intel i7 CPU with 16 GB main memory and an NVIDIA GTX Geforce Titan X GPU. Our prototype code is written in MATLAB 2015b including GPU implementation, and we used the author-provided MATLAB code for Caballero et al. [5]. As shown in Table 1, we observed that our CPU-based method is about $54\times$ to $73\times$, or about two orders of magnitude, faster than the stage-of-the-art DL-based CS-MRI reconstruction method for 100 epochs (i.e., the number of learning iterations). In addition, our GPU-based accelerated implementation also outperforms the CPU version about $1.25\times$ to $3.82\times$, which is greatly reduced to a level closer to be ready for clinical application. We expect that the performance of our method can improve further by using CUDA C/C++ without MATLAB.

Table 1. Reconstruction times of learning-based methods (100 epochs)

	2ch	4ch	sax
Caballero et al. [5]	558 Min	475 Min	427 Min
Our method (CPU)	7.67 Min	7.73 Min	7.94 Min
Our method (GPU)	6.14 Min	2.70 Min	2.08 Min

Quality Evaluation: Figure 2 visualizes the reconstruction errors compared to the full reconstruction of each method, respectively. As can be seen, our approach generated less error compared to the stage-of-the-art method of [5] and conventional CS-reconstruction using wavelet and TV energy [10]. Their glitches on the temporal profile are clearly observed since total variation along time axis may smooth out the temporal features that move quickly, especially near the heart boundary. In our case, the learned atoms are in 3D with larger supports, which helps to capture the time trait better even under fast motion and reduces errors in the reconstructed images. In addition, shift-invariance of CSC helps to generate more compact filters compared to the patch-based method.

Figure 3 shows the achieved Peak Signal-To-Noise-Ratios (PSNRs) measured between the CS-reconstruction results and the full reconstruction. As shown in

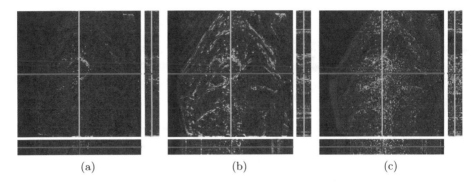

(a)   (b)   (c)

Fig. 2. Error plots (red: high, blue: low) between full reconstruction and the result from (a) the proposed method, (b) the DL-based method [5], and (c) wavelet and total variation energy method [10]. (Color figure online)

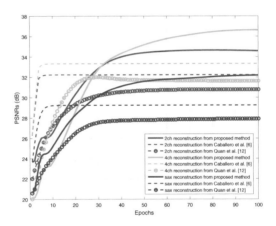

Fig. 3. Convergence rate evaluation based on PSNRs.

this figure, our method requires more iterations (epochs) to converge to the steady state, but the actual running time is much faster than the others due to GPU acceleration. In the mean time, our method can reach much higher PSNRs.

4   Conclusion

In this paper, we introduced an efficient CS-MRI reconstruction method based on pure 3D convolutional sparse coding where shift-invariant 3D filters can represent the temporal features of the MRI data. The proposed numerical solver is derived under the ADMM framework by leveraging the Fourier convolution theorem, which can be effectively accelerated using GPUs. As a result, we achieved faster running time and higher PSNRs compared to the state-of-the-art CS-MRI reconstruction methods, such as using a patch-based dictionary learning and conventional wavelet and total variation energy. In the future, we plan to conduct a proper controlled-study of tuning-parameters and assess its feasibility in clinical applications.

Acknowledgments. This work was partially supported by the 2016 Research Fund (1.160047.01) of UNIST, the R&D program of MOTIE/KEIT (10054548), the Basic Science Research Program through the National Research Foundation of Korea (NRF) funded by the Ministry of Education (NRF-2014R1A1A2058773) and the Bio & Medical Technology Development Program of the NRF funded by the Korean government, MSIP (NRF-2015M3A9A7029725).

References

1. Data science bowl cardiac challenge data (2015). https://www.kaggle.com/c/second-annual-data-science-bowl/data
2. Aharon, M., Elad, M., Bruckstein, A.: K-SVD: an algorithm for designing overcomplete dictionaries for sparse representation. IEEE Trans. Signal Process. **54**(11), 4311–4322 (2006)
3. Awate, S., DiBella, E.: Spatiotemporal dictionary learning for undersampled dynamic MRI reconstruction via joint frame-based and dictionary-based sparsity. In: 2012 9th IEEE International Symposium on Biomedical Imaging (ISBI), pp. 318–321, May 2012
4. Bristow, H., Eriksson, A., Lucey, S.: Fast convolutional sparse coding. In: 2013 IEEE Conference on Computer Vision and Pattern Recognition (CVPR), pp. 391–398, June 2013
5. Caballero, J., Price, A., Rueckert, D., Hajnal, J.: Dictionary learning and time sparsity for dynamic MR data reconstruction. IEEE Trans. Med. Imaging **33**(4), 979–994 (2014)
6. Caballero, J., Rueckert, D., Hajnal, J.V.: Dictionary learning and time sparsity in dynamic MRI. In: Ayache, N., Delingette, H., Golland, P., Mori, K. (eds.) MICCAI 2012, Part I. LNCS, vol. 7510, pp. 256–263. Springer, Heidelberg (2012)
7. Jung, H., Sung, K., Nayak, K.S., Kim, E.Y., Ye, J.C.: k-t FOCUSS: a general compressed sensing framework for high resolution dynamic MRI. Magn. Reson. Med. **61**(1), 103–116 (2009)
8. Lustig, M., Donoho, D., Santos, J., Pauly, J.: Compressed sensing MRI. IEEE Signal Process. Mag. **25**(2), 72–82 (2008)
9. Otazo, R., Cands, E., Sodickson, D.K.: Low-rank plus sparse matrix decomposition for accelerated dynamic MRI with separation of background and dynamic components. Magn. Reson. Med. **73**(3), 1125–1136 (2015)
10. Quan, T.M., Han, S., Cho, H., Jeong, W.-K.: Multi-GPU reconstruction of dynamic compressed sensing MRI. In: Navab, N., Hornegger, J., Wells, W.M., Frangi, A.F. (eds.) MICCAI 2015. LNCS, vol. 9351, pp. 484–492. Springer, Heidelberg (2015). doi:10.1007/978-3-319-24574-4_58
11. Ravishankar, S., Bresler, Y.: MR image reconstruction from highly undersampled k-space data by dictionary learning. IEEE Trans. Med. Imaging **30**(5), 1028–1041 (2011)
12. Tremoulhac, B., Dikaios, N., Atkinson, D., Arridge, S.R.: Dynamic MR image reconstruction; separation from undersampled (k-t)-space via low-rank plus sparse prior. IEEE Trans. Med. Imaging **33**(8), 1689–1701 (2014)

13. Wohlberg, B.: Efficient convolutional sparse coding. In: 2014 IEEE International Conference on Acoustics, Speech and Signal Processing (ICASSP), pp. 7173–7177, May 2014

14. Yao, J., Xu, Z., Huang, X., Huang, J.: Accelerated dynamic MRI reconstruction with total variation and nuclear norm regularization. In: Navab, N., Hornegger, J., Wells, W.M., Frangi, A.F. (eds.) MICCAI 2015. LNCS, vol. 9350, pp. 635–642. Springer, Heidelberg (2015). doi:10.1007/978-3-319-24571-3_76

Dynamic Volume Reconstruction from Multi-slice Abdominal MRI Using Manifold Alignment

Xin Chen[✉], Muhammad Usman, Daniel R. Balfour, Paul K. Marsden,
Andrew J. Reader, Claudia Prieto, and Andrew P. King

Division of Imaging Sciences and Biomedical Engineering,
King's College London, London, UK
xin.chen@kcl.ac.uk

Abstract. We present a novel framework for retrospective dynamic 3D volume reconstruction from a multi-slice MRI acquisition using manifold alignment. K-space data are continuously acquired under free breathing using a radial golden-angle trajectory in a slice-by-slice manner. Non-overlapping consecutive profiles that were acquired within a short time window are grouped together. All grouped profiles from all slices are then simultaneously embedded using manifold alignment into a common manifold space (MS), in which profiles that were acquired at similar respiratory states are close together. Subsequently, a 3D volume can be reconstructed at each of the grouped profile MS positions by combining profiles that are close in the MS. This enables the original multi-slice dataset to be used to reconstruct a dynamic 3D sequence based on the respiratory state correspondences established in the MS. Our method was evaluated on both synthetic and *in vivo* datasets. For the synthetic datasets, the reconstructed dynamic sequence achieved a normalised cross correlation of 0.98 and peak signal to noise ratio of 26.64 dB compared with the ground truth. For the *in vivo* datasets, based on sharpness measurements and visual comparison, our method performed better than reconstruction using an adapted central k-space gating method.

Keywords: Manifold alignment · Respiratory motion estimation · MRI · Dynamic 3D volume reconstruction

1 Introduction

Dynamic magnetic resonance imaging (MRI) involves imaging a region of interest ideally with high temporal resolution, and is useful in many applications in which knowledge of motion (e.g. respiratory motion) is of interest. However, the acquisition speed of MRI is not sufficiently fast to permit enough data to be acquired quickly enough to reconstruct fully sampled images with high temporal resolution, especially for 3D imaging. This problem can be tackled by using under-sampled reconstruction schemes such as compressed sensing (CS) [1], but such techniques typically involve a complex optimisation which can be time-consuming for large amounts of dynamic MRI data. Another approach is to use a gating technique, which involves the retrospective combination of imaging data that were acquired at different times but similar motion states.

© Springer International Publishing AG 2016
S. Ourselin et al. (Eds.): MICCAI 2016, Part III, LNCS 9902, pp. 493–501, 2016.
DOI: 10.1007/978-3-319-46726-9_57

The term 'self-gating' refers to performing this gating using the acquired data itself. A common self-gating approach for radial acquisitions is to use the magnitude of the centre of k-space which is acquired in every radial profile as the self-gating signal [2]. A key weakness of this approach is the simplicity of the gating signal – gating using a scalar value necessarily causes complex intra- and inter-cycle variations in respiratory motion to be averaged out.

Alternative self-gating methods that are based on manifold learning (ML) have been reported [3–7]. The intuition behind such methods is that respiratory motion is pseudo-repetitive in nature, and can therefore be represented by a small number of motion variables. Usman et al. [7] applied Laplacian Eigenmaps to estimate respiratory motion from the central intersection region of a number of consecutive profiles using a radial golden-angle acquisition (RGA) [8]. Similarly, Bhatia et al. [5] used Laplacian Eigenmaps to estimate cardiac motion from repetitively sampled central k-space lines using a Cartesian acquisition. However, both methods estimated only 1D signals (i.e. scalar values over time) for self-gating and also only worked for 2D images. It would be nontrivial to extend these approaches to reconstruction of 3D volume. In [3, 4], Baumgartner et al. proposed a method for MRI self-gating using manifold alignment (MA) of 2D reconstructed image slices acquired at different anatomical positions. However, [3, 4] are image-based self-gating methods that assumed there was no motion within each of the fully sampled 2D image acquisitions (~ 300 ms per image), which may not be true for fast motion. The use of images for self-gating also limits the achievable temporal resolution to the time taken to acquire enough data to reconstruct the entire image.

In this paper, we propose to retrospectively reconstruct 3D dynamic volume sequences from k-space data acquired using a multiple 2D slice (M2D) acquisition. The proposed framework provides a number of advantages over other methods in the literature: (1) In contrast to the central k-space gating (CKG) method, instead of using a 1D gating signal, the proposed method allows the use of a larger k-space region to estimate a multi-dimensional gating signal to better capture intra-cycle and inter-cycle motion variations. (2) Different from [3, 4], we perform MA directly on k-space profiles rather than reconstructed images. This enables our technique to achieve higher temporal resolution. (3) Compared to the 2D ML methods in [5, 7], our method works for reconstruction of 3D dynamic volumes. To the authors' knowledge, no work has been reported in the literature for reconstructing high temporal resolution dynamic 3D MRI sequences based on k-space data from a M2D acquisition.

2 Methodology

As illustrated in Fig. 1, the proposed framework consists of k-space data acquisition, manifold alignment and image reconstruction, which are described in the following subsections.

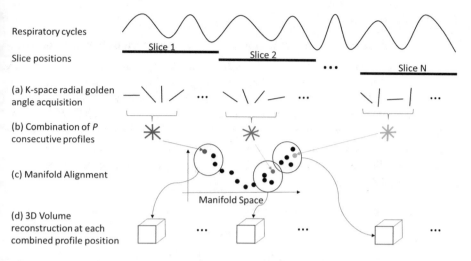

Fig. 1. Overview of the proposed framework.

2.1 K-Space Data Acquisition and Pre-processing

Data acquisition is performed under free breathing using a RGA trajectory (Fig. 1(a)), in which the angle between each two consecutive profiles is 111.25°. This enables a uniform coverage of k-space with high temporal incoherence for any arbitrary number of consecutive profiles.

M profiles are acquired at each slice position, followed by M profiles at the next slice position, and so on (see Fig. 1(a)). We denote the k-space data for each slice by $X_n = [x_{n,1}, \dots, x_{n,M}]$ ($n \in \{1, 2, \dots, N\}$ is the slice number), where the columns $x_{n,m}$ are k-space profiles. As reported in [7], using a larger central k-space region rather than the single sample of the k-space centre can produce more reliable estimation of respiratory motion. Therefore, since it takes only about 3 ms to acquire a single profile, we combine P consecutive profiles (Fig. 1(b)), and assume that no significant motion within this short time period occurred. Combination of profiles in this way enables a larger k-space central region to be used for respiratory self-gating. Since the radial profiles are sampled at non-uniform k-space positions, the convolutional gridding method [9] is applied to re-sample the non-uniform data to a Cartesian grid. Finally, the central $S \times S$ k-space region is used for the subsequent MA (see Sect. 2.2). After the profile combination and central region extraction, the original k-space data X_n are re-organised as $A_n = [a_{n,1}, \dots, a_{n,L}]$. L is the quotient of M/P, and the remaining profiles after the $L \times P^{th}$ profile are not used. The columns $a_{n,l}$ are the vector representations of the $S \times S$ central k-space region. To reduce sensitivity to noise, we applied a 1D Gaussian smoothness filter ($\sigma = 15$ ms) along the temporal direction for each element in $a_{n,l}$.

2.2   Manifold Alignment

The k-space dataset $A_1, \ldots, A_N$, now consists of N groups, each of which represents a different slice, where each group contains L vectors with S^2 elements each. The MA method is used to simultaneously reduce the dimensionality ($\mathbb{R}^{S \times S}$) of each group and align all groups of profiles into a common MS (with dimensionality $d < S \times S$), in which profiles acquired at similar respiratory states are close together (Fig. 1(c)). The dimensionality reduction and alignment of the groups is performed using the MA scheme proposed in [3]. Therefore, we briefly review this technique here. The MA scheme estimates the low dimensional embeddings $Y_n = \left[y_1^{(n)}, \ldots, y_L^{(n)} \right]$ of the input high dimensional data by minimising a joint cost function:

$$\emptyset_{total}\left(Y_1 \ldots Y_N \right) = \sum_{n=1}^{N} \varphi_n\left(Y_n \right) + \frac{\mu}{2} \sum_{\substack{n=1, m=1, \\ m \neq n}}^{N} \sum_{l,j}^{L} U_{lj}^{(nm)} ||y_l^{(n)} - y_j^{(m)}||^2 \tag{1}$$

The first term φ_n is the locally linear embedding (LLE) cost function [10], which represents the intra-group embedding errors. LLE forms the low-dimensional MS by preserving locally linear relations derived from the original high-dimensional data A_n. These relations at the lth high dimensional data vector are represented by a weighted ($W_{lj}^{(n)}$) linear combination of its K^{LLE} nearest neighbours with indices j ($j \in \eta(l)$), i.e.

$$\varphi_n\left(Y_n \right) = \sum_l ||y_l - \sum_{j \in \eta(l)} W_{lj}^{(n)} y_j||^2 = Tr(YMY^T) \tag{2}$$

$Tr(\bullet)$ is the trace operator, and the centred reconstruction weight matrix M is calculated as $M = (I - W)^T (I - W)$. Note that $W_{lj}^{(n)}$ are computed from the high dimensional data A_n.

The second term in Eq. (1) represents the inter-group cost function. $y_l^{(n)}$ represents the MS coordinates of vector $a_{n,l}$. μ is a weighting parameter that balances the intragroup and inter-group terms. $U^{(nm)}$ is an inter-group similarity kernel derived from intragroup comparisons of the high-dimensional data $A_1, \ldots, A_N$. This is achieved by deriving a feature descriptor for each vector $a_{n,l}$ using the concept of random walks from graph theory. This feature descriptor allows the relationships between vectors from the same group to be preserved and uniquely represented, which permits the inter-group similarity to be robustly measured without inter-group comparisons of the original high-dimensional data. For us, the groups represent k-space data acquired from different slices, which are not directly comparable since they encode the frequency properties of different anatomical regions. For more details of the MA process please refer to [3].

2.3   3D Dynamic Sequence Reconstruction

As illustrated in Fig. 1(c), after the MA process, all of the combined profiles (CPs) from different slice positions are embedded into a common MS. (The CPs refer to the combined consecutive profiles as described in Sect. 2.1.) The CPs that were acquired at similar respiratory states should be close together in the MS, even though they belong to different slice positions. Image reconstruction is subsequently performed by grouping the G CPs for each slice that have the closest Euclidean distances (in MS) to the current CPs (Fig. 1(d)). G is determined by the total number of profiles (T) which is required for reconstruction of each slice, divided by P (the number of combined profiles). Since a RGA acquisition is used, this ensures the selected profiles are approximately evenly distributed in k-space. Using a multi-slice reconstruction, a 3D volume can be reconstructed at each of the L respiratory states for each of the N slice positions. This enables the original multi-slice dataset to be used to reconstruct a dynamic 3D sequence. For the reconstruction, the non-uniform Fast Fourier Transform [9] is applied to reconstruct the final image from the selected radial k-space profiles.

3   Experiments and Results

The proposed method was evaluated on both synthetic and *in vivo* datasets. The synthetic datasets were used to establish a ground truth for quantitative evaluation. We also demonstrated the practical feasibility of our technique using 3D *in vivo* datasets, and the results were compared with an adapted CKG method.

3.1   Materials

Synthetic Dataset Generation: To mimic the M2D acquisition, we generated high temporal resolution 3D synthetic datasets, based on image registration of a respiratory gated high resolution (RGHR) 3D MRI volume to a dynamic 3D low-resolution (DLR) MRI sequence. The RGHR volume had 120 sagittal slices and was acquired at the end-exhale position, with TR = 4.4 ms, TE = 2.2 ms, flip angle = 90°, and acquired voxel size $2.19 \times 2.19 \times 2.74$ mm^3 with matrix size 160×120. The DLR sequences comprised 35 dynamics acquired under free-breathing using cardiac gating at late diastole. 20 slices were acquired for each volume using 3D TFEPI with TR = 10 ms, TE = 4.9 ms, flip angle 20°, acquired voxel size $2.7 \times 3.6 \times 8.0$ mm^3, acquired matrix size 128×77, TFE factor 26, EPI factor 13, TFE acquisition time 267.9 ms. The region-of-interest focused on the right lung and liver region. In order to generate a large amount of realistic synthetic high spatial/temporal resolution volumes, the following steps were followed.

(a)   The RGHR volume was deformed to align with the corresponding end-exhale DLR volume using B-spline deformable image registration [11].

(b)   The end-exhale DLR volume was registered with all other DLR volumes.

(c)   The DLR volumes were grouped into three different respiratory groups (inhale, exhale and mid-inhale), according to their head-foot diaphragm positions in the central slice. We then randomly selected one volume from each of the inhale and exhale groups, and two volumes from the mid-inhale group. Extra volumes were interpolated between these four volumes using B-spline registrations over a complete breathing cycle. In our experiments, 60 such breathing cycles were generated. Each breathing cycle lasted approximately 5 s and the interpolated volumes had a temporal resolution of ~ 3.2 ms.

(d) The RGHR volume was warped to each of the DLR positions based on the corresponding registration results, resulting in about 90000 high spatial/temporal resolution dynamics containing realistic intra-cycle and inter-cycle variations.

(e) One k-space profile was extracted from each of the synthetic volumes at the corresponding slice position. Approximately 9000 profiles were extracted for each slice before moving to the next slice position. We generated 6 (1 for parameter optimisation and 5 for validation) such highly realistic synthetic sequences to validate our method against known gold-standard volumes.

***In vivo* Dataset Acquisition:** A M2D acquisition with RGA trajectory was employed for data acquisition in the liver and lung region of five healthy volunteers. For each volunteer, $M = 9000$ profiles were acquired using the RGA trajectory in sagittal view at each slice position before moving to the next slice. Data with 8 slices were acquired on a Philips 1.5T scanner using a 28 channel-coil. The settings were TR = 3.2 ms, TE = 1.58 ms, flip angle = 70°, and acquired voxel size $2.0 \times 2.0 \times 8.0$ mm^3 with acquired matrix size of 160×160 for 8 slices. For each volunteer, a total of 72000 radial profiles were acquired under free-breathing in approximately 4 min.

3.2   Results

All free parameters were tuned using a parameter sweep based on a single synthetic dataset (which was not used for validation) and consistently applied to the remaining synthetic and *in vivo* datasets. The parameters were set as $S = 9$, $P = 20$, $\mu = 10^{-5}$, $d = 3$ and $T = 200$ for the following experiments.

Synthetic Dataset: The manifold embedding for one of the synthetic datasets is shown in Fig. 2 (left). The colours represent the normalised head-foot diaphragm position of the ground truth. Similar coloured points grouping together indicates a good manifold alignment. The larger distances between the red points in the MS are due to larger respiratory variations in the end inhale positions. The reconstructed image quality was quantitatively measured for all 5 datasets based on normalised cross correlation (NCC) and peak signal-to-noise ratio (PSNR), against the ground truth. Example ground truth and

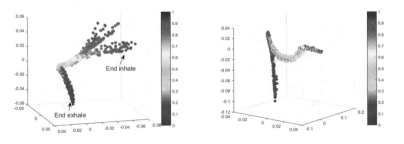

Fig. 2. Manifold embeddings for a synthetic dataset (left) and an *in vivo* dataset (right).

corresponding reconstructed images of 3 different sagittal slices, and coronal views at 4 different respiratory positions are shown in Fig. 3. The mean and standard deviation of NCC and PSNR values for all corresponding volumes of 5 synthetic datasets were 0.9801 ± 0.0057 and 26.64 ± 0.88 dB respectively.

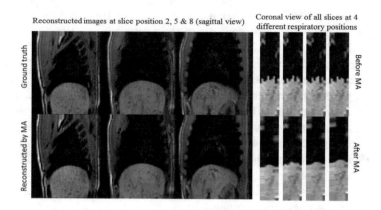

Fig. 3. Reconstructed volumes using MA and the corresponding ground truth of a synthetic dataset.

***In vivo* Dataset:** Due to the lack of ground truth and comparative techniques for the *in vivo* datasets, we adapted the CKG method (ACKG) for comparison. The central k-space magnitudes of each slice were normalised to the range of 0 to 1. Correspondences

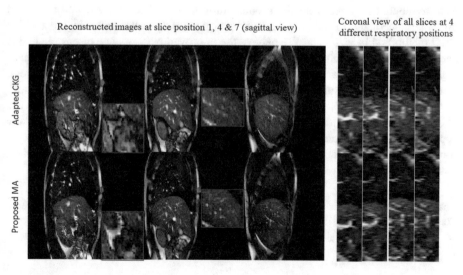

Fig. 4. Examples of reconstructed images using adapted CKG (top row) and the proposed MA method (bottom row) at different slice positions and different respiratory positions. (Color figure online)

across slices were then established by searching the same value of the normalised k-space magnitudes. To reconstruct a gated 3D volume for a specific profile, a gating window (0.05) was set around the current profile magnitude for each slice. Any profiles (T^{all}) with a magnitude within the gating window represent similar respiratory positions, and only the T temporally closest profiles were selected for image reconstruction. If $T^{all} < T$, the gating window was iteratively increased by 0.005 until $T^{all} \geq T$. Subsequently, the reconstructed slices were stacked into a volume.

The manifold embeddings for one of the *in vivo* datasets is shown in Fig. 2 (right). The colours represent the normalised k-space magnitude. A sharpness measurement was used as a quantitative measure of image quality. Sharpness was measured by the average of the image gradient magnitude in the liver and liver-lung boundary. Over all five *in vivo* datasets, the mean and standard deviation of the sharpness measure for our method was 0.0587 ± 0.0069. This was statistically significantly ($p < 0.01$) higher than the ACKG method (0.0559 ± 0.0071), based on two-sided Wilcoxon signed rank test of the paired datasets. Figure 4 shows examples of the reconstructed images using the ACKG method and our method, at different sagittal slice positions, and coronal views at 4 respiratory positions. Sharper organ details (red boxes) and more accurate slice alignment (red arrows) can be observed using our method.

4   Conclusion and Discussion

We have presented a novel framework that is able to reconstruct high temporal resolution dynamic 3D MRI sequences using manifold alignment of k-space data from M2D acquisitions. Based on synthetic datasets, our method achieved high NCC and PSNR measurements compared with the ground truth. Our method also showed improved image sharpness and visual image quality over images reconstructed using an adapted CKG method on *in vivo* data. We believe the improved performance of our method is due to the fact that a multi-dimensional gating signal is extracted from a larger k-space region. However, similar to the CKG method, the MA method cannot achieve a good reconstruction if an insufficient number of profiles is available at similar respiratory positions. It is possible that such a limitation may be addressed by the subsequent use of CS techniques. High temporal resolution 3D motion information will be useful in any application for which retrospective motion estimations are required, such as motion correction of positron emission tomography (PET) data in a simultaneous PET-MR scenario, or motion-correction of the MR data.

Acknowledgements. This work was funded by the Engineering and Physical Sciences Research Council (Grant EP/M009319/1).

References

1. Lustig, M., Donoho, D., Pauly, J.: Sparse MRI: the application of compressed sensing for rapid MR imaging. Mag. Res. Med. **58**(6), 1182–1195 (2007)
2. Larson, A., White, R., Laub, G., McVeigh, E., Li, D., Simonetti, O.: Self-gated cardiac cine MRI. Mag. Res. Img. **51**(1), 93–102 (2004)
3. Baumgartner, C.F., Gomez, A., Koch, L.M., Housden, J.R., Kolbitsch, C., McClelland, J.R., Rueckert, D., King, A.P.: Self-aligning manifolds for matching disparate medical image datasets. In: Ourselin, S., Alexander, D.C., Westin, C.-F., Cardoso, M. (eds.) IPMI 2015. LNCS, vol. 9123, pp. 363–374. Springer, Heidelberg (2015)
4. Baumgartner, C., Kolbitsch, C., Balfour, D., Marsden, P., McClelland, J., Rueckert, D., King, A.: High-resolution dynamic MR imaging of the thorax for respiratory motion correction of PET using groupwise manifold alignment. Med. Img. Anal. **18**, 939–952 (2014)
5. Bhatia, K.K., Caballero, J., Price, A.N., Sun, Y., Hajnal, J.V., Rueckert, D.: Fast reconstruction of accelerated dynamic MRI using manifold kernel regression. In: Navab, N., Hornegger, J., Wells, W.M., Frangi, A.F. (eds.) MICCAI 2015, Part III. LNCS, vol. 9351, pp. 510–518. Springer, Heidelberg (2015). doi:10.1007/978-3-319-24574-4_61
6. Usman, M., Atkinson, D., Kolbitsch, C., Schaeffter, T., Prieto, C.: Manifold learning based ECG-Free free-breathing cardiac CINE MRI. Mag. Res. Img. **41**, 1521–1527 (2015)
7. Usman, M., Vaillant, G., Atkinson, D., Schaeffter, T., Prieto, C.: Compressive manifold learning: estimating one-dimensional respiratory motion directly from undersampled k-space data. Mag. Res. Med. **72**, 1130–1140 (2014)
8. Winkelmann, S., Schaeffter, T., Koehler, T., Eggers, H., Doessel, O.: An optimal radial profile order based on the golden ratio for time-resolved MRI. IEEE Trans. Med. Img. **26**(1), 68–76 (2007)
9. Greengard, L., Lee, J.-Y.: Accelerating the nonuniform fast fourier transform. SIAM Rev. **46**(3), 443–454 (2006)
10. Roweis, S., Saul, L.: Nonlinear dimensionality reduction by locally linear embedding. Science **290**, 2323–2326 (2000)
11. Rueckert, D., Sonoda, L., Hayes, C., Hill, D., Leach, M., Hawkes, D.: Nonrigid registration using free-form deformations: application to breast MR images. IEEE Trans. Med. Img. **18**(8), 712–721 (1999)

Fast and Accurate Multi-tissue Deconvolution Using SHORE and H-psd Tensors

Michael Ankele[1], Lek-Heng Lim[2], Samuel Groeschel[3], and Thomas Schultz[1]([⊠])

[1] University of Bonn, Bonn, Germany
[2] University of Chicago, Chicago, IL, USA
schultz@cs.uni-bonn.de
[3] Experimental Pediatric Neuroimaging and Department of Pediatric Neurology and Developmental Medicine, University Children's Hospital Tübingen, Tübingen, Germany

Abstract. We propose a new regularization for spherical deconvolution in diffusion MRI. It is based on observing that higher-order tensor representations of fiber ODFs should be H-psd, i.e., they should have a positive semidefinite (psd) matrix H_T. We show that this constraint is stricter than the currently more widely used non-negativity, and that it can be enforced easily using quadratic cone programming. We demonstrate its use in a multi-tissue deconvolution framework that models the different tissue types in the continuous SHORE basis and can therefore be applied to data with multiple b values that are not organized on shells, such as in Diffusion Spectrum Imaging. Experiments on simulated fiber crossings, data from the Human Connectome Project, and clinical data, demonstrate the improved speed and accuracy of this new method.

1 Introduction

Spherical deconvolution [14] is widely used to analyze white matter (WM) in high angular resolution diffusion imaging (HARDI). Recently, it has been shown that, when HARDI data is available on multiple shells, parameters related to the volume fractions of gray matter (GM) and corticospinal fluid (CSF) can be added to the deconvolution model [3,5]. An important advantage of this is increased accuracy in voxels with partial voluming between different tissue types.

We present a novel method for multi-tissue deconvolution that makes two main contributions: First, non-negativity constraints have long been recognized as an indispensible regularization in deconvolution, and are most frequently

S. Groeschel—This work was supported by the DFG under grant SCHU 3040/1-1. LHL is supported by AFOSR FA9550-13-1-0133, DARPA D15AP00109, NSF IIS 1546413, DMS 1209136, and DMS 1057064. Parts of the data ("clin-dsi") were provided by Katrin Sakreida and Georg Neuloh (RWTH Aachen University Hospital), and by the HCP, WU-Minn Cons. (PIs: D. Van Essen and K. Ugurbil; 1U54MH091657) funded by the 16 NIH Institutes and Centers that support the NIH Blueprint for Neuroscience Research; and by the McDonnell Center for Systems Neuroscience at Washington U.

© Springer International Publishing AG 2016
S. Ourselin et al. (Eds.): MICCAI 2016, Part III, LNCS 9902, pp. 502–510, 2016.
DOI: 10.1007/978-3-319-46726-9_58

enforced at a set of discrete points on the sphere [14,16]. In contrast, we derive a positive definiteness constraint from a higher-order tensor representation of the fiber orientation distribution function (fODF) which implies non-negativity everywhere on the sphere. It can be implemented easily using quadratic cone programming, and can be combined both with multi-tissue and traditional single-shell single-tissue deconvolution.

Second, many dMRI acquisition schemes do not use a shell structure. This includes Diffusion Spectrum Imaging [15], which uses a Cartesian grid, and some recently proposed schemes that distribute samples freely in Q-space [7,9]. Our approach improves upon previous multi-tissue deconvolution methods, which have modeled the signal on each shell separately [3,5], by instead estimating the tissue response as a continuous function in Q-space, using the SHORE basis functions [8]. This allows us to work with data that is not organized on shells.

In a direct comparison between our approach and a state-of-the-art alternative [5], we demonstrate that ours is more well-conditioned, more accurate at small angles, and faster.

2 Related Work

Our approach extends previous work that has used higher-order Cartesian tensors to represent fiber ODFs [6,11,13,16] by the ability to handle data acquired at multiple b-values and by modeling multiple tissue types.

Our H-psd constraint is new, and stronger than the non-negativity constraints used previously when estimating higher-order diffusion tensors [1,4], or in the non-negative spherical deconvolution (NNSD) [2] approach. In addition, in contrast to NNSD, our method can be implemented using standard convex cone optimization packages rather than requiring a custom implementation of a computationally expensive Riemannian gradient descent.

3 Fiber ODFs are H-psd Tensors

Our approach extends previous work [13], which has proposed to describe fODFs f by fully symmetric fourth order tensors:

$$f(\mathbf{v}) = T(\mathbf{v}) = \sum_{i,j,k,l=1}^{3} T_{ijkl}\, v_i v_j v_k v_l, \quad \mathbf{v} \in \mathbb{S}^2 \tag{1}$$

Such fODF tensors T are obtained by deconvolution in the Spherical Harmonics basis and a subsequent change to the monomial basis, which spans the same space of functions. However, there are two important differences to standard spherical deconvolution [14]: First, the deconvolution step is constructed so that it maps the single fiber response in direction $\mathbf{v}$ to a symmetric rank-one tensor $\mathbf{v} \otimes \mathbf{v} \otimes \mathbf{v} \otimes \mathbf{v}$, rather than to a truncated delta peak. Second, principal fODF directions for fiber tractography are found using a low-rank approximation of the fODF tensor, rather than peaks in the fODF function.

The set of symmetric three-dimensional fourth-order tensors will be denoted by $S_{3,4}$. The subset of positive semidefinite tensors is

$$P_{3,4} = \{T \in S_{3,4} : T(\mathbf{v}) \geq 0 \quad \forall \mathbf{v} \in \mathbb{S}^2\}. \tag{2}$$

As pointed out in Chap. 5 of [10], $T \in S_{3,4}$ has an associated matrix

$$H_T = \begin{pmatrix} T_{xxxx} & T_{xxxy} & T_{xxxz} & T_{xxyy} & T_{xxyz} & T_{xxzz} \\ T_{xxxy} & T_{xxyy} & T_{xxyz} & T_{xyyy} & T_{xyyz} & T_{xyzz} \\ T_{xxxz} & T_{xxyz} & T_{xxzz} & T_{xyyz} & T_{xyzz} & T_{xzzz} \\ T_{xxyy} & T_{xyyy} & T_{xyyz} & T_{yyyy} & T_{yyyz} & T_{yyzz} \\ T_{xxyz} & T_{xyyz} & T_{xyzz} & T_{yyyz} & T_{yyzz} & T_{yzzz} \\ T_{xxzz} & T_{xyzz} & T_{xzzz} & T_{yyzz} & T_{yzzz} & T_{zzzz} \end{pmatrix} \tag{3}$$

that represents T's action on the six-dimensional space of symmetric products $\mathbf{v} \otimes \mathbf{v}$. We will denote the subset of tensors with a positive semidefinite matrix H_T as

$$P_H = \{T \in S_{3,4} : H_T \text{ is psd}\} \tag{4}$$

and call these tensors H-psd.

P_H is closely related to decomposable tensors. To show this, let

$$Q_{3,4} = \{T \in S_{3,4} : T(\mathbf{v}) = \sum_{i=1}^{k} \langle \alpha_i, \mathbf{v} \rangle^4\} \tag{5}$$

$$\Sigma_{3,4} = \{T \in S_{3,4} : T(\mathbf{v}) = \sum_{i=1}^{k} h_i^2(\mathbf{v})\} \tag{6}$$

be the subsets of tensors that are sums of fourth powers and sums of squares, respectively. Due to their geometric structure, these sets are called cones. They obey

$$Q_{3,4} \subsetneq \Sigma_{3,4} \subseteq P_{3,4}. \tag{7}$$

Obviously, sums of squares and sums of fourth powers are positive semidefinite. In fact, a result by Hilbert, which has been applied to enforce non-negativity of fourth-order diffusion tensors [1,4], states that $P_{3,4} = \Sigma_{3,4}$. In contrast, not every tensor in $P_{3,4}$ can be written as a sum of fourth powers [10].

The dual of a cone C is defined as $C^* = \{y \in C : \langle x, y \rangle \geq 0 \ \forall x \in C\}$ and, in [10], it is shown that

$$\Sigma_{3,4}^\star = P_H \quad \text{and} \quad P_{3,4}^\star = Q_{3,4}. \tag{8}$$

Combining these dualities with the dual of the result by Hilbert yields

$$Q_{3,4} = P_{3,4}^\star = \Sigma_{3,4}^\star = P_H, \tag{9}$$

i.e., a tensor in $S_{3,4}$ can be written as a sum of fourth powers or, equivalently, decomposed into symmetric rank-1 terms, if and only if it is H-psd.

For spherical deconvolution, this has the following implications: First, fODF tensors arise from a mixture of an unknown number of single-fiber compartments, each of which is represented as a symmetric rank-1 tensor. Therefore, any valid fODF tensor must be decomposable. Second, decomposability can be checked easily by positive semidefiniteness of Eq. (3) (H-psd). Third, as Eq. (7) shows, H-psd is a stronger condition than simple non-negativity, as it has been imposed previously on fODFs [2,14], or on fourth-order diffusion tensors [1,4].

4   Using SHORE for Multi-tissue Deconvolution

Multi-tissue deconvolution requires modelling the dMRI response of all tissue types. Previous approaches [3,5] do so separately for each shell. To avoid dependence on a shell structure, we instead create a continuous model of functions $f(\mathbf{q} = q\mathbf{u})$ in Q-space using the SHORE basis functions [8]

$$\phi_{lnm}(\mathbf{q}) = \left[\frac{2(n-l)!}{\zeta^{3/2}\Gamma(n+3/2)} \right]^{1/2} \left(\frac{q^2}{\zeta} \right)^{l/2} \exp\left(\frac{-q^2}{2\zeta} \right) L_{n-l}^{l+1/2}\left(\frac{q^2}{\zeta} \right) Y_l^m(\mathbf{u}) \quad (10)$$

with the associated Laguerre polynomials L_n^α, the real Spherical Harmonics Y_l^m and a radial scaling factor ζ.

Let $K(\mathbf{q}) = \sum_{ln} K_{ln} \phi_{ln0}(\mathbf{q})$ be the white matter single-fiber response, with $m = 0$ due to cylinder symmetry. The signal from an fODF f is then modeled by a convolution on the sphere, $S(\mathbf{q}) \approx K \star_{\mathbb{S}^2} f$ [2]. For a given K and signal vector $S_i = S(\mathbf{q}_i)$, finding the Spherical Harmonics coefficients f via deconvolution then becomes a linear least squares problem with a nonlinear constraint:

$$\operatorname{argmin}_f \|Mf - S\|^2 \quad \text{subject to} \quad f \in P_H \quad (11)$$

with convolution matrix

$$M_{(i)(lm)} = \sum_n \frac{1}{\alpha_l} K_{ln} \phi_{lnm}(\mathbf{q}_i). \quad (12)$$

As in [13], the α_l are the Spherical Harmonics coefficients of the unit rank-1 tensor along the z-axis.

The problem is equivalent to the quadratic cone program (QCP)

$$\operatorname{argmin}_f \frac{1}{2}\langle f, Pf \rangle + \langle q, f \rangle \quad \text{subject to} \quad (Gf)\,\text{psd} \quad (13)$$

with $P = M^T M$, $q = -M^T S$, and a matrix G that first maps f from Spherical Harmonics to the monomial basis, and then to its H_T matrix, $Gf = H_f$. This QCP can be solved efficiently using CVXOPT (cvxopt.org).

Multi-tissue support is added by concatenating individual tissue matrices

$$M = [M_{\mathrm{CSF}}, M_{\mathrm{GM}}, M_{\mathrm{WM}}], \quad f = \begin{bmatrix} f_{\mathrm{CSF}} \\ f_{\mathrm{GM}} \\ f_{\mathrm{WM}} \end{bmatrix}. \quad (14)$$

Since CSF and GM are isotropic, M_{CSF} and M_{GM} are single-column matrices. In the QCP, non-negativity constraints are enforced for f_{GM} and f_{CSF}.

5 Results

5.1 Condition and Computational Efficiency

We compared our method to the approach of Jeurissen et al. [5], using CVXOPT in both cases. We used data provided by the Human Connectome Project (HCP) with 270 DWIs, 90 each at $b \approx \{1000, 2000, 3000\}$ s/mm^2, and a two-shell clinical data set ("clin-2-sh") with 94 DWIs, 30 at $b = 700$ and 64 at $b = 2000$. We also show results on another clinical data set ("clin-dsi") with 128 DWIs, acquired on a Cartesian grid with $b_{\max} = 3000$. The approach in [5] cannot be applied to this data, since it includes many different b values with few directions each.

Tissue response functions were estimated as described previously [5], based on tissue segmentation of a coregistered T_1 image, and FA thresholds (FA > 0.7 for white matter, FA < 0.2 for CSF), except that we model the responses in the SHORE basis as described in Sect. 4.

The processing time (on a single CPU core) as well as the condition number of the matrix P in the quadratic program are listed in Table 1. The fact that we use fourth-order fODFs makes the problem much better conditioned. Our method is also significantly faster, despite the fact that we guarantee nonnegativity everywhere, instead of enforcing it only at discrete points. We will now demonstrate that, when combined with tensor approximation [13], order 4 is sufficient to resolve crossings, and even more accurate at smaller angles.

Table 1. Our approach is much better conditioned than the traditional one, and requires less computation. Unlike the existing method, it is applicable also to DSI data

	cond(P)			Optimization time		
	HCP	clin-2-sh	clin-dsi	HCP	clin-2-sh	clin-dsi
SHORE order 4, H-psd	290	1 545	889	51 m 10 s	11 m 02 s	8 m 58 s
SH order 8, non-neg [5]	619 063	8 999 150	N/A	239 m 53 s	21 m 27 s	N/A

5.2 Accuracy on Simulated Data

Evaluating the accuracy of our method requires data for which volume fractions and orientations of crossing fiber compartments are known. From an HCP data set, we extracted the signal from voxels believed to contain a single fiber of white matter, i.e., being within the white matter mask and having FA > 0.7. The fiber direction for each voxel was estimated by fitting the diffusion tensor model and finding the eigenvector to the highest eigenvalue. Every voxel of simulated data was created by randomly choosing several single fiber voxels and a voxel with FA < 0.2 from either the grey matter or the CSF mask, and adding their signals with random volume fractions.

For comparison, we evaluated the original method by Jeurissen et al. [5], our proposed method, as well as a hybrid, which uses our novel regularization and tensor decomposition, but models the response functions using Spherical Harmonics for each shell, rather than SHORE.

The accuracy of estimated fiber directions and volume fractions on simulated data containing two fibers can be seen in Fig. 1. They demonstrate that, for crossing angles below 60°, order-4 tensor approximation reconstructs the fibers much more accurately than finding peaks in order-8 fODFs. The theoretical advantage of H-psd being stricter than non-negativity becomes relevant for small angles, starting around 40°. Our simulated data includes the noise from the HCP data from which it was generated. We tried adding more noise, and observed that this increased the advantage of using the H-psd constraint.

Practically no difference is visible when replacing SHORE with Spherical Harmonics models on each shell. This demonstrates that, while SHORE is more flexible in that it does not assume a multi-shell structure, it does not decrease accuracy when data is given on shells.

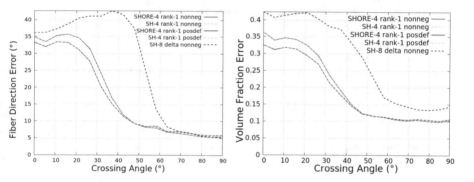

Fig. 1. On simulated two-fiber crossings with variable amounts of GM and CSF, our method estimates fiber directions and volume fractions with improved accuracy.

5.3   Results on Real Data

On the two-shell clinical data, our method and the state-of-the-art approach by Jeurissen et al. [5] produced similar results. The estimated directions of up to three fibers with volume fractions above 0.1 are shown on a map of white matter volume fractions in Fig. 2(a/b), and exhibit little difference.

Averaged over the brain mask, the absolute deviation between tissue volume fractions estimated by the two methods was only 0.005 (CSF), 0.022 (GM), and 0.027 (WM). Averaged over the white matter, the angular deviation of fiber directions, weighted by their volume fractions, was 7.98°, which is comparable to our simulation-based estimate of accuracy.

Since the true fiber directions are unknown in this case, we cannot be sure which method is more accurate in practice. However, a clear practical benefit of

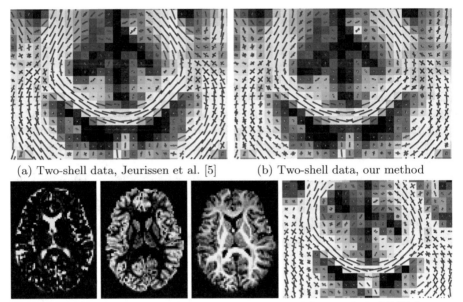

(a) Two-shell data, Jeurissen et al. [5]   (b) Two-shell data, our method

(c) Volume fraction maps and fiber directions estimated from a clinical DSI data set

Fig. 2. On two-shell clinical data, similar results were obtained using a state-of-the-art approach (a) and ours (b), which is faster and can also be applied to DSI data, as demonstrated in (c).

our method is its increased speed, and the fact that it can also be applied to data that has multiple b values, but no shell structure, as the DSI clinical data, for which results are shown in Fig. 2(c).

6   Conclusion

We introduced H-psd, a new positive definiteness constraint for spherical deconvolution, and showed that it is more stringent than usual non-negativity. It can be combined with all deconvolution methods, multi-tissue as well as the more widely used single-shell single-tissue variant [14]. We showed that the H-psd constraint increases accuracy at small angles, and is easy to enforce using convex cone programming libraries.

We also demonstrated that SHORE can be used as an extension of multi-tissue deconvolution [5]. This allowed us to apply multi-tissue deconvolution to DSI data, without sacrificing accuracy when working with data on shells.

Our method relies on the use of fourth-order tensors to describe fODFs. However, it is clear from the results (and was observed previously in [13]) that fourth-order is enough even for low angles and three-way crossings if we combine it with low-rank tensor approximation.

In the future, we will apply the H-psd constraint in the context of adaptive deconvolution [12] to improve per-voxel estimations of fiber response in patients with demyelinating disease. We expect that this will result in more accurate maps of tissue properties, and more reliable tractography.

References

1. Barmpoutis, A., Jian, B., Vemuri, B.C., Shepherd, T.M.: Symmetric positive 4th order tensors & their estimation from diffusion weighted MRI. In: Karssemeijer, N., Lelieveldt, B. (eds.) IPMI 2007. LNCS, vol. 4584, pp. 308–319. Springer, Heidelberg (2007)
2. Cheng, J., Deriche, R., Jiang, T., Shen, D., Yap, P.T.: Non-negative spherical deconvolution (NNSD) for estimation of fiber orientation distribution function in single-/multi-shell diffusion MRI. NeuroImage **101**, 750–764 (2014)
3. Christiaens, D., Maes, F., Sunaert, S., Suetens, P.: Convex non-negative spherical factorization of multi-shell diffusion-weighted images. In: Navab, N., Hornegger, J., Wells, W.M., Frangi, A.F. (eds.) MICCAI 2015. LNCS, vol. 9349, pp. 166–173. Springer, Heidelberg (2015). doi:10.1007/978-3-319-24553-9_21
4. Ghosh, A., Deriche, R., Moakher, M.: Ternary quartic approach for positive 4th order diffusion tensors revisited. In: Proceedings of IEEE International Symposium on Biomedical Imaging, pp. 618–621 (2009)
5. Jeurissen, B., Tournier, J.D., Dhollander, T., Connelly, A., Sijbers, J.: Multi-tissue constrained spherical deconvolution for improved analysis of multi-shell diffusion MRI data. NeuroImage **103**, 411–426 (2014)
6. Jiao, F., Gur, Y., Johnson, C.R., Joshi, S.: Detection of crossing white matter fibers with high-order tensors and rank-k decompositions. In: Székely, G., Hahn, H.K. (eds.) IPMI 2011. LNCS, vol. 6801, pp. 538–549. Springer, Heidelberg (2011)
7. Knutsson, H., Westin, C.-F.: Tensor metrics and charged containers for 3D Q-space sample distribution. In: Mori, K., Sakuma, I., Sato, Y., Barillot, C., Navab, N. (eds.) MICCAI 2013, Part I. LNCS, vol. 8149, pp. 679–686. Springer, Heidelberg (2013)
8. Merlet, S.L., Deriche, R.: Continuous diffusion signal, EAP and ODF estimation via compressive sensing in diffusion MRI. Med. Image Anal. **17**, 556–572 (2013)
9. Paquette, M., Merlet, S., Gilbert, G., Deriche, R., Descoteaux, M.: Comparison of sampling strategies and sparsifying transforms to improve compressed sensing diffusion spectrum imaging. Magn. Reson. Med. **73**(1), 401–416 (2015)
10. Reznick, B.: Sums of Even Powers of Real Linear Forms. American Mathematical Society, Providence (1992)
11. Schultz, T., Fuster, A., Ghosh, A., Deriche, R., Florack, L., Lim, L.H.: Higher-order tensors in diffusion imaging. In: Westin, C.F., Vilanova, A., Burgeth, B. (eds.) Visualization and Processing of Tensors and Higher Order Descriptors for Multi-Valued Data. Mathematics and Visualization, pp. 129–161. Springer, Heidelberg (2014)
12. Schultz, T., Groeschel, S.: Auto-calibrating spherical deconvolution based on ODF sparsity. In: Mori, K., Sakuma, I., Sato, Y., Barillot, C., Navab, N. (eds.) MICCAI 2013, Part I. LNCS, vol. 8149, pp. 663–670. Springer, Heidelberg (2013)
13. Schultz, T., Seidel, H.P.: Estimating crossing fibers: a tensor decomposition approach. IEEE Trans. Vis. Comput. Graph. **14**(6), 1635–1642 (2008)
14. Tournier, J.D., Calamante, F., Connelly, A.: Robust determination of the fibre orientation distribution in diffusion MRI: non-negativity constrained super-resolved spherical deconvolution. NeuroImage **35**, 1459–1472 (2007)

15. Wedeen, V.J., Hagmann, P., Tseng, W.Y.I., Reese, T.G., Weisskoff, R.M.: Mapping complex tissue architecture with diffusion spectrum magnetic resonance imaging. Magn. Reson. Med. **54**(6), 1377–1386 (2005)
16. Weldeselassie, Y.T., Barmpoutis, A., Atkins, M.S.: Symmetric positive semi-definite cartesian tensor fiber orientation distributions (CT-FOD). Med. Image Anal. **16**(6), 1121–1129 (2012)

Optimisation of Arterial Spin Labelling Using Bayesian Experimental Design

David Owen[1(✉)], Andrew Melbourne[1], David Thomas[1,2], Enrico De Vita[3,4], Jonathan Rohrer[2], and Sebastien Ourselin[1]

[1] Translational Imaging Group, University College London, London, UK
david.owen.14@ucl.ac.uk
[2] Dementia Research Centre, Institute of Neurology, University College London, London, UK
[3] Neuroradiology, National Hospital for Neurology and Neurosurgery, London, UK
[4] Academic Neuroradiological Unit, UCL Institute of Neurology, London, UK

Abstract. Large-scale neuroimaging studies often use multiple individual imaging contrasts. Due to the finite time available for imaging, there is intense competition for the time allocated to the individual modalities; thus it is crucial to maximise the utility of each method given the resources available. Arterial Spin Labelled (ASL) MRI often forms part of such studies. Measuring perfusion of oxygenated blood in the brain is valuable for several diseases, but quantification using multiple inversion time ASL is time-consuming due to poor SNR and consequently slow acquisitions. Here, we apply Bayesian principles of experimental design to clinical-length ASL acquisitions, resulting in significant improvements to perfusion estimation. Using simulations and experimental data, we validate this approach for a five-minute ASL scan. Our design procedure can be constrained to any chosen scan duration, making it well-suited to improve a variety of ASL implementations. The potential for adaptation to other modalities makes this an attractive method for optimising acquisition in the time-pressured environment of neuroimaging studies.

1 Introduction

Arterial Spin Labelling (ASL) can be used to characterise the perfusion of oxygenated blood in the brain. Multiple inversion time (multi-TI) ASL is used to simultaneously estimate perfusion, f, and arterial transit time, Δt. These are promising biomarkers for many neurological diseases such as stroke and dementia [1,2]. However, ASL acquisitions are time-consuming and have low SNR, necessitating a large number of measurements. This can make them unsuitable for large neuroimaging studies with competing requirements from other MR modalities such as diffusion and functional MRI, and often only a short period of time is devoted to ASL. Here, we develop a general Bayesian design approach to optimise multi-TI ASL scans of any chosen duration, and show that it can be used to optimise the ASL acquisition in the clinically-limited setting where information from ASL must be acquired in only a few minutes.

© Springer International Publishing AG 2016
S. Ourselin et al. (Eds.): MICCAI 2016, Part III, LNCS 9902, pp. 511–518, 2016.
DOI: 10.1007/978-3-319-46726-9_59

In ASL, blood is magnetically tagged at the neck, and then allowed to perfuse into the brain before acquiring an MR image. The inversion times (TIs) at which the MR images are acquired can make a significant difference to the quality of the perfusion and arterial transit time estimates in both pulsed and pseudo-continuous ASL [3]. Previous work has attempted to optimise the selection of TIs [4]. However, these have been optimised only for a fixed number of TIs, ignoring the impact of these TIs on the total scan duration.

Here, we examine the more realistic situation in which there is a fixed amount of scanner time available, and the task of experimental design is to select the best possible ASL measurements that can fit within this time. Such measurements are characterised by the set of TIs used, and here they are jointly optimised within a novel Bayesian experimental design framework. We show results from numerical simulations and experimental results from four healthy volunteers. We demonstrate that our framework improves parameter estimation in ASL, compared to a more conventional multi-TI experiment, and when optimised for a five-minute acquisition we obtain significant improvements in f estimation.

2   Methods

2.1   Arterial Spin Labelling

In ASL, blood is magnetically tagged before entering the brain. Images are acquired repeatedly, with and without this tagging, and the *difference images* between them are used to fit a kinetic model. When images are acquired at several different inversion times, this allows the simultaneous estimation of perfusion (the amount of blood perfusing through the tissue) and arterial transit time (the time taken for blood to reach a given voxel from the labelling plane) [3].

Throughout this work, the single-compartment kinetic model of Buxton *et al.* [3] is used to describe the pulsed ASL (PASL) signal:

$$\Delta M(t) = \begin{cases} 0, & 0 < t < \Delta t \\ 2M_{0b}f(t - \Delta t)e^{-t/T_{1b}}q_p(t) & \Delta t < t < \tau + \Delta t \\ 2M_{0b}f\tau e^{-t/T_1'}q_p(t) & \tau + \Delta t < t \end{cases}$$

$$q_p(t) = \begin{cases} \frac{e^{kt}(e^{-k\Delta t} - e^{-kt})}{k(t - \Delta t)} & \Delta t < t < \tau + \Delta t \\ \frac{e^{-k\Delta t} - e^{-k(\tau + \Delta t)}}{k\tau} & \tau + \Delta t < t \end{cases}$$

$$k = \frac{1}{T_{1b}} - \frac{1}{T_1'} \qquad \frac{1}{T_1'} = \frac{1}{T_1} + \frac{f}{\lambda} \tag{1}$$

where $\Delta M(t)$ is the demagnetisation response, equal to the difference image; t is the inversion time at which the signal is measured; T_1 and T_{1b} are decay constants for magnetisation of water, in tissue and blood respectively; f is perfusion magnitude; Δt is the transit delay from the labelling plane to the voxel of interest; τ is the bolus temporal length; and λ is the blood-tissue partition coefficient. All constants, where not stated, use the recommended values given in [2]. The methods herein are equally applicable to pseudo-continuous ASL (PCASL), the only difference being the use of a slightly different kinetic model [3].

2.2   Bayesian Design Theory

The guiding principle of Bayesian experimental design is to maximise the expected information gain from a set of experiments. Experiments consist of a set of measured data points, y_i, which are related to the parameters to be estimated, θ, and the design parameters, η, by a forward model, $y_i = g(\theta; \eta) + e$. In multi-TI ASL, $\theta = (f \ \Delta t)^T$, and $g(\theta)$ is the Buxton model of Sect. 2.1, with $g(\theta; \eta) = \Delta M(\eta; f, \Delta t)$. η here are the inversion times, t_i. Because the noise model is Gaussian, maximisation of the information gain for a given θ is approximately equivalent to maximisation of the Fisher information matrix [5]:

$$u(\theta, \eta) = det \sum_i \begin{pmatrix} \frac{\partial^2 g_i}{\partial \theta_1^2} & \frac{\partial^2 g_i}{\partial \theta_1 \theta_2} & \cdots \\ \frac{\partial^2 g_i}{\partial \theta_2 \theta_1} & \frac{\partial^2 g_i}{\partial \theta_2^2} & \cdots \\ \vdots & \vdots & \ddots \end{pmatrix} \tag{2}$$

It is unclear, however, what value of θ to use when evaluating this utility function. θ is not known *a priori* – it is θ that we seek to estimate. In a Bayesian approach, we should marginalise the utility function over our prior for θ [5]:

$$U(\eta) = \int_\theta \log u(\theta, \eta) \, p(\theta) d\theta = \int_f \int_{\Delta t} \log u(f, \Delta t) p(f) p(\Delta t) \, d\Delta t \, df \tag{3}$$

In the early Bayesian experimental design literature, to avoid the computationally demanding step of evaluating the *expected* Fisher information, the Fisher information was merely evaluated once at a representative point estimate of parameter values [5]. Subsequent work improved on this by sampling from the θ prior, and then optimising for each sample, making the assumption that the distribution of point-wise optimal designs reflects the optimal design for that prior [4]. This assumption is only approximately true, however, and cannot be used when there are constraints (in this work, scan duration) on η. Consequently, we use a numerical approach to approximate Eq. 3, allowing us to find the true solution and respect feasibility constraints on η.

2.3   Computationally Tractable Optimal Design Solutions

In order to evaluate the expected utility for a given design, an adaptive quadrature technique [6] is used to approximate Eq. 3. In this high-performance C++ implementation of the TOMS algorithm, the parameter space is iteratively divided into subregions, over which the integral is approximated. Subregions are refined preferentially when they have larger error, leading to highly accurate approximations of the overall integral. This estimate of the expected utility is then used as the utility function by which η is selected.

Throughout this work, $p(\theta)$ is assumed to be a normal distribution, with $f \sim N(100, 30) \, \text{ml}/100 \, \text{g/min}$ and $\Delta t \sim N(0.8, 0.3) \, \text{s}$. These distributions were chosen to be broadly representative of physiologically-plausible f and Δt across the whole population [2], ensuring the optimised design works over a wide range of values. If more information were known *a priori*, such as reference values for a specific clinical population [4] or pre-existing measurements from a given patient, then this could be used instead, and would further improve the design optimisation. In particular, the prior on f is set to be very broad, and includes values much higher than typical perfusion – this is to ensure the optimised design is capable of measuring hyperperfusion, hypoperfusion and normal perfusion.

Performing an exhaustive search for the optimal solution is impractical, as there are many inversion times in a typical scan duration – in this work, 28–32 such inversion times. In a naive exhaustive search, each inversion time is an additional dimension over which to search, and the curse of dimensionality means this search cannot be performed on a realistic timescale. Fortunately, there is a simplifying symmetry in the utility function: when η is restricted to the inversion times, $U(\eta)$ does not depend upon the order of elements in η. This follows from Eq. 2: overall utility is a function of the sum of individual utilities, making it commutative under reordering of inversion times. Thus, with no loss of generality, t can be constrained to be in increasing order. Such a constraint lends itself to solution by a coordinate exchange algorithm [4], in which each inversion time is optimised separately, bounded between its neighbouring inversion times. Although there is no theoretical guarantee of global optimality, the coordinate exchange results show good agreement with more time-consuming heuristic solutions such as controlled random search with local mutation [7,8].

2.4   Constrained Optimal Design

Much of the experimental design literature concerns experiments with a fixed number of measurements. In ASL, and medical imaging more generally, this often is not the case. Instead, there is a fixed amount of time available in which to acquire data. Different acquisition parameters will result in a given measurement taking more or less time, and this constraint changes the optimal solution. Hence, in addition to the constraint that TIs are ordered, we impose a duration constraint, for our experiments here requiring that the whole ASL acquisition last no longer than five minutes. To calculate the duration, we set an experimentally-determined "cool-down" period (0.5 s here) to wait after every TI, which allows the experiment to comply with MR Specific Absorption Rate limits. We also enforce that f and Δt must be positive – effectively truncating their Gaussian priors. The optimisation is performed in parallel over a range of TI list lengths, and the resulting design with the highest utility is selected.

2.5   Synthetic Data

Synthetic data were generated from the Buxton model with additive Gaussian noise, with the SNR representative of real ASL data at $\sigma \approx M_0/100$ [4]. Simulations, to assess performance across parameter space, were implemented by dividing the parameter space into a grid (f: 0 to 200 ml/100 g/min, Δt: 0 to 4.0 s) and simulating 1000 noisy ASL signals at each point, for optimised and reference designs. Least-squares fitting was subsequently used on each dataset to estimate parameters for both designs. Finally, to estimate performance, we used these estimated values and the priors of Sect. 2.2 to calculate the expected root mean square error (RMSE) and coefficient of variation (CoV).

2.6 Experimental Data

Experimental ASL data were acquired from four healthy subjects (ages 24–34, two male) using a 3T Siemens Trio scanner at resolution $3.75 \times 3.75 \times 4.5$ mm. PASL labelling was used, with Q2TIPS to fix the bolus length to 0.8 s. Here, a two-segment 3D-GRASE readout was used, although the optimal design approach would be applicable to any readout. No motion correction or smoothing were performed, and f and Δt were estimated using variational inference [9]. Scan duration was fixed at 5 min for both optimal and reference scans. Each of the optimised and reference scans was acquired twice, to allow for reproducibility comparisons. To minimise the effects of subject motion and small drifts in perfusion values, measurements were acquired in an interleaved fashion, alternating between optimised and reference TIs. MPRAGE T_1-weighted structural scans and inversion-recovery (1 s, 2 s, 5 s) calibration images were acquired in the same session, to allow for gray matter masking and absolute quantification of f.

3 Results

3.1 Proposed Design

The more conventional reference design used 28 TIs, equally spaced between 0.5 s and 3 s. The optimised design used 32 TIs, which tend to cluster between 1 s and 1.5 s. This makes intuitive sense, as the Buxton model predicts higher signal magnitudes near $t \approx \Delta t$. However, accounting for the effect of TI choice on scan duration, as done here, discourages longer, time-consuming TIs. This trade-off explains why the TIs are shorter than those in the reference scan. It also illustrates the value of this approach: the optimised scan not only chooses more informative TIs, but was able to fit in more TIs than the reference scan. To some extent, it is preferable to use many shorter TIs, rather than a smaller number of longer TIs, and this is reflected in the optimised design (Fig. 1).

3.2 Synthetic Results

Table 1 summarises the expected improvement from the optimised design, compared to the reference. This is expressed through the root mean square error

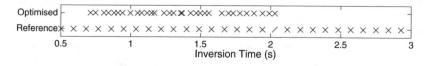

Fig. 1. Optimised design and reference design.

(RMSE) and the expected coefficient of variation (CoV), which are evaluated at each pair of parameter values based upon the 1000 estimates: $CoV_{f=f_0, \Delta t = \Delta t_0} = \frac{\sigma}{\mu}$. A better design produces less variable estimates of the parameters, hence $\Delta CoV = CoV^{Ref} - CoV^{Opt}$ and $\Delta RMSE = RMSE^{Ref} - RMSE^{Opt}$ should be positive where the optimised design outperforms the reference. P values are calculated using nonparametric Kruskal-Wallis tests for the equivalence of distributions: values below the significance threshold indicate significant differences between the distributions of optimised and reference values.

As expected, the performance is best near the prior's mean, and falls as it is evaluated over the whole parameter space. Over the entire parameter space, these results suggest there should be a large improvement in f estimation, and a slight worsening of Δt estimation. The design optimisation is a trade-off between the two parameters, to some extent: if Δt were the main parameter of interest, the problem could be recast to improve Δt estimation, at a cost to f estimation.

Table 1. Synthetic results, evaluated within 1 and 2 prior deviations and the whole space. Positive CoV/RMSE indicate better performance in the new design

	f			Δt		
	ΔCoV (%)	ΔRMSE (%)	P	ΔCoV (%)	ΔRMSE (%)	P
1SD	24.9	20.2	$< 1 \times 10^{-3}$	7.7	12.0	0.059
2SD	18.5	18.8	$< 1 \times 10^{-3}$	−3.7	−1.4	0.007
Whole space	13.7	11.7	$< 1 \times 10^{-3}$	−6.2	−2.1	$< 1 \times 10^{-3}$

3.3   Experimental Results

Per-slice test-retest correlation coefficients are shown for f and Δt, in all subjects, in Fig. 2. P values are calculated using nonparametric Kruskal-Wallis tests, with the approximation that per-slice coefficients are independent. For f, these results show good agreement with the simulations: test-retest correlation coefficients are reliably higher for f in the optimised experiment. For Δt, there is no clear trend, and KW tests do not suggest significant differences in the correlations. Although simulations suggest that Δt estimation is slightly worse in the optimised experiment, the difference is small, and it is unsurprising that it cannot be seen in the experiments. Moreover, simulations do not account for the increase in robustness against outliers, for example due to motion or hardware instability. The optimised acquisition has more TIs, so it is more robust against outliers, and might be expected to perform even better than simulations suggest.

Example parameter estimates are shown in Fig. 3. The optimised f image is smoother than the reference image, suggesting greater consistency in estimated results. This interpretation is supported by the higher test-retest coefficient. There is no appreciable difference in the smoothness of the Δt images, which similarly agrees with simulation-based predictions and test-retest statistics.

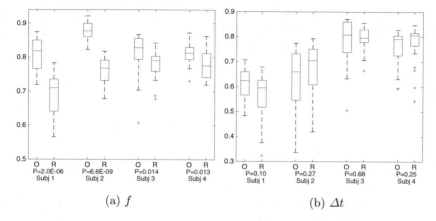

(a) f (b) Δt

Fig. 2. Distribution of per-slice test-retest correlation coefficients, in all subjects, for optimised (O) and reference (R) acquisitions.

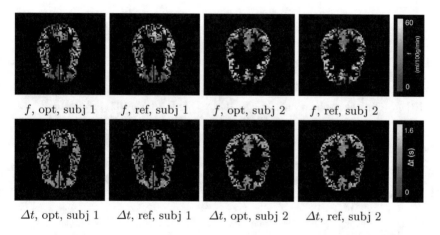

f, opt, subj 1 f, ref, subj 1 f, opt, subj 2 f, ref, subj 2

Δt, opt, subj 1 Δt, ref, subj 1 Δt, opt, subj 2 Δt, ref, subj 2

Fig. 3. Parameter maps for subjects 1 and 2, optimised and reference designs.

4   Discussion

The optimal design approach in this work has demonstrated effectiveness in significantly improving ASL estimation of perfusion, with little effect on Δt estimation. The optimisation, for this five-minute ASL experiment, leads to a coefficient of variation reduction of approximately 10 %, with corresponding improvement in test-retest correlation coefficients. There is good agreement between simulations and experimental results, which demonstrates the validity of this model-based optimisation approach. Moreover, optimisation with a constrained scan duration allows for additional TIs to be used in the acquisition, which can improve robustness of the experiment. Reducing the time needed for ASL experiments (or, equivalently, obtaining better perfusion estimates from experiments of the same duration) may increase uptake of ASL in research studies and in clinical trials. The long duration of the scan is often given as a major weakness of ASL [2], and this work directly improves on this.

Future work will jointly optimise inversion times and label durations, allowing even more efficient use of scanner time. Moreover, there is the prospect of using population-specific or subject-specific priors, adapting the acquisition for maximum experimental efficiency. This general optimisation framework is applicable to other imaging modalities, and we will also examine how it affects other time-constrained MR acquisitions, such as relaxometry or diffusion imaging.

Acknowledgments. We would like to acknowledge the MRC (MR/J01107X/1), the National Institute for Health Research (NIHR), the EPSRC (EP/H046410/1) and the National Institute for Health Research University College London Hospitals Biomedical Research Centre (NIHR BRC UCLH/UCL High Impact Initiative BW.mn.BRC10269). This work is supported by the EPSRC-funded UCL Centre for Doctoral Training in Medical Imaging (EP/L016478/1) and the Wolfson Foundation.

References

1. Detre, J., Wang, J., Wang, Z., Rao, H.: Arterial spin-labeled perfusion MRI in basic and clinical neuroscience. Curr. Opin. Neurol. **22**(4), 348–355 (2009)
2. Alsop, D., et al.: Recommended implementation of arterial spin-labeled perfusion MRI for clinical applications. Magn. Reson. Med. **73**(1), 102–116 (2015)
3. Buxton, R., Frank, L., Wong, E., Siewert, B., Warach, S., Edelman, R.: A general kinetic model for quantitative perfusion imaging with arterial spin labeling. Magn. Reson. Med. **40**(3), 383–396 (1998)
4. Xie, J., Gallichan, D., Gunn, R., Jezzard, P.: Optimal design of pulsed arterial spin labeling MRI experiments. Magn. Reson. Med. **59**(4), 826–834 (2008)
5. Chaloner, K., Verdinelli, I.: Bayesian experimental design: a review. Stat. Sci. **10**, 273–304 (1995)
6. Hahn, T.: Cuba - a library for multidimensional numerical integration. Comput. Phys. Commun. **168**(2), 78–95 (2005)
7. Johnson, S.: The NLopt nonlinear-optimization package (2014). http://ab-initio.mit.edu/nlopt
8. Kaelo, P., Ali, M.: Some variants of the controlled random search algorithm for global optimization. J. Optim. Theory Appl. **130**(2), 253–264 (2006)
9. Chappell, M., Groves, A., Whitcher, B., Woolrich, M.: Variational Bayesian inference for a nonlinear forward model. IEEE Trans. Signal Process. **57**(1), 223–236 (2009)

4D Phase-Contrast Magnetic Resonance CardioAngiography (4D PC-MRCA) Creation from 4D Flow MRI

Mariana Bustamante[1,2]([✉]), Vikas Gupta[1,2], Carl-Johan Carlhäll[1,2,3], and Tino Ebbers[1,2]

[1] Division of Cardiovascular Medicine, Department of Medical and Health Sciences, Linköping University, Linköping, Sweden
mariana.bustamante@liu.se
[2] Center for Medical Image Science and Visualization (CMIV), Linköping University, Linköping, Sweden
[3] Department of Clinical Physiology, Department of Medical and Health Sciences, Linköping University, Linköping, Sweden

Abstract. MR angiography (MRA) and phase-contrast MRA (PC-MRA) generation methods that facilitate blood flow assessment in the heart and thoracic vessels typically lead to the compression of data from all the timeframes of a cardiac cycle into one 2D or 3D image. This process, however, results in information loss from individual timeframes. We propose a new method for PC-MRA data generation from 4D flow MRI, which uses registration between the timeframes of the 4D acquisition to create a "four-dimensional PC-MR CardioAngiography (4D PC-MRCA)" that retains vascular and cardiac blood flow information over the entire cardiac cycle.

When evaluated on 10 4D flow MRI datasets, 4D PC-MRCA outperformed 3D PC-MRA, especially when cardiac or vessel motion was present. Consequently, the proposed method improves the existing PC-MRA generation techniques by effectively utilizing spatial as well as temporal blood flow information on both the heart and thoracic vasculature from 4D flow MR images.

1 Introduction

Three-dimensional (3D), time-resolved Phase-Contrast Magnetic Resonance Imaging with three-directional velocity encoding (4D flow MRI) is an MRI technique commonly used to evaluate blood flow in the heart and great thoracic vessels over the cardiac cycle [1]. For visualization and analysis, anatomical data is often generated from the 4D flow MRI acquisition, which has large similarities to the data obtained using phase-contrast Magnetic Resonance Angiography (PC-MRA) acquisitions.

Vascular assessment for the detection of pathologies such as stenoses, aneurysms, or anomalies is typically performed using conventional MRA, which

© Springer International Publishing AG 2016
S. Ourselin et al. (Eds.): MICCAI 2016, Part III, LNCS 9902, pp. 519–526, 2016.
DOI: 10.1007/978-3-319-46726-9_60

relies on an external agent for contrast enhancement. In PC-MRA, however, contrast is obtained using phase differences in the MR signal, where high intensities correspond to high velocities. PC-MRA data are typically acquired without cardiac gating in a breath hold. Therefore, the resulting image represents an average view of the cardiovascular system over the cardiac cycle. The heart and large arteries change location and expand during the cycle, but the resulting changes are averaged, and moving structures are consequently difficult to perceive.

In 4D flow MRI, data is acquired using cardiac electrocardiography (ECG) gating. Consequently, the resulting images contain information about the specific motion of the heart and vessels during the cardiac cycle.

Generation of 3D PC-MRA data from 4D flow MRI is typically accomplished by combining the blood flow velocity information and the magnitude data. The velocity information provides higher intensities to the resulting image in areas of high blood flow velocity, while the magnitude signal adds morphological information to the images and mitigates noise in areas of very low signal (e.g., lungs) [2,3].

The 3D PC-MRA data can be used to visualize the lumen using MIP visualization, volume rendering, or shaded surface rendering. Moreover, this data can also be used during post-processing to segment the blood lumen, necessary for further analyses (e.g. wall shear stress estimation [4]). It will also have the same advantages and disadvantages as a standard PC-MRA, such as smoothing of moving structures. This hampers visualization of the heart chambers, as well as the computation of parameters in the large arteries that rely on segmentation, such as wall shear stress. The distension and recoil of the aorta over the cardiac cycle results in some movement of the wall, which is not accounted for in the wall shear stress estimation, as the wall is obtained from a time-averaged PC-MRA [5].

The goal of this study is to present a new technique for the creation of PC-MRA data that utilizes the full potential of 4D flow MRI, facilitating better depiction of moving structures, and allowing for the creation of a temporally resolved Phase-Contrast Magnetic Resonance CardioAngiography (4D PC-MRCA) that includes the geometry of the lumen of the vessels, as well as the heart over the cardiac cycle.

2 Materials and Methods

2.1 Creation of a 3D Phase-Contrast Magnetic Resonance Angiography (3D PC-MRA)

3D PC-MRA data was created for this study using a variation of the method presented in [6], as follows:

1. The velocity and magnitude data of the 4D flow MRI were combined for each timeframe t, as shown in (1). In this equation, V_x, V_y and V_z are the averages of the blood flow velocity components in three spatial directions, and M is the magnitude of the signals acquired during the 4D flow MRI acquisition.

$$\text{3D PC-MRA}(t) = M(t) * \sqrt{V_x^2(t) + V_y^2(t) + V_z^2(t)} \tag{1}$$

The resulting four-dimensional image contains information about the locations of high blood flow at each timeframe.

2. 3D PC-MRA data was created by calculating a Maximum Intensity Projection (MIP) of the data over the cardiac cycle, in order to include spatial as well as temporal blood flow information into one image, as shown in Fig. 1.

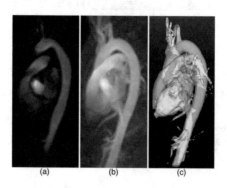

Fig. 1. 3D PC-MRA data created from a 4D flow MRI dataset. (a) 2D coronal slice of the volume. (b) Maximum intensity projection. (c) 3D shaded surface display.

2.2 Creation of a 4D Phase-Contrast Magnetic Resonance CardioAngiography (4D PC-MRCA)

Steps for 4D PC-MRCA generation were as follows:

1. PC-MRA data was generated using the 4D flow MRI dataset as described in Sect. 2.1. In this case, however, the final MIP step is skipped in order to still retain the information specific to each timeframe of the cardiac cycle. Additionally, gamma correction of 0.4 was used on the speed calculation.
2. All the timeframes of the MRI magnitude image were registered to one specific timeframe in diastasis (mid-diastole), when the heart is at an "intermediate" position between early and late ventricular diastole. This resulted in N transformations, B_i, each corresponding to one timeframe, i (Fig. 2).
3. Each timeframe, i, of the previously created PC-MRA was transformed using the corresponding transformation, B_i, to produce a set of images with intensities that depend on the blood flow patterns at each timeframe, but with the shape and morphology expected in the chosen diastasis timeframe.
4. A 3D PC-MRCA was calculated as an MIP of these images over time. This image contains high contrast in all sections of the cardiovascular system where high blood flow takes place at least once during the heartbeat, and morphologically corresponds to one specific timeframe of the cardiac cycle.
5. A new set of registrations were executed where the magnitude image of the chosen diastasis timeframe was registered to all the other available timeframes. The result was N transformations, F_i, one for each timeframe, i, that were then applied to the 3D PC-MRCA in order to obtain a time-resolved 4D PC-MRCA.

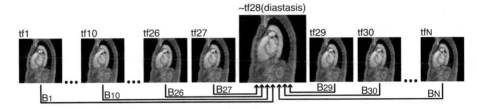

Fig. 2. Registration of every timeframe of the average magnitude image to a timeframe in diastasis, resulting in N transformations, B_i.

The non-rigid registration method used during this study was based on the Morphon algorithm [7], together with diffeomorphic field accumulation and both fluid and elastic regularization of the displacement fields [8]. The 4D PC-MRCA tool was implemented using MATLAB, Release 2015b (The MathWorks, Inc., Natick, Massachusetts, United States).

2.3   Experimental Setup

Evaluation of the proposed method was performed on 10 4D flow MRI datasets acquired from healthy volunteers with no prior history of cardiovascular disease. 4D flow MRI examinations were performed on a clinical 3T Philips Ingenia scanner (Philips Healthcare, Best, the Netherlands) and were acquired during free-breathing, using a navigator gated gradient-echo pulse sequence with interleaved three-directional flow-encoding and retrospective vector cardiogram controlled cardiac gating. All subjects were injected with a Gd contrast agent (Magnevist, Bayer Schering Pharma AG) prior to the acquisition for a late-enhancement study. Scan parameters included: Candy cane view adjusted to cover both ventricles, velocity encoding (VENC) 120 cm/s, flip angle 10°, echo time 2.6 ms, repetition time 4.4 ms, parallel imaging (SENSE) speed up factor 3 (AP direction), k-space segmentation factor 3, acquired temporal resolution of 52.8 ms, spatial resolution $2.7 \times 2.7 \times 2.8$ mm^3, elliptical k-space acquisition. The typical scan time was 7–8 min excluding and 10–15 min including the navigator efficiency.

The 4D flow MRI data were corrected for concomitant gradient fields on the scanner. Offline processing corrected for phase wraps using a temporal phase unwrapping method [9], and background phase errors were corrected using a weighted 2nd order polynomial fit to the static tissue [10].

The generation of one 4D PC-MRCA took on average twenty minutes without any user interaction on a computer with 64 GB RAM and a 6-core 3.5 GHz processor. The current implementation included parallel execution of multiple registrations. Further improvements to the running time can be achieved by using GPU programming.

4D PC-MRCA and 3D PC-MRA data were generated for each dataset and shaded surface visualizations of each method were used to assess the resulting images.

The main regions of the cardiovascular system visible in the angiographies were evaluated and scored independently based on visual agreement with the magnitude signal of the 4D flow MRI at two representative timeframes during the heart cycle (mid-systole and end-diastole). A value was given as the agreement score based on the following scale: 1 = unacceptable size, unacceptable position; 2 = unacceptable position, acceptable size; 3 = unacceptable size, acceptable position; 4 = acceptable size, acceptable position.

3   Results

Figure 3 shows different visualization methods applied to a 4D PC-MRCA. 3D PC-MRAs and 4D PC-MRCAs for two datasets are shown in Fig. 4, only three different timeframes of the 4D image are shown due to space constraints.

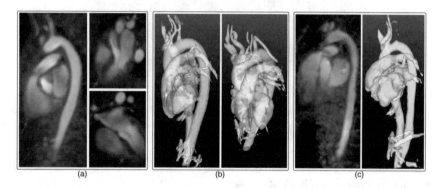

Fig. 3. 4D PC-MRCA visualization. (a) Coronal (left), three-chambers (top right), and four-chambers (bottom right) slices at mid-diastole. Arrows point to areas of slow blood flow where visibility was improved. (b) Isosurfaces from two points of view at end-diastole. (c) 4D PC-MRCA of a 4D flow MRI acquired without contrast agent.

Resulting scores for the visual comparison of 3D PC-MRA versus 4D PC-MRCA at two different timeframes can be seen in Table 1. Note that the 3D PC-MRA data is not time-resolved; consequently, the same surface was used for the two timeframes evaluated.

4   Discussion and Conclusion

The proposed method provides the ability to analyze the whole cardiovascular system from several viewpoints, together with the possibility of observing the motion of the heart and vessels during the entire cardiac cycle. This constitutes an improvement over 3D PC-MRA generation techniques and presents an advantage in the clinical setting, particularly when the type of problem being assessed is influenced by cardiac motion.

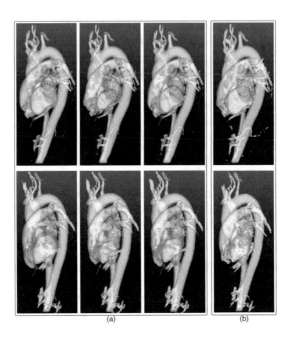

Fig. 4. Isosurfaces generated for two 4D flow MRI datasets (top and bottom). (a) 4D PC-MRCAs at three timeframes of the cardiac cycle (end-diastole, systole, mid-diastole). The arrows point to the left ventricles, where cardiac motion is visible. (b) 3D PC-MRAs.

Table 1. Number of datasets that received the indicated score during visual evaluation of the PC-MRA and PC-MRCA at two timeframes: mid-systole and end-diastole. Scale: 1 = unacceptable size, unacceptable position; 2 = unacceptable position, acceptable size; 3 = unacceptable size, acceptable position; 4 = acceptable size, acceptable position

Region	3D PC-MRA (mid-systole)				4D PC-MRCA (mid-systole)			
	Score:1	Score:2	Score:3	Score:4	Score:1	Score:2	Score:3	Score:4
Aorta	0	0	3	7	0	0	0	10
Pulmonary arteries	0	0	2	8	0	0	0	10
Pulmonary veins	0	0	0	10	0	0	0	10
Caval veins	0	1	1	8	0	1	3	6
Left ventricle and atrium	1	2	7	0	0	0	4	6
Right ventricle and atrium	0	0	8	2	0	0	6	4
Carotid arteries	0	0	0	10	0	0	0	10
Region	3D PC-MRA (end-diastole)				4D PC-MRCA (end-diastole)			
	Score:1	Score:2	Score:3	Score:4	Score:1	Score:2	Score:3	Score:4
Aorta	9	1	0	0	0	0	1	9
Pulmonary artery	5	0	4	1	0	0	0	10
Pulmonary veins	0	0	9	1	0	0	5	5
Caval veins	1	4	1	4	2	4	1	3
Left ventricle and atrium	0	0	5	5	0	0	4	6
Right ventricle and atrium	1	1	6	2	0	0	6	4
Carotid arteries	0	9	0	1	0	1	2	7

It is important to note that the goal of the proposed method is not to substitute the existing contrast enhanced angiography and phase-contrast angiography generation techniques used commonly in the clinical setting. Instead, it aims to improve the way that geometrical data is generated specifically from 4D flow MRI by adequately using all the information available in this type of acquisition.

Although the time required to generate a 4D PC-MRCA is longer than that of creating a 3D PC-MRA from a 4D flow MRI dataset, the method is completely automatic. As a result, it can be easily added to the existing post-processing framework for 4D flow MRI acquisitions that includes algorithms such as background correction and phase unwrapping.

The first registration series could also be applied to each timeframe in order to create a timeframe-specific PC-MRCA for all possible configurations of the heart and vessels during the cardiac cycle. This could produce a slightly more robust version of the MRCA, but it will require a much larger number of registrations, and consequently longer computation times.

In visual evaluation, 4D PC-MRCA outperformed 3D PC-MRA mainly for the heart and vessels at end-diastole. This was due to the fact that vessel motion is not accounted for when using 3D PC-MRA. Disagreements were especially visible in the 3D PC-MRA in the ascending aorta, pulmonary arteries, and carotid arteries at this timeframe. Although the motion of the myocardium is not thoroughly followed by the 4D PC-MRCA, it better represented the position and size of the ventricles and atria, particularly in systole, since the cardiac motion is included in the angiography. The pulmonary veins seem to be considerably stable during the course of the cardiac cycle, which generated mostly stable scores for the methods at both timeframes. The caval veins are usually located very close to the borders of the 4D flow MRI image, and are consequently prone to be affected by registration issues. Because of this, they were scored lower than the rest of the evaluated regions for the 4D PC-MRCA.

The acquisition protocol of the 4D flow MRI images in this study included the injection of an extracellular contrast agent, which was injected for viability studies. Traces of the contrast agent were present during the 4D flow MRI acquisitions, which improved the contrast between the blood and the remaining tissues. The presented method was not tested in depth on images without any contrast agent. However, since a significant part of the contrast on the final image comes from the phase signal, a 4D PC-MRCA with acceptable levels of contrast would still be expected as a result.

A recent study showed promising results using atlas-based segmentation on 4D flow MRI to automatically segment and analyze the flow on the major vessels surrounding the heart [11]. The proposed method, together with atlas-based segmentation, could be used to automatically segment more challenging regions of the cardiovascular system such as the cardiac ventricles and atria using 4D flow MRI. The resulting four-dimensional segmentation could be used not only to visualize the entire cardiovascular system, but also to analyze the flow of blood in the different vessels and chambers of the heart.

In conclusion, the proposed technique generates a four-dimensional phase-contrast Magnetic Resonance CardioAngiography that includes the heart and thoracic vasculature using a 4D flow MRI acquisition as input. This represents a considerable improvement for visualization and analysis of 4D flow MRI data.

References

1. Markl, M., Kilner, P., Ebbers, T.: Comprehensive 4D velocity mapping of the heart and great vessels by cardiovascular magnetic resonance. J Cardiovasc. Magn. Reson. **13**, 7 (2011)
2. Bock, J., Frydrychowicz, A., Stalder, A.F., Bley, T.A., Burkhardt, H., Hennig, J., Markl, M.: 4D phase contrast MRI at 3 T: effect of standard and blood-pool contrast agents on SNR, PC-MRA, and blood flow visualization. Magn. Reson. Med. **63**, 330–338 (2010)
3. Markl, M., Harloff, A., Bley, T., Zaitsev, M., Jung, B., Weigang, E., Langer, M., Hennig, J., Frydrychowicz, A.: Time-resolved 3D MR velocity mapping at 3T: improved navigator-gated assessment of vascular anatomy and blood flow. J. Magn. Reson. Imaging **25**, 824–831 (2007)
4. Harloff, A., Nubaumer, A., Bauer, S., Stalder, A., Frydrychowicz, A., Weiller, C., Hennig, J., Markl, M.: In vivo assessment of wall shear stress in the atherosclerotic aorta using flow-sensitive 4D MRI. Magn. Reson. Med. **63**, 1529–1536 (2010)
5. Petersson, S., Dyverfeldt, P., Ebbers, T.: Assessment of the accuracy of MRI wall shear stress estimation using numerical simulations. J. Magn. Reson. Imaging **36**, 128–138 (2012)
6. Bock, J., Wieben, O., Johnson, K.M., Hennig, J., Markl, M.: Optimal processing to derive static PC-MRA from time-resolved 3D PC-MRI data. Proc. Intl. Soc. Mag. Reson. Med. **16**, 3053 (2008)
7. Knutsson, H., Andersson, M.: Morphons: segmentation using elastic canvas and paint on priors. ICIP II-1226-9 (2005)
8. Forsberg, D., Andersson, M., Knutsson, H.: Non-rigid diffeomorphic image registration of medical images using polynomial expansion. In: Campilho, A., Kamel, M. (eds.) ICIAR 2012, Part II. LNCS, vol. 7325, pp. 304–312. Springer, Heidelberg (2012)
9. Xiang, Q.S.: Temporal phase unwrapping for CINE velocity imaging. J Magn. Reson. Imaging **5**, 529–534 (1995)
10. Ebbers, T., Haraldsson, H., Dyverfeldt, P., Sigfridsson, A., Warntjes, M., Wigström, L.: Higher order weighted least-squares phase offset correction for improved accuracy in phase-contrast MRI. Proc. Intl. Soc. Mag. Reson. Med. **16**, 1367 (2008)
11. Bustamante, M., Petersson, S., Eriksson, J., Alehagen, U., Dyverfeldt, P., Carlhäll, C.-J., Ebbers, T.: Atlas-based analysis of 4D flow CMR: automated vessel segmentation and flow quantification. J Cardiovasc. Magn. Reson. **17**, 1–12 (2015)

Joint Estimation of Cardiac Motion and T_1^* Maps for Magnetic Resonance Late Gadolinium Enhancement Imaging

Jens Wetzl[1,2]([✉]), Aurélien F. Stalder[3], Michaela Schmidt[3], Yigit H. Akgök[1],
Christoph Tillmanns[4], Felix Lugauer[1], Christoph Forman[3],
Joachim Hornegger[1,2], and Andreas Maier[1,2]

[1] Pattern Recognition Lab, FAU Erlangen-Nürnberg, Erlangen, Germany
jens.wetzl@fau.de
[2] Graduate School in Advanced Optical Technologies (SAOT), Erlangen, Germany
[3] Siemens Healthcare GmbH, Diagnostic Imaging, MR, Erlangen, Germany
[4] Diagnostikum Berlin, Berlin, Germany

Abstract. In the diagnosis of myocardial infarction, magnetic resonance imaging can provide information about myocardial contractility and tissue characterization, including viability. In current clinical practice, separate scans are required for each aspect. A recently proposed method showed how the same information can be extracted from a single, short scan of 4 s, but made strong assumptions about the underlying cardiac motion. We propose a fixed-point iteration scheme that retains the benefits of their approach while lifting its limitations, making it robust to cardiac arrhythmia. We compare our method to the state of the art using phantom data as well as data from 11 patients and show a consistent improvement of all evaluation criteria, e.g. the end-diastolic Dice coefficient of an arrythmic case improves from 86 % (state-of-the-art method) to 94 % (proposed method).

1 Introduction

Magnetic resonance imaging (MRI) can be used for the comprehensive diagnosis of myocardial infarction. Three important aspects are: Time-resolved cardiac imaging (*CINE imaging*) allows contractility assessment of the myocardium [2]. Myocardial viability can be assessed with *late gadolinium enhancement (LGE) imaging*, which visualizes scar tissue [6]. T_1 *mapping* can be used for the diagnosis of diffuse myocardial fibrosis [1,11]. In current clinical practice, separate scans are performed for each aspect. For the case of LGE imaging, an additional pre-scan is required for the a-priori selection of a parameter called *inversion time (TI)*, which ensures that the LGE scan suppresses signal from healthy myocardium while highlighting scar tissue (see Fig. 1).

A recent method [10] allows the acquisition of a series of images from which all of the above information can be extracted from a single measurement. After an inversion pulse, 4 s or ~4 cardiac cycles of real-time images are

© Springer International Publishing AG 2016
S. Ourselin et al. (Eds.): MICCAI 2016, Part III, LNCS 9902, pp. 527–535, 2016.
DOI: 10.1007/978-3-319-46726-9_61

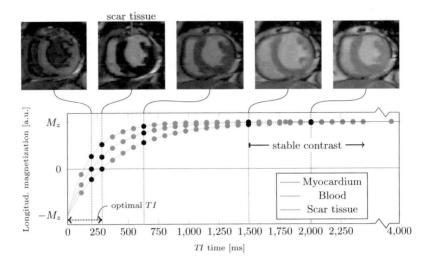

Fig. 1. Example images from the acquired series and corresponding points on the T_1 recovery curve of different tissues. After inversion, longitudinal magnetization starts at the negative maximum value, $-M_z$, and then recovers back to M_z. Most notably, the 2nd image from the left shows the optimal TI time for scar visualization, because the myocardium is black and the scar tissue is hyperintense compared to the blood.

acquired. This leads to an image series where both the image contrast and cardiac motion state change over time (see Fig. 1). The contrast change is related to the tissue-dependent time constant for longitudinal magnetization recovery, T_1, and the time between inversion and acquisition of each image, TI. Simultaneously acquired ECG data allows the segmentation of the series into cardiac cycles. Detsky *et al.* [2] also measure viability and contractility in one scan, but use a longer, segmented acquisition, and don't jointly estimate both parameters.

Related to the three aspects mentioned above, CINE imaging is provided by the last cardiac cycle in the series, where the image contrast has already stabilized. An image with optimal TI for scar visualization can be selected retrospectively in the first cardiac cycle. For T_1^* mapping, the approach in [10] is to estimate cardiac motion by image registration of the last cardiac cycle. Under the assumption that motion is identical in the first and last cardiac cycles, this estimate is then used to transform the first cardiac cycle into a consistent motion state to perform pixel-wise least-squares regression of measured values to a signal model [8]. Additionally, a joint scar tissue and contractility visualization is generated by animating the image with optimal TI contrast with the motion estimate to show how wall motion abnormalities relate to scar tissue. The limitations of this method are the assumption of identical motion in the first and last cardiac cycles, and the use of just the first cardiac cycle for T_1^* mapping.

We propose an iterative approach to jointly estimate cardiac motion for all cardiac cycles and utilize all available data for T_1^* mapping, retaining the advantages of a-posteriori TI selection and combined contractility and scar visualization, while removing the limitations of the previous approach and improving robustness. We tested our method with phantom data and 11 patient data sets.

2   Materials and Methods

If the motion between cardiac phases is known, i.e. we have deformation fields $d_{i \to j}(x)$ such that an image $m_i(x)$ in one cardiac phase $i \in [0, M[$, where M is the total number of images, can be transformed as $m_i(x + d_{i \to j}(x))$ to match the cardiac phase j in image $m_j(x)$, then pixel-wise T_1^* mapping is possible using images transformed to a common reference phase. Conversely, given a T_1^* mapping of an image series, cardiac motion can be estimated using intensity-based registration, similar to the use in [12] for imperfect breath-hold correction.

We propose a fixed-point iteration scheme which alternately improves T_1^* mapping results and motion estimates:

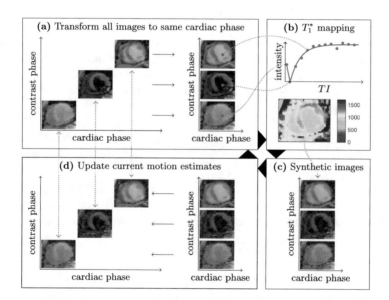

Fig. 2. Overview of the iterative estimation: The measured image series is transformed to a common cardiac phase using the current motion estimate (a), followed by pixelwise T_1^* mapping (b). From the T_1^* map, synthetic images at the same TI times as the measured images are generated (c), which are then transformed to the different cardiac phases, followed by pair-wise registration of the measured image series and current synthetic image series to update the current motion estimate (d).

1. Compute initial motion estimate from last cardiac cycle (see Sect. 2.1)
2. Iteratively update T_1^* map and motion parameter estimates (see Fig. 2)
    (a) Transform the originally acquired image series to a single cardiac phase using the current motion estimate

(b) Compute pixel-wise T_1^* parameter estimates (see Sect. 2.2)
(c) Using the resulting parameters, compute synthetic images corresponding to the inversion times of the acquired image sequence
(d) Update the motion estimate by performing image registration between the original and synthetic images (see Sect. 2.3)
3. Compute the true T_1 map from the final T_1^* map (see Sect. 2.2)

2.1   Initial Motion Estimation

The first motion estimate is computed with intensity-based registration of the last cardiac cycle of the acquisition. The first frame of the last cycle $m_f(\boldsymbol{x})$ is selected as the reference frame, so we obtain deformation fields $\boldsymbol{d}_{i \to f}(\boldsymbol{x})$ for $i \in [f, M[$. Non-rigid registration based on the `elastix` toolbox [5] with these components is used: the transform model is uniform cubic B-splines with a 16 mm isotropic control point spacing, the similarity metric is cross-correlation, optimized with the L-BFGS algorithm on a 3-level multi-resolution pyramid.

Deformation fields for the other cardiac cycles are then determined by linear interpolation of those from the last cardiac cycle, as we no longer assume that cardiac cycles are of the same length. For the initial motion estimation, we assume that there is no motion between the first images of each cardiac cycle. Thus, a deformation field $\boldsymbol{d}_{i \to f_i}(\boldsymbol{x})$, where f_i is the first frame of the cardiac cycle containing image i, can also be used as a deformation field $\boldsymbol{d}_{i \to 0}(\boldsymbol{x})$ to transform image i to the cardiac state of the very first frame. This allows us to transform all images $i \in [0, M[$ into a reference cardiac phase for T_1^* mapping.

2.2 T_1^* Mapping and T_1 Correction

For T_1^* mapping, the current motion estimate $\boldsymbol{d}_{i \to 0}(\boldsymbol{x})$ ($i \in [0, M[$) is used to transform all images $m_i(\boldsymbol{x})$ to the cardiac phase of the first image:

$$m_i'(\boldsymbol{x}) = m_i(\boldsymbol{x} + \boldsymbol{d}_{i \to 0}(\boldsymbol{x})). \tag{1}$$

The $m_i'(\boldsymbol{x})$ now only differ in their contrast, which is dependent on TI_i, the inversion time of image i, as well as tissue-dependent parameters $a(\boldsymbol{x})$, $b(\boldsymbol{x})$ and $T_1^*(\boldsymbol{x})$, which can be determined by a pixel-wise non-linear least-squares fit [8]:

$$\min_{a(\boldsymbol{x}),\ b(\boldsymbol{x}),\ T_1^*(\boldsymbol{x})} \sum_{i=0}^{M-1} (m_i'(\boldsymbol{x}) - |a(\boldsymbol{x}) + b(\boldsymbol{x}) \cdot \exp(-\tfrac{TI_i}{T_1^*(\boldsymbol{x})})|)^2. \tag{2}$$

Unlike [10], all cardiac cycles are considered for the fit, not just the first one, to increase robustness. The residual error of this fit is due to noisy measurements and errors due to misalignment, which can be reduced by improving motion estimates in each iteration. As the MRI measurement influences the longitudinal magnetization recovery, this does not yield the true T_1 value, but an "apparent" T_1 called T_1^*. A correction from T_1^* to T_1 maps can then be computed [7,8].

2.3 Motion Estimate Updating

The current set of parameters $a(x)$, $b(x)$ and $T_1^*(x)$ can be used to generate a synthetic image series $s_i'(x)$ in the reference cardiac phase as

$$s_i'(x) = |a(x) + b(x) \cdot \exp(-\tfrac{TI_i}{T_1^*(x)})| \tag{3}$$

and transformed to the cardiac phase it was acquired in:

$$s_i(x) = s_i'(x + d_{i\to 0}^{-1}(x)). \tag{4}$$

Pairwise registration between originally measured images $m_i(x)$ and corresponding synthetic images $s_i(x)$ then yields the error $e_{m_i\to s_i}(x)$ of the current motion estimate $d_{i\to 0}(x)$, so the motion estimate is updated by concatenation:

$$d_{i\to 0}^{(\text{new})} = d_{i\to 0}^{(\text{old})} \circ e_{m_i\to s_i}. \tag{5}$$

As this step considers each cardiac cycle individually, errors of the initial motion estimate will be corrected at this stage.

2.4 Experiments

Phantom data. A cardiac T_1 map, acquired from a patient with a dedicated T_1 mapping protocol, was used to generate different phantom data sets for the same *TI* times a real acquisition would use. This allowed to evaluate the algorithm against ground truth motion and T_1 values. Phantom deformation fields mimicking 3 cardiac cycles were generated to simulate contraction of the heart. The resulting magnitude images were distorted with Rician noise [4], the appropriate distribution for magnitude MRI images. The noise parameter was chosen as 5 % of the maximum magnitude. Figure 3 shows examples of the phantom image series.

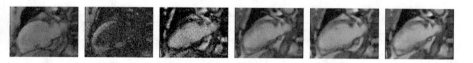

Fig. 3. Phantom images for different *TI* times and cardiac states.

Different datasets for the following 3 scenarios were simulated, with the last two simulating arrhythmia: (i) Same cardiac motion in all cardiac cycles, the ideal case assumed in method [10], (ii) Deviation of the magnitude of cardiac motion, (iii) Deviation of the position of end-systole within the cardiac cycle. For the quantitative evaluation of the T_1 mapping step, the root-mean-squared error (RMSE) of estimated T_1 maps to ground truth and the residual of the least-squares parameter estimation were computed. To evaluate the quality of the motion estimate, the blood pool of the heart was manually segmented in one cardiac phase. The resulting mask was transformed to all other cardiac phases using the ground truth deformation fields as well as the estimated deformation field. Finally, they were compared using Dice [3] and Hausdorff [9] coefficients.

Patient data. Data acquisition as described in [10] was performed in 11 patients (age 63±10, 4 female) with known or suspected status post myocardial infarction on a 3 T clinical scanner (MAGNETOM Skyra, Siemens Healthcare, Erlangen, Germany). Prototype sequence parameters include: 4 s breath-hold acquisition, 192×150 matrix size, $(1.9\,\text{mm})^2$ in-plane, 8 mm slice, 33 ms temporal resolution.

For T_1 mapping evaluation, the residual was computed. To evaluate the motion estimates, the blood pool of the heart was manually segmented for each end-diastolic (ED) and end-systolic (ES) frame. The last ED frame is also the reference frame for registration. The resulting mask for the reference frame was transformed to all other segmented frames using the motion estimates, and compared to the manual segmentations using the Dice and Hausdorff coefficients.

3   Results and Discussion

Phantom data. Figure 4 plots the Dice coefficients for data sets (i)–(iii) for all images in the series without and with initial motion correction (corresponding to method [10]), and after 1 and 2 fixed-point iterations, after which the mean magnitude of motion estimate updates dropped below 0.2 px and no more substantial changes were observed. Table 1 lists T_1 mapping RMSE, residual, and the mean Dice and Hausdorff coefficients over all images. The mean Pearson correlation between T_1 mapping RMSE and residual over all data sets is 0.98 ± 0.01.

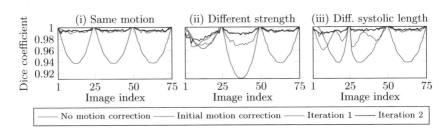

Fig. 4. Plots of Dice coefficients for all images in all phantom data sets with the same motion in all cardiac cycles (left), different motion strength in each cardiac cycle (middle), and different positions of end-systole (right). Results without motion correction represent the baseline, followed by initial motion correction using motion information from the last cardiac cycle, and two iterations of the joint T_1^* and motion estimation.

For phantom data set (i), the prerequisites of method [10] are met and fixed-point iteration shows no benefit. For the cases of simulated cardiac arrhythmia (ii) and (iii), our method improves the T_1 mapping RMSE and residual as well as the Dice and Hausdorff coefficients compared to [10], in terms of both mean and standard deviation. The non-zero RMSE using ground truth motion is due to interpolation. The correlation between T_1 mapping RMSE and residual suggests that we can use the latter as a surrogate to evaluate the quality of T_1 maps for patient data, where no ground truth exists.

Table 1. Quantitative results for phantom data sets for different stages of motion correction. For the evaluation of the T_1 maps, the RMSE compared to ground truth and residual error of least-squares estimation are given. For the evaluation of the motion estimates, mean Dice and Hausdorff coefficients of all images are given

Data set	Motion correction	Mapping RMSE [ms]	Mapping residual [a.u.]	Dice coefficient [%]	Hausdorff coefficient [px]
(i) Same motion	No motion corr.	40.9	184 ± 111	96.1 ± 2.1	2.6 ± 1.23
	Initial motion corr.	23.3	123 ± 15	99.1 ± 0.3	1.0 ± 0.26
	Iteration 1	23.4	123 ± 14	99.2 ± 0.3	1.0 ± 0.25
	Iteration 2	24.0	123 ± 14	99.4 ± 0.3	0.9 ± 0.24
	Ground truth motion	21.0	122 ± 12	100.0 ± 0.0	0.0 ± 0.00
(ii) Diff. strength	No motion corr.	60.0	205 ± 136	96.0 ± 2.7	2.6 ± 1.51
	Initial motion corr.	38.4	146 ± 66	98.2 ± 1.0	1.3 ± 0.53
	Iteration 1	35.4	126 ± 17	98.7 ± 0.9	1.2 ± 0.41
	Iteration 2	31.6	125 ± 16	98.9 ± 0.8	1.2 ± 0.34
	Ground truth motion	22.9	124 ± 12	100.0 ± 0.0	0.0 ± 0.00
(iii) Diff. sys. length	No motion corr.	42.5	185 ± 111	96.4 ± 2.2	2.4 ± 1.34
	Initial motion corr.	32.4	143 ± 57	98.3 ± 1.0	1.3 ± 0.51
	Iteration 1	27.0	124 ± 17	99.1 ± 0.5	1.1 ± 0.29
	Iteration 2	26.6	123 ± 16	99.1 ± 0.4	1.0 ± 0.23
	Ground truth motion	22.2	123 ± 16	100.0 ± 0.0	0.0 ± 0.0

Patient data. Table 2 lists mean T_1^* mapping residuals over all patients and mean ED and ES Dice and Hausdorff coefficients without and with initial motion correction (as in method [10]), and after 1 and 5 fixed-point iterations, after which the mean magnitude of motion estimate updates dropped below 0.4 px and no more substantial changes were observed. One patient data set contained a premature ventricular contraction (PVC), where the Dice coefficient of ED phase between normal systole and PVC systole using initial motion correction was 86 % and after 5 iterations was 94 %. Our website[1] contains visual results.

For patient data, fixed-point iteration improves all quality measures compared to [10], most notably also the standard deviations. The appearance of

Table 2. Quantitative results of patient data evaluation for different stages of motion correction. For the evaluation of the T_1 maps, the residual error of least-squares estimation is given. For the quality of the motion estimates, Dice and Hausdorff coefficients of all ED and ES images are given

Motion correction	Mapping resid. [a.u.]	ED Dice coeff. [%]	ES Dice coeff. [%]	ED Hausd. coeff. [px]	ES Hausd. coeff. [px]
No motion corr.	151 ± 99	96.1 ± 4.2	77.5 ± 8.4	1.1 ± 0.71	6.3 ± 0.53
Init. motion corr.	140 ± 68	96.1 ± 4.2	86.1 ± 5.3	1.1 ± 0.85	3.8 ± 1.64
Iteration 1	124 ± 48	96.9 ± 2.6	89.3 ± 4.5	1.1 ± 0.84	2.6 ± 0.86
Iteration 5	120 ± 45	97.0 ± 2.5	89.4 ± 4.3	1.1 ± 0.85	2.5 ± 0.67

[1] http://www5.cs.fau.de/our-team/wetzl-jens/suppl-material/miccai-2016/

papillary muscles near the endocardial boundary rendered blood pool segmentation in ES ambiguous, which could explain the comparatively lower ES Dice coefficients. The assumption that there is no motion between the first frames of each cardiac cycle (which are ED frames) is shown to be reasonable by the ED Dice coefficient without motion correction of 96 %. The results for ED Dice coefficients without and with initial motion correction are necessarily identical due to this assumption. However, cardiac arrhythmia violates the assumption, as demonstrated by the PVC case. Still, the T_1^* mapping step is robust to some images being misaligned, with only 3 parameters fitted to ~ 100 observations. Thus, fixed-point iteration is able to correct the misalignment and substantially raise the Dice coefficient closer to the mean level for ED. While its application to 2-D imaging is susceptible to through-plane motion artifacts, our proposed algorithm is equally applicable to 3-D data, which would eliminate this problem.

4   Conclusion

Our proposed method provides joint contractility and scar tissue visualization as well as T_1 mapping for the comprehensive assessment of myocardial infarction patients. Evaluations on phantom and patient data show substantial improvements to the state of the art, most notably robustness to cardiac arrhythmia, which is common in this patient population.

Acknowledgments. The authors gratefully acknowledge funding of the Erlangen Graduate School in Advanced Optical Technologies (SAOT) by the German Research Foundation (DFG) in the framework of the German excellence initiative.

References

1. Burt, J.R., Zimmerman, S.L., Kamel, I.R., Halushka, M., Bluemke, D.A.: Myocardial T1 mapping: techniques and potential applications. RadioGraphics **34**(2), 377–395 (2014)
2. Detsky, J., Stainsby, J., Vijayaraghavan, R., Graham, J., Dick, A., Wright, G.: Inversion-recovery-prepared SSFP for cardiac-phase-resolved delayed-enhancement MRI. Magn. Reson. Med. **58**(2), 365–372 (2007)
3. Dice, L.R.: Measures of the amount of ecologic association between species. Ecology **26**(3), 297–302 (1945)
4. Gudbjartsson, H., Patz, S.: The rician distribution of noisy MRI data. Magn. Reson. Med. **34**(6), 910–914 (1995)
5. Klein, S., Staring, M., Murphy, K., Viergever, M.A., Pluim, J.P.W.: elastix: a toolbox for intensity-based medical image registration. IEEE Trans. Med. Imaging **29**(1), 196–205 (2010)
6. Li, W., Li, B.S., Polzin, J.A., Mai, V.M., Prasad, P.V., Edelman, R.R.: Myocardial delayed enhancement imaging using inversion recovery single-shot steady-state free precession: initial experience. J. Magn. Reson. Imaging **20**(2), 327–330 (2004)
7. Marty, B., Vignaud, A., Greiser, A., Robert, B., de Sousa, P.L., Carlier, P.G.: Bloch equations-based reconstruction of Myocardium T1 maps from modified look-locker inversion recovery sequence. PLoS ONE **10**(5), 1–17 (2015)

8. Messroghli, D.R., Radjenovic, A., Kozerke, S., Higgins, D.M., Sivananthan, M.U., Ridgway, J.P.: Modified look-locker inversion recovery (MOLLI) for high-resolution T1 mapping of the heart. Magn. Reson. Med. **52**(1), 141–146 (2004)
9. Rockafellar, R.T., Wets, R.J.B.: Variational Analysis. Springer, Heidelberg (2009)
10. Stalder, A.F., Speier, P., Zenge, M., Greiser, A., Tillmanns, C., Schmidt, M.: Cardiac multi-contrast CINE: real-time inversion-recovery balanced steady-state free precession imaging with compressed-sensing and motion-propagation. In: Proceedings of the 22nd Annual Meeting of ISMRM (2014). abstract 5667
11. Treibel, T., White, S., Moon, J.: Myocardial tissue characterization: histological and pathophysiological correlation. Curr. Cardiovasc. Imaging Rep. **7**(3), 1–9 (2014)
12. Xue, H., Shah, S., Greiser, A., Guetter, C., Littmann, A., Jolly, M.P., Arai, A.E., Zuehlsdorff, S., Guehring, J., Kellman, P.: Motion correction for myocardial T1 mapping using image registration with synthetic image estimation. Magn. Reson. Med. **67**(6), 1644–1655 (2012)

Correction of Fat-Water Swaps in Dixon MRI

Ben Glocker[1(✉)], Ender Konukoglu[2], Ioannis Lavdas[3], Juan Eugenio Iglesias[4,5],
Eric O. Aboagye[3], Andrea G. Rockall[3], and Daniel Rueckert[1]

[1] Biomedical Image Analysis Group, Imperial College London, London, UK
b.glocker@imperial.ac.uk
[2] Computer Vision Laboratory, ETH Zurich, Zürich, Switzerland
[3] Comprehensive Cancer Imaging Centre, Imperial College London, London, UK
[4] Translational Imaging Group, UCL, London, UK
[5] BCBL, Donostia, Spain

Abstract. The Dixon method is a popular and widely used technique
for fat-water separation in magnetic resonance imaging, and today, nearly
all scanner manufacturers are offering a Dixon-type pulse sequence that
produces scans with four types of images: in-phase, out-of-phase, fat-
only, and water-only. A natural ambiguity due to phase wrapping and
local minima in the optimization problem cause a frequent artifact of
fat-water inversion where fat- and water-only voxel values are swapped.
This artifact affects up to 10 % of routinely acquired Dixon images, and
thus, has severe impact on subsequent analysis. We propose a simple yet
very effective method, *Dixon-Fix*, for correcting fat-water swaps. Our
method is based on regressing fat- and water-only images from in- and
out-of-phase images by learning the conditional distribution of image
appearance. The predicted images define the unary potentials in a globally optimal maximum-a-posteriori estimation of the swap labeling with
spatial consistency. We demonstrate the effectiveness of our approach on
whole-body MRI with various types of fat-water swaps.

1 Introduction

Reliable fat-water separation in magnetic resonance imaging (MRI) has a wide
range of clinical applications [1]. As the fat signal has a relatively short T1
relaxation time, its bright appearance, without separation or suppression, can
obscure pathological structures and patterns of edema, inflammation, or enhancing tumors [1]. Additionally, if separated, the fat signal can highlight pathologies
such as fatty tumors. The quantification of the amount of visceral adipose tissue
is another example requiring reliable separation of water from fat. There are
several techniques for fat suppression and fat-water imaging in MRI, and among
these chemical shift based fat-water separation is one of the most popular and
widely used ones [2]. This is also referred to as the Dixon method [3], originally developed as a simple spectroscopic imaging technique using two images I
and O with a modified spin echo pulse sequence from which fat- and water-only
images F and W are derived. The images I and O are acquired at time points
where the fat and water signal are *in-phase*, i.e. $I = W + F$, and *out-of-phase*,

© Springer International Publishing AG 2016
S. Ourselin et al. (Eds.): MICCAI 2016, Part III, LNCS 9902, pp. 536–543, 2016.
DOI: 10.1007/978-3-319-46726-9_62

i.e. $O = W - F$. Theoretically, fat- and water-only signals can be recovered by $F = \frac{1}{2}(I - O)$ and $W = \frac{1}{2}(I + O)$. The original approach is sensitive to B_0 inhomogeneities, and hence, many improvements had been suggested, including three- and multi-point Dixon methods [4] which overcome the limitation of an inherent ambiguity in the fat and water signal. A breakthrough has been achieved by employing mathematical optimization for iterative decomposition, known as IDEAL [5]. Nowadays, all major scanner manufacturers offer one or multiple variants of a Dixon-based sequence for routine, clinical fat-water imaging.

Still, inherent to all Dixon methods is an artifact that causes fat-water swaps due to a natural ambiguity in the phase encoding and convergence of the employed optimization method to local minima. Even with sophisticated unwrapping algorithms this artifact cannot be completely avoided [1]. If undetected, those swaps can severely impact subsequent processing and analysis steps, for example, yielding wrong estimates of body fat. In a recent study, the impact of fat-water inversion has been investigated in the context of PET/MR, where Dixon images are used for attenuation correction [6]. The study found that 8 % (23 of 283) of the images were affected by fat-water swaps. The average fraction of fat in the brain calculated from images with no fat-water swap was 13 %, and 56 % in the scans with inversions demonstrating the severe impact that this artifact can have on analysis. In our own database consisting of 46 subjects with whole-body Dixon MRI we found 10 cases exhibiting various types of fat-water swaps. Visual examples are shown in Fig. 1. While in smaller studies, visual quality control can be established to detect (and possibly discard) affected scans, this is not possible in large-scale studies with many hundreds or even thousands of subjects. Automated methods for detecting whether fat-water swaps are present are required. Furthermore, due to the high costs for imaging it is desirable to be able to include as many subjects as possible for further analysis, and thus, a method that can not only detect but correct fat-water swaps is needed.

1.1 Related Work

Robust estimation of the inherent fat-water separation is an active field of research, and an overview is provided in [7]. There are several extensions [8] and alternatives to the original IDEAL method, including graph-cut formulations [7] and other discrete optimization approaches [9,10]. All require access to the original echo sequences or a B0 field map [11] as part of their optimization procedure. However, these data are not available after the scanning has been completed. In fact, most Dixon protocols yield exactly four types of images, irrespective of the underlying sequence, optimization procedure and number of echo times. The in-phase, out-of-phase, fat- and water-only images are what is accessible once the data have been reconstructed and stored in the imaging archive. To the best of our knowledge, there exist no technique that allows correction of fat-water swaps retrospectively based on just those derived images. Such a technique, however, would be very valuable as it can be applied to already acquired datasets, in particular in clinical studies, where the presence of fat-water swaps is often only detected during subsequent analysis. Being able to correct such

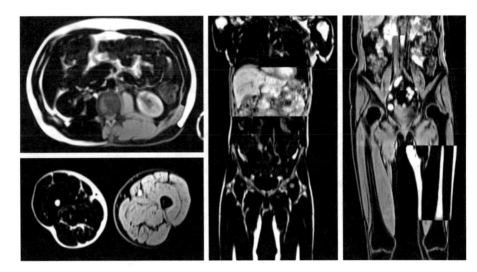

Fig. 1. Examples of different types of fat-water swaps in Dixon MRI. Swaps can affect local regions as seen in on the axial slices on the left for kidneys and legs. In whole-body MRI, entire stations can be affected as seen in the middle image, or partially affected, as seen for the lower extremities on the right.

corrupted data is important in clinical research as data are expensive to acquire and samples sizes are calculated tightly to reduce scanning time and costs.

1.2   Contribution

We propose a simple yet very effective approach for correcting fat-water swaps that can be applied retrospectively on already acquired data taking only the four derived images, in-phase, out-of-phase, fat- and water-only, as input. Our method makes use of image synthesis, i.e., a regression problem dealing with the prediction of images of a certain modalities, given input image(s) of other modalities. In our case, we learn the conditional distribution of image appearance of the fat- and water-only images given the in- and out-of-phase images. We utilize a training database of fat-water swap-free Dixon images. The predicted fat- and water-only images yield a noisy, but swap-free estimate that is employed in a voxel-wise energy term within a swap-labeling problem that is solved via graph-cuts. The details of our method are given in the following.

2   Dixon-Fix: Correction of Fat-Water Swaps

The core of our method for detecting and correcting fat-water swaps in Dixon MRI is based on an image synthesis component for predicting fat- and water-only images, F and W, from the in-phase and out-of-phase images, I and O. Given a training database $T = \{\mathcal{D}_i\}_{i=1}^m$ of m Dixon MRIs $\mathcal{D}_i = \{I_i, O_i, F_i, W_i\}$ where

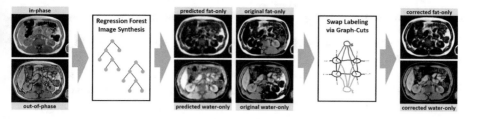

Fig. 2. Overview of the Dixon-Fix pipeline with the two main components of image synthesis to predict swap-free fat- and water-only images, and the swap labeling solved with graph-cuts that yields the corrected images.

(F_i, W_i) are known to be swap-free, we can learn the conditional distribution $p(F, W | I, O)$. For a set of test images $(I_{\text{test}}, O_{\text{test}})$, we can then predict a potentially noisy, but swap-free estimation $(F_{\text{test}}^{\star}, W_{\text{test}}^{\star})$ by inferring the most likely images according to $(F_{\text{test}}^{\star}, W_{\text{test}}^{\star}) = \arg\max_{(F,W)} p(F, W | I_{\text{test}}, O_{\text{test}})$. For learning this conditional distribution, we employ Regression Forests which have been shown to yield good synthesis results in the context of diffusion MRI [12,13]. Using the predicted fat- and water-only images, we then formulate a binary labeling task in terms of an energy minimization problem of a pairwise Markov random field (MRF). Both, the image synthesis based on Regression Forests and the MRF labeling formulation are detailed in the following. Figure 2 provides an overview of the whole processing pipeline for correcting fat-water swaps.

2.1 Prediction of Swap-Free Fat- and Water-only Images

Regression Forests are an attractive choice for image synthesis as they can efficiently handle the multivariate, high-dimensional input data and yield a probabilistic, joint estimate of the fat- and water-only voxel values. Additionally, it is straightforward to incorporate both local and contextual information based on the popular, randomized, offset box-features which are efficiently implemented using integral images. We follow the basic Regression Forest methodology as described in [14]. We employ a leaf node predictor model based on multivariate Gaussians which summarize the statistics over the incoming training data. This model then yields predictions for every voxel v of the fat- and water-only values corresponding to the means $F_{\mu}^{\star}(v)$ and $W_{\mu}^{\star}(v)$, together with an estimate of the uncertainty corresponding to the standard deviations $F_{\sigma}^{\star}(v)$ and $W_{\sigma}^{\star}(v)$. The greedy learning procedure during which the randomized decision trees are constructed is driven by an objective function that aims to minimize the variance in each internal split node. Those split nodes are associated with binary tests applied on the most discriminate feature responses. At test time, the predictions from individual trees are aggregated by averaging.

2.2   Estimation of Swap-Labeling using Graph-Cuts

The image synthesis yields a swap-free estimate for the fat- and water-only images, denoted as $(F^{\star}_{\text{test}}, W^{\star}_{\text{test}})$. To determine which voxels in the original images $(F_{\text{test}}, W_{\text{test}})$ need to be swapped, we formulate a binary labeling problem as a Markov random field where each voxel v is associated with a binary random variable x_v that takes values $\{0, 1\}$, with *zero* meaning 'no-swap', and *one* meaning 'swap'. The probability of a voxel being swapped $p(x_v | F(v), W(v), F^{\star}(v), W^{\star}(v))$ given the original and predicted fat- and water-only voxel values $F(v), W(v), F^{\star}(v), W^{\star}(v)$ is defined with respect to similarities between those values. We are omitting the $_{\text{test}}$ subscript to avoid clutter. Mathematically, this can be defined as an MRF unary potential function as

$$\psi_v(x_v) = \begin{cases} \dfrac{|F(v) - F^{\star}_{\mu}(v)|}{F^{\star}_{\sigma}(v)} + \dfrac{|W(v) - W^{\star}_{\mu}(v)|}{W^{\star}_{\sigma}(v)} & \text{if } x_v = 0 \\[2ex] \dfrac{|F(v) - W^{\star}_{\mu}(v)|}{W^{\star}_{\sigma}(v)} + \dfrac{|W(v) - F^{\star}_{\mu}(v)|}{F^{\star}_{\sigma}(v)} & \text{if } x_v = 1 \end{cases} . \tag{1}$$

The potential function is a robust version of an intensity difference term that takes the voxel-wise uncertainty, $F^{\star}_{\sigma}(v)$ and $W^{\star}_{\sigma}(v)$, from the image synthesis into account. The potential function determines the cost of assigning 'non-swap' $(x_v = 0)$ and 'swap' $(x_v = 1)$ labels depending on whether the original voxel values are closer to the predicted fat- or water-only voxel values. To encourage spatial consistency, we add a simple pairwise potential function based on the Potts model which is defined for neighboring voxels (v, w) in a 6-neighborhood as $\psi_{vw}(x_v, x_w) = \lambda \cdot \mathbb{1}_{x_v \neq x_w}$. The pairwise function returns a penalty λ if the label assignments to voxels v and w are different, i.e. $x_v \neq x_w$, and it returns a zero-penalty otherwise. The total MRF energy for a swap-labeling $\mathbf{x}$ is then defined as the sum of the unary and pairwise potentials, $E(\mathbf{x}) = \sum_v \psi_v(x_v) + \sum_{(v,w)} \psi_{vw}(x_v, x_w)$. The globally optimal solution in terms of the maximum-a-posteriori estimate $\hat{\mathbf{x}} = \arg\max_{\mathbf{x}} E(\mathbf{x})$ is efficiently computed using graph-cuts.

3   Experiments

To evaluate the effectiveness of our correction method, we utilize a database of whole-body Dixon MRIs from 46 subjects. The data have been visually inspected and 10 cases have been identified with fat-water swaps. We normalize for intensity variation by matching intensity means to a fixed value. From the 36 swap-free cases, we randomly select 23 for training the Regression Forest with 50 trees, maximum depth 30, and a minimum of 4 samples per leaf as stopping criterion. A large pool of box-feature parameters $(n = 10,000)$ is randomly generated. Parameters include the image channels, allowing cross-channel box difference features, and the side lengths and offsets of the 3D cuboids. We evaluate 200 randomly selected features on-the-fly for all incoming training samples at each split node. Ten equidistant thresholds in the interval defined by the minimum and maximum feature response are tested, and the overall best feature/threshold

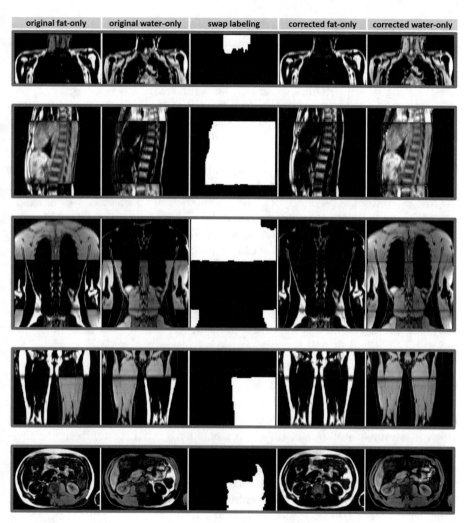

Fig. 3. Visual results of successful fat-water swap correction for five different cases. **First row** illustrates a case with a fat-water swap in the head/neck area. **Second row** shows a case of a whole station swap that is common in whole-body Dixon MRI. **Third row** shows a case with a mix of whole station swap and local swaps in the lower arm region. **Fourth row** shows successful correction of a left/right image swap, while the **last row** shows a challenging case of local, complex swaps of internal anatomical structures. Note that horizontal stripy artifacts are results of the stitching method used for generating whole-body images from individual stations, and not a result of the fat-water swap correction.

pair yielding largest decrease of the trace of the covariance matrix over the two-dimensional target variable is selected. This greedy, randomized optimization has shown to yield decision trees with good generalization ability.

Given a multi-channel input with in- and out-of-phase images, the forest predicts jointly the appearance of swap-free fat- and water-only images. The swap labeling is determined efficiently through multi-resolution graph-cuts. A dense 3D MRF is defined first on low resolution images with 6 mm voxel spacing. The resulting labeling defines the region for a full resolution non-regular, sparse MRF with nodes corresponding to voxels labeled as 'swap' in the first stage. The result of the second stage is an accurate swap labeling map used to generate the corrected fat- and water-only images. In all experiments, we fix the regularization parameter $\lambda = 5$, empirically chosen, and its optimal value depends on the range of MR intensities. The average running time of the synthesis is about 10 min for a whole-body scan, and the multi-resolution graph-cut takes less than 5 s. The fat-water swaps in all 10 cases are successfully corrected. Visual examples with original, corrupted images, swap labeling maps, and corrected images are shown in Fig. 3. The examples illustrate the variety of swaps that can be handled, including one case with multiple swaps across the whole-body image. When tested on the 13 swap-free images, we find that in all cases some voxels are incorrectly predicted as 'swap'. Thus, with the current approach it is not possible to confirm whether an image is swap-free. The incorrectly labeled voxels, however, either correspond to background regions or form small patches in noisy, unstructured and less important areas which both appear dark in the fat- and water-only images and therefore cause confusion in the MRF unaries.

4 Conclusion

The Dixon-Fix method provides an effective way for correcting fat-water swaps which is demonstrated qualitatively on whole-body MRI. Quantitative evaluation is difficult due to unknown ground truth. In future work synthesized swaps will be considered for this purpose, however, it should be noted that generating realistic swaps is difficult as the underlying process that causes these artifacts is quite complex. As our test cases exhibit a large variety of swaps in different areas, such as head/neck, upper and lower extremities, and internal organs, it is expected that the method works well in other applications, such as spine and brain. The two main components of our pipeline are based on established techniques, Regression Forests and graph-cuts. Others could be considered, in particular, for the synthesis, which is an active area of research with many recently proposed methods (see [15] for an overview). Probabilistic approaches might be considered in particular, as the predictions should come with confidence estimates for integration into the MRF energy. A direction for future work concerns the regularization term. The location-agnostic Potts model with a global weighting factor might not be optimal for all cases of fat-water swaps. A learned prior that takes contextual information and expected size and shape of the swap area into account could be explored. This might also provide effective means of removing the false positive swap predictions in swap-free images. To facilitate further development, the source code of our Dixon-Fix implementation is made publicly available on http://biomedia.doc.ic.ac.uk/software/.

Acknowledgments. This work is supported by the NIHR (EME Project: 13/122/01). JEI is funded by a Marie Curie fellowship (654911 - THALAMODEL).

References

1. Bley, T.A., Wieben, O., François, C.J., Brittain, J.H., Reeder, S.B.: Fat and water magnetic resonance imaging. J Magn. Reson. Imaging **31**(1), 4–18 (2010)
2. Ma, J.: Dixon techniques for water and fat imaging. J Magn. Reson. Imaging **28**(3), 543–558 (2008)
3. Dixon, W.T.: Simple proton spectroscopic imaging. Radiology **153**(1), 189–194 (1984)
4. Glover, G.H.: Multipoint dixon technique for water and fat proton and susceptibility imaging. J Magn. Reson. Imaging **1**(5), 521–530 (1991)
5. Reeder, S.B., Pineda, A.R., Wen, Z., Shimakawa, A., Yu, H., Brittain, J.H., Gold, G.E., Beaulieu, C.H., Pelc, N.J.: Iterative decomposition of water and fat with echo asymmetry and least-squares estimation (IDEAL): application with fast spin-echo imaging. MR Med. **54**(3), 636–644 (2005)
6. Ladefoged, C.N., Hansen, A.E., Keller, S.H., Holm, S., Law, I., Beyer, T., Højgaard, L., Kjær, A., Andersen, F.L.: Impact of incorrect tissue classification in dixon-based MR-AC: fat-water tissue inversion. EJNMMI Phys. **1**(1), 101 (2014)
7. Hernando, D., Kellman, P., Haldar, J., Liang, Z.P.: Robust water/fat separation in the presence of large field inhomogeneities using a graph cut algorithm. MR Med. **63**(1), 79–90 (2010)
8. Sharma, S.D., Artz, N.S., Hernando, D., Horng, D.E., Reeder, S.B.: Improving chemical shift encoded water-fat separation using object-based information of the magnetic field inhomogeneity. MR Med. **73**(2), 597–604 (2015)
9. Berglund, J., Ahlström, H., Johansson, L., Kullberg, J.: Two-point dixon method with flexible echo times. MR Med. **65**(4), 994–1004 (2011)
10. Berglund, J., Kullberg, J.: Three-dimensional water/fat separation and T2* estimation based on whole-image optimization: application in breathhold liver imaging at 1.5T. MR Med. **67**(6), 1684–1693 (2012)
11. Narayan, S., Kalhan, S.C., Wilson, D.L.: Recovery of chemical estimates by field inhomogeneity neighborhood error detection (REFINED): fat/water separation at 7 tesla. J. Magn. Reson. Imaging **37**(5), 1247–1253 (2013)
12. Jog, A., Roy, S., Carass, A., Prince, J.L.: Magnetic resonance image synthesis through patch regression. In: 2013 IEEE 10th International Symposium on Biomedical Imaging (ISBI), pp. 350–353. IEEE (2013)
13. Alexander, D.C., Zikic, D., Zhang, J., Zhang, H., Criminisi, A.: Image quality transfer via random forest regression: applications in diffusion MRI. In: Golland, P., Hata, N., Barillot, C., Hornegger, J., Howe, R. (eds.) MICCAI 2014, Part III. LNCS, vol. 8675, pp. 225–232. Springer, Heidelberg (2014)
14. Criminisi, A., Shotton, J., Konukoglu, E.: Decision forests: a unified framework for classification, regression, density estimation, manifold learning and semi-supervised learning. Found. Trends Comput. Graph. Vis. **7**(2–3), 81–227 (2012)
15. Vemulapalli, R., Van Nguyen, H., Kevin Zhou, S.: Unsupervised cross-modal synthesis of subject-specific scans. In: Proceedings of the IEEE International Conference on Computer Vision, pp. 630–638 (2015)

Motion-Robust Reconstruction Based on Simultaneous Multi-slice Registration for Diffusion-Weighted MRI of Moving Subjects

Bahram Marami, Benoit Scherrer, Onur Afacan, Simon K. Warfield,
and Ali Gholipour[✉]

Boston Children's Hospital, Harvard Medical School, Boston, MA, USA
ali.gholipour@childrens.harvard.edu

Abstract. Simultaneous multi-slice (SMS) echo-planar imaging has had
a huge impact on the acceleration and routine use of diffusion-weighted
MRI (DWI) in neuroimaging studies in particular the human connectome
project; but also holds the potential to facilitate DWI of moving subjects,
as proposed by the new technique developed in this paper. We present a
novel registration-based motion tracking technique that takes advantage
of the multi-plane coverage of the anatomy by simultaneously acquired
slices to enable robust reconstruction of neural microstructure from SMS
DWI of moving subjects. Our technique constitutes three main components: (1) motion tracking and estimation using SMS registration, (2)
detection and rejection of intra-slice motion, and (3) robust reconstruction. Quantitative results from 14 volunteer subject experiments and the
analysis of motion-corrupted SMS DWI of 6 children indicate robust
reconstruction in the presence of continuous motion and the potential to
extend the use of SMS DWI in very challenging populations.

Keywords: Simultaneous multi-slice · Diffusion-weighted MRI · Motion

1 Introduction

Diffusion-weighted magnetic resonance imaging (DWI) is the technique of choice
for the analysis of neural microstructure and structural connectivity in the brain.
While early works focused on a diffusion tensor imaging (DTI) model to describe
major fiber bundles, models and techniques have evolved to characterize the
complex underlying structure of the neural anatomy including crossing fibers and
free water compartments [1,2]. Fitting more complex models requires relatively
dense q-space sampling which can be extremely time consuming. Acceleration
through simultaneous multi-slice (SMS) acquisition with multiband excitation
and controlled aliasing [3] has played a significant role in routine use of these
techniques in large-scale projects such as the human connectome project [4].

A. Gholipour—This study was supported in part by NIH grants R01EB018988,
R01EB019483, R01 NS079788, and U01 NS082320; and Intel(C) IPCC.

S. Ourselin et al. (Eds.): MICCAI 2016, Part III, LNCS 9902, pp. 544–552, 2016.
DOI: 10.1007/978-3-319-46726-9_63

Accelerations of a factor of two or more are achieved by SMS DWI, but these scans are still lengthy and generate loud noise and vibration that is not easily tolerated by non-cooperative patients, children, and newborns, who may move continuously during a DWI scan. Extensive research has been done on motion-robust sequences and motion correction methods in MRI [5], but the use of these methods is limited by the the type and amount of motion that can be corrected, and the challenges in implementation or setup. Motion correction in DWI is currently performed at the volume level either retrospectively using volume-to-volume registration [6] or prospectively using navigators [7]. These techniques are slow and do not perform well when motion is continuous and fast.

There has been some promising work on slice-level motion correction in DWI to deal with continuous motion [8–11]. While robust motion estimation is a challenge in these techniques, SMS DWI, which is being increasingly used, holds the potential to facilitate slice-level motion correction by the novel approach proposed in this paper. We achieve this by (1) integrating a model of motion with image registration that particularly takes advantage of rigidly-coupled simultaneously acquired multiple slices to strengthen slice-level motion tracking and estimation; (2) detecting and rejecting intra-slice motion; and (3) robust reconstruction of multi-compartment models from motion-corrected SMS DWI data. This work extends our earlier work on motion-robust DTI reconstruction [11].

2 Materials and Methods

An SMS DWI scan is performed by interleaved 2D echo-planar imaging with M_B multi-band excitations. Therefore, at the smallest time step, k-space data is acquired for M_B slices simultaneously from multiple receiver coils and is used to reconstruct slice images through unaliasing. Subject motion can occur between excitations (i.e. inter-slice motion) or within excitation-sampling (i.e. intra-slice motion). The latter results in signal loss or distortion in all M_B slices. Our approach constitutes tracking the dynamics of motion through slice-level image registration, and detecting and excluding slices corrupted by intra-slice motion.

2.1 Slice-Level Motion Tracking and Estimation

Slice-to-volume registration, used previously for inter-slice motion correction and image reconstruction, is often initialized by volume-to-volume registration. This is suboptimal and is not robust. In contrast, we introduce the notion of slice-level motion tracking, where image registration is used to capture the dynamics of motion. We formulate the problem as a dynamic state-space model estimation where slices, as observations, are used in image registration to estimate motion parameters considered to be the hidden states. We take advantage of slice timing profile and the 3D coverage of the anatomy provided by multiple slices acquired simultaneously in an SMS acquisition (see Fig. 1a).

Assuming that one set of simultaneous slices $\mathbf{y}_k = \{y_1, y_2, ..., y_{M_B}\}$ are acquired at a time k, we show the relative position of the head at time k by

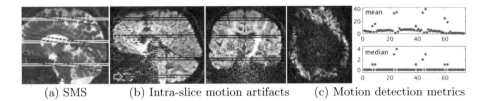

(a) SMS   (b) Intra-slice motion artifacts   (c) Motion detection metrics

Fig. 1. (a) Three slices are acquired simultaneously by a 3-band SMS DWI: as compared to a single slice, these rigidly-coupled slices provide multi-plane (3D) coverage of the anatomy, therefore they mitigate the ill-posed problem of slice-to-volume registration. (b) Pairs of arrows point at intra-slice motion artifacts seen in simultaneously acquired slices in a 2-band axial SMS DWI. Partial signal loss is observed in a corrupted axial slice on the right. (c) Outliers of the proposed mean and median metrics on a difference filtered image are used to detect intra-slice motion (x-axis is the slice number).

the hidden states $\mathbf{x}_k$, where $\mathbf{x}_k$ in this case is a vector of 6 rigid transformation parameters. Given a finite sequence of observations (slice acquisitions), our goal is to estimate the states $\mathbf{x}_k$ of motion dynamics governed by a stochastic equation:

$$\mathbf{x}_k = \mathbf{x}_{k-1} + \omega_{k-1} \quad , \quad \mathbf{y}_k = \mathrm{H}(\mathbf{x}_k) + \nu_k \qquad (1)$$

where ω_k and ν_k are the process and measurement noise and represent uncertainty in the modeling of motion dynamics and measurements, respectively. H is a function that relates states $\mathbf{x}_k$ to the measurements $\mathbf{y}_k$. In other words, H is a generative function for the slices $\mathbf{y}_k$ acquired at time k at head position $\mathbf{x}_k$.

We aim to use Kalman filter for state estimation, so we separate the nonlinear output model from the filtering process, rewrite it as $\mathbf{z}_k = \mathbf{x}_k + \nu_k$, and integrate it with image registration that estimates $\mathbf{z}_k$ by matching the observations (as target) and the reference image (as source) transformed by $\mathbf{p}$; i.e. $\mathbf{z}_k = \underset{\mathbf{p}}{\mathrm{argmax}}\, Sim\,(\mathrm{H}(\mathbf{p}), \mathbf{y}_k)$, where $Sim(.)$ is a similarity metric between the set of M_B slices $(\mathbf{y}_k)$ and the transformed source image. Simultaneous slices in $\mathbf{y}_k$ are in maximum distance to each other and provide 3D multi-plane coverage of the anatomy, thus enable 3D image-based navigation as opposed to a single slice that only provides a single-plane coverage. Image registration based on $\mathbf{y}_k$ is thus much more robust than slice-to-volume registration based on a single slice. The output of image registration is $\mathbf{z}_k$, which is then used in state estimation.

For robust state estimation in the presence of nonlinearity and registration errors, we use an outlier-robust Kalman filter [12], which assumes a Gaussian distribution for the process noise, i.e. $\omega_k \sim \mathcal{N}(0, Q)$, but updates the measurement noise $(\nu_k \sim \mathcal{N}(0, S_k))$ based on sequential observations by estimating its covariance S_k at time k. S_k is sampled from a Wishart distribution as $S_k^{-1} \sim \mathcal{W}\left(R^{-1}/s, s\right)$, where $\Lambda \succ 0$ is a precision matrix with s degrees of freedom. The prior mean of $\mathcal{W}(\Lambda, s)$ is $s\Lambda$ where s quantifies the concentration of the distribution around its mean [12]. Algorithm 1 shows the pseudo code of the entire process.

Algorithm 1. Pseudo-code of the slice-level motion estimation algorithm

---

Input: H, $\mathbf{y}_k = \{y_1, y_2, ..., y_{M_B}\}$, $\hat{\mathbf{x}}_{k-1}$

Output: $\hat{\mathbf{x}}_k$

1: *register source to simultaneous slices:* $\mathbf{z}_k \leftarrow \max_{\mathbf{p}} Sim\,(\mathrm{H}(\mathbf{p}), \mathbf{y}_k)$; $\mathbf{p}_0 = \hat{\mathbf{x}}_{k-1}$

2: *predict states:* $\hat{\mathbf{x}}_k^- \leftarrow \hat{\mathbf{x}}_{k-1}$, $\hat{\mathbf{x}}_k \leftarrow \hat{\mathbf{x}}_k^-$; $\mathrm{P}_k^- \leftarrow \mathrm{P}_{k-1} + \mathrm{Q}$, $\mathrm{P}_k \leftarrow \mathrm{P}_k^-$

3: **repeat**

4:    *update noise:* $\delta = \mathbf{z}_k - \hat{\mathbf{x}}_k$; $\Lambda_k = (s\mathrm{R} + \delta\delta^T + \mathrm{P}_k)/(s+1)$

5:    *update states:* $\mathrm{K}_k = (\mathrm{P}_k^- + \Lambda_k)^{-1}\mathrm{P}_k^-$; $\hat{\mathbf{x}}_k = \hat{\mathbf{x}}_k^- + \mathrm{K}_k^T(\mathbf{z}_k - \hat{\mathbf{x}}_k^-)$

6:                  $\mathrm{P}_k = \mathrm{K}_k^T\Lambda_k\mathrm{K}_k + (\mathrm{H} - \mathrm{K}_k)^T\mathrm{P}_k^-(\mathrm{H} - \mathrm{K}_k)$

7: **until** converged

8: **return** $\hat{\mathbf{x}}_k$

2.2 Intra-slice Motion Detection and Rejection

Intra-slice motion at time k results in signal loss and distortion in all slices that are acquired at k. Figure 1b shows an example. To detect it, we rely on the fact that SMS DWI slices are acquired in an interleaved manner and fast intra-slice motion occurs occasionally. As such, we use inter-slice intensity discontinuity [13] to detect motion-corrupted slices. In this approach, we compute an intensity difference image I_d by subtracting the image from a filtered version of it based on a morphological closing filter. We use robust statistics to detect intra-slice motion; i.e. a slice is considered to be affected by intra-slice motion if its median in I_d is greater than 0 or its mean is an outlier (Fig. 1c) [11]. When intra-slice motion is detected at time k, all M_B slices acquired at that time, are rejected.

2.3 Model Reconstruction from Motion-Corrected Data

We aim to fit a model to motion-corrected DWI data from non-diffusion weighted scans S_0 and diffusion-weighted scans S_i ($b_i \neq 0$) with gradients g_i and b values b_i. We formulated the problem based on a ball-and-stick model [1] (but a similar approach can be used for other multi-compartment models and DTI):

$$S_i = S_0 \sum_{j=0}^{N} f_j e^{-b_i g_i^T \mathbf{D}_j g_i}, \tag{2}$$

where $\mathbf{D}_j$s are 3×3 symmetric positive definite (SPD) matrices, and $f_j \in [0, 1]$ are sum-of-unity fractions of occupancy. This model assumes that all $\mathbf{D}_j$s have equal first eigenvalues (λ_1), a single ball compartment quantifies isotropic water fraction, and the stick compartments quantify fibers. The model has $3N + 1$ degrees-of-freedom. To ensure estimation of SPD matrices we parameterized the tensors $\mathbf{D}_j$ in the log-domain by setting $\mathbf{L} = (log(\mathbf{D}_1), ..., log(\mathbf{D}_N))$.

To estimate model parameters, we used maximum a posteriori (MAP) estimation at the voxel level, i.e. $\{\hat{\mathbf{L}}, \hat{\mathbf{f}}\} = \underset{\mathbf{L}, \mathbf{f}}{\operatorname{argmax}}\, p(\mathbf{L}, \mathbf{f}|\mathbf{S_i})$, where $\mathbf{f} = (f_1, ..., f_N)$

is the vector of the compartment fractions. The issue here is that due to motion and slice-level motion correction, voxels from S_0 and S_i slices are not spatially aligned and are scattered in 3D space; therefore, the q-space is differently sampled at every voxel. To handle this, we built a 3D high-resolution vector-class image in the space of S_0 (i.e. V_0) from motion-corrected DWI slices. Each voxel of this image ($v \in V_0$) is a variable-length vector (of length M_v) of a class that contains the intensity values (C_is), g_is corrected by the estimated rotation matrices (from estimated slice motion parameters), b_is, and finally the physical coordinates and direction, of all M_v DWI voxels mapped to the neighborhood (one-voxel radius) of v after motion correction. We assumed a uniform distribution for the *a priori* probability distribution functions and a zero-mean normal distribution with variance σ^2 around the unknown modeled signal S_i:

$$P(\mathbf{C}|\mathbf{L}, \mathbf{f}) = \prod_{v \in V_0} \frac{1}{\sigma\sqrt{2\pi}} \exp\left(\frac{-\sum_{i=1}^{M_v} w_i \|S_i(e^{\mathbf{L}_v}, \mathbf{f}_v) - C_i\|^2}{2\sigma^2}\right) \qquad (3)$$

The weights (w_i) are calculated by the distance between neighborhood voxels and the reference voxel by a Gaussian kernel that models the point-spread-function of the DWI slice acquisition. We used numerical optimization [14] and gradually increased the complexity of the model from a single stick to the ball-and-stick.

3   Experimental Results

For quantitative evaluation, first we performed 14 volunteer subject motion experiments with different amounts and types of head motion up to 30° rotation in 2 volunteers; we also acquired 3 motion-free DWI scans for each volunteer, which were used as gold standard (GS). Each DWI scan involved 6 $b = 0$ and 30 $b \neq 0$ volumes, and a multi-band factor of 2, for which we fit a DTI model. We used normalized cross correlation similarity metric for slice-level motion estimation in both $b = 0$ and $b \neq 0$ images, and mutual information to register the reconstructed S_0 and S_i images. The amount of motion was estimated for each experiment using $d = \sqrt{x^2 + y^2 + z^2 + (cr)^2}$, where x, y and z are the translation parameters, $c = 50\,\mathrm{mm}$, and r is the Euler angle of the estimated motion, which is computed from 3 rotation angles based on Euler's rotation theorem.

We compared the performance of our motion tracking based on simultaneous multi-slice registration (MT-SMR) to the original reconstruction without motion correction (Orig), reconstruction with volume-to-volume registration (VVR) [6], and slice-to-volume registration (SVR) initialized by VVR [8]. Figure 2 shows sample DTI results: color-coded fractional anisotropy (FA) maps. We calculated the difference in FA values (Δ_{FA}), mean diffusivity (Δ_{MD}), and angular difference of first eigenvectors (Δ_{Dir}) between each method and the GS in four regions-of-interest (ROIs): corpus callosum (CC), cingulum (Cin), limbs of the internal capsule (LIC), and the lateral ventricles (Vent). The average results, given in Table 1, show consistently lower errors by MT-SMR compared to the other methods. We plotted Δ_{FA} in the CC and Cin ROIs vs. the estimated

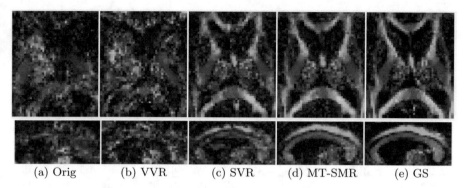

(a) Orig   (b) VVR   (c) SVR   (d) MT-SMR   (e) GS

Fig. 2. Axial (top) and sagittal (bottom) views of color FA in a volunteer. MT-SMR generated FA very similar to the GS (motion-free) and outperformed other methods.

Table 1. The mean of Δ_{FA}, Δ_{Dir} and Δ_{MD} error metrics in corpus callosum (CC), cingulum (Cin), limbs of the internal capsule (LIC) and ventricles (Vent) regions. MT-SMR consistently generated the lowest errors in all regions (highlighted in bold).

	Δ_{FA}				Δ_{Dir}				$\Delta_{MD}(\times 10^3)$			
	Orig	VVR	SVR	SMR	Orig	VVR	SVR	SMR	Orig	VVR	SVR	SMR
CC	0.41	0.32	0.15	**0.12**	0.75	0.76	0.36	**0.30**	0.38	0.24	0.17	**0.15**
Cin	0.34	0.27	0.18	**0.12**	0.93	0.92	0.53	**0.36**	0.22	0.27	0.15	**0.09**
LIC	0.26	0.23	0.11	**0.10**	0.54	0.56	0.30	**0.27**	0.27	0.19	0.09	**0.08**
Vent	0.13	0.11	0.08	**0.07**	0.87	0.86	0.83	**0.82**	0.91	0.72	0.25	**0.22**

amount of motion in Fig. 3. While the errors were high in VVR, SVR, and Orig, MT-SMR generated lower errors in a robust manner regardless of the amount of motion.

Next, we applied our method to multi b-value, 90-direction, motion-corrupted DWI scans of 6 children (between 3 and 14 years old), who significantly moved during DWI scans. We fit a single tensor model as well as a ball-and-stick model with $N = 3$. Based on a single tensor model, we calculated FA in the CC, Cin, and LIC ROIs. Motion blurs the images and reduces FA in these fiber-rich regions. On the other hand, if motion is corrected and FA is robustly reconstructed, we expect high FA in these regions. Figure 4 shows boxplot analysis of the results, which indicates superior performance of MT-SMR compared to the other methods. Figure 5 shows multiple fascicles and isotropic water fraction compartments detected by different methods from motion-corrupted DWI of a 5 year old child. The structure and direction of crossing fibers is correctly identified by MT-SMR.

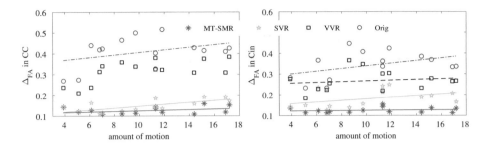

Fig. 3. FA value differences (Δ_{FA}) between the gold-standard (GS) and each motion-correction method in the CC and Cin ROIs based on the amount of motion (mm). Regardless of the amount of motion, MT-SMR generated low errors in all experiments.

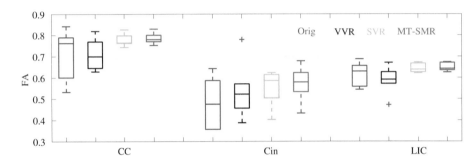

Fig. 4. Boxplot analysis of the FA of 4 methods in 3 ROIs (CC, Cin, LIC) using DWI of 6 children who moved during scans. The high FA values with low variance by MT-SMR in these fiber-rich ROIs indicate robust reconstruction in the presence of motion.

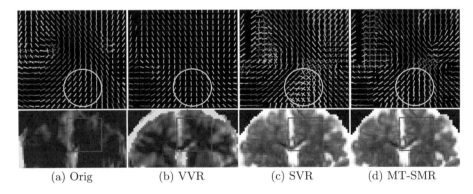

Fig. 5. Top: multiple fascicles, and bottom: isotropic water fraction, detected by the ball-and-stick model by different methods. The results from MT-SMR (d) comply with our knowledge of the anatomy in this region where fascicles from CC, corticospinal tracts, and the superior longitudinal fasciculus cross. Orig and VVR generated blurred, inaccurate isotropic water fraction maps, and failed to find crossing fibers in many regions, and SVR (c) generated wrong angles in the ROI highlighted by circles.

4   Discussions and Conclusion

We developed a slice-level motion tracking and estimation technique that takes advantage of the 3D coverage of the anatomy at multiple image planes provided by simultaneously acquired slices in SMS DWI. We showed that this technique outperforms slice-to-volume registration as it performs 3D registration based on data from multiple planes rather than a single plane. This technique also outperforms the current routinely-used volume-to-volume registration techniques as it enables faster motion tracking which results in more efficient use of DWI data. In this work, we reported retrospective analysis of motion-corrupted data, but our motion tracking and estimation system is causal, therefore, with sufficient computation power it can be implemented and used in real-time for prospective motion tracking and correction. This technique can extend the use of SMS DWI to populations that move near continuously during lengthy DWI scans.

References

1. Behrens, T., Woolrich, M., Jenkinson, M., Johansen-Berg, H., Nunes, R., Clare, S., Matthews, P., Brady, J., Smith, S.: Characterization and propagation of uncertainty in diffusion-weighted MR imaging. Magn. Reson. Med. **50**, 1077–1088 (2003)
2. Scherrer, B., Schwartzman, A., Taquet, M., Sahin, M., Prabhu, S.P., Warfield, S.K.: Characterizing brain tissue by assessment of the distribution of anisotropic microstructural environments in diffusion-compartment imaging (DIAMOND). Magn. Reson. Med. **76**, 963–977 (2015)
3. Setsompop, K., Gagoski, B., Polimeni, J., Witzel, T., Wedeen, V., Wald, L.: Blipped-controlled aliasing in parallel imaging for simultaneous multislice echo planar imaging with reduced g-factor penalty. Magn. Reson. Med. **67**, 1210–1224 (2012)
4. Sotiropoulos, S.N., Jbabdi, S., Xu, J., Andersson, J.L., Moeller, S., Auerbach, E.J., Glasser, M.F., Hernandez, M., Sapiro, G., Jenkinson, M., et al.: Advances in diffusion MRI acquisition and processing in the human connectome project. Neuroimage **80**, 125–143 (2013)
5. Zaitsev, M., Maclaren, J., Herbst, M.: Motion artifacts in MRI: a complex problem with many partial solutions. J. Magn. Reson. Imaging **42**(4), 887–901 (2015)
6. Elhabian, S., Gur, Y., Vachet, C., Piven, J., Styner, M., Leppert, I.R., Pike, G.B., Gerig, G.: Subject-motion correction in HARDI acquisitions: choices and consequences. Front Neurol. **5**, 240 (2014)
7. Kober, T., Gruetter, R., Krueger, G.: Prospective and retrospective motion correction in diffusion magnetic resonance imaging of the human brain. Neuroimage **59**(1), 389–398 (2012)
8. Jiang, S., Xue, H., Counsell, S., Anjari, M., Allsop, J., Rutherford, M., Rueckert, D., Hajnal, J.: Diffusion tensor imaging of the brain in moving subjects: application to in-utero fetal and ex-utero studies. Magn. Reson. Med. **62**, 645–655 (2009)
9. Oubel, E., Koob, M., Studholme, C., Dietemann, J.L., Rousseau, F.: Reconstruction of scattered data in fetal diffusion MRI. Med. Image Anal. **16**(1), 28–37 (2012)
10. Fogtmann, M., Seshamani, S., Kroenke, C., Cheng, X., Chapman, T., Wilm, J., Rousseau, F., Studholme, C.: A unified approach to diffusion direction sensitive slice registration and 3-D DTI reconstruction from moving fetal brain anatomy. IEEE Trans. Med. Imaging **33**(2), 272–289 (2014)

11. Marami, B., Scherrer, B., Afacan, O., Erem, B., Warfield, S., Gholipour, A.: Motion-robust diffusion-weighted brain MRI reconstruction through slice-level registration-based motion tracking. IEEE Trans. Med. Imaging (2016, in press)
12. Agamennoni, G., Nieto, J., Nebot, E., et al.: Approximate inference in state-space models with heavy-tailed noise. IEEE Trans. Signal Process. **60**(10), 5024–5037 (2012)
13. Li, Y., Shea, S.M., Lorenz, C.H., Jiang, H., Chou, M.C., Mori, S.: Image corruption detection in diffusion tensor imaging for post-processing and real-time monitoring. PLOS ONE **8**(10), e49764 (2013)
14. Powell, M.J.: The BOBYQA algorithm for bound constrained optimization without derivatives. Cambridge NA report NA2009/06, University of Cambridge (2009)

Self Super-Resolution for Magnetic Resonance Images

Amod Jog[1(✉)], Aaron Carass[1,2], and Jerry L. Prince[1]

[1] Department of Electrical and Computer Engineering, Baltimore, USA
{amodjog,aaron_carass,prince}@jhu.edu
[2] Department of Computer Science, Johns Hopkins University, Baltimore, USA
http://www.iacl.ece.jhu.edu

Abstract. It is faster and therefore cheaper to acquire magnetic resonance images (MRI) with higher in-plane resolution than through-plane resolution. The low resolution of such acquisitions can be increased using post-processing techniques referred to as super-resolution (SR) algorithms. SR is known to be an ill-posed problem. Most state-of-the-art SR algorithms rely on the presence of external/training data to learn a transform that converts low resolution input to a higher resolution output. In this paper an SR approach is presented that is not dependent on any external training data and is only reliant on the acquired image. Patches extracted from the acquired image are used to estimate a set of new images, where each image has increased resolution along a particular direction. The final SR image is estimated by combining images in this set via the technique of Fourier Burst Accumulation. Our approach was validated on simulated low resolution MRI images, and showed significant improvement in image quality and segmentation accuracy when compared to competing SR methods. SR of FLuid Attenuated Inversion Recovery (FLAIR) images with lesions is also demonstrated.

Keywords: Super-resolution · MRI · Self-generated training data

1 Introduction

Spatial resolution is one of the most important imaging parameters for magnetic resonance imaging (MRI). The choice of spatial resolution in MRI is dictated by many factors such as imaging time, desired signal to noise ratio, and dimensions of the structures to be imaged. Spatial resolution—or simply, the resolution—of MRI is decided by the extent of the Fourier space acquired. Digital resolution is decided by the number of voxels that are used to reconstruct the image; it can be changed by upsampling via interpolation. However, interpolation by itself does not add to the frequency content of the image. Super-resolution (SR) is the process by which we can estimate high frequency information that is lost when a low resolution image is acquired.

MRI images are typically acquired with an anisotropic voxel size; usually with a high in-plane resolution (small voxel lengths) and a low through-plane

© Springer International Publishing AG 2016
S. Ourselin et al. (Eds.): MICCAI 2016, Part III, LNCS 9902, pp. 553–560, 2016.
DOI: 10.1007/978-3-319-46726-9_64

resolution (large slice thickness). Such images are upsampled to isotropic digital resolution using interpolation. Interpolation of low resolution images causes partial volume artifacts that affect segmentation and need to be accounted for [1]. SR for natural images has been a rich area of research in the computer vision community [3,11,14]. There has been a significant amount of research in SR for medical images, especially neuroimaging [7,8]. Since SR is an ill-posed problem, a popular way to perform SR in MRI is to use example-based super-resolution. Initially proposed by Rousseau [8], example-based methods leverage the high resolution information extracted from a high resolution (HR) image in conjunction with a low resolution (LR) input image to generate an SR version approximating the HR image. A number of approaches have followed up on this idea by using self-similarity [6] and a generative model [5]. However, these methods are reliant on external data that may not be readily available.

Single image SR methods [4] downsample the given LR image to create an even lower resolution image LLR and learn the mapping from the LLR image to the LR image. This mapping is then applied to the LR to generate an SR image. This approach has seen use in MRI [9] where HR and LR dictionaries were trained to learn the LR-HR mapping. However, even these methods depend on learning their dictionaries on external LR-HR training images and are not truly "single image" methods. They assume that the test LR image is a representative sample of the training data, which may not always be the case.

In this paper, we propose a method that only uses information from the available LR image to estimate its SR image. Our approach—called Self Superresolution (SSR)—takes advantage of the fact that in an anisotropic acquisition, the in-plane resolution is higher than the through-plane resolution. SSR comprises two steps: (1) We generate new additional images, each of which is LR along a certain direction, but is HR in the plane normal to it. Thus, each new image contributes information to a new region in the Fourier space. (2) We combine these images in the Fourier space via Fourier Burst Accumulation [2]. We describe the algorithm in Sect. 2. In Sect. 3 we validate SSR results using image quality and tissue classification. We also demonstrate SR on Magnetization Prepared Gradient Echo (MPRAGE) and FLAIR images and show visually improved image appearance and tissue segmentation in the presence of white matter lesions.

2   Method

Background: Fourier Burst Accumulation. The motivation for our approach is from a recent image deblurring method devised by Delbracio et al. [2] called Fourier Burst Accumulation (FBA). Given a series of images of the same scene acquired in the burst mode of a digital camera, FBA was used to recover a single high resolution image with reduced noise. Each of the burst images is blurred due to random motion blur introduced by hand tremors and the blurring directions are independent of each other. Let $\mathbf{x}$ be the true high resolution image of the scene. Let $\mathbf{y}_i$, $i \in \{1, \ldots, N\}$ be the ith observed image in the burst which is blurred in a random direction with kernel $\mathbf{h}_i$. The observation model for $\mathbf{y}_i$, is $\mathbf{y}_i = \mathbf{h}_i * \mathbf{x} + \boldsymbol{\sigma}_i$, where $\boldsymbol{\sigma}_i$ is the additive noise in the ith image. For a non-negative parameter p, the FBA estimate $\hat{\mathbf{x}}_p(j)$ at voxel j is obtained by,

$$\hat{\mathbf{x}}_p(j) = \mathcal{F}^{-1}\left[\sum_{i=1}^{N} \mathbf{w}_i(\omega)\mathbf{Y}_i(\omega)\right](j), \tag{1}$$

where $\mathbf{w}_i(\omega)$ are weights calculated for each frequency ω, and $\mathbf{Y}_i(\omega) = \mathcal{F}(\mathbf{y}_i)$ are the Fourier transforms of the observed burst images, $\mathbf{y}_i$. Simply put, the Fourier transform of the high resolution image $\mathbf{x}$ is a weighted average of the Fourier transforms $\mathbf{Y}_i(\omega)$ of the input burst images. The weights are given by,

$$\mathbf{w}_i(\omega) = \frac{|\mathbf{Y}_i(\omega)|^p}{\sum_{i=1}^{N} |\mathbf{Y}_i(\omega)|^p}, \tag{2}$$

which determines the contribution of $\mathbf{Y}_i(\omega)$ at the frequency ω. If the magnitude of $\mathbf{Y}_i(\omega)$ is large, it will dominate the summation. Thus, given LR images blurred independently from the same HR image, an estimate of the underlying HR can be calculated using FBA.

Our Approach: SSR. For the SR of MRI, the input is a LR image $\mathbf{y}_0$ and the expected output is the SR image $\hat{\mathbf{x}}$. We assume that $\mathbf{y}_0$ has low resolution in the through-plane (z) direction and has a higher spatial resolution in the in-plane. Let the spatial resolution of $\mathbf{y}_0$ be $p_x \times p_y \times p_z$ mm^3, and assume that $p_z > p_x = p_y$. In the Fourier space, the extent of the Fourier cube is $[-P_x, P_x]$, where $P_x = 1/2p_x$ mm^{-1} on the ω_x axis, $[-P_y, P_y]$, $P_y = 1/2p_y$ mm^{-1} on the ω_y axis, and $[-P_z, P_z]$ $P_z = 1/2p_z$ mm^{-1} on the ω_z axis. Clearly, $P_z < P_x = P_y$. To improve the resolution in the z direction, it is necessary to widen the Fourier limit on the ω_z axis by estimating the Fourier coefficients for frequencies that are greater than P_z. We use FBA for estimating the Fourier coefficients at these frequencies.

FBA requires multiple images as input and expects that some of the images have the Fourier coefficients in the desired region and uses those to fill in the missing Fourier information. It is impossible to perform FBA with just a single image $\mathbf{y}_0$ as there is no way to estimate the Fourier information outside of $[-P_z, P_z]$ on the ω_z axis. Thus, we need additional images that can provide higher frequency information on the ω_z axis. The first stage in our proposed SR algorithm is to create these additional images through synthesis given only $\mathbf{y}_0$.

Synthesize Intermediate Images: To gain Fourier information from frequencies greater than $|P_z|$, we need images that have non-zero Fourier magnitudes for frequencies that have the ω_z component greater than $|P_z|$. In other words, we need images that are higher resolution in any direction that has a non-zero z component. We propose to use rotated and filtered versions of the available $\mathbf{y}_0$ to generate these images. At the outset, we upsample $\mathbf{y}_0$ to an isotropic $p_x \times p_x \times p_x$ digital resolution using cubic b-spline interpolation. If $\mathbf{x}$ is the underlying true high resolution isotropic image, then we have, $\mathbf{y}_0 = \mathbf{h}_0 * \mathbf{x} + \boldsymbol{\sigma}_0$, where $\mathbf{h}_0$ is the smoothing kernel, which in 2D MRI acquisitions is the inverse Fourier transform of the slice selection pulse. In an ideal case, this is a rect function because the slice selection pulse is assumed to be a sinc function. However, in reality it is usually implemented in the scanner as a truncated sinc.

Given rotation matrices R_i, $i \in \{1, \ldots, N\}$ perform the following steps:

1. Consider an image $R_i(\mathbf{y}_0)$, which is $\mathbf{y}_0$ rotated by a rotation matrix R_i.
2. Next, apply the rotated kernel $R_i(\mathbf{h}_0)$ to $\mathbf{y}_0$ to create $\mathbf{y}_{a0}^i = R_i(\mathbf{h}_0) * \mathbf{y}_0$.
3. Finally, apply the kernel $\mathbf{h}_0$ to $R_i(\mathbf{y}_0)$ to form $\mathbf{y}_{s0}^i = \mathbf{h}_0 * R_i(\mathbf{y}_0)$.

For each rotation matrix R_i, we have two new images $\mathbf{y}_{a0}^i$ and $\mathbf{y}_{s0}^i$. From Step 2 and the definition of $\mathbf{y}_0$ (ignoring the noise), we know that $\mathbf{y}_{a0}^i = R_i(\mathbf{h}_0) * \mathbf{y}_0 = R_i(\mathbf{h}_0) * \mathbf{h}_0 * \mathbf{x}$. We use $\mathbf{y}_{a0}^i$ and $\mathbf{y}_0$ as training images by extracting features from $\mathbf{y}_{a0}^i$ and pairing them with corresponding patches in $\mathbf{y}_0$ and learn the transformation that essentially deconvolves $\mathbf{y}_{a0}^i$ to get $\mathbf{y}_0$. We need to learn this transformation so that we can apply it to $\mathbf{y}_{s0}^i$ and therefore deconvolve it to cancel the effect of convolution by $\mathbf{h}_0$. From Step 3 and the definition of $\mathbf{y}_0$ (ignoring the noise), we know that $\mathbf{y}_{s0}^i = \mathbf{h}_0 * R_i(\mathbf{y}_0) = \mathbf{h}_0 * R_i(\mathbf{h}_0 * \mathbf{x}) = \mathbf{h}_0 * R_i(\mathbf{h}_0) * R_i(\mathbf{x})$. Deconvolving $\mathbf{y}_{a0}^i$ to cancel the effects of $R_i(\mathbf{h}_0)$ is analogous to deconvolving $\mathbf{y}_{s0}^i$ to cancel the effects of $\mathbf{h}_0$, as $\mathbf{y}_{s0}^i$ is also rotated.

With the training pair $\mathbf{y}_{a0}^i$ and $\mathbf{y}_0$, and test image $\mathbf{y}_{s0}^i$, we use a single image SR approach known as Anchored Neighborhood Regression (ANR) [11] to learn the desired transformation. ANR was shown to be effective in 2D super-resolution of natural images with better results than some of the state-of-the-art methods [3,14]. ANR is computationally very fast as opposed to most other SR methods [11], which is a highly desirable feature in our setting. In brief, ANR creates training data from $\mathbf{y}_{a0}^i$ and $\mathbf{y}_0$ by calculating the first and the second gradient images of $\mathbf{y}_{a0}^i$ in all three directions using the Sobel and Laplacian filters respectively. At voxel location j a 3D patch is extracted from each of these gradient images and concatenated to form a feature vector $\mathbf{f}_j(\mathbf{y}_{a0}^i)$. ANR uses PCA to reduce the dimensionality of the feature to the order of $\sim 10^2$. In our case, we do not extract continuous voxels as the LR acquisition means neighboring voxels are highly correlated. Our patch dimensions are linearly proportional to the amount of relative blurring in the x, y, and z directions in $\mathbf{y}_0$. This means that patches are cuboids in shape and are longer in the dimension where the blurring is higher. We then calculate the difference image $\mathbf{y}_{a0d}^i = \mathbf{y}_0 - \mathbf{y}_{a0}^i$ and the extracted patch $\mathbf{g}_j(\mathbf{y}_{a0d}^i)$ and pair it with $\mathbf{f}_j(\mathbf{y}_{a0}^i)$ to create the training data. Next, ANR jointly learns paired high resolution and low resolution dictionaries, using the K-SVD algorithm. The atoms of the learned dictionary are regarded as cluster centers with each feature vector $\mathbf{f}_j(\mathbf{y}0_{a0}^i)$ being assigned to one based on the correlation between feature vectors and centers. Cluster centers and their associated feature vectors are used to estimate a projection matrix P_k for every cluster k, by solving a least squares problem such that, $P_k \mathbf{f}_j(\mathbf{y}_{a0}^i) = \mathbf{g}_j(\mathbf{y}_{a0d}^i)$. Given an input test image, $\mathbf{y}_{s0}^i$, feature vectors $\mathbf{f}_j(\mathbf{y}_{s0}^i)$ are computed and a cluster center is assigned based on the arg max of the correlation, following which, the stored P_k is applied to estimate the patch $\hat{\mathbf{g}}_j$ at voxel j in the newly created image $\hat{\mathbf{y}}_i$. Overlapping patches are predicted and the overlapping voxels have

Algorithm 1. SSR

Data: LR image $\mathbf{y}_0$

Upsample $\mathbf{y}_0$ to isotropic digital resolution

Based on the spatial resolution of $\mathbf{y}_0$, calculate $\mathbf{h}_0$, the slice selection filter

for i=1:N **do**

    Construct a rotation matrix R_i and apply to $\mathbf{y}_0$ to form the rotated image $R_i(\mathbf{y}_0)$

    Apply R_i to $\mathbf{h}_0$ to form the rotated filter $R_i(\mathbf{h}_0)$

    Generate $\mathbf{y}^i_{a0} = R_i(\mathbf{h}_0) * \mathbf{y}_0$

    Generate $\mathbf{y}^i_{s0} = \mathbf{h}_0 * R_i(\mathbf{y}_0)$

    Use ANR to synthesize $\hat{\mathbf{y}}_i = \text{ANR}(\mathbf{y}^i_{a0}, \mathbf{y}_0, \mathbf{y}^i_{s0})$

end for

Apply FBA to get, $\hat{\mathbf{x}}_p = \text{FBA}(\mathbf{y}_0, R_1^{-1}(\hat{\mathbf{y}}_1), \ldots, R_N^{-1}(\hat{\mathbf{y}}_N), p)$

---

their intensities averaged to produce the final output $\hat{\mathbf{y}}_i$. This modified ANR is carried out to estimate each $\hat{\mathbf{y}}_i$ where the rotation matrices can be chosen intelligently to cover the Fourier space. ANR on its own can only add information in a single direction of the Fourier domain. However, when run in multiple directions, we are able to add coefficients for more frequencies in the Fourier space. We rotate $\hat{\mathbf{y}}_i$ back to their original orientation to get them in the same reference frame. We can now use FBA on the set $\{\mathbf{y}_0, R_1^{-1}(\hat{\mathbf{y}}_1), \ldots, R_N^{-1}(\hat{\mathbf{y}}_N)\}$ to estimate the SR result $\hat{\mathbf{x}}$ that accumulates Fourier information from all these images to enhance the resolution. Our algorithm is summarized in Algorithm 1.

3   Results

Validation: Super-resolution of T_1***-weighted Images.*** Our dataset consists of T_1-weighted MPRAGE images from 20 subjects of the Neuromorphometrics dataset. The resolution of images in this dataset is 1 mm^3 isotropic and we consider this our HR dataset. We create LR images by modeling a slice selection filter ($\mathbf{h}_0$) based on a slice selection pulse modeled as a truncated sinc function. The slice selection filter itself looks like a jagged rect function. We create LR datasets with slice thicknesses of 2 and 3 mm. The in-plane resolution remains 1×1 mm^2.

Using these LR datasets, we generated SR images and evaluated their quality using peak signal to noise ratio (PSNR) that directly compares them with the original HR images. We also evaluated the sharpness in the SR images by calculating a sharpness metric known as S3 [13]. We compare our algorithm against trilinear and cubic b-spline interpolation, ANR, and non-local means (NLM)-based upsampling [7].

For our algorithm, we use a base patch-size of $4 \times 4 \times 4$, which is multiplied by the blurring factor in each dimension to create a different-sized patch for each direction. We have used $N = 9$ rotation matrices ($\Rightarrow$ 9 synthetic LR images in a particular direction which are HR in the perpendicular plane). The number of dictionary elements used in ANR was 128. Table 1 details the comparison done using the PSNR metric calculated over 20 subjects. As can be seen, our algorithm

Table 1. Mean PSNR values (dB).

LR (mm)	Lin.	BSP	ANR	NLM	SSR
2	35.64	35.99	36.55	36.21	37.98*
3	31.20	31.98	26.80	32.71	33.49*

Table 2. Mean S3 values.

Lin.	BSP	ANR	NLM	SSR	HR
0.43	0.39	0.47	0.49	0.65*	0.81
0.40	0.39	0.48	0.45	0.61*	0.81

The '*' indicates that SSR results are statistically significantly greater than all the methods using a one-tailed t-test and Wilcoxon rank-sum tests for PSNR and S3 metrics.

Table 3. Mean Dice overlap scores with ground truth HR classifications for WM, GM, CSF, and ventricles, over 20 subjects.

LR (mm)	Method	Mean tissue dice coefficients			
		WM	GM	CSF	Ven.
2	BSP	0.960	0.949	0.950	0.941
	ANR	0.926	0.795	0.396	0.881
	NLM	0.921	0.791	0.391	0.871
	SSR	0.973*	0.960*	0.957*	0.959*
3	BSP	0.891	0.773	0.405	0.832
	ANR	0.877	0.782	0.490	0.846
	NLM	0.898	0.773	0.379	0.843
	SSR	0.916*	0.811*	0.510*	0.875*

The '*' indicates that SSR results are statistically significantly greater than all the methods using a one-tailed t-test and Wilcoxon rank-sum tests for PSNR and S3 metrics.

outperforms the interpolation methods and ANR statistically significantly (using one-tailed t-test and Wilcoxon rank sum tests) in all the LR datasets. Table 2 shows the S3 values which are the highest for SSR.

In the second part of this experiment, we performed segmentation of the HR, LR, and, SR images. In the absence of HR data, we want to show that it is beneficial to apply our algorithm and use the SR images for further processing. We use an in-house implementation of the atlas-based EM algorithm for classification proposed by Van Leemput et al. [12], that we refer to as AtlasEM, which provides white matter (WM), gray matter (GM), sulcal cerebrospinal fluid (CSF), and ventricles (Ven). For each of the 2 and 3 mm LR datasets, we run AtlasEM on (1) cubic b-spline interpolated images, (2) SR images produced by ANR, NLM, and SSR, and (3) available HR images. The HR classifications are used as ground truth against which we compare other results using Dice overlap coefficients. Our observations are recorded in Table 3.

For each of the tissues we demonstrate a significant increase in the Dice, for both LR datasets. The HR, BSP, and different SR results for both the datasets are shown in the top row of Fig. 1. The SSR results are visually sharper as the fine details on the cortex and the tissue boundaries are more apparent. The classifications are shown in the bottom row of Fig. 1. The classification near the cortex and tissue boundaries is better in the SR image than the rest.

HR	BSP (2 mm)	ANR (2 mm)	NLM (2 mm)	SSR (2 mm)

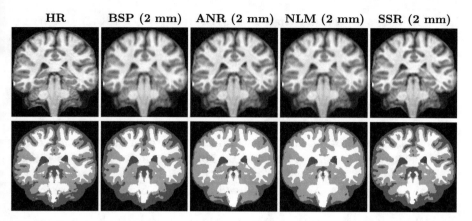

Fig. 1. On the top row from left to right are coronal views of the original HR image, cubic bspline (BSP) interpolated image of the 2 mm LR image, ANR, NLM, and our SSR results. In the bottom row are their respective tissue classifications.

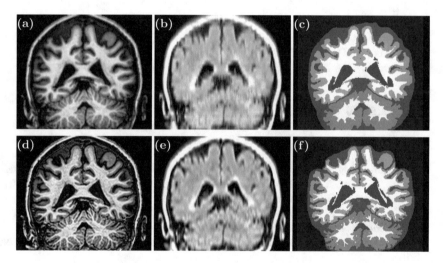

Fig. 2. (a) Interpolated MPRAGE, (b) Interpolated FLAIR, (c) segmentation of interpolated images, (d) SSR MPRAGE, (e) SSR FLAIR, and (f) segmentation of SSR images.

SR of MPRAGE and FLAIR Images. In this section, we describe an application where we use SSR to improve the resolution of FLAIR images that were acquired in a 2D acquisition with a slice thickness of 4.4 mm whereas the axial resolution was 0.828×0.828 mm^3. The MPRAGE images were also anisotropic with a resolution of $0.828 \times 0.828 \times 1.17$ mm^3. These FLAIR images were acquired on multiple sclerosis subjects that present with white matter lesions that appear hyperintense. We generated isotropic SSR MPRAGE (Fig. 2(d)) and SSR FLAIR (Fig. 2(e)). In Figs. 2(a) and (b) are their interpolated counterparts.

The SSR images are visually sharper than the interpolated LR images. We ran a brain and lesion segmentation algorithm [10] that shows a crisper cortex and lesion segmentation for the SSR images, but we cannot validate these results due to lack of ground truth data.

4   Discussion and Conclusions

We have described SSR, an MRI super-resolution approach that uses the existing high frequency information in the given LR image to estimate Fourier coefficients of higher frequency ranges where it is absent. SSR is fast (15 mins) and needs minimal preprocessing. We have validated SSR terms of image quality metrics and segmentation accuracy. We have also demonstrated an application of FLAIR and MPRAGE SR that can potentially improve segmentation in the cortex and lesions. It is therefore an ideal replacement for interpolation.

References

1. Ballester, M.A.G., et al.: Estimation of the partial volume effect in MRI. Med. Image Anal. **6**(4), 389–405 (2002)
2. Delbracio, M., Sapiro, G.: Removing camera shake via weighted fourier burst accumulation. IEEE Trans. Image Proc. **24**(11), 3293–3307 (2015)
3. Freeman, W.T., et al.: Example-based super-resolution. IEEE Comput. Graph. Appl. **22**(2), 56–65 (2002)
4. Huang, J.B., et al.: Single image super-resolution from transformed self-exemplars. In: IEEE Conference on Computer Vision and Pattern Recognition) (2015)
5. Konukoglu, E., van der Kouwe, A., Sabuncu, M.R., Fischl, B.: Example-based restoration of high-resolution magnetic resonance image acquisitions. In: Mori, K., Sakuma, I., Sato, Y., Barillot, C., Navab, N. (eds.) MICCAI 2013, Part I. LNCS, vol. 8149, pp. 131–138. Springer, Heidelberg (2013)
6. Manjón, J.V., et al.: MRI superresolution using self-similarity and image priors. Int. J. Biomed. Imaging **425891**, 11 (2010)
7. Manjón, J.V., et al.: Non-local MRI upsampling. Med. Image Anal. **14**(6), 784–792 (2010)
8. Rousseau, F.: Brain hallucination. In: Forsyth, D., Torr, P., Zisserman, A. (eds.) ECCV 2008, Part I. LNCS, vol. 5302, pp. 497–508. Springer, Heidelberg (2008)
9. Rueda, A., et al.: Single-image super-resolution of brain MR images using over-complete dictionaries. Med. Image Anal. **17**(1), 113–132 (2013)
10. Shiee, N., et al.: A topology-preserving approach to the segmentation of brain images with multiple sclerosis lesions. Neuroimage **49**(2), 1524–1535 (2010)
11. Timofte, R., et al.: Anchored neighborhood regression for fast example-based super-resolution. ICCV **2013**, 1920–1927 (2013)
12. Van Leemput, K., et al.: Automated model-based tissue classification of MR images of the brain. IEEE Trans. Med. Imag. **18**(10), 897–908 (1999)
13. Vu, C.T., et al.: S3: a spectral and spatial measure of local perceived sharpness in natural images. IEEE Trans. Image Proc. **21**(3), 934–945 (2012)
14. Yang, J., et al.: Image super-resolution via sparse representation. IEEE Trans. Image Proc. **19**(11), 2861–2873 (2010)

Tight Graph Framelets for Sparse Diffusion MRI q-Space Representation

Pew-Thian Yap[1(✉)], Bin Dong[2], Yong Zhang[3], and Dinggang Shen[1]

[1] Department of Radiology and BRIC,
University of North Carolina, Chapel Hill, USA
ptyap@med.unc.edu
[2] Beijing International Center for Mathematical Research,
Peking University, Beijing, China
[3] Department of Psychiatry and Behavioral Sciences,
Stanford University, Stanford, USA

Abstract. In diffusion MRI, the outcome of estimation problems can often be improved by taking into account the correlation of diffusion-weighted images scanned with neighboring wavevectors in q-space. For this purpose, we propose in this paper to employ tight wavelet frames constructed on non-flat domains for multi-scale sparse representation of diffusion signals. This representation is well suited for signals sampled regularly or irregularly, such as on a grid or on multiple shells, in q-space. Using spectral graph theory, the frames are constructed based on quasi-affine systems (i.e., generalized dilations and shifts of a finite collection of wavelet functions) defined on graphs, which can be seen as a discrete representation of manifolds. The associated wavelet analysis and synthesis transforms can be computed efficiently and accurately without the need for explicit eigen-decomposition of the graph Laplacian, allowing scalability to very large problems. We demonstrate the effectiveness of this representation, generated using what we call *tight graph framelets*, in two specific applications: denoising and super-resolution in q-space using ℓ_0 regularization. The associated optimization problem involves only thresholding and solving a trivial inverse problem in an iterative manner. The effectiveness of graph framelets is confirmed via evaluation using synthetic data with noncentral chi noise and real data with repeated scans.

1 Introduction

Diffusion-weighted MR signals, in addition to the diffusion time, are controlled by a quantity called wavevector. The wavevector is dependent on the length, strength, and orientation of the gradient pulses during the measurement sequence. It is often denoted as vector $\mathbf{q}$, which can be separated into a scalar wavenumber $|\mathbf{q}|$ and a diffusion encoding direction $\hat{\mathbf{q}} = \mathbf{q}/|\mathbf{q}|$. The effects of

---

This work was supported in part by NIH grants (NS093842, EB006733, EB008374, EB009634, AG041721, and MH100217).

S. Ourselin et al. (Eds.): MICCAI 2016, Part III, LNCS 9902, pp. 561–569, 2016.
DOI: 10.1007/978-3-319-46726-9_65

both diffusion time, t, and wavenumber are summarized using a quantity called b-value, which is defined as $b = t|\mathbf{q}|^2$. A diffusion MRI protocol normally acquires multiple diffusion-weighted images, each corresponding to a wavevector $\mathbf{q}$ in q-space. For example, in shell acquisition schemes, b is fixed by fixing both t and $|\mathbf{q}|$ and only the gradient direction varies among measurements. This can be extended to multi-shell acquisition, where the measurements are collected at shells of different b-values. These images afford microstructural information that can be harnessed for tissue characterization and axonal tracing.

Due to the noisy nature of diffusion MRI, it is often beneficial to leverage the correlation between diffusion-weighted images acquired with neighboring wavevectors in q-space for improving estimation robustness in applications such as denoising and compressed-sensing reconstruction. To achieve this, a common practice is by fitting a diffusion model to the data, concurrently taking into account all q-space measurements at each voxel. Such approach, however, is dependent on specific assumptions the model makes regarding the data. For example, the diffusion tensor model assumes that the signals at each voxel reflect only axon bundles that are aligned in one coherent direction, hence falling short in capturing the complexity of the water diffusion patterns in the human brain.

In this paper, we take a wavelet-based approach, which is less dependent on specific biophysical assumptions, to constructing sparse representations for diffusion signals. To cater to the fact that q-space sampling schemes can differ significantly, ranging from Cartesian sampling in diffusion spectrum imaging (DSI) to multi-shell sampling with multiple distinct b-values, we propose to represent the q-space signals using tight wavelet frames defined on graphs [1, 2], which can be flexibly adapted to different sampling domains. The power of tight wavelet frames lies in their ability to sparsely approximate piecewise smooth functions and the existence of fast decomposition and reconstruction algorithms associated with them. A wide range of tight wavelet frames can be generated conveniently using the unitary extension principle (UEP) [3]. We use the term *tight graph framelets* to denote basic functions that, when dilated and shifted, form tight wavelet frames on graphs. Tight graph framelets have compact support, are not restricted to signals of a certain shape (e.g., the "donut" [4]), and provide a natural bridge between continuous and discrete representations [1].

We demonstrate the utility and effectiveness of tight graph framelets in two specific applications: denoising and super-resolution reconstruction in q-space. To take advantage of the high redundancy of graph framelets, we regularize the associated problems using a sparse-inducing norm. Instead of the more conventional ℓ_1 regularization, which has been shown in the theory of compressed sensing to produce sparse solutions, we opted to use the ℓ_0-"norm". In [5], both iterative soft and hard thresholding algorithms were adopted and the latter was found to achieve better image quality. In [6], wavelet frame based ℓ_0 regularization also shows better edge-preserving quality compared with the conventional ℓ_1 regularization. Evaluation performed using synthetic data with noncentral chi signal distribution as well as real data with repeated scans indicates that the proposed method is superior to denoising and interpolation using spherical radial basis functions (sRBF) [7].

2 Approach

2.1 Graph Framelets

In q-space, sampling points and their relationships can be encoded, respectively, using vertices and edges of a graph. We denote a graph by $\mathcal{G} := \{\mathcal{E}, \mathcal{V}, w\}$, where $\mathcal{V} := \{v_k \in \mathcal{M} : k = 1, \ldots, K\}$ is a set of vertices representing points on a manifold $\mathcal{M}$, $\mathcal{E} \subset \mathcal{V} \times \mathcal{V}$ is a set of edges relating the vertices, and $w : \mathcal{E} \mapsto \mathbb{R}^+$ is a weight function. The associated adjacency matrix $\mathcal{A} := (w_{k,k'})$ is symmetric with $w_{k,k'} > 0$ if v_k and $v_{k'}$ are connected by an edge in $\mathcal{E}$; otherwise $w_{k,k'} = 0$. Given the degree matrix $D := \mathrm{diag}\{d[1], d[2], \ldots, d[K]\}$, where $d[k] := \sum_{k'} w_{k,k'}$, the graph Laplacian, defined as $\mathcal{L} := D - W$, is consistent with the Laplace-Beltrami operator of the manifold [8]. Denote by $\{\lambda_k, u_k\}_{k=0}^{K-1}$ the pairs of eigenvalues and eigenvectors of $\mathcal{L}$ with $0 = \lambda_0 \leq \lambda_1 \leq \lambda_2 \leq \ldots \leq \lambda_{K-1} = \lambda_{\max}$. The eigenvectors form an orthonormal basis for all functions on the graph: $\langle u_k, u_{k'} \rangle := \sum_{n=1}^{K} u_k[n] u_{k'}[n] = \delta_{k,k'}$. The Fourier transform of a function $f_\mathcal{G} : \mathcal{V} \mapsto \mathbb{R}$ on the graph $\mathcal{G}$ is given by $\widehat{f_\mathcal{G}}[k] := \sum_{n=0}^{K-1} f_\mathcal{G}[n] u_k[n]$.

Table 1. Framelet masks.

Haar	Linear	Quadratic
$\widehat{a}_0(\xi) = \cos(\xi/2)$	$\widehat{a}_0(\xi) = \cos^2(\xi/2)$	$\widehat{a}_0(\xi) = \cos^3(\xi/2)$
$\widehat{a}_1(\xi) = \sin(\xi/2)$	$\widehat{a}_1(\xi) = \frac{1}{\sqrt{2}} \sin(\xi)$	$\widehat{a}_1(\xi) = \sqrt{3} \sin(\xi/2) \cos^2(\xi/2)$
	$\widehat{a}_2(\xi) = \sin^2(\xi/2)$	$\widehat{a}_2(\xi) = \sqrt{3} \sin^2(\xi/2) \cos(\xi/2)$
		$\widehat{a}_3(\xi) = \sin^3(\xi/2)$

The key idea involved in constructing wavelet frames on a graph is to view eigenvectors of the graph Laplacian as Fourier basis on graphs and the associated eigenvalues as frequency components [1,2]. One then slices the frequency spectrum in a multi-scale fashion by using a set of masks $\{\widehat{a}_r(\cdot) : r = 0, \ldots, R\}$, where $\widehat{a}_0(\cdot)$ acts as a low-pass filter and $\widehat{a}_r(\cdot)$ with $0 < r \leq R$ as band-pass or high-pass filters. More specifically, the graph framelet analysis transform is defined as $\mathbf{W} f_\mathcal{G} := \{W_{l,r} f_\mathcal{G} : (l, r) \in \mathcal{B}_L\}$, with $\mathcal{B}_L := \{(1,1), (1,2), \ldots, (1,R), (2,1), \ldots, (L,R)\} \cup \{(L,0)\}$ and

$$\widehat{W_{l,r} f_\mathcal{G}}[k] := \begin{cases} \widehat{a}_r(\gamma^{-L+1}\tilde{\lambda}_k)\widehat{f_\mathcal{G}}[k] & l = 1, \\ \widehat{a}_r(\gamma^{-L+l}\tilde{\lambda}_k)\widehat{a}_0(\gamma^{-L+l-1}\tilde{\lambda}_k) \cdots \widehat{a}_0(\gamma^{-L+1}\tilde{\lambda}_k)\widehat{f_\mathcal{G}}[k] & 2 \leq l \leq L, \end{cases} \tag{1}$$

where $\tilde{\lambda}_k = \lambda_k/\lambda_{\max}$ and $\gamma > 1$ is the dilation factor. Noting the eigen-decomposition $\mathcal{L} = U \Lambda U^\top$, where $\Lambda = \mathrm{diag}\{\lambda_0, \lambda_1, \ldots, \lambda_{K-1}\}$, we have

$$W_{l,r} := \begin{cases} U \widehat{\Omega}_r(\gamma^{-L+1}\tilde{\Lambda}) U^\top & l = 1, \\ U \widehat{\Omega}_r(\gamma^{-L+l}\tilde{\Lambda}) \widehat{\Omega}_0(\gamma^{-L+l-1}\tilde{\Lambda}) \cdots \widehat{\Omega}_0(\gamma^{-L+1}\tilde{\Lambda}) U^\top & 2 \leq l \leq L, \end{cases} \tag{2}$$

where $\tilde{\Lambda} = \mathrm{diag}\{\tilde{\lambda}_0, \tilde{\lambda}_1, \ldots, \tilde{\lambda}_{K-1}\}$ and

$$\hat{\Omega}_r(\beta\tilde{\Lambda}) = \mathrm{diag}\{\hat{a}_r(\beta\tilde{\lambda}_0), \hat{a}_r(\beta\tilde{\lambda}_1), \ldots, \hat{a}_r(\beta\tilde{\lambda}_{K-1})\}. \tag{3}$$

Letting $\boldsymbol{\alpha} := \mathbf{W}f_{\mathcal{G}} := \{\alpha_{r,l} := W_{l,r}f_{\mathcal{G}} : (l,r) \in \mathcal{B}_L\}$ and if the masks satisfy $\sum_{r=0}^{R} |\hat{a}_r(\xi)|^2 = 1$, which is one of the requirements of the unitary extension principle (UEP) [1,3]), it is easy to show that the synthesis transform $\mathbf{W}^\top\boldsymbol{\alpha}$ gives $\mathbf{W}^\top\boldsymbol{\alpha} = \mathbf{W}^\top\mathbf{W}f_{\mathcal{G}} = If_{\mathcal{G}} = f_{\mathcal{G}}$. To avoid explicit decomposition of a potentially large Laplacian matrix, we approximate the masks using Chebyshev polynomials, i.e., $\hat{a}_r(\xi) = \mathcal{T}_r^n(\xi)$, where $\mathcal{T}_r^n(\xi) = \frac{1}{2}c_{r,0} + \sum_{k=1}^{n-1} c_{r,k}T_k(\xi)$ with $T_k(\xi)$ being the k-th order Chebyshev polynomial and

$$c_{r,k} = \frac{2}{\pi} \int_0^\pi \cos(k\theta)\hat{a}_r\left(\frac{\pi}{2}(\cos\theta + 1)\right) d\theta. \tag{4}$$

Equation (2) can be shown to be equivalent to

$$W_{r,l} := \begin{cases} \mathcal{T}_r^n(\gamma^{-L+1}\mathcal{L}) & l = 1, \\ \mathcal{T}_r^n(\gamma^{-L+l}\mathcal{L})\mathcal{T}_r^n(\gamma^{-L+l-1}\mathcal{L})\cdots\mathcal{T}_r^n(\gamma^{-L+1}\mathcal{L}) & 2 \le l \le L. \end{cases} \tag{5}$$

Note the interchange between scalar-valued and matrix-valued polynomials. See [1,2] for more details. Some examples of framelet masks are shown in Table 1.

2.2   Sparse Recovery

Given the observation vector $f \in \mathbb{R}^{K'}$, we are interested in recovering $u \in \mathbb{R}^K$ by solving the following problem:

$$\min_u \left\{ \phi(u) = \|Au - f\|_{2,\mathcal{G}}^2 + \sum_{(l,r)\in\mathcal{B}_L} \lambda_{l,r} \|W_{l,r}u\|_{0,\mathcal{G}} \right\}, \tag{6}$$

where $\|\bullet\|_{2,\mathcal{G}}^2 := \sum_i^{K'} (\bullet[i])^2 d[k_i]$ and $\|\bullet\|_{0,\mathcal{G}} := \sum_{k=1}^{K} \mathcal{I}(\bullet[k])d[k]$ with $\mathcal{I}(z)$ being an indicator function that returns 1 when $z \neq 0$ or 0 otherwise. Here, u is defined on $\mathcal{G}$ with degree matrix $D := \mathrm{diag}\{d[1], d[2], \ldots, d[K]\}$. The observation vector f is defined in relation to a subset of vertices of $\mathcal{G}$, indexed by $\{k_i : i = 1, \ldots, K'\}$. We let $D' := \mathrm{diag}\{d[k_1], d[k_2], \ldots, d[k_{K'}]\}$. K' and K are in general not necessarily equal. We require $K' \le K$.

The problem (6) can be solved effectively using penalty decomposition (PD) [6,9]. Defining auxiliary variables $v := (v_{l,r}) := (W_{l,r}u)$, this amounts to minimizing the following objective function with respect to u and v:

$$L_\mu(u,v) = \|Au - f\|_{2,\mathcal{G}}^2 + \sum_{(l,r)\in\mathcal{B}_L} \lambda_{l,r} \|v_{l,r}\|_{0,\mathcal{G}} + \frac{\mu}{2} \sum_{(l,r)\in\mathcal{B}_L} \|W_{l,r}u - v_{l,r}\|_2^2. \tag{7}$$

In PD, we (i) alternate between solving for u and v using block coordinate descent (BCD). Once this converges, we (ii) increase $\mu > 0$ by a multiplicative factor that is greater than 1 and repeat step (i). This is repeated until increasing μ does not result in further changes to the solution [6,9].

First Subproblem: We solve for v in the first problem, i.e., $\min_v L_\mu(u,v)$:

$$\min_v \sum_{(l,r)\in\mathcal{B}_L} \left\{ \frac{\lambda_{l,r}}{\mu} \|v_{l,r}\|_{0,\mathcal{G}} + \frac{1}{2}\|W_{l,r}u - v_{l,r}\|_2^2 \right\}. \tag{8}$$

The solution can be obtained via hard thresholding [10,11]:

$$v_{l,r}[k] = \begin{cases} (W_{l,r}u)[k] & ((W_{l,r}u)[k])^2 \geq \frac{2\lambda_{l,r}d[k]}{\mu}, \\ 0 & \text{otherwise.} \end{cases} \tag{9}$$

Second Subproblem: By taking the partial derivative of $L_\mu(u,v)$ with respect to u, the solution to the second subproblem, i.e., $\min_u L_\mu(u,v)$, is

$$\left(A^\top D'A + \frac{\mu}{2} \sum_{(l,r)\in\mathcal{B}_L} W_{l,r}^\top W_{l,r} \right) u = A^\top D'f + \frac{\mu}{2} \sum_{(l,r)\in\mathcal{B}_L} W_{l,r}^\top v_{l,r}. \tag{10}$$

Since $\sum_{(l,r)\in\mathcal{B}_L} W_{l,r}^\top W_{l,r} = \mathbf{W}^\top\mathbf{W} = I$, the problem can be simplified to become

$$\left(A^\top D'A + \frac{\mu}{2}I \right) u = A^\top D'f + \frac{\mu}{2} \sum_{(l,r)\in\mathcal{B}_L} W_{l,r}^\top v_{l,r}, \tag{11}$$

which is a set of linear equations that can be solved, for example, using the conjugate gradient method.

2.3 Denoising and Super-Resolution

We are interested in the super-resolution problem of recovering signals when given only a subset of noisy measurements. We partition u as $u = [u_1; u_2] \in \mathbb{R}^K$, where $u_1 \in \mathbb{R}^{K'}$ is defined on vertices whose observed values are given by $f \in \mathbb{R}^{K'}$. No observed values are available for u_2. To recover u, we set in (6) $A = [I_{K'\times K'}\ 0] \in \mathbb{R}^{K'\times K}$, where $I_{K'\times K'}$ is an identity matrix of size $K' \times K'$. When $K' = K$, i.e., $u = u_1$ and $A = I_{K'\times K'}$, the problem reduces to a denoising problem, where we are interested in recovering the noiseless version of f. Since

$$A^\top D'A = [I_{K'\times K'}\ 0]^\top D'[I_{K'\times K'}\ 0] = \begin{bmatrix} D' & 0 \\ 0 & 0 \end{bmatrix}, \tag{12}$$

the resulting matrix on the left of (11) is diagonal and the solution can hence be obtained easily without matrix inversion.

3 Experiments

3.1 Parameter Settings

For all experiments, we used the quadratic masks, set the decomposition level to $L = 5$, and set the maximum order of Chebyshev polynomials to $n = 8$. No significant gain in improvement was obtained beyond these values. The dilation factor was set to a standard value $\gamma = 2$. The tuning parameters for the sparse recovery problem were set as

$$\lambda_{l,r} = \begin{cases} \eta^{-l+1}\lambda & 1 \le l \le L, \ r \ne 0, \\ 0 & l = L, \ r = 0, \end{cases} \tag{13}$$

with $\eta = 0.75$ and $\lambda = \sigma_{\text{noise}}^2 \log(K|\mathcal{B}_L|)$ (i.e., the universal penalty level [12]). We define the adjacency matrix $\mathcal{A} := (w_{k,k'})$ of the q-space samples by letting

$$w_{k,k'} = \exp\left\{ -\frac{3(1 - \hat{\mathbf{q}}_k^\top \hat{\mathbf{q}}_{k'})}{(1 - \cos^2(\theta))} \right\} \exp\left\{ -\frac{(b_{k'} - b_k)^2}{2\sigma_b^2} \right\}, \tag{14}$$

where $\sigma_b = 10$ and θ is set to the maximum of the angles between neighboring gradient directions.

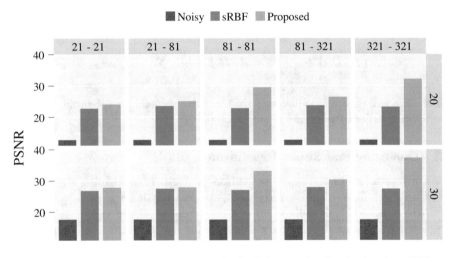

Fig. 1. Performance evaluation in terms of PSNR for two levels of noise, i.e., SNR=20 and 30. We have used here the notation $K' - K$, where K' and K are the numbers of input and output gradient directions, respectively. The standard errors are negligible and are hence not shown here.

3.2   Results

Synthetic Data: We generated a synthetic dataset consisting of a set of voxels with white matter (WM), gray matter (GM), and cerebrospinal fluid (CSF) signal profiles. Combinations of these signal profiles were also included to simulate partial volume effects. To generate the WM signal profiles, mixtures of up to two tensor models were used. The diffusivities for WM, GM, and CSF are respectively $[1.7, 0.3, 0.3] \times 10^{-3} \ \text{mm}^2/\text{s}$, $0.9 \times 10^{-3} \ \text{mm}^2/\text{s}$, and $2.5 \times 10^{-3} \ \text{mm}^2/\text{s}$. The

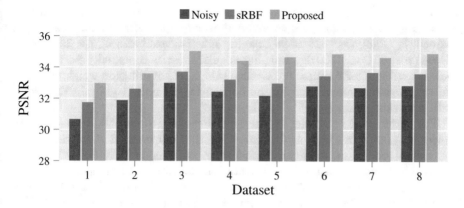

Fig. 2. Performance statistics of the denoising of the real data consisting of 8 repeated sets of diffusion-weighted images.

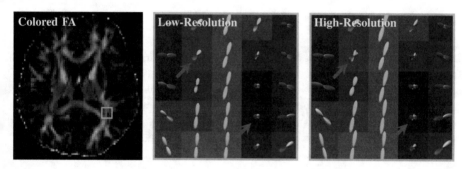

Fig. 3. Fiber ODFs of the low-angular-resolution data with 48 gradient directions and high-angular resolution data with 81 gradient directions. Visible improvements in resolving crossing fibers are marked by the red arrows. (Color figure online)

number of non-collinear gradient directions were 21, 81, and 321, each generated by subdividing the faces of an icosahedron a number of times. Three shells were generated, i.e., $b = 1000, 2000, 3000\,\text{s/mm}^2$. For evaluation, two levels of 32-channel noncentral chi noise [13] was added, corresponding to SNR = 20 and 30 with respect to the non-diffusion-weighted signal of WM.

Results for denoising $(21 - 21, 81 - 81, 321 - 321)$ and super-resolution $(21 - 81, 81 - 321)$, averaged over 10 realizations of noise, are shown in Fig. 1. The comparison baseline is the spherical radial basis function (sRBF) method described in [7]. This basically amounts to weighted averaging of signals on the shells using the weights given by (14). The results confirm that our method yields consistent PSNR improvements. Note that, for both synthetic and real data, noncentral chi bias was removed from the solution of (6) using the method described in [13].

Real Data: The real datasets were acquired using Siemens 3T TRIO MR scanner with $b = 2000 \, \text{s/mm}^2$ and 48 non-collinear gradient directions. The imaging protocol is as follows: 128×96 imaging matrix, voxel size of $2 \times 2 \times 2 \, \text{mm}^3$, TE = 97 ms, TR = 11,300 ms. Imaging acquisition was repeatedly performed on the same subject for 8 times. We averaged the 8 sets of diffusion-weighted images and removed the bias caused by the noncentral chi noise to obtain the ground truth for evaluation.

The performance statistics for the denoising of the 8 sets of diffusion-weighted images are shown in Fig. 2, again confirming that our method yields results that are in close agreement with the ground truth with higher PSNRs. We also show in Fig. 3 the white matter fiber orientation distribution functions (ODFs) to demonstrate the benefit of q-space super-resolution. We used the measurements from the original 48 gradient directions to generate the data for 81 directions. It can be observed from the figure that increasing the angular resolution helps resolve some fiber crossings.

4   Conclusion

In this paper, we present preliminary results confirming that tight graph framelets can be employed for sparse representation of diffusion signals in q-space. The effectiveness of this representation is demonstrated with applications involving denoising and super-resolution. Future work will be directed to incorporating this representation with spatial framelet representation to obtain a joint representation for both spatial and wavevector dimensions.

References

1. Dong, B.: Sparse representation on graphs by tight wavelet frames and applications. Applied and Computational Harmonic Analysis (2015)
2. Hammond, D.K., Vandergheynst, P., Gribonval, R.: Wavelets on graphs via spectral graph theory. Appl. Comput. Harmonic Anal. **30**(2), 129–150 (2011)
3. Ron, A., Shen, Z.: Affine systems in $L_2(\mathbb{R}^d)$: the analysis of the analysis operator. J. Funct. Anal. **148**(2), 408–447 (1997)
4. Michailovich, O., Rathi, Y.: On approximation of orientation distributions by means of spherical ridgelets. IEEE Trans. Image Process. **19**(2), 461–476 (2010)
5. Chan, R.H., Chan, T.F., Shen, L., Shen, Z.: Wavelet algorithms for high-resolution image reconstruction. SIAM J. Sci. Comput. **24**(4), 1408–1432 (2003)
6. Zhang, Y., Dong, B., Lu, Z.: ℓ_0 minimization for wavelet frame based image restoration. Math. Comput. **82**, 995–1015 (2013)
7. Tuch, D.S.: Q-ball imaging. Magn. Reson. Med. **52**, 1358–1372 (2004)
8. Belkin, M., Niyogi, P.: Towards a theoretical foundation for laplacian-based manifold methods. In: Auer, P., Meir, R. (eds.) COLT 2005. LNCS (LNAI), vol. 3559, pp. 486–500. Springer, Heidelberg (2005)
9. Lu, Z., Zhang, Y.: Sparse approximation via penalty decomposition methods. SIAM J. Optim. **23**(4), 2448–2478 (2013)
10. Lu, Z.: Iterative hard thresholding methods for l_0 regularized convex cone programming. Math. Prog. Ser. A B **147**(1–2), 125–154 (2014)

11. Yap, P.-T., Zhang, Y., Shen, D.: Diffusion compartmentalization using response function groups with cardinality penalization. In: Navab, N., Hornegger, J., Wells, W.M., Frangi, A.F. (eds.) MICCAI 2015. LNCS, vol. 9349, pp. 183–190. Springer, Heidelberg (2015). doi:10.1007/978-3-319-24553-9_23

12. Donoho, D.L.: De-noising by soft-thresholding. IEEE Trans. Inf. Theor. **41**(3), 613–627 (1995)

13. Koay, C.G., Özarslan, E., Basser, P.J.: A signal transformational framework for breaking the noise floor and its applications in MRI. J. Magn. Reson. **197**, 108–119 (2009)

A Bayesian Model to Assess T_2 Values and Their Changes Over Time in Quantitative MRI

Benoit Combès[1]([⊠]), Anne Kerbrat[2], Olivier Commowick[1], and Christian Barillot[1]

[1] Inria, INSERM, VisAGeS U746 Unit/Project, 35042 Rennes, France
benoit.combes@irisa.fr
[2] Service de Neurologie, Rennes, France

Abstract. Quantifying T_2 and T_2^* relaxation times from MRI becomes a standard tool to assess modifications of biological tissues over time or differences between populations. However, due to the relationship between the relaxation time and the associated MR signals such an analysis is subject to error. In this work, we provide a Bayesian analysis of this relationship. More specifically, we build posterior distributions relating the raw (spin or gradient echo) acquisitions and the relaxation time and its modifications over acquisitions. Such an analysis has three main merits. First, it allows to build hierarchical models including prior information and regularisations over voxels. Second, it provides many estimators of the parameters distribution including the mean and the α-credible intervals. Finally, as credible intervals are available, testing properly whether the relaxation time (or its modification) lies within a certain range with a given credible level is simple. We show the interest of this approach on synthetic datasets and on two real applications in multiple sclerosis.

1 Introduction

Relaxometry imaging provides a way to quantify modifications of biological tissues over time or differences between different populations. In this context, the problem of estimating T_2 values from echo train acquisitions is discussed in many works [10–12]. Since we deal with quantitative values, being able to then detect and assess significant differences and changes seems an important goal to achieve. However, to our knowledge, there is still a lack of statistical method to analyse such data. In this work, we focus on the analysis of the T_2 or T_2^* modification between two time-points (*e.g.* baseline versus 3 months later or pre versus post contrast agent injection) for a given subject. A naive approach to perform such a task consists in first computing the T_2 maps for the pre and post acquisitions using an optimisation algorithm and then in comparing the variation level inside a region of interest -typically multiple sclerosis lesions- to the variation inside the normal appearing white matter (NAWM). However, this solution may drive to important issues. The reproducibility error of T_2 and T_2^* maps is indeed significantly smaller in the NAWM than in regions with higher intensities. This

S. Ourselin et al. (Eds.): MICCAI 2016, Part III, LNCS 9902, pp. 570–578, 2016.
DOI: 10.1007/978-3-319-46726-9_66

makes the task, in the best case, complex and, in the worst, error prone with many false positive detections in the higher intensities regions.

In fact, due to the form of the relationship relating the MR signal and the relaxation time, the uncertainty of estimation increases with the relaxation time (see [7] for illustrating experiments on phantoms). In this work, we provide a Bayesian analysis of this relationship. More specifically, we build posterior distributions relating the raw (spin or gradient echo) acquisitions and the relaxation time and its modification over time. These posterior distributions extract the relevant information from the data and provide complete and coherent characterisations of the parameters distribution. Our approach has three main advantages over the existing T_2 and T_2^* estimation methods. First, it allows to build complex models including prior belief on parameters or regularisations over voxels. Second, it provides many estimators of the parameters distribution including the mean and α-credible highest posterior density (HPD) intervals. Finally, once the credible intervals estimated, testing properly whether the relaxation time (or its modification) lies to a certain range given a credible level becomes simple.

The article is organized as follows. In Sect. 2, we describe a set of models to analyse the T_2 and T_2^* relaxation times. More specifically, in Sect. 2.1, we give a posterior for the T_2 (or T_2^*) estimation. In Sect. 2.2, we give a procedure to assess differences of T_2 in a voxel between two time points at a given credible level. Then, in Sect. 2.3, we slightly modify the posterior so that the estimation is not anymore performed voxel-wise but region-wise leading to non-independent multivariate estimations and testings. In Sect. 2.4, we propose a prior to use the extended phase graph function instead of the exponential decay function used in the previous models. Then, in Sect. 3, we assess our method on synthetic data. In Sect. 4, we provide two examples of applications on Multiple Sclerosis data. Finally, in Sect. 5, we discuss this work and give perspectives.

2 Models

2.1 Bayesian Analysis of T_2 Relaxometry

For a given voxel in a volume, the MR signal S_i for a given echo time τ_i can be related to the two (unknown) characteristics of the observed tissue T_2 and M (where M accounts for a combination of several physical components) through:

$$S_i | T_2 = t_2, M = m, \boldsymbol{\sigma} = \sigma \sim N(f_{t_2,m}(\tau_i), \sigma^2), \tag{1}$$

where $f_{t_2,m}(\tau_i) = m \cdot \exp\left(-\frac{\tau_i}{t_2}\right)$ and $N(\mu, \sigma^2)$ is the normal distribution with mean μ and variance σ^2. The Gaussian error term allows to account for measurement noise as well as for model inadequacy (due to e.g. multi exponential decay of the true signal, partial volumes or misalignment). Then we consider that for all $i \neq j$ $(S_i | t_2, m, \sigma) \perp (S_j | t_2, m, \sigma)$ ($\perp$ standing for independence).

The associated reference prior [1] for σ and (M, T_2) in different groups writes:

$$\Pi_1(t_2, m, \sigma) = \Pi_{T_2}(t_2) \cdot \Pi_M(m) \cdot \Pi_{\boldsymbol{\sigma}}(\sigma) \tag{2}$$

$$\propto \left(\frac{l_0(t_2) \cdot l_2(t_2) - l_1^2(t_2)}{t_2^2} \cdot 1_{[t_{2min}, t_{2max}]}(t_2) \right) \cdot \left(m \cdot 1_{[m_{min}, m_{max}]}(m) \right) \cdot \left(\frac{1}{\sigma} 1_{\mathbb{R}^+}(\sigma) \right),$$

where $l_k(t_2) = \sum_i \tau_i^k \exp(-2\frac{\tau_i}{t_2})$ for $k = 0, 1, 2$ and where $1_A(x) = 1$ if $x \in A$ and 0 elsewhere. Notice that the upper limit for M and positive lower limit for T_2 in the prior support are needed to ensure posterior properness. This prior leads to invariance of the inference under reparametrisation of the exponential decay function. Moreover, as it will be shown in Sect. 2.1, it provides satisfying performances whatever the actual values of T_2 (so, under normal and pathological conditions). Estimators for the resulting marginal posterior $p(T_2|(s_i))$ can then be computed using a Markov Chain Monte Carlo algorithm (details in Sect. 3).

2.2 Bayesian Analysis of T_2 Modification

We are now concerned with the following question: how to assess that the T_2 value associated to a given voxel has changed between two acquisitions with a given minimal credible level. Let call X_a the random variable associated to a quantity for the pre acquisitions and X_b for the post acquisitions. We assume that the volumes are aligned and model for the pre acquisition:

$$S_{a,i}|t_2, m_a, \sigma_a \sim N(f_{t_2, m_a}(\tau_i), \sigma_a^2), \tag{3}$$

and introduce C as the T_2 modification between the two acquisitions through:

$$S_{b,i}|t_2, c, m_b, \sigma_b \sim N(f_{t_2+c, m_b}(\tau_i), \sigma_b^2), \tag{4}$$

where (additionally to above independences) for all i, j $(S_{b,i}|t_2, c, m_b, \sigma_b) \perp (S_{a,j}|t_2, m_a, \sigma_a)$. From Eq. 2 we can define the prior:

$$\Pi_2(c, t_2, m_a, m_b, \sigma_a, \sigma_b) \propto \Pi_{T_2}(t_2 + c)\Pi_{T_2}(t_2)\Pi_M(m_a)\Pi_M(m_b)\Pi_{\boldsymbol{\sigma}}(\sigma_a)\Pi_{\boldsymbol{\sigma}}(\sigma_b), \tag{5}$$

that defines, with Eqs. 3 and 4, the marginal posterior for (among others) the T_2 modification $p(C|(s_{a,i}), (s_{b,i}))$. Then a voxel can be defined as negatively (resp. positively) altered at α level, if the α-credible HPD interval for C does not contain any positive (resp. negative) value (see [8] for a testing perspective).

The previous model of variation $T_{2b} = T_{2a} + C$ was dedicated to T_2 modification. Another important alternative model of variation states that when adding a contrast agent to a biological tissue the effect on its T_2 property is additive with the rate $1/T_2$: $1/T_{2b} = 1/T_{2a} + C_R$ and that C_R (we use this notation to distinguish it from the above C) is proportional to the contrast agent concentration. From the posterior of T_2 and C designed above, its posterior writes:
$p(C_R = c_R|(s_{a,i}), (s_{b,i})) = p(\frac{-C}{T_2(C+T_2)} = c_R|(s_{a,i}), (s_{b,i}))$.

2.3   Region-Wise Analysis

The models proposed previously allow a voxel-wise analysis where each voxel is processed independently from others. Performing a grouped inference for all the voxels of a given region (*e.g.* lesion) can be performed by adding a supplemental layer to the model. Let us use j to index voxels, then one can replace each prior $\Pi_2(c^j)$ by for example: $\Pi_2(c^j|\mu_C, \sigma_C) = \psi_N(\mu_C - c^j, \sigma_C^2)(\psi_N$ being the Normal kernel). We then assume that $\forall i_1, i_2$ and $j_1 \neq j_2, (S_{i_1}^{j_1}|t_2^{j_1}, m^{j_1}, \sigma^{j_1}) \perp (S_{i_2}^{j_2}|t_2^{j_2}, m^{j_2}, \sigma^{j_2})$ (in particular, we consider the errors as independent between voxels). For the two hyperparameters μ_C and σ_C, we use the weakly informative priors (see [5] for details) $\mu_C \sim N(0, 10^6)$ (approximating the uniform density over $\mathbb{R}$) and $\sigma_C \sim \text{Cauchy}(x_0 = 0, \gamma = 100)I_{\mathbb{R}+}$ (allowing σ_C to go well below 400ms), where $I_{\mathbb{R}+}$ denotes a left-truncation. Such a model allows the set of inferences over the (C^j) to be performed not independently thus dealing in a natural way with multiple comparisons by shrinking exceptional C^j toward its estimated region-wise distribution [6] and improving the overall inference. Depending on the expected regularity of the C^j within the regions, we can alternatively opt for a Cauchy density and/or add an informative prior for the error variances $\sigma_{a,i}^2$ and $\sigma_{b,i}^2$ to favour goodness of the fit. Similarly, a spatial Markovian regularisation can also be considered.

2.4   Using the Extended Phase Graph

When the signals $(s_i)_{i=1:N}$ are obtained using sequences of multiple echoes spin echoes (*e.g.* CMPG sequence), the exponential decay function is only a rough approximation of the relation between T_2 and the MR signals. Some solutions to adapt it to this situation exist [10] and could be easily added to our model. In the following, we propose a broader solution that consists in replacing the exponential decay by the Extended Phase Graph function (EPG) [9] that relates the signal S_i to two other quantities (additionally to T_2 and M) so that $(S_i) = EPG(T_2, M, T_1, B_1, (\tau_i)) + \epsilon$ (T_1 being the spin-lattice relaxation time, B_1 the field inhomogeneity *i.e.* multiplicative departure from the nominal flip angle and ϵ representing the noise term of Eq. 1). This function is complicated (product of N 3×3 matrices involving non-linearly the different parameters) and derivating a dedicated reference prior would be cumbersome. Nevertheless, it consists of small departures from the exponential function and mainly depends on M and T_2. Thus a reasonable choice consists in using the same priors as those derived for the exponential function. Then, an informative prior is designed for B_1. In practice, B_1 typically takes 95 % of its values in $[0.4, 1.6]$ (we deliberatively use this symmetric form to avoid $B_1 = 1$ to be a boundary of the prior support) so we set $B_1 \sim \text{Gamma}(k = 8.5, \theta = 0.1)$. We did the same for T_1 by choosing a gamma distribution with 95 % of its density in $[20, 2000](T_1 \sim \text{Gamma}(2.3, 120))$. In practice, T_1 has a very small impact on the EPG and on the inference. Then the EPG model can be used by simply replacing $f_{t_2, m}(\tau_i)$ by $EPG(t_2, m, t_1, b_1, (\tau_i))$ (prior sensitivity analyses for T_1 and B_1 give satisfying results).

3   Results on Synthetic Data

3.1   Implementation, Datasets and Convergence Diagnosis

For the sake of concision, for the previous models, we only exhibited the likelihoods, the priors and the independence assumptions. The resulting posteriors can be obtained using the Bayes rule. Then for each marginal posterior $p(T_2|(s_i))$ (Sect. 2.1), $p(C|(s_{a,i}),(s_{b,i}))$ (Sect. 2.2) and $p((C^j)|(s^j_{a,i}),(s^j_{b,i}))$ (Sect. 2.3), we get its statistics using the "logarithm scaling" adaptive one variable at a time Metropolis-Hastings algorithm [13]. We used 10k samples (40k for the region-wise model) after discarding the first 5k (20k for the region-wise model). Convergence has been assessed using the Geweke score [2].

The data we use in this section are numerically generated T_2 spin echo acquisitions with 7 echo times τ equally spaced by 13.8 ms and a repetition time of 1 s. Since the $EPG(t_2, t_1, b_1, (\tau_i))$ function is time consuming and many function calls are needed, it is tabulated on a fine grid for different values of t_2, t_1 and b_1. All the results given below are those using the EPG (for both generating data and inference), those obtained using the exponential decay are slightly better and lead to the same conclusion.

3.2   Results

T_2 **estimation:** We run 400 estimations for different configurations of T_2 and σ (realistic values are randomly given to T_1, B_1 and M). Results are summarized in Table 1 and illustrate how the length of the credible intervals increases as expected with T_2 and σ. Moreover, these intervals exhibit excellent coverage properties, illustrating the interest of the derived priors in the absence of prior information for T_2. Notice that other choices of prior such as the reference prior with σ and M as nuisance parameters [1] do not lead us to analytical solutions.

Table 1. Mean 0.05-credible interval length and coverage properties (*i.e.* percentage of intervals containing the true value of T_2) using 400 simulations for each configuration

T_2/σ	50/5	80/5	120/5	200/5	300/5	50/10	80/10	120/10	200/10	300/10
Mean interval length	4.95	8.63	14.54	35.85	71.17	10.08	17.40	28.27	72.30	154.89
Coverage	0.97	0.96	0.98	0.95	0.96	0.96	0.97	0.96	0.97	0.98

C **estimation:** For different configurations of T_2, σ and C, we analyse the specificity (denoted p^-) and sensitivity (denoted p^+) of the estimator for C modification (Sect. 2.2) for $\alpha=0.05$. Results are summarized in Table 2 and illustrate that for the used acquisition protocol, detecting low T_2 modifications in high values is limited with a 0.95 specificity level. Such simulations can be used to design decision rules providing an optimized specificity/sensitivity trade-off for given T_2/C values by adjusting α. We also observe that the region-wise model can lead to strong improvements of the performances.

Table 2. Specificity and sensitivity for $\alpha = 0.05$ for different $\sigma/T_2/C$ configurations (using 400 simulations). The region-wise analysis is performed with regions of 16 voxels with C values drawn from a Cauchy density (to deviate from the chosen model) with mean $1.1 \cdot C$ (C being the value for the voxel of interest) and scale parameter 10

	T_2/σ	80/5	120/5	200/5	300/5	80/10	120/10	200/10	300/10
Voxel-wise	$C = 0, p^-$	0.96	0.97	0.97	0.95	0.96	0.96	0.97	0.95
	$C = 30, p^+$	1	1	0.78	0.43	0.98	0.96	0.55	0.29
	$C = 60, p^+$	1	1	1	0.86	1	1	0.88	0.64
Region-wise	$C = 0, p^-$	1	0.99	0.98	0.98	1	0.99	0.99	0.98
	$C = 30, p^+$	1	1	0.96	0.92	1	0.98	0.80	0.57
	$C = 60, p^+$	1	1	1	0.97	1	1	0.93	0.88

4   Two Applications on Real Data

The present method has been developed in a clinical context including a dataset of about 50 pre/post acquisitions from relapsing-remitting multiple sclerosis patients. In this section, we exemplified applications of our method on a few data from this study. Data are acquired on a 3T Verio MRI scanner (Siemens Healthcare, 32-channel head coil) and consists of volumes of $192 \times 192 \times 44$ voxels of size $1.3 \times 1.3 \times 3 \, \text{mm}^3$. The sequence parameters are the same as those used in Sect. 3. For each patient, all volumes are rigidly co-registered using a robust block-matching method [3]. No other preprocessing is applied.

4.1   Assessing USPIO Enhancement in MS Lesion

Ultra small superparamagnetic iron oxide (USPIO) is a contrast agent used to assess macrophagic activity that reduces the T_2 relaxation of the surrounding tissues [4]. We use, in this section, sets of pre-post injection acquisitions to detect the presence of USPIO in MS lesions using our model. Figure 1 displays detection with a 5 % level for a patient acquired twice without USPIO injection and for a patient with potentially active lesions. The pre-post T_2 relaxation maps illustrate the difficulty to label the lesions as enhanced or not by simply using the point estimates. The map for the patient without USPIO injection, for which our method does not detect any voxels, highlights this point. More generally, on this data we never detected more than 5 % of the voxels. For the active patient with USPIO injection, the method detects lesion 1 -for which we have independent clues that it is effectively active (*i.e.* high variation of MTR, FA and ADC values between baseline and acquisitions 3 months later)- as enhanced. By contrast, lesion 2 -for which we had no initial clue that it was actually active- is not detected as enhanced, while it shows a substantially positive pre-post signal.

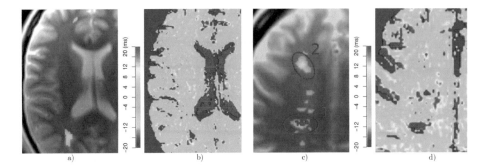

Fig. 1. Pictures (a) and (b): acquisitions performed without USPIO injection (so all lesions should be detected as negative). (a) superposition of a T_2 weighted image, the lesion segmentation mask (white patches) and the enhanced voxels (red) for the 5 % level and (b) the pre-post T_2 relaxation map (using ML estimates). **Pictures (c) and (d): an active patient.** Same displays than for (a) and (b) (Color figure online)

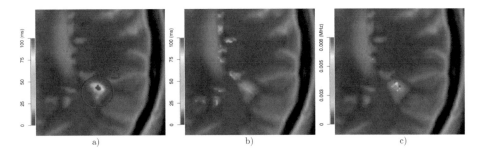

Fig. 2. Recovery assessment in MS lesions. From left to right: (a) *Minimal T_2* recovered value for $[m_3, m_0]$ (admissible with $\alpha = 0.05$), (b) *Maximal T_2* recovered value for the next time $[m_3, m_6]$ and (c) *Minimal* USPIO concentration C_R at m_0

4.2   Assessing T_2 Recovery in an Active MS Lesion

In this section, we use our model to assess the evolution of the T_2 associated to a MS lesion just after its emergence (m_0) and 3 (m_3) and 6 (m_6) months after. To illustrate the interest of the credible intervals, we display the minimal plausible C values for the 0.05 level *i.e.* the lower bound of the 0.05-credible interval for $[m_3, m_0]$ (Fig. 2.a) and the upper one for $[m_6, m_3]$ (Fig. 2.b). Notice that, for a sake of clarity, we quantify here differences from m_3 to m_0 so that expected difference C (a decrease of the T_2 signals over time) is positive (and similarly for m_3 and m_6). These maps offer a quantitative scale to compare lesions recovery among and within patient. More precisely, for lesion 3, the minimal admissible C is positive for $[m_3, m_0]$ (thus the interval does not contain 0) demonstrating that the lesion is recovering during this period. By contrast, this is not the case for the other lesions of the slice and for lesion 3 at $[m_6, m_3]$ (not displayed): it cannot be excluded with a 5 % level that the recovering process is finished.

Moreover, the *maximal* admissible value for $[m_6, m_3]$ (Fig. 2.b) is far lower than the *minimal* one for $[m_3, m_0]$. We also give the *minimal* USPIO concentration *i.e.* C_R changes for the 5 % level (Fig. 2.c): we observe a good adequacy between USPIO concentration and T_2 change for $[m_0, m_3]$.

5   Discussion and Conclusion

In this paper, we proposed a Bayesian analysis of T_2/T_2^* relaxation time assessment and modification. Then, we showed the interesting properties of our models on synthetic datasets. Finally, we exemplified the interest of the obtained credible intervals with two applications. As illustrated, when available, *interval* estimates can be more powerful than *point* ones to address naturally complex issues in medical imaging. Moreover, this work can be extended in several ways:

– It can be used as a basis for the development of more informative hierarchical models (this is a motivation for considering a Bayesian setting). For example, the B_1^js are spatially correlated. This could be accounted for adding a supplemental layer to the model (similarly to what proposed in Sect. 2.3). An informative prior for σ^j could also be of interest to get less conservative intervals.
– In this work, we considered the errors (modelled by the error term of Eq. 1 or Eqs. 3 and 4) as not correlated between voxels and modelling correlated errors (with unknown structure) would be of interest and is a challenge to meet.
– The method is computationally intensive (about 2 s per voxel for the EPG region-wise approach) and for more demanding applications, other strategies *e.g.* maximisation over nuisance parameters could be investigated.

More generally, we think there is room for potential applications of interval estimation in *e.g.* T_1 or DTI and hope this work will encourage such development.

References

1. Berger, J.O., et al.: The formal definition of reference priors. Ann. Stat. **37**(2), 905–938 (2009)
2. Brooks, S., et al.: Handbook of Markov Chain Monte Carlo. Chapman & Hall/CRC Handbooks of Modern Statistical Methods. CRC Press, Boca Raton (2011)
3. Commowick, O., et al.: Block-matching strategies for rigid registration of multimodal medical images. In: ISBI, pp. 700–703, May 2012
4. Corot, C., et al.: Recent advances in iron oxide nanocrystal technology for medical imaging. Adv. Drug Deliv. Rev. **58**(14), 1471–1504 (2006)
5. Gelman, A.: Prior distributions for variance parameters in hierarchical models. Bayesian Anal. **1**(3), 515–534 (2006)
6. Gelman, A., et al.: Why we (usually) don't have to worry about multiple comparisons. J. Res. Educ. Effectiveness **5**(2), 189–211 (2012)
7. Kjos, B.O., et al.: Reproducibility of T1 and T2 relaxation times calculated from routine mr imaging sequences: phantom study. Am. J. Neuroradiol. **6**(2), 277–283 (1985)

8. Kruschke, J.K.: Bayesian assessment of null values via parameter estimation and model comparison. Perspect. Psychol. Sci. **6**(3), 299–312 (2011)
9. Matthias, W.: Extended phase graphs: dephasing, RF pulses, and echoes - pure and simple. J. Magn. Reson. Imaging **41**(2), 266–295 (2015)
10. Milford, D., et al.: Mono-exponential fitting in T2-relaxometry: relevance of offset and first echo. PLoS ONE **10**(12), e0145255 (2015). Fan X Editor
11. Neumann, D., et al.: Simple recipe for accurate T2 quantification with multi spin-echo acquisitions. Magn. Reson. Mater. Phys. Biol. Med. **27**(6), 567–577 (2014)
12. Petrovic, A., et al.: Closed-form solution for T2 mapping with nonideal refocusing of slice selective CPMG sequences. Magn. Reson. Med. **73**, 818–827 (2015)
13. Roberts, G.O., Rosenthal, J.S.: Examples of adaptive MCMC. J. Comput. Graph. Stat. **18**(2), 349–367 (2009)

Simultaneous Parameter Mapping, Modality Synthesis, and Anatomical Labeling of the Brain with MR Fingerprinting

Pedro A. Gómez[1,2,4]([✉]), Miguel Molina-Romero[1,2,4], Cagdas Ulas[1,2],
Guido Bounincontri[3], Jonathan I. Sperl[2], Derek K. Jones[4], Marion I. Menzel[2],
and Bjoern H. Menze[1]

[1] Computer Science, Technische Universität München, Munich, Germany
pedro.gomez@tum.de
[2] GE Global Research, Munich, Germany
[3] INFN Pisa, Pisa, Italy
[4] CUBRIC School of Psychology, Cardiff University, Cardiff, UK

Abstract. Magnetic resonance fingerprinting (MRF) quantifies various properties simultaneously by matching measurements to a dictionary of precomputed signals. We propose to extend the MRF framework by using a database to introduce additional parameters and spatial characteristics to the dictionary. We show that, with an adequate matching technique which includes an update of selected fingerprints in parameter space, it is possible to reconstruct parametric maps, synthesize modalities, and label tissue types at the same time directly from an MRF acquisition. We compare (1) relaxation maps from a spatiotemporal dictionary against a temporal MRF dictionary, (2) synthetic diffusion metrics versus those obtained with a standard diffusion acquisition, and (3) anatomical labels generated from MRF signals to an established segmentation method, demonstrating the potential of using MRF for multiparametric brain mapping.

1 Introduction

Magnetic resonance fingerprinting (MRF) is an emerging technique for the simultaneous quantification of multiple tissue properties [7]. It offers absolute measurements of the T1 and T2 relaxation parameters (opposed to traditional weighted imaging) with an accelerated acquisition, leading to efficient parameter mapping. MRF is based on matching measurements to a dictionary of precomputed signals that have been generated for different parameters. Generally, the number of atoms in the dictionary is dictated by the amount of parameters, and the range and density of their sampling. As an alternative to continuous sampling of the parameter space, one could use measured training examples to learn the dictionary, reducing the number of atoms to only feasible parameter combinations [2]. In this work, we propose to use a database of multi-parametric datasets to create the dictionary, presenting two new features of MRF that can be achieved simultaneously with relaxation mapping: modality synthesis and automatic labeling of the corresponding tissue.

© Springer International Publishing AG 2016
S. Ourselin et al. (Eds.): MICCAI 2016, Part III, LNCS 9902, pp. 579–586, 2016.
DOI: 10.1007/978-3-319-46726-9_67

In this extended application of MRF towards image synthesis and segmentation, we follow a direction that has recently gained attention in the medical image processing literature [1,3,5,6,9,10]. The working principle behind these methods is similar: given a source image and a multi-contrast database of training subjects, it is possible to generate the missing contrast (or label) of the source by finding similarities within the database and transferring them to create a new image. The search and synthesis strategy can take several forms: it could be iterative to incorporate more information [10]; can be optimized for multiple scales and features [1]; may include a linear combination of multiple image patches [9]; or be configured to learn a nonlinear transform from the target to the source [5]. There have been several applications of synthetic contrasts, including inter-modality image registration, super-resolution, and abnormality detection [3,5,6,9,10]. Furthermore, in addition to the creation of scalar maps in image synthesis, similar techniques can be used for mapping discrete annotations; for example, in the segmentation of brain structures [1].

Inspired by these ideas, we present a method for synthesizing modalities and generating labels from magnetic resonance fingerprints. It relies on the creation of a spatiotemporal dictionary [2] and its mapping to different parameters. Specifically, in addition to the physics-based mapping of MRF signals to the T1 and T2 relaxation parameters, we train empirical functions for a mapping of the signals to diffusion metrics and tissue probabilities. We show that we can achieve higher efficiency relaxation mapping, and demonstrate how the use of a spatiotemporal context improves the accuracy of synthetic mapping and labeling.

We see three main contributions to our work. (1) We present a framework for creating a spatiotemporal MRF dictionary from a multi-parametric database (Sect. 2.1). (2) We generalize fingerprint matching and incorporate a data-driven update to account for correlations in parameter space, allowing for the simultaneous estimation of M different parameters from any fingerprinting sequence (Sect. 2.2). (3) Depending on the nature of the m-th parameter, we call it a mapping, synthesis, or labeling, and show results for all three applications (Sect. 3.1). This is the first attempt - to the best of our knowledge - to simultaneously map parameters, synthesize diffusion metrics, and estimate anatomical labels from MR fingerprints.

2 Methods

Let $\mathcal{Q} = \{Q_s\}_{s=1}^S$ represent a database of spatially aligned parametric maps for S subjects, where each subject $Q_s \in \mathbb{R}^{N \times M}$ contains a total of $N = N_i \times N_j \times N_k$ voxels and M maps. Every map represents an individual property, and can originate from a different acquisition or modality, or even be categorical. Our database includes the quantitative relaxation parameters T1 and T2; a non-diffusion weighted image (S0); the diffusion metrics mean diffusivity (MD), radial diffusivity (RD), and fractional anisotropy (FA); and probability maps for three tissue classes: gray matter (GM), white matter (WM), and cerebrospinal fluid (CSF). Thus, for every subject $Q_s = \{T1, T2, S0, MD, RD, FA, GM, WM, CSF\}$. We use this database to create a spatiotemporal MRF dictionary as follows.

2.1 Building a Spatiotemporal MRF Dictionary

With the relaxation parameters T1 and T2 and knowledge of the sequence variables, it is possible to follow the extended phase graph (EPG) formalism to simulate the signal evolution of a *fast imaging with steady state precession MRF* (FISP-MRF) pulse sequence [4]. In EPG the effects of a sequence on a spin system are represented by operators related to radio-frequency pulses, relaxation, and dephasing due to gradient moments. Therefore, for every voxel in all subjects, application of the EPG operators leads to a dictionary $D \in \mathbb{C}^{NS \times T}$ with a total of T temporal points (see Fig. 1).

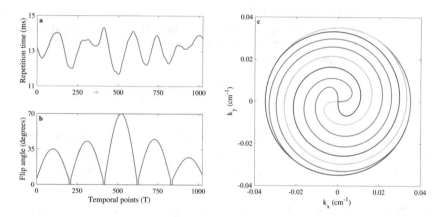

Fig. 1. FISP-MRF acquisition sequence. **a**, Repetition times following a Perlin noise pattern. **b**, Flip angles of repeating sinusoidal curves. **c**, k-space trajectory of four different spiral interleaves, 32 interleaves are required for full k-space coverage.

We further process the dictionary to incorporate spatial information by expanding each voxel with its 3D spatial neighborhood of dimension $P = P_i \times P_j \times P_k$ and compressing the temporal dimension into its first V singular vectors [8]. This results in a compressed spatiotemporal dictionary $\tilde{D} \in \mathbb{C}^{NS \times PV}$. Finally, we define a search window $W_n = W_i \times W_j \times W_k$ around every voxel n, limiting the dictionary per voxel to $\tilde{D}_n \in \mathbb{C}^{W_n S \times PV}$. The choice for a local search window has a two-fold motivation: it reduces the number of computations by decreasing the search space and it increases spatial coherence for dictionary matching [10].

Applying subject concatenation, patch extraction, and search window reduction on the database $\mathcal{Q}$ leads to a voxel-wise spatio-parametric matrix $\tilde{R}_n \in \mathbb{R}^{W_n S \times PM}$. For simplicity, we will use D and R instead of $\tilde{D}_n$ and $\tilde{R}_n$, where every dictionary entry $d_c \in \mathbb{C}^{PV}$ has its corresponding matrix entry $r_c \in \mathbb{R}^{PM}$.

2.2 Dictionary Matching and Parameter Estimation

MRF aims to simultaneously estimate several parametric maps from undersampled data. This is achieved by reconstructing an image series and matching it to the dictionary. We reconstruct V singular images [8] and extract 3D patches from them to create the patch-based matrix $X \in \mathbb{C}^{N \times PV}$. At every voxel x_n, we find the set $\mathcal{M}_n$ of the C highest correlated dictionary entries d_c, $c = 1, .., C$, by:

$$\mathcal{M}_n = \{d_c \in D : \rho(x_n, d_c) > \tau_C\} \tag{1}$$

with the threshold value τ_C such that $|\mathcal{M}| = C$ and

$$\rho(x, d) = \frac{\langle x, d \rangle}{\|x\|_2 \|d\|_2}. \tag{2}$$

Making use of the selected entries d_c and the corresponding parametric vectors r_c, an estimated value $\tilde{q}_{n,m}$ at voxel location n in map m is determined by the weighted average of the correlation between every entry d_c and the signals x_p within Ω_n, the spatial neighborhood of n:

$$\tilde{q}_{n,m} = \frac{\sum_{p \in \Omega_n} \sum_c \rho(x_p, d_c) r_{c,pm}}{P \sum_c \rho(x_p, d_c)}, \tag{3}$$

where $r_{c,pm}$ indexes the quantitative value of voxel p centered around atom c in map m. Repeating this procedure for every voxel creates an estimate $\tilde{Q}$ of all of the parametric maps, including synthetic modalities and anatomical labels.

Data-Driven Updates. Ye et al. [10] proposed the use of intermediate results to increase spatial consistency of the synthetic maps. We take a similar approach, and define a similarity function relating image space and parameter space:

$$f(x, d, r, q, \alpha) = (1 - \alpha)\rho(x, d) + \alpha\rho(q, r) \tag{4}$$

where α controls the contributions of the correlations in image and parameter space. The selected atoms are now determined by

$$\mathcal{M}_n = \{d_c \in D, r_c \in R : f(x_n, d_c, \tilde{q}_n, r_c, \alpha) > \tau_C\}. \tag{5}$$

In the first iteration $\alpha = 0$ as we have no information on the map $\tilde{Q}$ for our subject. In a second iteration we increase α, adding weight to the similarities in parameter space and compute Eq. 5 again to find a new set of dictionary atoms. The final version of the maps is given by a modified version of Eq. 3:

$$\hat{q}_{n,m} = \frac{\sum_{p \in \Omega_n} \sum_c f(x_p, d_c, \tilde{q}_n, r_c, \alpha) r_{c,pm}}{P \sum_c f(x_p, d_c, \tilde{q}_n, r_c, \alpha)}. \tag{6}$$

This procedure is essentially a 3D patch-match over a V-dimensional image space and M-dimensional parameter space, where the matching patches are combined by their weighted correlation to create a final result.

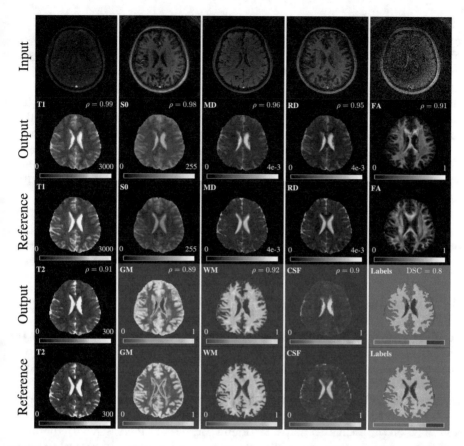

Fig. 2. Exemplary results of one test subject with $P = 3 \times 3 \times 3$. The upper row displays the first five singular images; while the second and fourth row show the output for different parametric maps and the correlation to the reference image, displayed in the third and fifth row, respectively. Additionally, the last column in rows four and five shows labels obtained from selecting the tissue class with highest probability and the dice similarity coefficient (DSC) from the output labels to the reference. The bar underneath represents, from left to right, background, GM, WM, and CSF; and the DSC was computed from the GM, WM, and CSF labels. T1 and T2 scale is displayed in ms; S0 is qualitatively scaled to 255 arbitrary units; MD and RD are in mm^2/s; FA, GM, WM, and CSF are fractional values between zero and one.

2.3 Data Acquisition and Pre-processing

We acquired data from six volunteers with a FISP-MRF pulse sequence [4] on a 3T GE HDx MRI system (GE Medical Systems, Milwaukee, WI) using an eight channel receive only head RF coil. After an initial inversion, a train of $T = 1024$ radio-frequency pulses with varying flip angles and repetition times following a Perlin noise pattern [4] was applied (see Fig. 1). We use one interleave of a zero-moment compensated variable density spiral trajectory per repetition, requiring

32 interleaves to sample a 22×22 cm field of view (FOV) with 1.7 mm isotropic resolution. We acquired 10 slices per subject with a scan time of 13.47 seconds per slice, performed a gridding reconstruction onto a 128×128 Cartesian grid, projected the data into SVD space, and truncated it to generate $V = 10$ singular images. The choice of $V = 10$ was motivated by the energy ratio, as this was the lowest rank approximation which still yielded an energy ratio of 1.0 [8]. The singular images were matched to a MRF dictionary comprising of T1 values ranging from 100 to 6,000 ms; and T2 values ranging from 20 ms to 3,000 ms.

In addition, we scanned each volunteer with a diffusion weighted imaging (DWI) protocol comprising of 30 directions in one shell with $b = 1000$ s/mm^2. The FOV, resolution, and acquired slices were the same as with MRF-FISP, resulting in a 15 min scan. We applied FSL processing to correct for spatial distortions derived from EPI readouts, skull strip, estimate the diffusion tensor and its derived metrics MD, RD, and FA; and used the non-diffusion weighted image S0 to compute probability maps of three tissue types (GM, WM, CSF) using [11]. Finally, we applied registration across all subjects to create the database.

3   Experiments and Results

For every subject, we performed a leave-one-out cross validation, wherein the dictionary was constructed from five subjects and the remaining subject was used as a test case. Following the procedure described in Sect. 2.2, we created a database of nine parametric maps (T1,T2,S0,MD,RD,FA,GM,WM,CSF) and compared the estimated metrics to the reference by their correlation.

We explored the influence of the window size W_n, the number of entries C, and the α on the estimated maps. We found correlations increased with diminishing returns as W_n increased, while adding more entries yielded smoother maps. Correlations were higher after a second iteration of data-driven updates with $\alpha > 0$, irrespective of the value of α. Nonetheless, variations of these parameters didn't have a significant effect on the overall results. To investigate the impact of using spatial information, we repeated the experiment for spatial patch sizes of $P = 1 \times 1 \times 1$, $3 \times 3 \times 3$, and $5 \times 5 \times 5$. For these experiments we used $W_n = 11 \times 11 \times 11$, $C = 5$, $\alpha = 0.5$, and two iterations.

3.1   Results

The reference T1 and T2 maps were estimated from a FISP-MRF sequence with a temporal dictionary, while we used a spatiotemporal dictionary with varying spatial patches. Estimated T1 and T2 maps were consistent with the reference, with increasing spatial smoothness for larger spatial patches. This also lead to a decrease in correlation to the reference, most notably in T2 estimation (see Fig. 3a–b), which could also be attributed noisier T2 estimates. In future experiments we will rely on standard relaxation mapping for reference comparison.

The synthetic S0 and diffusion metrics MD, RD, and FA show spatial coherence, achieving correlation values over 0.90 with respect to a standard DWI

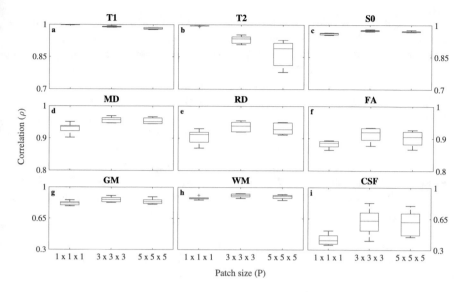

Fig. 3. Correlation as a function of spatial patches for all subjects. **a–b**, T1 and T2 parameter mapping. **c–f**, Synthesis of S0 and diffusion metrics. **g–i**, Tissue labeling.

acquisition (Fig. 2). Similar to [10], we found that FA maps were generally the least correlated to the reference. This is due to the fact that diffusion encoding in DWI acts as a proxy for underlying tissue anisotropy, whereas the measured fingerprints are not diffusion sensitive, failing to exactly recover directionality present in FA. In fact, the higher the directionality encoded in a given modality, the lower the correlation to the reference ($\overline{\rho_{S0}} > \overline{\rho_{MD}} > \overline{\rho_{RD}} > \overline{\rho_{FA}}$). Furthermore, for all cases in modality synthesis, incorporating spatial information generated increased consistency and higher correlated results (Fig. 3c–f).

Figure 2 shows the visual similarity between tissue probability maps obtained directly as an output from matching and those computed with [11] and the labels obtained by selecting the class with the highest probability. As with modality synthesis, anatomical labels improved when spatial information was taken into account (Fig. 3g–i). Particularly in CSF, incorporation of spatial information eliminated false positives, yielding better quality maps. On the other hand, thresholding of probability maps lead to an overestimation of GM labels, notably at tissue boundaries. Labeling at tissue boundaries could benefit from higher resolution scans and a multi-channel reference segmentation.

4   Discussion

This work proposes to replace a simulated temporal MRF dictionary with a spatiotemporal dictionary that can be learnt from data, increasing the efficiency of relaxation parameter mapping, and enabling the novel applications of modality synthesis and anatomical labeling. In terms of methodology, we borrow concepts such as the search window and parameter space regularization from the image segmentation and synthesis literature [1,3,10], but change the input to a V-dimensional image space and the output to an M-dimensional parameter space, making it applicable to MRF. Moreover, our framework is valid for any MR sequence, provided signal evolutions can be computed from the training data.

Results indicate that it is possible to use MRF to simultaneously map T1 and T2 parameters, synthesize modalities, and classify tissues with high consistency with respect to established methods. While our method allows us to circumvent post-processing for diffusion metric estimation and tissue segmentation, it is important to note that changes in synthetic diffusion maps can only be propagated from the information available in the database. Therefore, creating the dictionary from pathology and exploring advanced learning techniques capable of capturing these changes is the subject of future work.

Acknowledgments. With the support of the Technische Universität München Institute for Advanced Study, funded by the German Excellence Initiative and the European Commission under Grant Agreement Number 605162.

References

1. Giraud, R., Ta, V.T., Papadakis, N., et al.: An optimized PatchMatch for multi-scale and multi-feature label fusion. NeuroImage **124**, 770–782 (2016)
2. Gómez, P.A., Ulas, C., Sperl, J.I., et al.: Learning a spatiotemporal dictionary for magnetic resonance fingerprinting with compressed sensing. In: MICCAI Patch-MI Workshop, vol. 9467, pp. 112–119 (2015)
3. Iglesias, J.E., Konukoglu, E., Zikic, D., et al.: Is synthesizing MRI contrast useful for inter-modality analysis? MICCAI **18**(9), 1199–1216 (2013)
4. Jiang, Y., Ma, D., Seiberlich, N., et al.: MR fingerprinting using fast imaging with steady state precession (FISP) with spiral readout. MRM **74**(6), 1621–1631 (2014)
5. Jog, A., Carass, A., Roy, S., et al.: MR image synthesis by contrast learning on neighborhood ensembles. Med. Image Anal. **24**(1), 63–76 (2015)
6. Konukoglu, E., van der Kouwe, A., Sabuncu, M.R., Fischl, B.: Example-based restoration of high-resolution magnetic resonance image acquisitions. In: Mori, K., Sakuma, I., Sato, Y., Barillot, C., Navab, N. (eds.) MICCAI 2013, Part I. LNCS, vol. 8149, pp. 131–138. Springer, Heidelberg (2013)
7. Ma, D., Gulani, V., Seiberlich, N., et al.: Magnetic resonance fingerprinting. Nature **495**, 187–192 (2013)
8. McGivney, D., Pierre, E., Ma, D., et al.: SVD compression for magnetic resonance fingerprinting in the time domain. IEEE TMI **0062**, 1–13 (2014)
9. Roy, S., Carass, A., Prince, J.L.: Magnetic resonance image example based contrast synthesis. IEEE TMI **32**(12), 2348–2363 (2013)
10. Ye, D.H., Zikic, D., Glocker, B., et al.: Modality propagation: coherent synthesis of subject-specifc scans with data-driven regularization. MICCAI **8149**, 606–613 (2013)
11. Zhang, Y., Brady, M., Smith, S.: Segmentation of brain MR images through a hidden Markov random field model and the expectation-maximization algorithm. IEEE TMI **20**, 45–57 (2001)

XQ-NLM: Denoising Diffusion MRI Data via x-q Space Non-local Patch Matching

Geng Chen[1,2], Yafeng Wu[1], Dinggang Shen[2], and Pew-Thian Yap[2(✉)]

[1] Data Processing Center, Northwestern Polytechnical University, Xi'an, China
[2] Department of Radiology and BRIC, University of North Carolina,
Chapel Hill, USA
ptyap@med.unc.edu

Abstract. Noise is a major issue influencing quantitative analysis in diffusion MRI. The effects of noise can be reduced by repeated acquisitions, but this leads to long acquisition times that can be unrealistic in clinical settings. For this reason, post-acquisition denoising methods have been widely used to improve SNR. Among existing methods, non-local means (NLM) has been shown to produce good image quality with edge preservation. However, currently the application of NLM to diffusion MRI has been mostly focused on the spatial space (i.e., the x-space), despite the fact that diffusion data live in a combined space consisting of the x-space and the q-space (i.e., the space of wavevectors). In this paper, we propose to extend NLM to both x-space and q-space. We show how patch-matching, as required in NLM, can be performed concurrently in x-q space with the help of azimuthal equidistant projection and rotation invariant features. Extensive experiments on both synthetic and real data confirm that the proposed x-q space NLM (XQ-NLM) outperforms the classic NLM.

1 Introduction

Diffusion MRI suffers from low signal-to-noise ratio (SNR), especially when the diffusion weighting (i.e., b-value) is high. To improve SNR, a common approach is to repeat the acquisition multiple times so that repeated measurements can be averaged to reduce noise and enhance SNR. However, this approach is time consuming and is oftentimes prohibitive in clinical settings.

Post-acquisition denoising methods [1–3] have been shown to be a viable alternative in improving SNR without resorting to repeating acquisitions. Among existing methods, the non-local means (NLM) [4] algorithm has been shown to offer particularly good performance in edge-preserving denoising. The key feature that distinguishes NLM from the other methods is its ability to increase significantly the information available for denoising by going beyond the local neighborhood and allowing non-local or spatially distant information to be involved

This work was supported in part by NIH grants (NS093842, EB006733, EB008374, EB009634, AG041721, and MH100217).

S. Ourselin et al. (Eds.): MICCAI 2016, Part III, LNCS 9902, pp. 587–595, 2016.
DOI: 10.1007/978-3-319-46726-9_68

in denoising. Self-similar information is gathered via a patch matching mechanism where voxels with similar neighborhoods are given greater weights and those with dissimilar neighborhoods are given lesser weights in denoising. The effectiveness of NLM stems from the fact that the non-local nature of the algorithm allows significantly more information to be available for denoising than local methods.

In particular, NLM has been applied to removing noise in diffusion-weighted (DW) images [1,2]. Using NLM, the DW images can be denoised as individual images, as a multi-spectral vector image, or as parametric maps given by a diffusion model [1]. However, existing methods are mainly focused on neighborhood matching in the spatial domain (i.e., x-space). While effective, this approach might not perform as well in regions with highly curved white matter structures, resulting in averaging over disparate axonal directions and failing to make full use of information from differentially oriented structures.

In this paper, we show that improved denoising performance can be attained by extending the NLM algorithm beyond x-space to include q-space. The advantage afforded by this extension is twofold: (i) Non-local information can now be harnessed not only across x-space, but also across measurements in q-space; and (ii) In white matter regions with high curvature, q-space neighborhood matching corrects for such non-linearity so that information from structures oriented in different directions can be used more effectively for denoising without introducing artifacts. To allow NLM to be carried out in x-q space, the patch for neighborhood similarity evaluation is defined in q-space. This involves mapping a spherical neighborhood in q-space to a disc and then computing a set of rotation invariant features from the disc for patch matching.

2   Methods

2.1 x-q Space Non-local Means

Our method utilizes neighborhood matching in both x-space and q-space for effective denoising. For each voxel at location $\mathbf{x}_i \in \mathbb{R}^3$, the diffusion-attenuated signal measurement $S(\mathbf{x}_i, \mathbf{q}_k)$ corresponding to wavevector $\mathbf{q}_k \in \mathbb{R}^3$ is denoised by averaging over non-local measurements that have similar q-neighborhoods. We estimate the denoised signal $\mathrm{NL}(S)(\mathbf{x}_i, \mathbf{q}_k)$ as

$$\mathrm{NLM}(S)(\mathbf{x}_i, \mathbf{q}_k) = \sum_{(\mathbf{x}_j, \mathbf{q}_l) \in \mathcal{V}_{i,k}} w_{i,k;j,l}[S(\mathbf{x}_j, \mathbf{q}_l) + c_{i,k;j,l}], \tag{1}$$

where $\mathcal{V}_{i,k}$ is the search neighborhood in x-q space associated with $S(\mathbf{x}_i, \mathbf{q}_k)$, $c_{i,k;j,l}$ is a variable used to compensate for differences in signal levels due to spatial intensity inhomogeneity and signal decay in q-space, $w_{i,k;j,l}$ is the weight indicating the similarity between $S(\mathbf{x}_i, \mathbf{q}_k)$ and $S(\mathbf{x}_j, \mathbf{q}_l)$.

Instead of restricting neighborhood matching to x-space, we introduce x-q space neighborhood matching by defining a patch in q-space. For each point in x-q space, $(\mathbf{x}_i, \mathbf{q}_k)$, we define a spherical patch, $\mathcal{N}_{i,k}$, centered at $\mathbf{q}_k$ with fixed $q_k = |\mathbf{q}_k|$ and subject to a neighborhood angle α_p. The samples on this spherical patch are mapped to a disc using azimuthal equidistant projection (AEP, Sect. 2.2) before computing rotation invariant features via polar complex exponential transform (PCET, Sect. 2.3) for patch matching. Figure 1 illustrates the concept of patch matching in *x-q* space. The search radius in *x*-space is s and the search angle in *q*-space is α_s. Matching between different shells is allowed.

To deal with the fact that *q*-space is not always sampled in a shell-like manner, we project the samples in the neighbor of the spherical patch radially onto the spherical patch and weight them accordingly. For instance, we project measurement $S(\mathbf{x}_i, \mathbf{q}_{k'})$ to the shell, i.e.,

$$S\left(\mathbf{x}_i, \frac{|\mathbf{q}_k|}{|\mathbf{q}_{k'}|}\mathbf{q}_{k'}\right) = S(\mathbf{x}_i, \mathbf{q}_{k'}) \exp\left\{-\frac{(\sqrt{b_{k'}} - \sqrt{b_k})^2}{h_{\text{projection}}^2}\right\}. \tag{2}$$

where $b_k = t|\mathbf{q}_k|^2$ and $b_{k'} = t|\mathbf{q}_{k'}|^2$ are the respective *b*-values and t is the diffusion time. $\mathcal{N}_{i,k}$ is then constructed using the projected measurements.

The diffusion-weighted signal can vary due to inhomogeneity or natural signal decay in *q*-space when the *b*-value is increased. This difference in signal level is compensated using $c_{i,k;j,l}$, defined as the mean difference between two patches, i.e., $c_{i,k;j,l} = \overline{\mathbf{S}(\mathcal{N}_{i,k})} - \overline{\mathbf{S}(\mathcal{N}_{j,l})}$, where $\bar{\cdot}$ denotes the mean and $\mathbf{S}(\mathcal{N}_{i,k})$ is a vector containing the values of all diffusion signals in $\mathcal{N}_{i,k}$. Before feature computation for patch matching, we centralize the signal vector as $\widehat{\mathbf{S}}(\mathcal{N}_{i,k}) = \mathbf{S}(\mathcal{N}_{i,k}) - \overline{\mathbf{S}(\mathcal{N}_{i,k})}$.

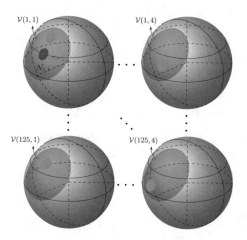

Fig. 1. Patch Matching in *x-q* Space. Patch matching involving 4 shells in *q*-space and a search radius of 2 voxels in *x*-space. The search neighborhood $\mathcal{V}$ is a combination of the sub-neighborhoods $\{\mathcal{V}(j,r)\}$ (blue) associated with different locations, $\{\mathbf{x}_j\}$, and *b*-values, $\{b_r\}$, i.e., $\mathcal{V} = \cup_{j,r}\mathcal{V}(j,r)$, where $\mathcal{V}(j,r) \equiv \mathcal{V}(\mathbf{x}_j, b_r)$. The total number of sub-neighborhoods is $4 \times (2 \times 2 + 1)^3 = 500$. The reference patch is marked by red and the search patches are marked by orange. (Color figure online)

2.2   Azimuthal Equidistant Projection (AEP)

AEP [5] maps the coordinates on a sphere to a plane where the distances and azimuths of points on the sphere are preserved with respect to a reference point [5]. This provides a good basis for subsequent computation of invariant features for matching. The reference point, which in our case corresponds to the center of the spherical patch, will project to the center of a circular projection. Viewing the reference point as the 'North pole', all points along a given azimuth, θ, will project along a straight line from the center. In the projection plane, this line subtends an angle θ with the vertical. The distance from the center to another projected point is given as ρ. We represent the reference point $\hat{\mathbf{q}}_0 = \frac{\mathbf{q}_0}{|\mathbf{q}_0|}$ as spherical coordinates (ϕ_0, λ_0), with ϕ referring to latitude and λ referring to longitude. We project (ϕ, λ) to a corresponding point (ρ, θ) in a 2D polar coordinate system, where ρ is the radius and θ is the angle. Based on [5], the relationship between (ϕ, λ) and (ρ, θ) is as follows:

$$\cos \rho = \sin \phi_0 \sin \phi + \cos \phi_0 \cos \phi \cos(\lambda - \lambda_0), \tag{3a}$$

$$\tan \theta = \frac{\cos \phi \sin(\lambda - \lambda_0)}{\cos \phi_0 \sin \phi - \sin \phi_0 \cos \phi \cos(\lambda - \lambda_0)}. \tag{3b}$$

The projection can be described as a two-step mapping:

$$\mathbf{q} \longrightarrow (q, \phi, \lambda) \longrightarrow (q, \rho, \theta). \tag{4}$$

Note that extra care needs to be taken when using the above equations to take into consideration the fact that diffusion signals are antipodal symmetric. Prior to performing AEP, we map antipodally all the points on the sphere to the hemisphere where the reference point is located. AEP maps a q-space spherical patch $\mathcal{N}$ to a 2D circular patch $\widehat{\mathcal{N}}$. Note that AEP changes only the coordinates but not the actual values of the signal vector, i.e., $\mathbf{S}(\widehat{\mathcal{N}}) = \mathbf{S}(\mathcal{N})$.

2.3   Polar Complex Exponential Transform (PCET)

After AEP, we proceed with the computation of rotation invariant features. We choose to use the polar complex exponential transform (PCET) [6] for its computation efficiency. Denoting an element of $\widehat{\mathbf{S}}(\widehat{\mathcal{N}})$ as $\widehat{S}(\mathbf{x}, q, \rho, \theta)$, the PCET of order n, $|n| = 0, 1, 2, \ldots, \infty$, and repetition l, $|l| = 0, 1, 2, \ldots, \infty$, is defined as

$$M_{n,l}(\widehat{\mathcal{N}}) = \frac{1}{\pi} \int_{(\mathbf{x}, q, \rho, \theta) \in \widehat{\mathcal{N}}} [H_{n,l}(\rho, \theta)]^* \widehat{S}(\mathbf{x}, q, \rho, \theta) \rho \, d\rho \, d\theta, \tag{5}$$

where $[\cdot]^*$ denotes the complex conjugate and $H_{n,l}(\rho, \theta)$ is the basis function defined as $H_{n,l}(\rho, \theta) = e^{i2\pi n \rho^2} e^{il\theta}$. It can be easily verified that $|M_{n,l}(\widehat{\mathcal{N}})|$ is invariant to rotation [6]. $|M_{n,l}(\widehat{\mathcal{N}})|$'s up to maximum order m, i.e., $-m \leq l, n \leq m$, are concatenated into a feature vector $\mathbf{M}(\widehat{\mathcal{N}})$.

2.4 Patch Matching

If $\mathbf{M}(\widehat{\mathcal{N}}_{i,k})$ is the feature vector of the projected patch $\widehat{\mathcal{N}}_{i,k}$, the matching weight $w_{i,k;j,l}$ is defined as

$$w_{i,k;j,l} = \frac{1}{Z_{i,k}} \exp\left\{-\frac{\|\mathbf{M}(\widehat{\mathcal{N}}_{i,k}) - \mathbf{M}(\widehat{\mathcal{N}}_{j,l})\|_2^2}{h_{\mathbf{M}}^2(i,k)}\right\} \exp\left\{-\frac{(\sqrt{b_k} - \sqrt{b_l})^2}{h_b^2}\right\}, \quad (6)$$

where $Z_{i,k}$ is a normalization constant to ensure that the weights sum to one:

$$Z_{i,k} = \sum_{(\mathbf{x}_j,\mathbf{q}_l)\in\mathcal{V}_{i,k}} \exp\left\{-\frac{\|\mathbf{M}(\widehat{\mathcal{N}}_{i,k}) - \mathbf{M}(\widehat{\mathcal{N}}_{j,l})\|_2^2}{h_{\mathbf{M}}^2(i,k)}\right\} \exp\left\{-\frac{(\sqrt{b_k} - \sqrt{b_l})^2}{h_b^2}\right\}.$$
$$(7)$$

Here $h_{\mathbf{M}}(i,k)$ is a parameter controlling the attenuation of the first exponential function. As in [7], we set $h_{\mathbf{M}}(i,k) = \sqrt{2\beta\hat{\sigma}_{i,k}^2 |\mathbf{M}(\widehat{\mathcal{N}}_{i,k})|}$, where β is a constant [7] and $\hat{\sigma}_{i,k}^2$ is the estimated noise standard deviation, which can be computed globally as shown in [8] or spatial-adaptively as shown in [7]. The former is used in this paper. Similarly, $h_b = \sqrt{2}\sigma_b$ controls the attenuation of the second exponential function, where σ_b is a scale parameter. $|\mathbf{M}(\widehat{\mathcal{N}}_{i,k})|$ denotes the length of the vector $\mathbf{M}(\widehat{\mathcal{N}}_{i,k})$.

2.5 Adaption to Noncentral Chi Noise

The classic NLM is designed to remove Gaussian noise and needs to be modified for the noncentral Chi noise distribution typical in parallel MRI, which uses multiple receiver coils. Based on [9], we define the unbiased denoised signal $\text{UNLM}(S)(\mathbf{x}_i, \mathbf{q}_k)$ as

$$\text{UNLM}(S)(\mathbf{x}_i, \mathbf{q}_k) = \sqrt{\sum_{(\mathbf{x}_j,\mathbf{q}_l)\in\mathcal{V}_{i,k}} w_{i,k;j,l}[S(\mathbf{x}_j, \mathbf{q}_l) + c_{i,k;j,l}]^2 - 2N\sigma^2}, \quad (8)$$

where σ is the Gaussian noise standard deviation that can be estimated from the image background [8], N is the number of receiver coils. When there is only one coil (i.e., $N = 1$), the noncentral Chi distribution reduces to a Rician distribution.

3 Experiments

3.1 Datasets

Synthetic Data: A synthetic multi-shell dataset of a spiral was generated for the quantitative evaluation of the proposed method. The parameters used in synthetic data simulation were consistent with the real data described next: $b = 1000, 2000, 4000, 6000\,\text{s/mm}^2$, 81 gradient directions, 128×128 voxels with

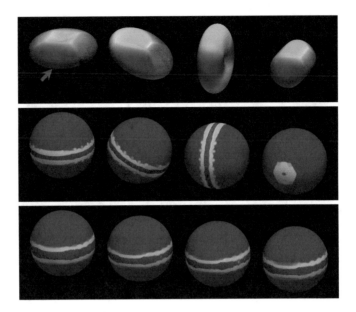

Fig. 2. q-Space Patch Matching. Two cases of q-space patch matching: (middle row) variation of fiber orientations and (bottom row) variation of b-values. The top row shows the profiles of the diffusion signals. Patch matching is performed using the point marked by the red arrow as the reference. The middle row shows the matching results of signal profiles in different orientations. Warm colors indicate greater agreement, cool colors indicate otherwise. The bottom row shows the matching results for different b-values (i.e., 1000, 2000, 3000, 4000 s/mm²), based on the leftmost signal profile. (Color figure online)

resolution 2×2 mm². Four levels of Rician noise (3 %, 9 %, 15 %, and 21 %) were added to the resulting ground truth data. Rician noise was generated by adding Gaussian noise with distribution $\mathcal{N}(0, v(p/100))$ in the complex domain of the signal with noise variance determined based on noise-level percentage p and maximum signal value v (150 in our case) [7].

Real Data: The real dataset was acquired using the same gradient directions and b-values as the synthetic dataset. A Siemens 3T TRIO MR scanner was used for data acquisition. The imaging protocol is as follows: 96×128 imaging matrix, $2 \times 2 \times 2$ mm³ resolution, TE=145 ms, TR = 12, 200 ms, 32 receiver coils.

3.2 Results

In all experiments, we set $s = 2$ voxels, $\beta = 0.1$, $\sigma_b = 5$, $\alpha_p = 30°$, $\alpha_s = 30°$ and $m = 4$. The dataset is acquired using spherical sampling, therefore we set $h_{\text{projection}}$ to a small value to disable the signal projection described in (2). We use peak-to-signal-ratio (PSNR) as the metric for performance evaluation.

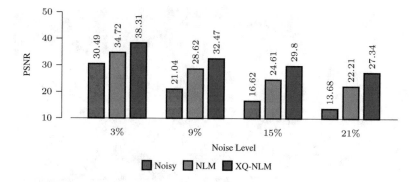

Fig. 3. PSNR Comparison. Performance comparison between NLM and XQ-NLM using the synthetic dataset

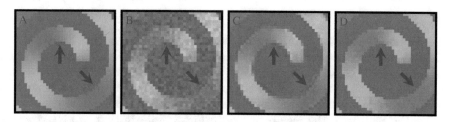

Fig. 4. DW Images – Synthetic Data. (A) Ground truth DW image; (B) Image with 3% noise; (C) NLM-denoised image; (D) XQ-NLM-denoised image

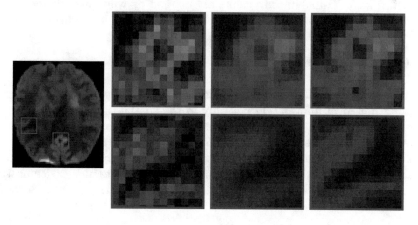

Fig. 5. DW Images – Real Data. The reference DW image is shown on the far left. Close-up views of (left) noisy DW image, (middle) NLM-denoised image, and (left) XQ-NLM-denoised image

Figure 2 indicates that the new patch matching scheme is robust to the variation of fiber orientations and *b*-values. This allows our method, XQ-NLM, to use information from differentially oriented signal profiles for effective denoising. For

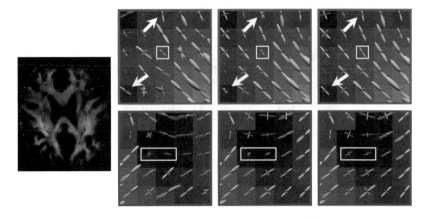

Fig. 6. Fiber ODFs. White matter fiber ODFs shown in order identical to Fig. 5

different noise levels, the PSNR results shown in Fig. 3 indicate that XQ-NLM significantly improves the PSNR. The largest improvement over NLM is 5.19 dB when the noise level is 15 %. The denoised DW images, shown in Fig. 4, indicate that XQ-NLM is able to preserve sharp edges and effectively remove noise, thanks to the robust q-space patch matching mechanism, as demonstrated in Fig. 2.

For the real data, the results shown in Fig. 5 indicate that XQ-NLM yields markedly improved edge-preserving results in cortical regions. The influence of denoising on the white matter fiber orientation distribution functions (ODFs) is shown in Fig. 6. Visible improvements are marked by white arrows and rectangles, indicating that XQ-NLM yields cleaner results with less spurious peaks.

4   Conclusion

We have extended NLM beyond x-space to include q-space, allowing denoising using non-local information not only in the spatial domain but also in the wavevector domain. Our method allows information from highly curve white matter structures to be used effectively for denoising. The synthetic data experiments show that our method increases the PSNR markedly and yields improved results, especially at boundaries. The real data experiments further demonstrate that our method gives cleaner white matter fiber ODF with less spurious peaks.

References

1. Wiest-Daesslé, N., Prima, S., Coupé, P., Morrissey, S.P., Barillot, C.: Non-local means variants for denoising of diffusion-weighted and diffusion tensor MRI. In: Ayache, N., Ourselin, S., Maeder, A. (eds.) MICCAI 2007, Part II. LNCS, vol. 4792, pp. 344–351. Springer, Heidelberg (2007)

2. Descoteaux, M., Wiest-Daesslé, N., Prima, S., Barillot, C., Deriche, R.: Impact of rician adapted non-local means filtering on HARDI. In: Metaxas, D., Axel, L., Fichtinger, G., Székely, G. (eds.) MICCAI 2008, Part II. LNCS, vol. 5242, pp. 122–130. Springer, Heidelberg (2008)

3. Chen, G., Zhang, P., Wu, Y., Shen, D., Yap, P.T.: Denoising magnetic resonance images using collaborative non-local means. Neurocomputing **177**, 215–227 (2016)

4. Buades, A., Coll, B., Morel, J.M.: A review of image denoising algorithms, with a new one. Multiscale Model. Simul. **4**(2), 490–530 (2005)

5. Wessel, P., Smith, W.H.: The generic mapping tools. http://gmt.soest.hawaii.edu

6. Yap, P.T., Jiang, X., Kot, A.C.: Two-dimensional polar harmonic transforms for invariant image representation. IEEE Trans. Pattern Anal. Mach. Intell. **32**(7), 1259–1270 (2010)

7. Coupé, P., Yger, P., Prima, S., Hellier, P., Kervrann, C., Barillot, C.: An optimized blockwise nonlocal means denoising filter for 3-D magnetic resonance images. IEEE Trans. Med. Imaging **27**(4), 425–441 (2008)

8. Manjón, J.V., Carbonell-Caballero, J., Lull, J.J., García-Martí, G., Martí-Bonmatí, L., Robles, M.: MRI denoising using non-local means. Med. Image Anal. **12**(4), 514–523 (2008)

9. Koay, C.G., Özarslan, E., Basser, P.J.: A signal transformational framework for breaking the noise floor and its applications in MRI. J. Magn. Reson. **197**(2), 108–119 (2009)

Spatially Adaptive Spectral Denoising for MR Spectroscopic Imaging using Frequency-Phase Non-local Means

Dhritiman Das[1,3]([envelope]), Eduardo Coello[2,3], Rolf F. Schulte[3],
and Bjoern H. Menze[1]

[1] Department of Computer Science, Technical University of Munich,
Munich, Germany
dhritiman.das@tum.de

[2] Department of Physics, Technical University of Munich, Munich, Germany

[3] GE Global Research, Munich, Germany

Abstract. Magnetic resonance spectroscopic imaging (MRSI) is an imaging modality used for generating metabolic maps of the tissue in-vivo. These maps show the concentration of metabolites in the sample being investigated and their accurate quantification is important to diagnose diseases. However, the major roadblocks in accurate metabolite quantification are: low spatial resolution, long scanning times, poor signal-to-noise ratio (SNR) and the subsequent noise-sensitive non-linear model fitting. In this work, we propose a frequency-phase spectral denoising method based on the concept of non-local means (NLM) that improves the robustness of data analysis and scanning times while potentially increasing spatial resolution. We evaluate our method on simulated data sets as well as on human in-vivo MRSI data. Our denoising method improves the SNR while maintaining the spatial resolution of the spectra.

1 Introduction

Magnetic Resonance Spectroscopic imaging (MRSI), also known as chemical shift imaging, is a clinical imaging modality for studying tissues in-vivo to investigate and diagnose neurological diseases. More specifically, this modality can be used in non-invasive diagnosis and characterization of patho-physiological changes by measuring specific tissue metabolites in the brain. Accurate metabolite quantification is a crucial requirement for effectively using MRSI for diagnostic purposes. However, a major challenge with MRSI is the long scanning time required to obtain spatially resolved spectra due to abundance of metabolites that have a concentration which is approximately 10,000 times smaller than water. Current acquisition techniques such as Parallel Imaging [13] and Echo-Planar Spectroscopic Imaging [9] focus on accelerated scanning times combined with reconstruction techniques to improve the SNR of the spectral signal. Despite this, further accelerated acquistions are desirable. Furthermore, an improved SNR is needed as the non-linear voxel-wise fitting to noisy data leads to a high amount of local minima and noise amplification resulting in poor spatial resolution [7].

© Springer International Publishing AG 2016
S. Ourselin et al. (Eds.): MICCAI 2016, Part III, LNCS 9902, pp. 596–604, 2016.
DOI: 10.1007/978-3-319-46726-9_69

The SNR of the signal can be improved by post-processing methods such as denoising algorithms [8], apodization (Gaussian/Lorentzian), filter-based smoothing and transform-based methods [3]. However, these methods reduce resolution and remove important quantifiable information by averaging out the lower-concentration metabolites. Recently, data-dependent approaches such as the Non-local Means (NLM), which use the redundancy inherent in periodic images, are being used extensively for denoising [3]. In the case of MRS, this periodicity implies that the spectra in any voxel may have similar spectra in other voxels in the frequency-phase space. Therefore, it carries out a weighted average of the voxels in this space, depending on the similarity of the spectral information of their neighborhoods to the neighborhood of the voxel to be denoised.

Our Contribution. *In this work, we propose a method for spectrally adaptive denoising of MRSI spectra in the frequency-phase space based on the concept of Non-local Means.* Our method compensates for the lack of phase-information in the acquired spectra by implementing a dephasing approach on the spectral data. In the next section, we introduce the experimental methods beginning with the concept of NLM in the frequency-phase space followed by the spectral dephasing and rephasing approach. Our proposed method is then validated quantitatively and qualitatively using simulated brain data and human in-vivo MRSI data sets to show the improvements in SNR and spatial-spectral resolution of MRSI data.

2 Methods

MR Spectroscopy. Magnetic resonance spectroscopy is based on the concept of nuclear magnetic resonance (NMR). It exploits the resonance frequency of a molecule, which depends on its chemical structure, to obtain information about the concentration of a particular metabolite [12]. The time-domain complex signal of a nuclei is given by: $S(t) = \int p(\omega)\exp(-i\Phi)\exp(-t/T_2^*)dw$. The frequency-domain signal is given by $S(\omega)$, T_2^* is the magnetization decay in the transverse plane due to magnetic field inhomogeneity and $p(\omega)$ comprises of Lorentzian absorption and dispersion line-shapes function having the spectroscopic information about the sample. Φ represents the phase, $(\omega t + \omega_0)$, of the acquired signal where ωt is the time-varying phase change and ω_0 is the initial phase. For the acquired MRSI data, I, Φ is unknown. This process allows generation of metabolic maps through non-linear fitting to estimate concentration of metabolites such as N-acetyl-aspartate (NAA), Creatine (Cr) and Choline (Cho).

2.1 Non-local Means (NLM) in Frequency-Phase Space

As proposed by Buades et al. [3], the Non-local Means (NLM) method restores the intensity of voxel x_{ij} by computing a similarity-based weighted average of all the voxels in a given image. In the following, we adapt NLM to the MRSI data: let us suppose that we have complex data, $I : \Omega^3 \longmapsto \mathbb{C}$ of size $M \times N$ and noisy spectra $S_{ij}(\omega)$, where $(x_{ij}|i \in [1, M], j \in [1, N])$ and Ω^3 is the frequency-phase grid. Using NLM for denoising, the restored spectra $\hat{S}_{ij}(\omega)$ is computed as the weighted average of all other spectra in the frequency-phase space defined as:

$$\hat{S}_{ij}(\omega) = \sum_{x_{kl} \in \Omega^3} w(x_{ij}, x_{kl}) S_{kl}(\omega) \tag{1}$$

As a probabilistic interpretation, spectral data $S_{11}(\omega), ..., S_{MN}(\omega)$ of voxels $x_{11}, ..., x_{MN}$ respectively are considered as MN random variables X_{ij} and the weighted average estimate $\hat{S}_{ij}(\omega)$ is the maximum likelihood estimate of $S_{ij}(\omega)$.
$N_{ij} = (2p+1)^3$, $p \in \mathbb{N}$ is the cubic neighborhood of voxel x_{ij} within the search volume $V_{ij} = (2R+1)^3$ around x_{ij} along the frequency, phase and spatial directions. $R \in \mathbb{N}$, where R is the radius of search centered at the voxel x_{ij}. The weight $w(x_{ij}, x_{kl})$ serves as a quantifiable similarity metric between the neighborhoods N_{ij} and N_{kl} of the voxels x_{ij} and x_{kl} provided $w(x_{ij}, x_{kl}) \in [0, 1]$ and $\sum w(x_{ij}, x_{kl}) = 1$. The Gaussian-weighted Euclidean distance is computed between $S(N_{ij})$ and $S(N_{kl})$ as shown below:

$$w(x_{ij}, x_{kl}) = \frac{1}{Z_{ij}} e^{-\frac{\|S(N_{ij}) - S(N_{kl})\|_2^2}{h^2}} \tag{2}$$

where Z_{ij} serves as the normalization constant such that $\sum_j w(x_{ij}, x_{kl}) = 1$, $S(N_{ij})$ and $S(N_{kl})$ are vectors containing the spectra of neighborhoods N_{ij} and N_{kl} of voxels x_{ij} and x_{kl} respectively and h serves as a smoothing parameter [5].
To increase the robustness of our method for MRSI data, in the next section we propose a dephasing approach tailored for use in the frequency-phase NLM.

2.2   Spectral Dephasing

For the acquired data I, as the spectral phase $\Phi(I)$ is unknown, the probability of finding a similar neighborhood spectra are very low. To counter this effect, a dephasing step is performed to consider a wide range of possible phase variations in the pattern analysis. For each voxel x_{ij}, the complex time-domain signal $S_{ij}(t)$ is shifted by a set of phase angles Θ. This is given by $S_{ij}^\Theta(t) = S_{ij}(t).e^{-(i\Theta)}$, where $\Theta \in [-n_1\pi, (n_2+2)\pi]$, $\{n_1, n_2 \in \mathbb{R} \mid n_1, n_2 \geq 0\}$. Θ here is defined to be the range of angles through which the spectrum can be shifted. The dephased signal is transformed into the frequency-domain, $S_{ij}^\Theta(t) \xrightarrow{\mathscr{F}} S_{ij}^\Theta(\omega)$, following which its real component, $\mathbb{R}(S_{ij}^\Theta(\omega))$, is taken to generate a 2D spectral-phase matrix. Note that in this 2D matrix generated, for each voxel x_{ij}, the imaginary part at a given Θ is $\mathbb{I}(\Theta) = \mathbb{R}(\Theta + \pi/2)$. This approach is illustrated in Fig. 1.
Repeating this step for all MN voxels gives us a 3-D dataset on which the NLM is implemented to give the denoised spectra $\hat{S}_{ij}^\Theta(\omega) \in \mathbb{R}$. Our approach has 2 key innovations: the denoising method is (i) robust to phase shifts as the range of angles considered varies from 0 to 2π periodically for all spectral signals, and is (ii) adaptive to the imaging sequence as the spectrum is denoised by relying on similar signals in the given data and not on predefined prior assumptions.

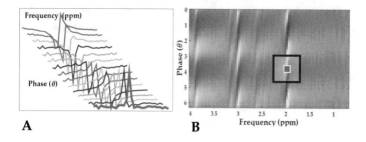

Fig. 1. MRSI data dephasing shown here for a sample voxel: (A) Changes in spectral pattern as it is shifted by different phase angles. (B) Corresponding 2D frequency-phase image space generated for the voxel. A sample patch (black box) is selected and then denoised by the NLM-based matching in the frequency-phase space.

Algorithm 1. Frequency-Phase NLM denoising for MRSI

$\quad$ **MRSI Input** $I : \Omega^3 = (S(\omega) \times M \times N) \longmapsto \mathbb{C}$
$\quad$ **Define Phase Angle range** $\Theta : [-n_1\pi : (n_2 + 1)\pi] \ \{n_1, n_2 \in \mathbb{R} \mid n_1, n_2 \geq 0\}$
$\quad$ **Spectral Dephasing:**
$\quad$ $S_{ij}(t) = \mathcal{F}^{-1}(S_{ij}(\omega))$: for each voxel $ij \in (M \times N)$
$\quad$ $S_{ij}^{\Theta}(\omega) = \mathcal{F}(S_{ij}(t).e^{(-i\Theta)})$: Phase shift by Θ
$\quad$ **NLM:** $\hat{S}_{ij}/^{\Theta}(\omega) = NLM[\mathbb{R}(S_{ij}^{\Theta}(\omega)) \times MN]$: $\forall$ voxels
$\quad$ **Spectral Rephasing:**
$\quad$ $\mathbb{C}(\hat{S}_{ij}^{\Theta}(t)) = \mathcal{F}^{-1}[\mathbb{R}(\hat{S}_{ij}^{\Theta}(\omega)) + \mathbb{I}(\hat{S}_{ij}^{\Theta}(\omega))]$: Re-generate complex data for all Θ
$\quad$ $\mathbb{C}(\hat{S}_{ij}^{-\Theta}(\omega)) = \mathcal{F}(\mathbb{C}(\hat{S}_{ij}^{\Theta}(t)).e^{(i\Theta)})$: Rephase by $-\Theta$
$\quad$ **Frequency-Phase NLM Output:** $\mathbb{C}(\hat{S}_{ij}(\omega)) = mean(\mathbb{C}(\hat{S}_{ij}^{-\Theta}(\omega))) \ \forall \ \Theta$

2.3 Spectral Rephasing and Recombination

Post-NLM, $\hat{S}_{ij}^{\Theta}(\omega)$ is rephased in order to generate the denoised complex signal $\mathbb{C}(\hat{S}_{ij}(\omega))$. The complex spectral signal $\mathbb{C}(\hat{S}_{ij}^{\Theta}(\omega))$ is re-generated $\forall\Theta$ by combining $\mathbb{R}(\hat{S}_{ij}^{\Theta}(\omega))$ and $\mathbb{I}(\hat{S}_{ij}^{\Theta}(\omega))$ $(= \mathbb{R}(\hat{S}_{ij}^{\Theta+\pi/2}(\omega)))$. The equivalent time signal is obtained by $\mathbb{C}(\hat{S}_{ij}^{\Theta}(\omega)) \xrightarrow{\mathscr{F}^{-1}} \mathbb{C}(\hat{S}_{ij}^{\Theta}(t))$. After this, $\mathbb{C}(\hat{S}_{ij}^{\Theta}(t))$ undergoes an inverse phase shift by $-\Theta$ to remove the dephasing effect as given by $\mathbb{C}(\hat{S}_{ij}^{-\Theta}(t)) = \mathbb{C}(\hat{S}_{ij}^{\Theta}(t)).e^{(i\Theta)}$. This re-phased signal is transformed back to the spectral domain to obtain $\mathbb{C}(\hat{S}_{ij}^{-\Theta}(\omega))$. Thereafter, the $\mathbb{C}(\hat{S}_{ij}^{-\Theta}(\omega))$ are averaged over all Θ to generate a single complex spectra $\mathbb{C}(\hat{S}_{ij}(\omega))$. The entire pipeline for dephasing and rephasing the spectra is shown in Algorithm 1.

3 Experiments and Results

We performed two different experiments to test the improvement in SNR and metabolite quantification using our proposed denoising method. In the first experiment, we evaluate our method on the publicly available BrainWeb database [4], while in the second experiment we use human in-vivo MRSI data. The SNR of a metabolite was calculated by dividing the maximum value of the metabolite peak by the standard deviation of the spectral region having pure noise. For both experiments, we tested with different noise levels against a ground-truth data to assess the improvement in SNR and spatial-spectral resolution.

3.1   Data Acquisition

We used BrainWeb to simulate a brain MRSI image (size: 64×64 voxels, slice thickness $= 1\,mm$, noise level $= 3\,\%$) with segmented tissue types, namely White Matter (WM), Grey Matter (GM) and Cerebro Spinal Fluid (CSF) as shown in Fig. 2. In order to have a comparable spectrum with the in-vivo data, water was added to the signal and the main metabolites- NAA, Cho and Cr- were simulated using Priorset (Vespa) [1]. Metabolite concentrations for WM, GM and CSF were based on commonly reported literature values [10,14]. Next, Gaussian noise of levels 2 and 3 times the standard deviation, σ, of the original image data were added to the ground-truth signal.

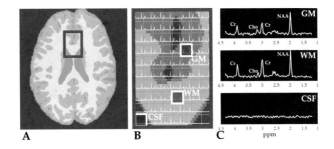

Fig. 2. Simulated brain MRSI dataset. (A) The simulated brain with the region of interest (red box). (B) Highlighted regions corresponding to GM, WM and CSF (c) Corresponding spectrum of GM, WM and CSF. Note that CSF has only water. (Color figure online)

In the case of in-vivo data, we acquired a 2D-MRSI data of the brain of a healthy human volunteer using a 3T-HDxt system (GE-Healthcare). PRESS localization [2], CHESS water suppression [6] and EPSI readout [9] were used as part of the sequence. The acquisition parameters were: Field of view (FOV) $= 160 \times 160 \times 10\,mm^3$, voxel size $= 10 \times 10 \times 10\,mm^3$, TE/TR$=35/2000\,ms$ and spectral bandwidth $= 1\,kHz$. The dataset was zero-filled and reconstructed to generate a grid of 32×32 voxels and 256 spectral points. 6 (**ground truth**), 3 and 1 averages were acquired with a total scan duration of 33 min (5.5 min per average). Figure 4(A) shows the in-vivo data acquired along with the entire field-of-view (white grid) and the corresponding spectra of a voxel (red box).

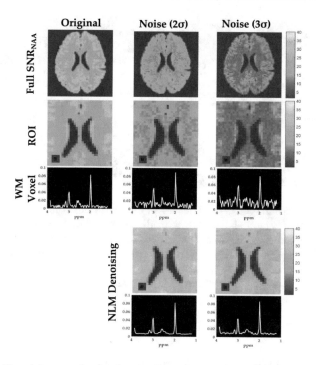

Fig. 3. NLM Denoising results in the simulated data. (From Top) Row 1 (L-R): Full SNR of NAA in – original data, with additive noise 2σ, and noise 3σ (σ is the standard deviation of the original data). Row 2 & 3: 32×32 Region of Interest (ROI) for applying the frequency-phase NLM: SNR of NAA in the original data, noise level 2σ, 3σ and the corresponding spectra of reference WM voxel (red box). Row 4 & 5 (L-R): Denoised SNR for noise level 2σ (SNR improvement = 2.9), for noise level 3σ (SNR improvement = 2.2), and the corresponding denoised spectrum. The SNR improves significantly while retaining the spatial-spectral resolution (seen by no voxel bleeding in the CSF). (Color figure online)

3.2 Results

Simulated data: In Fig. 3, we show the SNR improvement for NAA for data with noise levels 2σ and 3σ in a 32×32 region of interest. It is evident that while the spectral SNR improves significantly, the spatial resolution is preserved as the lower concentration metabolite peaks have only a small amount of smoothing and there is no voxel bleeding in the CSF (containing only water).

In-vivo data: Figure 4 reports the SNR improvement in NAA for the 3-averages and the 1-average data as compared to the ground-truth 6-averages data. The figure also presents the results from the LCModel [11] which is the gold stan- dard quantitation tool in MRS analysis. LCModel fits the spectral signal $S(\omega)$ using a basis set of spectra of metabolites acquired under identical acquisition conditions as the in-vivo data. As explained earlier for noisy data, the non-linear fitting leads to poor spatial resolution. Therefore, the LCModel can be used to

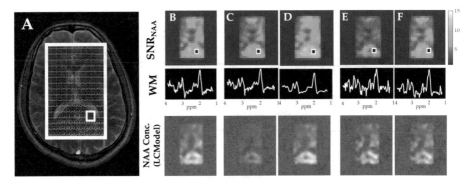

Fig. 4. Denoising results for in-vivo data. (A) Original human in-vivo brain MRSI data with the excitation region shown (white grid). (From Top) Row 1 & 2: SNR of NAA and the corresponding WM voxel spectra in: (B) 6-averages data **(ground-truth)**, (C) 3-averages data (original) and (D) denoised, (E) single-scan data (original) and (F) denoised with corresponding spectra. Row 3: LCModel based absolute concentration estimate of NAA in: 6-averages data, 3-averages data (original) and denoised, 1-average data (original) and denoised. The NAA concentration estimate and spectral SNR improve considerably as seen in columns D (SNR = 23.29) and F (SNR = 11.38) against the ground-truth (SNR = 11.44).

Table 1. SNR and LCM Quantification results for NAA, Cho and Cr before and after using frequency-phase NLM on in-vivo MRSI data. Mean SNR for the denoised data is comparable or better than the ground-truth data while the FWHM of the water peak is lower than the ground-truth data thereby preserving spatial-spectral resolution.

Data	Mean SNR (NAA)	SNR improvement (NAA)	Mean SNR (Cho)	SNR (Cho)	Mean SNR (Cr)	SNR improvement (Cr)	FWHM
1-average	5.70	–	3.74	–	4.04	–	0.125
3-averages	8.82	–	5.59	–	5.97	–	0.135
6-averages (ground-truth)	11.44	–	6.96	–	7.61	–	0.135
Single scan (NLM)	**11.38**	1.98	**6.89**	1.82	**7.78**	1.90	**0.130**
3-averages (NLM)	**23.29**	2.63	**14.08**	2.48	**15.59**	2.57	**0.134**

assess the improvement in spatial resolution through a better fit. Due to space constraints, we present the results for NAA only and mention the SNR values for Cho and Cr. LCModel quantification (Fig. 4) shows that the absolute concentration estimation of NAA in the denoised data improves significantly. The Full-Width Half Maximum (FWHM) shows information about the water peak – a narrow peak gives a better spatial resolution. As shown in Table 1, the FWHM of the denoised 1- and 3-averages data is lower than the 6-averages data while the corresponding mean SNR improves considerably. Therefore, we observe here that our method can accelerate MRSI data acquisition by almost 2 times by reducing the number of scans acquired.

4   Conclusion

In this work, we proposed a novel frequency-phase NLM-based denoising method for MRS Imaging to improve the SNR and spatial resolution of the metabolites. A spectral dephasing approach is promoted to compensate for the unknown phase information of the acquired data. To the best of our knowledge, this is a novel application of the concept of NLM and has been validated on both simulated and in-vivo MRSI data.

In particular, we assessed the effect of our method on metabolites such as NAA, Cho and Cr and obtained a visible improvement in SNR while the spatial resolution was preserved which, subsequently, led to a better estimation of the absolute concentration distribution of NAA. This has direct benefits as it would accelerate data acquisition by taking fewer scan averages. Future work would involve using a more robust metabolite-specific search in the given dataset with less smoothing. This can be coupled with optimal computational efficiency and better estimation of the in-vivo metabolites.

Acknowledgments. The research leading to these results has received funding from the European Union's H2020 Framework Programme (H2020-MSCA-ITN-2014) under grant agreement no 642685 MacSeNet.

References

1. Vespa project (Versatile simulation, pulses and analysis). https://scion.duhs.duke.edu/vespa/project
2. Bottomley, P.A.: Spatial localization in NMR spectroscopy in vivo. Ann. N. Y. Acad. Sci. **508**, 333–348 (1987). doi:10.1111/j.1749-6632.1987.tb32915.x
3. Buades, A., Coll, B.: A non-local algorithm for image denoising. Comput. Vis. Pattern **2**(0), 60–65 (2005)
4. Collins, D.L., Zijdenbos, P., Kollokian, V., Sled, J.G., Kabani, N.J., Holmes, C.J., Evans, C.: Design and construction of a realistic digital brain phantom. IEEE Trans. Med. Imaging **17**(3), 463–468 (1998)
5. Coupé, P., Yger, P., Prima, S., Hellier, P., Kervrann, C.: An optimized blockwise non local means denoising filter for 3D magnetic resonance images. IEEE Trans. Med. Imaging **27**(4), 425–441 (2008)
6. Haase, A., Frahm, J., Hänicke, W., Matthaei, D.: 1H NMR chemical shift selective (CHESS) imaging. Phys. Med. Biol. **30**(4), 341–344 (1985). http://stacks.iop.org/0031-9155/30/i=4/a=008
7. Kelm, B.M., Kaster, F.O., Henning, A., Weber, M.A., Bachert, P., Boesiger, P., Hamprecht, F.A., Menze, B.H.: Using spatial prior knowledge in the spectral fitting of MRS images. NMR Biomed. **25**(1), 1–13 (2012)
8. Nguyen, H.M., Peng, X., Do, M.N., Liang, Z.: Spatiotemporal denoising of MR spectroscopic imaging data by low-rank approximations. IEEE ISBI: From Nano to Macro **0**(3), 857–860 (2011)
9. Posse, S., DeCarli, C., Le Bihan, D.: Three-dimensional echo-planar MR spectroscopic imaging at short echo times in the human brain. Radiology **192**(3), 733–738 (1994). http://pubs.rsna.org/doi/abs/10.1148/radiology.192.3.8058941

10. Pouwels, P.J.W., Frahm, T.: Regional metabolite concentrations in human brain as determined by quantitative localized proton MRS. Magn. Reson. Med. **39**(1), 53–60 (1998)
11. Provencher, S.W.: Estimation of metabolite concentrations from localized in vivo proton NMR spectra. Magn. Reson. Med. **30**(6), 672–679 (1993). http://www.ncbi.nlm.nih.gov/pubmed/8139448
12. de Graaf, R.A.: In Vivo NMR Spectroscopy: Principles and Techniques, 2nd edn. Wiley, Hoboken (2013)
13. Schulte, R.F., Lange, T., Beck, J., Meier, D., Boesiger, P.: Improved two-dimensional J-resolved spectroscopy. NMR Biomed. **19**(2), 264–270 (2006)
14. Wang, Y., Li, S.: Differentiation of metabolic concentrations between gray matter and white matter of human brain by in vivo ' h magnetic resonance spectroscopy. Magn. Reson. Med. **39**(1), 28–33 (2005)

Beyond the Resolution Limit: Diffusion Parameter Estimation in Partial Volume

Zach Eaton-Rosen[1]([✉]), Andrew Melbourne[1], M. Jorge Cardoso[1],
Neil Marlow[2], and Sebastien Ourselin[1]

[1] Translational Imaging Group, Centre for Medical Image Computing,
University College London, London, UK
rmapzea@ucl.ac.uk
[2] Academic Neonatology, EGA UCL Institute for Women's Health, London, UK

Abstract. Diffusion MRI is a frequently-used imaging modality that can infer microstructural properties of tissue, down to the scale of microns. For single-compartment models, such as the diffusion tensor (DT), the model interpretation depends on voxels having homogeneous composition. This limitation makes it difficult to measure diffusion parameters for small structures such as the fornix in the brain, because of partial volume. In this work, we use a segmentation from a structural scan to calculate the tissue composition for each diffusion voxel. We model the measured diffusion signal as a linear combination of signals from each of the tissues present in the voxel, and fit parameters on a per-region basis by optimising over all diffusion data simultaneously. We test the proposed method by using diffusion data from the Human Connectome Project (HCP). We downsample the HCP data, and show that our method returns parameter estimates that are closer to the high-resolution ground truths than for classical methods. We show that our method allows accurate estimation of diffusion parameters for regions with partial volume. Finally, we apply the method to compare diffusion in the fornix for adults born extremely preterm and matched controls.

1 Introduction

Diffusion imaging is a vital tool for probing the microstructure of *in-vivo* tissue. Parametric models of diffusion offer an informative way to summarise the information from many different b-values and gradient directions. The model parameters are often averaged over a region, under the reasonable assumption that tissue within a structure will have similar diffusion properties. This approach works well in large regions, where we can erode a probabilistic segmentation to obtain voxels that are fully within the tissue. But, the diffusion parameters within structures such as the fornix—a narrow white matter structure, surrounded by cerebrospinal fluid—might not be measured well by this approach, especially at typical diffusion resolutions [1]. Because of the large scale of diffusion MRI voxels relative to the fornix many, and perhaps all, voxels will contain partial volume. This partial volume affects the ability to interpret

© Springer International Publishing AG 2016
S. Ourselin et al. (Eds.): MICCAI 2016, Part III, LNCS 9902, pp. 605–612, 2016.
DOI: 10.1007/978-3-319-46726-9_70

the parameters of diffusion parameter models. For instance, the size of the fornix may confound parameter estimation by introducing varying amounts of partial volume in different subjects or at different timepoints (for example, due to atrophy). In order for the measured diffusion parameters to accurately represent microstructure, we must remove the confound of partial volume.

In this work, we extend the calculation of a region's parameters to include information from all voxels in the region *during* the model-fitting, instead of fitting voxel-wise and then averaging. While there has been work on eliminating the contribution of free water to diffusion parameter estimates [2], our proposed approach directly estimates the diffusion parameters of all tissue types within the image, without relying on *a priori* diffusion models or values. In the proposed framework, we use a probabilistic segmentation as weights for canonical diffusion signals, optimised for each segmentation class or tissue (we use the terms interchangeably). The modelled signal in a voxel is calculated as a weighted sum of each tissue present in the voxel, where the weights are given by the segmentation probabilities (which represent the proportion of each tissue type present).

We first validate the method on *in-vivo* diffusion data from the Human Connectome Project [3]. By using such high-resolution data, we can measure diffusion parameters in the fornix directly, using hand-drawn regions of interest. By downsampling this data, we simulate a more typical diffusion acquisition, and are able to test whether our approach retrieves the correct parameter values. After validating our approach, we apply it to adults born extremely preterm, comparing the diffusion within the fornix to that of term-born controls. The comparison is interesting as the patient group has pervasive differences in brain morphology and function, including memory (associated with the fornix).

This framework presented is similar to [4] in its use of multi-modal imaging to make a diffusion mixture model. This work differs in that there is no requirement of multiple shells of diffusion data, an important advantage for using this method in older data.

2   Methods

2.1   Theory

In this work we attempt to measure diffusion parameters from below the resolution at which they were obtained. If we imagine a voxel at a higher resolution (for example, the T_1-weighted scan) being downsampled to a lower resolution (the diffusion scans), the proportion of the tissue in a voxel of diffusion space will be reduced. Even in a best case scenario, the probability of there being at least a threshold T% of the tissue within a voxel depends on the position of the tissue relative to the voxel borders. Our approach eliminates the dependence of measured parameters on the precise voxel boundaries, by using all diffusion information within the region of interest.

In diffusion MRI, the diffusion of water within is summarised with a mathematical model. Within a given voxel, the water diffusion from several microstructural environments is measured together. A voxel's signal, S, in the diffusion tensor (DT) model, is given by:

$$\frac{S}{S_0} = e^{-b\mathbf{g}^T \mathbf{D} \mathbf{g}} \tag{1}$$

where S_0 is the diffusion signal with zero diffusion weighting, b are the b-values, $\mathbf{g}$ are the gradient directions and $\mathbf{D}$ is the second-rank diffusion tensor.

In our approach, we aim to obtain $\mathbf{D}$ for each of the k tissue classes (in the case of the fornix, white matter and CSF). In a given voxel, we model the signal as being represented as a weighted sum of each of the tissue classes that are present:

$$S = S_0 \sum_{j=1}^{k} p_j e^{-b\mathbf{g}^T \mathbf{D}_j \mathbf{g}} \tag{2}$$

$\mathbf{D_j}$ is now the diffusion tensor for a given region or tissue. The p_j are non-negative, and constrained between 0 and 1. The $\mathbf{D_j}$ are unknown parameters that are optimised to best fit the data. This is a mixture-model approach, that generates the diffusion parameter estimates for the entire volume simultaneously, instead of per voxel. For the case of two tissue classes, this reduces to the signal model in [1].

In order for a single DT to represent the diffusion properties in different voxels, we must account for different orientation in different parts of the same tissue. Conventionally, we would use the same b-matrix for each voxel in the image. However, we are mainly interested in orientationally-independent measurements, such as the fractional anisotropy (FA). In this work, we redefine the gradient-directions for each voxel, so that the principal directions of all voxels in the image align. The gradient directions at each voxel are calculated by first, performing a tensor-fit to the voxel and establishing $\mathbf{v}_1$ and $\mathbf{v}_2$, the first and second eigenvectors of $\mathbf{D}$. We then calculate the rotation matrix R such that $\mathbf{v}_1$ and $\mathbf{v}_2$ align with [1,0,0] and [0,1,0]. Our vector for the ith voxel then becomes $\mathbf{g}_i = R\mathbf{g}$.

After calculating principal diffusion directions in every voxel, and the S_0, with a weighted-least-squares tensor fit, we initialise a $3 \times k$ matrix with identical diffusivities in each of the tissue classes. At each iteration of the optimisation, we calculate the signal for the entire volume simultaneously, before the $3k$ diffusion parameters are updated. We fit using Matlab 2014b, using non-linear optimisation [5].

3 Experiments and Results

3.1 MRI Data

To test the proposed approach, we use data from the HCP [3]. The diffusion data has a resolution of $1.25^3 \, \text{mm}^3$, with 108 volumes with $b \approx 1000 \, \text{s.mm}^{-2}$ (including reference volumes). The T_1-weighted MRI is at resolution $0.70^3 \, \text{mm}^3$.

For the experiments on adult subjects, we collected MRI data at 19 years of age from 15 adolescents. Eight (4 Male) of these were born extremely preterm (fewer than 26 weeks completed gestation) and seven (3 Male) were recruited as matched controls. We acquired 3D T1-weighted volume at 1 mm isotropic resolution (TR/TE = 6.78/3.06 ms) for segmentation and diffusion MRI with the following characteristics: four b-values at b = (0, 300, 700, 2000) s.mm^{-2} with n = (4, 8, 16, 32) directions respectively at TE=70 ms (2.5 × 2.5 × 3.0 mm). For the fitting, we discarded the highest shell of b-values. All data was acquired using a Philips 3T Achieva. For the segmentations, we manually drew the fornix on a T_1-weighted segmentation and also labelled the surrounding tissue using multi-atlas label propagation and fusion [6] based on the Neuromorphometrics, Inc. labels.

3.2 Validating Method Using HCP Data

We used the high resolution of the HCP data to determine pseudo ground-truth values for diffusion parameters in the column, the crus and the body of the fornix. Each of these regions is hand-drawn onto the subject's T_1-weighted MRI. We downsample the segmentation from categorical labels into a probabilistic diffusion segmentation, where the probabilities represent fractions of the tissue in that diffusion voxel. We varied the downsampling to achieve voxels of isotropic dimension from 1.25 mm to 3.5 mm. In order to use HCP data as a model for a more typical diffusion acquisition, we adjust it in the following ways. We added rician noise to the downsampled data, to bring the data to a clinically realistic SNR. We only use one shell of the acquired data, to ignore effects that are not modelled with the DT. For each experiment, we used a subset of the 108 volumes. We tested the performance of our algorithm with between 12 and 60 of these volumes.

We compare three approaches for analysing average parameter values:

M1 For each region, we identify voxels where the membership to that region is above the threshold and average their values.

M2 We resample the downsampled DWI to high-resolution HCP space before fitting the DT model and, again, averaging the values for each region. For this, we use 7th-order b-splines, as recommended in [7].

M3 (proposed): We calculate parameter values for each region, explicitly accounting for partial volume. The p are given by downsampling labels from the T_1-weighted segmentation into diffusion space.

3.3 Results

In Fig. 1 we test approach M1. As the threshold changes, so do the results for the classical approach. At a resolution of 2 mm isotropic, all fornix tissue has partial volume, so we would be unable to use a threshold of 90 % even at this good resolution. However, as we decrease the threshold, increasing the voxel dimension results in decreasing FA, as CSF partial volume contaminates the

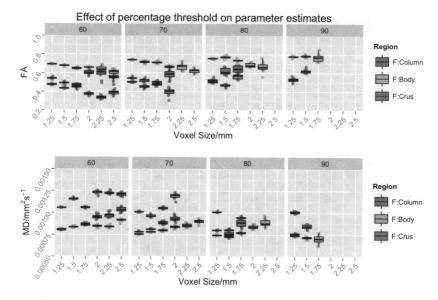

Fig. 1. In this graph, we see the effect of downsampling the resolution (x axis) on parameter estimates from a threshold-based approach. As the voxel dimension increases, the parameter estimation is less reliable and at some point stops, as there are no more supra-threshold voxels to sample. The choice of the threshold will influence the measured parameter value

estimates. For the body of the fornix, the measured FA decreases by up to 13 % by changing the thresholding, and when downsampled to 2.5 mm, the measured FA is up to 25 % lower than the pseudo-gold-standard.

In approach M2, we use the segmentation at the HCP resolution. After downsampling the data and adding noise, we interpolate the diffusion data back to the HCP resolution in order to fit the diffusion tensor and average the results over the ROI. These results are displayed in Fig. 2. The measured diffusion parameters diverge from their 'true' values as we interpolate data of lower resolution. With no downsampling, the values of nearby white matter, the column and the crus of the fornix are similar. However, as the downsampling increases, the FA estimates decrease due to the partial volume. This means that parameter values that should be similar are diverging because of local surroundings.

With the proposed method, the FA in the column and crus of the fornix is constant (Fig. 2). The body of the fornix has an increasing FA. The mean diffusivities are more constant in the proposed method than with the classical.

3.4 Comparison of Preterm-Born and Term-Born Young Adults

We compare fornix DTI parameters as calculated with M2 (upsampling DWI to T_1-space and fitting the tensor) and M3 (proposed) in Fig. 3. The MD in the fornix is higher in general for the classical approach compared to ours. In the

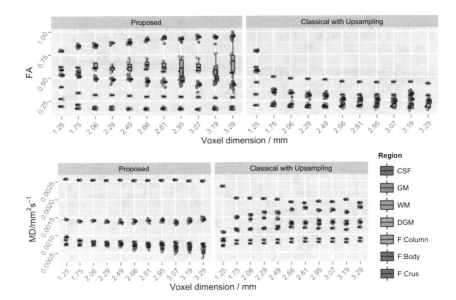

Fig. 2. In our method (left), the diffusion parameters in the fornix are fairly consistent with downsampling. While the results for larger regions match the classical approach, we improve for the fornix. We present the results for a thresholding approach *with* prior upsampling of the data (right). The results here, for diffusion parameters of the fornix, show a divergence of the diffusion parameter readings depending on their surrounding tissue. The scale factor is the factor by which we've downsampled the volume. In these experiments, we used 12 diffusion readings, 2 of which were reference volumes

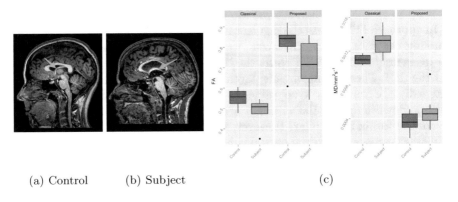

(a) Control   (b) Subject   (c)

Fig. 3. In a–b the fornix is highlighted with an arrow in a control and a preterm subject. The preterm-born subject has noticeable abnormalities in the corpus callosum, and enlarged ventricles. In c, we display the measured parameters using our proposed approach vs the classical.

classical approach, there is a significant difference in the MD with the subject group having higher MD (p ≤ 0.0005), which does not appear with the proposed method. Both approaches measure higher mean FA in the control group, but neither is significant when accounting for multiple comparisons. The fitting took less than a minute for each subject.

4 Discussion

Our method achieves consistent and accurate parameter estimates for small regions in partial volume. Although interpolating data reveals some details that are hidden at low resolution [7], interpolation of downsampled HCP data biased the results of the measured diffusion parameters in the fornix. FA values in all parts of the fornix tended to be underestimated and diverged from FA estimates in other white matter regions. This means that the local surroundings of the fornix biased the diffusion results, which our method was able to address.

There is promise in using this approach in subject groups, such as the preterm-born young adults in this study. Our approach reduces the impact of partial volume on measuring the properties of the fornix. The lower MD we measured for both subjects and controls is in accord with this. The higher FA values suggest that we are able to measure the diffusion in the highly-anisotropic region of the fornix with less impact from the surrounding cerebrospinal fluid. While this is not a conclusive result, due to the small number of subjects, it is a promising sign. There is some evidence from both methods that preterm-born adults have lower FA in the fornix than controls, which is congruent with the known result that preterm-born adults exhibit lower FA values in white matter.

While there are a range of biophysical compartment models in use in diffusion imaging, most of these rely on multi-shell data to fit compartments in each voxel, or else have to heavily restrict the available parameters. We circumvent this by fitting on a per-tissue basis, by using information from a structural segmentation.

Another way to calculate diffusion parameters would be using super-resolution techniques. Image Quality Transfer [8] uses a machine-learning approach to super-resolve the diffusion data from diffusion tensors. For this particular method, it is unclear how generalisable the approach is without high-resolution training data from each scanner in use. Our validation only used 12 diffusion volumes, and no training data, which renders the method suitable to past datasets.

We show that it is feasible and possible to estimate diffusion parameters for regions that are small on the scale of diffusion MRI. In large, contiguous regions we achieved the same results as for the classical approach, of thresholding and averaging. We used the fornix as a region of interest to show that our approach was able to recover diffusion parameter estimates consistently, when the classical approach failed. Although results were good in the fornix, the model would have to be extended significantly to cope with geometry such as crossing fibres.

The presented approach achieves close-to gold-standard results with minimal processing time and requirements for the diffusion acquisition. This is because we aggregate data from all voxels in which a particular tissue is present, even in part. This type of approach fits conceptually with more sophisticated, multi-compartment models, in its representation of a voxel's signal as coming from multiple sources.

In this work, we proposed a method to extract diffusion tensor parameters from tissue that has partial volume. We have validated the method using high-quality data from the HCP, and applied it in a new cohort of clinical interest.

Acknowledgments. We would like to acknowledge the MRC (MR/J01107X/1), the National Institute for Health Research (NIHR), the EPSRC (EP/H046410/1) and the National Institute for Health Research University College London Hospitals Biomedical Research Centre (NIHR BRC UCLH/UCL High Impact Initiative BW.mn.BRC10269). This work is supported by the EPSRC-funded UCL Centre for Doctoral Training in Medical Imaging (EP/L016478/1).
HCP data were provided by the HCP, WU-Minn Consortium (PIs: David Van Essen and Kamil Ugurbil; 1U54MH091657) funded by NIH and Wash. U.

References

1. Metzler-Baddeley, C., O'Sullivan, M.J., Bells, S., Pasternak, O., Jones, D.K.: How and how not to correct for CSF-contamination in diffusion MRI. NeuroImage **59**(2), 1394–1403 (2012)
2. Pasternak, O., Sochen, N., Gur, Y., Intrator, N., Assaf, Y.: Free water elimination and mapping from diffusion MRI. Magn. Reson. Med. **62**(3), 717–730 (2009)
3. Van Essen, D.C., Ugurbil, K., Auerbach, E., Barch, D., Behrens, T.E.J., Bucholz, R., Chang, A., Chen, L., Corbetta, M., Curtiss, S.W., Della Penna, S., Feinberg, D., Glasser, M.F., Harel, N., Heath, A.C., Larson-Prior, L., Marcus, D., Michalareas, G., Moeller, S., Oostenveld, R., Petersen, S.E., Prior, F., Schlaggar, B.L., Smith, S.M., Snyder, A.Z., Xu, J., Yacoub, E.: The human connectome project: a data acquisition perspective. NeuroImage **62**(4), 2222–2231 (2012)
4. Eaton-Rosen, Z., Cardoso, M.J., Melbourne, A., Orasanu, E., Bainbridge, A., Kendall, G.S., Robertson, N.J., Marlow, N., Ourselin, S.: Fitting parametric models of diffusion MRI in regions of partial volume. In: Proceedings of SPIE, Medical Imaging: Image Processing, vol. 9784 (2016)
5. Coleman, T.F., Li, Y.: An interior trust region approach for nonlinear minimization subject to bounds. SIAM J. Optim. **6**(2), 418–445 (1996)
6. Cardoso, M.J., Modat, M., Wolz, R., Melbourne, A., Cash, D., Rueckert, D., Ourselin, S.: Geodesic information flows: spatially-variant graphs and their application to segmentation and fusion. IEEE Trans. Med. Imaging **34**, 1976–1988 (2015)
7. Dyrby, T.B., Lundell, H., Burke, M.W., Reislev, N.L., Paulson, O.B., Ptito, M., Siebner, H.R.: Interpolation of diffusion weighted imaging datasets. NeuroImage **103**, 202–213 (2014)
8. Alexander, D.C., Zikic, D., Zhang, J., Zhang, H., Criminisi, A.: Image quality transfer via random forest regression: applications in diffusion MRI. In: Golland, P., Hata, N., Barillot, C., Hornegger, J., Howe, R. (eds.) MICCAI 2014, Part III. LNCS, vol. 8675, pp. 225–232. Springer, Heidelberg (2014)

A Promising Non-invasive CAD System for Kidney Function Assessment

M. Shehata[1], F. Khalifa[1], A. Soliman[1], M. Abou El-Ghar[2], A. Dwyer[3],
G. Gimel'farb[4], R. Keynton[1], and A. El-Baz[1(✉)]

[1] Bioengineering Department, University of Louisville, Louisville, KY, USA
aselba01@louisville.edu
[2] Urology and Nephrology Center, Mansoura University, Mansoura, Egypt
[3] Kidney Transplantation Center, University of Louisville, Louisville, KY, USA
[4] Department of Computer Science, University of Auckland,
Auckland, New Zealand

Abstract. This paper introduces a novel computer-aided diagnostic (CAD) system for the assessment of renal transplant status that integrates image-based biomarkers derived from 4D (3D + b-value) diffusion-weighted (DW) MRI, and clinical biomarkers. To analyze DW-MRI, our framework starts with kidney tissue segmentation using a level set approach after DW-MRI data alignment to handle the motion effects. Secondly, the cumulative empirical distributions (i.e., CDFs) of apparent diffusion coefficients (ADCs) of the segmented DW-MRIs are estimated at low and high gradient strengths and duration (b-values) accounting for both blood perfusion and diffusion, respectively. Finally, these CDFs are fused with laboratory-based biomarkers (creatinine clearance and serum plasma creatinine) for the classification of transplant status using a deep learning-based classification approach utilizing a stacked non-negativity constrained auto-encoder. Using "leave-one-subject-out" experiments on a cohort of 58 subjects, the proposed CAD system distinguished non-rejection transplants from kidneys with abnormalities with a 95% accuracy (sensitivity = 95%, specificity = 94%) and achieved a 95% correct classification between early rejection and other kidney diseases. Our preliminary results demonstrate the promise of the proposed CAD system as a reliable non-invasive diagnostic tool for renal transplants assessment.

Keywords: DW-MRI · Clinical biomarkers · Deep learning · Kidney diseases

1 Introduction

Accurate assessment of the renal transplant function is of great importance for graft survival [1]. Although transplantation can improve a patient's wellbeing, there is a potential post-transplantation risk of kidney dysfunction that, if not

---

M. Shehata and F. Khalifa—Shared first authorship (equal contribution).

© Springer International Publishing AG 2016
S. Ourselin et al. (Eds.): MICCAI 2016, Part III, LNCS 9902, pp. 613–621, 2016.
DOI: 10.1007/978-3-319-46726-9_71

treated in a timely manner, can lead to the loss of the entire graft, and even patients death [2]. Thus, accurate assessment of renal transplant function is crucial for the identification of proper treatment. Traditional evaluation of renal transplant function is based on blood tests and urine sampling, e.g., plasma creatinine and creatinine clearance. However, a significant change in creatinine levels is only observable after 60 % loss of the kidney function due to the low sensitivity of indices [3]. Biopsy remains the gold standard, yet only as the last resort because of its invasiveness, high cost, and potential morbidity.

On the other hand, evaluation of renal transplant functions has been investigated in several studies using different imaging modalities, which are favorable as they provide information on each kidney separately. A quick overview of these imaging techniques is provided below and the reader is referred to [4] for more details about renal function assessment using diagnostic imaging. The most frequently used imaging technique, scintigraphy, has been clinically explored for its good functional information (e.g., [5]). However, radionuclide approaches indexing radioisotope activity versus time (renograms) involve radiation exposure, thereby limiting the applicability of these techniques. Ultrasound (US) imaging with Doppler interrogation was explored for renal assessment (e.g., [6,7]). However, US imaging suffers from low signal-to-noise ratios, shadowing artifacts, and speckles that greatly decrease image quality and diagnostic confidence. Dynamic contrast-enhanced magnetic resonance imaging (DCE-MRI) has been also exploited due to its ability to provide both anatomical and functional kidney information (e.g., [8,9]). However, dynamic MRI imaging involves contrast agents which may implicate nephrogenic systemic fibrosis [9]. BOLD-MRI, another imaging technique, has been also utilized to study renal function, using the amount of oxygen diffused blood to examine the proper functionality of the kidney (e.g., [1,10]). Furthermore, DW-MRI has emerged as an imaging technology for renal transplant assessment based on the measurement of water molecules inside soft tissue (e.g., [10–12]). Several studies have utilized DW-MRI for functional renal assessment by measuring the cortical and/or medullary apparent diffusion coefficient (ADC), but the results have varied [1]. Also, several of the DW-MRI studies performed only a statistical analysis to investigate the significant difference between pairs at certain b-values.

In addition to the previous limitations, none of the aforementioned studies integrates both image– and laboratory–based biomarkers. Moreover, image analysis in most of them employ manual delineations of the kidney and do not account for motion effects. To account for these challenges, we propose a computer-aided diagnostic (CAD) system, which utilizes the fusion between DW-MRI-derived biomarkers and clinical biomarkers for the assessment of transplant status. Details of the proposed framework are described in the following section.

2   Methods

In order to build a robust diagnostic framework, the proposed CAD system integrates both clinical and image-based biomarkers. The former are based on creatinine clearance and serum plasma creatinine laboratory measurement. In order to extract the image-based biomarkers, our CAD system performs the following DW-MRI processing steps: (i) motion correction of the DW-MRI data using nonrigid registration; (ii) kidney segmentation from surrounding abdominal structures using level sets; (iii) ADC estimation to construct the discriminatory features (i.e., CDFs–cumulative distribution functions) for transplant status classification; Then, both image and clinical biomarkers are fused together for the assessment of transplant status by cascading two-stages of stacked non-negativity constrained auto-encoders. The first stage distinguishes non-rejection from abnormal transplants and the second stage classifies these abnormal transplants as rejection or other kidney diseases.

2.1 3D Kidney Segmentation

The first step of our CAD is to segment the kidney tissue from 4D DW-MRI data. To achieve a more accurate segmentation, we initially applied an intensity histogram equalization and the nonparametric bias correction method proposed in [13] to reduce noise effects and DW-MRI heterogeneity. Then, a 3D B-splines based transformation is applied to handle kidney motions using the sum of squared difference similarity metric. Finally, the 3D geometric (level-set based) deformable model approach proposed in [14] is applied to extract the kidney from the co-aligned DW-MRI data. The evolving boundary is controlled by a voxel-wise stochastic speed function that combines an adaptive kidney shape prior and visual appearances of DW-MRI data (image intensities and spatial interactions) into a joint kidney-background Markov-Gibbs random field model. For more details about our segmentation method, please see [14].

2.2 Diffusion Parameters Estimation

Following the segmentation of the kidney, the next step is to estimate diffusion parameters that can be used to assess renal transplant status and to differentiate renal rejection from other diagnostic possibilities (e.g., ATN, acute tubular injury, graft amyloidosis, and tubular inflammation). In this paper, we used the apparent diffusion coefficient (ADC) for global transplant status assessment: $\text{ADC}_{\mathbf{p}} = \frac{1}{b_0 - b} \ln\left(\frac{g_{b:\mathbf{p}}}{g_{0:\mathbf{p}}}\right)$; where $\mathbf{p} = (x, y, z)$ denotes a voxel at position with discrete Cartesian coordinates (x, y, z), and the segmented DW-MR images $\mathbf{g}_0$ and $\mathbf{g}_b$ were acquired with the b_0 and a given different b-value (total of 11 b-values in our study), respectively.

Conventional classification methods dealing directly with voxel-wise ADCs of the entire kidney volume as discriminative features encounter two difficulties: (i) varying input data size requires either data truncation for large kidney volumes or zero padding for small ones and (ii) large data volumes lead to considerable time expenditures for training and classification. In order to overcome these challenges, we characterize the whole 3D ADC maps, collected for each subject at different b-values, by the CDFs of the ADCs, as shown in Fig. 1. These descriptors are independent of the initial data size and can be quantified in accord with the actual accuracy of the ADCs. It is worth mentioning that fixing the input data size to 11 such CDFs helps to overcome the above challenges of the original ADCs' arbitrary sizes and notably accelerates the classification. We divided the range between the minimum and maximum ADCs for all the input data sets into 100 steps to keep the ADC data well-presented without losing any information. The PDFs and then CDFs of the ADCs were constructed for these quantized values, see Fig. 1.

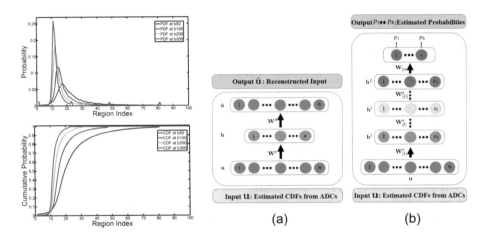

(a)

(b)

Fig. 1. Empirical ADC distributions and their CDFs for one subject at different b-values of (b_{50}, b_{100}, b_{200}, and b_{300}) s/mm^2.

Fig. 2. Block-diagram of an NCAE (a) and SNCAE (b) classifier.

2.3   Autoencoding and Deep Learning-Based Classifier

To classify the transplant status, our CAD employs a deep neural network with a stack of auto-encoders (AE) before the output layer that computes a softmax regression. Each AE compresses its input data to capture the most prominent variations and is built separately by greedy unsupervised pre-training [15]. The softmax output layer facilitates the subsequent supervised back-propagation-based fine tuning by minimizing the total loss (negative log-likelihood) for a given training labeled data. Using the non-negativity constraint AE (NCAE) [16] yields both more reasonable data codes (features) during its unsupervised pre-training and better classification performance after the supervised refinement.

Let $\mathbf{W} = \{\mathbf{W}_j^e, \mathbf{W}_i^d : j = 1, \ldots, s; i = 1, \ldots, n\}$ denote a set of column vectors of weights for encoding (e) and decoding (d) layers of a single AE in Fig. 2. Let T denote vector transposition. The AE converts an n-dimensional column vector $\mathbf{u} = [u_1, \ldots, u_n]^\mathsf{T}$ of input signals into an s-dimensional column vector $\mathbf{h} = [h_1, \ldots, h_s]^\mathsf{T}$ of hidden codes (features, or activations and $s \ll n$) by a uniform nonlinear transformation of s weighted linear combinations of signals:

$$h_j = \sigma\left((\mathbf{W}_j^\mathrm{e})^\mathsf{T}\mathbf{u}\right) \equiv \sigma\left(\sum_{i=1}^{n} w_{j:i}^\mathrm{e} u_i\right)$$

where $\sigma(\ldots)$ is a certain sigmoid. Unsupervised pre-training of the AE minimizes total deviations between each given training input vector $\mathbf{u}_k$; $k = 1, \ldots, K$, and the same-dimensional vector, $\widehat{\mathbf{u}}_{\mathbf{W}:k}$ reconstructed from its code, or activation vector, $\mathbf{h}_k$ (Fig. 2(a)). The total reconstruction error to compress and decompress the K training input vectors integrates the ℓ_2-norms of the deviations:

$$J_{\mathrm{AE}}(\mathbf{W}) = \frac{1}{2K}\sum_{k=1}^{K} \| \widehat{\mathbf{u}}_{\mathbf{W}:k} - \mathbf{u}_k \|^2 \tag{1}$$

To reduce the number of negative weights and enforce sparsity of the NCAE, Eq. (1) is appended, respectively, with quadratic negative weight penalties, $f(w_i) = (\min\{0, w_i\})^2$; $i = 1, \ldots, n$, and Kullback-Leibler (KL) divergence, $J_{\mathrm{KL}}(\mathbf{h}_{\mathbf{W}^\mathrm{e}}; \gamma)$, of activations, $\mathbf{h}_{\mathbf{W}^\mathrm{e}}$, obtained with the encoding weights $\mathbf{W}^\mathrm{e}$ for the training data, from a fixed small positive average value, γ, near 0:

$$J_{\mathrm{NCAE}}(\mathbf{W}) = J_{\mathrm{AE}}(\mathbf{W}) + \alpha\sum_{j=1}^{s}\sum_{i=1}^{n} f(w_{j:i}) + \beta J_{\mathrm{KL}}(\mathbf{h}_{\mathbf{W}^\mathrm{e}}; \gamma) \tag{2}$$

Here, the factors $\alpha \geq 0$ and $\beta \geq 0$ specify relative contributions of the non-negativity and sparsity constraints to the overall loss, $J_{\mathrm{NCAE}}(\mathbf{W})$, and

$$J_{\mathrm{KL}}(\mathbf{h}_{\mathbf{W}^\mathrm{e}}, \gamma) = \sum_{j=1}^{s} h_{\mathbf{W}^\mathrm{e}:j} \log\left(\frac{h_{\mathbf{W}^\mathrm{e}:j}}{\gamma}\right) + (1 - h_{\mathbf{W}^\mathrm{e}:j})\log\left(\frac{1 - h_{\mathbf{W}^\mathrm{e}:j}}{1 - \gamma}\right) \tag{3}$$

The classifier is built by stacking the NCAE layers with an output softmax layer, as shown in Fig. 2(b). Each NCAE is pre-trained separately in the unsupervised mode by using the activation vector of a lower layer as the input to the upper layer. In our case, we considered a two-layer SNCAE in which the bottom NCAE compresses the input vector to s_1 first-level activators, compressed by the next NCAE to s_2 second-level activators, which are reduced in turn by the output softmax layer to s° values. In our experiments, the SNCAE training parameters used to obtain all the results are shown in Table 1.

Separate pre-training of the first and second layers by minimizing the loss of Eq. (2) reduces the total reconstruction error, as well as increases sparsity of the extracted activations and numbers of the non-negative weights. The activations of the second NCAE layer, $\mathbf{h}^{[2]} = \sigma(\mathbf{W}_{[2]}^\mathrm{e}{}^\mathsf{T}\mathbf{h}^{[1]})$, are inputs of the softmax classification layer, as sketched in Fig. 2(b) to compute plausibility of a decision in favor of each particular output class, $c = 1, 2$:

$$p(c; \mathbf{W}_{\mathrm{o}:c}) = \frac{\exp(\mathbf{W}_{\mathrm{o}:c}^\mathsf{T}\mathbf{h}^{[2]})}{\exp(\mathbf{W}_{\mathrm{o}:1}^\mathsf{T}\mathbf{h}^{[2]}) + \exp(\mathbf{W}_{\mathrm{o}:2}^\mathsf{T}\mathbf{h}^{[2]})}; \ c = 1, 2; \ \sum_{c=1}^{2} p(c; \mathbf{W}_{\mathrm{o}:c}; \mathbf{h}^{[2]}) = 1.$$

Table 1. Two-stage SNCAE classifiers' training parameters, where n, s_1, s_2, s°, α, β, and γ stand for input signals (CDFs) size, 1st NCAE size, 2nd NCAE size, the softmax layer size, weight decay parameter, weight of sparsity penalty term, and desired activation of the hidden units, respectively.

	SNCAE Classifier Parameters						
	n	s_1	s_2	s°	α	β	γ
Stage 1	1100	22	5	2	$3 * 10^{-10}$	3	0.15
Stage 2	1100	22	5	2	$3 * 10^{-7}$	3	0.15

Its separate pre-training minimizes the total negative log-likelihood $J_\circ(\mathbf{W}_\circ)$ of the known training classes, appended with the negative weight penalties:

$$J_\circ(\mathbf{W}^o) = -\frac{1}{K}\sum_{k=1}^{K}\log p(c_k; \mathbf{W}_{\circ:c}) + \alpha \sum_{c=1}^{2}\sum_{j=1}^{s_2} w_{\circ:c:j} \qquad (4)$$

Finally, the entire stacked NCAE classifier (SNCAE) is fine-tuned on the labeled training data by the conventional error back-propagation through the network and penalizing only the negative weights of the softmax layer.

3   Experimental Results

The proposed CAD system has been tested on DW-MRI data collected from 58 subjects (47 male and 11 female with a mean age of 26 ± 10 years) that contains 16 non-rejection transplants and 42 transplant patients with abnormal kidneys, in which 37 cases are early rejection and 5 cases have other kidney diseases. All patients, as a part of post-transplantation routine medical care, were routinely assessed with serum creatinine laboratory values. Coronal DW-MRIs were acquired before any biopsy procedure using a 1.5 T scanner (SIGNA Horizon, General Electric Medical Systems, Milwaukee, WI) using a body coil and a gradient multi-shot spin-echo echo-planar sequence (TR/TE: 8000/61.2; bandwidth: 142 kHz; matrix: 1.25×1.25 mm^2; section thickness: 4 mm; intersection gap: 0 mm; FOV: 32 cm; signals acquired: 7; water signals acquired at different b-values of (b_0, b_{50}, and b_{100}–b_{1000} s/mm^2 with 100 increment). Approximately 50 sections have been obtained in 60–120 s to cover the whole kidney.

Since the segmentation is a key step in developing any CAD system to asses renal function, our segmentation approach was first evaluated on the collected DW-MRI data using the Dice coefficient (DC) [17], percentage volume difference (PVD), and the 95-percentile modified Hausdorff distance (MHD) [18] evaluation metrics. Our method achieved a mean DC, MHD, and PVD of 0.92 ± 0.02, 6.2 ± 2 mm, and $15 \pm 3\%$, respectively, compared to an MRI expert's ground truth maps. Also, comparisons between our method and the level-set approach by Chan and Vese (CV) [19] and the like boundary guided by combined intensity and spatial features (I+S) can be found in [14].

Following kidney segmentation, our system assesses the transplant status with a two-stage SNCAE-based classifier using the constructed CDFs and the clinical biomarkers. A leave-one-subject-out (LOSO) approach is applied to distinguish between (*i*) non-rejection (NR) and abnormal (AB) transplants and (*ii*) early rejection (ER) from other kidney diseases (OD). First, our system accuracy was evaluated using the clinical biomarkers alone. As demonstrated in Table 2, diagnostic accuracy using the clinical biomarkers only is very low due to the large overlap of these biomarkers between NR and AB groups. Secondly, we evaluated the overall accuracy using the image biomarkers (i.e. CDFs), see Table 2. Classification using image-derived biomarkers has higher accuracy compared to that based on clinical ones. To show the advantages of integrating both clinical and image biomarkers, the kidney status was also assessed using the same LOSO approach and an SNCAE classifier augmented with both biomarkers. As expected, the overall accuracy notably increases after fusion as shown in Table 2.

Table 2. Diagnostic accuracy (ACC), sensitivity (SENS), and specificity (SPEC) for our CAD system with the SNCAE classifier using clinical and image-driven biomarkers. Note that "NR", "AB", "ER", and "OD" stand for non-rejection, abnormal, early rejection and other diagnosis, respectively.

	Clinical biomarkers			Image biomarkers			Fused biomarkers		
	ACC%	SENS%	SPEC%	ACC%	SENS%	SPEC%	ACC%	SENS%	SPEC%
NR vs. AB	71	81	44	93	93	94	95	95	94
ER vs. OD	88	—	—	93	—	—	95	—	—

Table 3. Diagnostic accuracy (ACC), sensitivity (SENS), specificity (SPEC), and area under the curve (AUC) for the proposed CAD system with the SNCAE classifier and seven other classifiers from the Weka collection [20].

	K*	kNN	NBT	ADT	NNge	RT	RF	SNCAE
	Non-rejection (NR) vs. Abnormal (AB)							
ACC %	84	88	81	90	78	88	93	95
SENS %	95	93	83	93	90	93	98	95
SPEC %	56	75	75	81	37	75	81	94
AUC	0.82	0.84	0.81	0.89	0.67	0.84	0.92	0.93
	Early rejection (ER) vs. Other Diseases (OD)							
ACC %	52	76	88	76	88	74	88	95

To evaluate the capabilities of the SNCAE classifier, it has been compared with seven well-known learnable classifiers from the Weka collection [20]: K*, k-nearest neighbor (kNN), Naive Bayes tree (NBT), alternating decision tree (ADT), nearest neighbor with generalization (NNge), Random tree (RT), and

Random forest (RF). Table 3 presents their and our diagnostic accuracies in terms of the numbers of correctly classified cases with respect to the overall numbers of subjects. For the first stage (NR vs. AB), our classifier demonstrated the best total diagnostic accuracy of 95 %, or 15 correctly classified NR transplants out of the 16 subjects, and 40 correctly classified AB transplants out of the 42 subjects. Moreover, for the second stage (ER vs. OD), our classifier achieved a 95 % total diagnostic accuracy.

In addition, we tested the performance of the SNCAE compared to the chosen Weka classifiers using the receiver operating characteristics (ROC) [21] analysis. As shown in Table 3, the calculated area under the curve (AUC) is the highest for our classifier and approaches the top-most unit value. These initial diagnostic results confirm that the proposed CAD system holds promise as a reliable non-invasive diagnostic tool.

4 Conclusions

In total, we propose a CAD system for early assessment of renal transplant function from 4D DW-MRI data that combines deformable model segmentation, estimation of spatial diffusion parameters (ADCs), and a SNCAE classification of the transplant status using CDFs of the ADCs and clinical biomarkers as integral status descriptions. In a test on a biopsy-proven cohort of 58 participants, our system showed high diagnostic accuracy to distinguish non-rejection from abnormal transplants as well as to distinguish early rejection from other kidney dysfunction, which make our non-invasive CAD a reliable diagnostic tool. In the future, we intend to increase the test sets of both non-rejection and abnormal transplants in order to further validate the accuracy and robustness of our framework. Also, new kidney transplant data sets, which are acquired at lower b-values, will be used to explore the ability of our framework to determine the type of kidney rejection, i.e. anti-body mediated or T-cell rejection, or other causes of acute kidney dysfunction such as drug toxicity and viral infection.

References

1. Liu, G., et al.: Detection of renal allograft rejection using blood oxygen level-dependent and diffusion weighted magnetic resonance imaging: a retrospective study. BMC Nephrol. 15(1), 158 (2014)
2. Chon, W., et al.: Clinical manifestations and diagnosis of acute renal allograft rejection. UpToDate Version 21 (2014). http://www.uptodate.com/contents/clinical-manifestations-and-diagnosis-of-acute-renal-allograft-rejection
3. Katzberg, R.W., et al.: Functional, dynamic, and anatomic MR urography: feasibility and preliminary findings. Acad. Radiol. 8(11), 1083–1099 (2001)
4. Sharfuddin, A.: Renal relevant radiology: imaging in kidney transplantation. Clin. J. Am. Soc. Nephrol. 9(2), 416–429 (2014)
5. Dostbil, Z., et al.: Comparison of split renal function measured by ^{99m}Tc-DTPA, ^{99m}Tc-MAG3 and ^{99m}Tc-DMSA renal scintigraphies in paediatric age groups. Clin. Rev. Opinions 3(2), 20–25 (2011)

6. Tublin, M.E., et al.: The resistive index in renal doppler sonography: where do we stand? Am. J. Roentgenol. **180**(4), 885–892 (2003)
7. Chow, L., et al.: Power doppler imaging and resistance index measurement in the evaluation of acute renal transplant rejection. J. Clin. Ultrasound **29**(9), 483–490 (2001)
8. Khalifa, F., et al.: A comprehensive non-invasive framework for automated evaluation of acute renal transplant rejection using DCE-MRI. NMR Biomed. **26**(11), 1460–1470 (2013)
9. Hodneland, E., et al.: In vivo estimation of glomerular filtration in the kidney using DCE-MRI. In: IEEE International Symposium on Image and Signal, Processing and Analysis, pp. 755–761 (2011)
10. Sadowski, E.A., et al.: Blood oxygen level-dependent and perfusion magnetic resonance imaging: detecting differences in oxygen bioavailability and blood flow in transplanted kidneys. Magn. Reson. Med. **28**(1), 56–64 (2010)
11. Abou-El-Ghar, M., et al.: Role of diffusion-weighted MRI in diagnosis of acute renal allograft dysfunction: a prospective preliminary study. Br. J. Radiol. **85**(1014), 206–211 (2014)
12. Eisenberger, U., et al.: Evaluation of renal allograft function early after transplantation with diffusion-weighted MR imaging. Eur. Radiol. **20**(6), 1374–1383 (2010)
13. Tustison, N.J., et al.: N4ITK: improved N3 bias correction. IEEE Trans. Med. Iamging **29**(6), 1310–1320 (2010)
14. Shehata, M., et al.: A level set-based framework for 3D kidney segmentation from diffusion MR images. In: Proceedings of IEEE International Conference on Image Processing, pp. 4441–4445 (2015)
15. Bengio, Y., et al.: Greedy layer-wise training of deep networks. Adv. Neural Inf. Process. Syst. **19**, 153 (2007)
16. Hosseini-Asl, E., et al.: Deep learning of part-based representation of data using sparse autoencoders with nonnegativity constraints. IEEE Trans. Neural Netw. Learn. Syst. **PP**(99), 1–13 (2016). doi:10.1109/TNNLS.2015.2479223. e-publication ahead of print
17. Zou, K.H., et al.: Statistical validation of image segmentation quality based on a spatial overlap index. Acad. Radiol. **11**(2), 178–189 (2004)
18. Gerig, G., Jomier, M., Chakos, M.: Valmet: a new validation tool for assessing and improving 3D object segmentation. In: Niessen, W.J., Viergever, M.A. (eds.) MICCAI 2001. LNCS, vol. 2208, pp. 516–523. Springer, Heidelberg (2001)
19. Chan, T.F., Vese, L.A.: Active contours without edges. IEEE Trans. Image Process. **10**(2), 266–77 (2001)
20. Hall, M., et al.: The WEKA data mining software: an update. ACM SIGKDD Explor. Newsl. **11**(1), 10–18 (2009)
21. Fawcett, T.: An introduction to ROC analysis. Pattern Recogn. Lett. **27**(8), 861–874 (2006)

Comprehensive Maximum Likelihood Estimation of Diffusion Compartment Models Towards Reliable Mapping of Brain Microstructure

Aymeric Stamm[1,2]([⊠]), Olivier Commowick[3], Simon K. Warfield[2], and S. Vantini[1]

[1] MOX, Department of Mathematics, Politecnico di Milano, Milan, Italy
aymeric.stamm@polimi.it
[2] CRL, Harvard Medical School, Boston Children's Hospital, Boston, MA, USA
[3] VISAGES, INSERM U746, CNRS UMR6074, INRIA,
University of Rennes I, Rennes, France

Abstract. Diffusion MRI is a key in-vivo non invasive imaging capability that can probe the microstructure of the brain. However, its limited resolution requires complex voxelwise generative models of the diffusion. Diffusion Compartment (DC) models divide the voxel into smaller compartments in which diffusion is homogeneous. We present a comprehensive framework for maximum likelihood estimation (MLE) of such models that jointly features ML estimators of (i) the baseline MR signal, (ii) the noise variance, (iii) compartment proportions, and (iv) diffusion-related parameters. ML estimators are key to providing reliable mapping of brain microstructure as they are asymptotically unbiased and of minimal variance. We compare our algorithm (which efficiently exploits analytical properties of MLE) to alternative implementations and a state-of-the-art strategy. Simulation results show that our approach offers the best reduction in computational burden while guaranteeing convergence of numerical estimators to the MLE. In-vivo results also reveal remarkably reliable microstructure mapping in areas as complex as the centrum semiovale. Our ML framework accommodates any DC model and is available freely for multi-tensor models as part of the ANIMA software (https://github.com/Inria-Visages/Anima-Public/wiki).

1 Introduction

Diffusion MRI has raised a lot of interest over the past two decades as it provides an in-vivo non invasive mean for investigating the brain microstructure with great hopes of improved diagnosis, understanding and treatment of brain disorders. Current MR technologies however are limited in spatial resolution (finest resolution achieved so far in-vivo in diffusion is ~ 1.25 mm^3 [11]). Going further yields too long scans and too noisy data. Hence, brain microstructure is only accessible through careful modeling of the diffusion from which the MR signal arises. The coarser the resolution, the more heterogeneous the microstructure within the voxel and the more complex the voxelwise diffusion modeling.

© Springer International Publishing AG 2016
S. Ourselin et al. (Eds.): MICCAI 2016, Part III, LNCS 9902, pp. 622–630, 2016.
DOI: 10.1007/978-3-319-46726-9_72

Recently, there has been a growing interest in diffusion compartment models (DCM) [4,6]. Their strength lies in their biological interpretability in that each voxel compartment can be matched to an homogeneous biological substrate. Assuming Gaussian compartmental diffusion, the most complete microstructure mapping is given by the multi-tensor (MT) model [6], out of which several simplifications were devised in [4]. In essence, each compartment in the MT model is characterized by its diffusion tensor (DT). Current publicly available toolboxes for diffusion MRI processing often include multi-tensor ML estimation routines[1]. However, little attention has been paid to the actual numerical convergence to the ML estimate. We here propose a comprehensive maximum likelihood (ML) framework for the estimation of DCMs that aims at filling this gap. In effect, assuming identifiability of the unknown DCM, its ML estimator is guaranteed to be unbiased and of minimal variance as sample size increases. Our ML framework assumes that measurement error is modeled by white noise, which is fair for high signal-to-noise ratio (SNR) areas. Our ML framework is still valid for low SNR but a number of analytic properties of the likelihood used to improve time-efficiency do not hold anymore, which might lead to lengthier computations.

The contribution of this work is a comprehensive numerically convergent and massively fast framework for MLE of the MT model, provided that Gaussian homogeneous noise can be assumed. In Sect. 2.1, we briefly recall the definition of the MT model, propose a novel parametrization that features parameter-independent constraints, and formulate the derived maximization problem on a constrained domain. In Sect. 2.2, we provide analytic expressions of the ML estimators of the noise variance, the baseline MR signal and the compartment weights given the DTs and the number of compartments. In Sect. 2.3, we describe a time-efficient strategy for dealing with the constraints introduced in Sect. 2.1. In Sect. 2.4 we give the analytic expression of the log-likelihood depending on the unknown DTs exclusively and we derive the analytic expression of its Jacobian, which is key for time efficiency. Next, in Sect. 3, we present a simulation study whose goals are two-fold: (i) a mutual comparison of multiple algorithms for solving the maximization problem defined in Sect. 2.4 and (ii) a comparison with a reference estimation strategy [6]. We also describe our experiment on real data using a healthy subject from the Human Connectome Project (HCP) database [11]. Finally, Sect. 4 presents the results of both the simulation study and the experiment on real data and discuss our contribution.

2   ML Estimation of the Multi-Tensor Model

2.1   Description of the Problem

In the following, each voxel is considered independently. $\mathbf{y}$ is a set of N measured signals for pairs of b-values b_i and diffusion gradient directions $\mathbf{g}_i$, $\boldsymbol{\mu}$ is the set of corresponding signals generated by the DCM and τ^2 the noise inverse variance.

---

[1] http://fsl.fmrib.ox.ac.uk/fsl/fslwiki/,   http://camino.cs.ucl.ac.uk.

The Log-Likelihood. The Gaussian log-likelihood function ℓ reads:

$$\ell(\boldsymbol{\mu}, \tau^2; \mathbf{y}) = \frac{N}{2} \ln \left(\frac{\tau^2}{2\pi} \right) - \frac{\tau^2}{2} \|\mathbf{y} - \boldsymbol{\mu}\|^2 . \tag{1}$$

The MT Model. If the MT model with $C + 1$ compartments holds, the MR signal for a b-value b_i and direction $\mathbf{g}_i$ can be written in matrix form as:

$$\boldsymbol{\mu}(S_0, \mathbf{w}, \mathbf{D}) = S_0(\mathbf{a}(D_0) + \Phi(\mathbf{D})\mathbf{w}), \tag{2}$$

where S_0 is the baseline signal, $\mathbf{w} \in \mathbb{R}^C$ are the compartment weights, $\mathbf{D} \in \left[\mathcal{S}\left(\mathbb{R}^3\right) \right]^{C+1}$ are the DTs, $\mathbf{a}$ is an N-dimensional vector s.t. $a_i(D_j) = e^{-b_i \mathbf{g}_i^\top D_j \mathbf{g}_i}$ and Φ is an $N \times C$ matrix s.t. $\Phi_{ij} = a_i(D_j) - a_i(D_0)$.

Parametrization. We propose the following parametrization:

- S_0 is left as is with the constraint $S_0 \geq 0$ since MR signals are positive,
- τ^2 is left as is with the constraint $\tau^2 \geq 0$ since a variance is positive,
- $\mathbf{w}$ are fundamentally proportions, hence subject to $\mathbf{w} \geq \mathbf{0}$ and $\mathbf{1}^\top \mathbf{w} \leq 1$,
- $\mathbf{D}$ are 3D covariance matrices, i.e. positive definite symmetric matrices. Hence, we propose the following parametrization:

$$D_j = (d_{1j} + d_{2j})\mathbf{e}_{1j}\mathbf{e}_{1j}^\top + d_{2j}\mathbf{e}_{2j}\mathbf{e}_{2j}^\top + d_{3j}I_3, \tag{3}$$

where $\mathbf{e}_{kj}$ $(k = 1, 2, 3)$ are the 3 eigenvectors of D_j, parametrized by Euler angles $\theta_j \in [0, \pi]$, $\phi_j \in [0, 2\pi]$ and $\alpha_j \in [0, 2\pi]$ and respectively associated with the eigenvalues $\lambda_{1j} \geq \lambda_{2j} \geq \lambda_{3j} > 0$ such that $d_{1j} = \lambda_{1j} - \lambda_{2j} \geq 0$, $d_{2j} = \lambda_{2j} - \lambda_{3j} \geq 0$ and $d_{3j} = \lambda_{3j} > 0$.

Objective. To find the ML estimators of the parameters $\mathbf{w}$, $\mathbf{D}$, S_0, and τ^2, i.e., to maximize Eq. (1) plugged-in with Eq. (2) subject to the constraints above.

2.2   Complete Solution for a Known Number of Compartments

We propose to maximize Eq. (1) in a stepwise fashion solving maximization subproblems over a subset of the parameters in terms of the others:

Estimation of τ^2. Solving the partial derivative equation (PDE) in τ^2 yields:

$$\widehat{\tau^2}^{-1}(\mathbf{w}, \mathbf{D}, S_0) = N^{-1} \|\mathbf{y} - S_0\mathbf{a}(D_0) - S_0\Phi(\mathbf{D})\mathbf{w}\|^2 . \tag{4}$$

Since the right hand-side is always positive, Eq. (4) defines the MLE of τ^2.

Estimation of $\mathbf{w}$. Plugging Eqs. (2) and (4) into Eq. (1) turns the problem into a least squares problem linear in the compartment weights. As in [1], we resort to the method of variable projection (VP) to get the weights estimates:

$$\widehat{\mathbf{w}}(\mathbf{D}, S_0) = \left[\Phi^\top(\mathbf{D})\Phi(\mathbf{D}) \right]^{-1} \Phi^\top(\mathbf{D}) \left[S_0^{-1}\mathbf{y} - \mathbf{a}(D_0) \right], \tag{5}$$

In this section, the number of compartments is known which implies, in particular, that there are no pairs of compartments with equal diffusion distributions. Hence, the $C \times C$ matrix $\Phi^\top \Phi$ is invertible and Eq. (5) is the MLE of $\mathbf{w}$, provided that it satisfies the constraints $\widehat{\mathbf{w}} \geq 0$ and $\mathbf{1}^\top \widehat{\mathbf{w}} \leq 1$.

Estimation of S_0. Plugging Eqs. (2), (4) and (5) into Eq. (1) and solving the PDE in S_0 yields:

$$\widehat{S_0}(\mathbf{D}) = \frac{< \mathbf{a}(D_0), P_\Phi^\perp(\mathbf{D})\mathbf{y} >}{< \mathbf{a}(D_0), P_\Phi^\perp(\mathbf{D})\mathbf{a}(D_0) >}, \tag{6}$$

where $P_\Phi^\perp = I_N - \Phi(\Phi^\top\Phi)^{-1}\Phi^\top$ is the $N \times N$ projector on the orthogonal complement of the column space of Φ and $<\cdot,\cdot>$ is the inner product in $\mathbb{R}^N$. Equation (6) is the MLE of S_0 which is automatically positive since $\mathbf{y} \geq \mathbf{0}$.

Estimation of D. Maximizing Eq. (1) finally boils down to maximizing numerically the following log-likelihood function w.r.t. the DTs (obtained by plugging Eqs. (2) and (4) to (6) into Eq. (1)):

$$\ell(\mathbf{D}; \mathbf{y}) = -\frac{N}{2}\left[1 + \ln\left(\frac{2\pi}{N}\left(\left\|P_\Phi^\perp(\mathbf{D})\mathbf{y}\right\|^2 - \frac{<\mathbf{a}(D_0), P_\Phi^\perp(\mathbf{D})\mathbf{y}>}{\left\|P_\Phi^\perp(\mathbf{D})\mathbf{a}(D_0)\right\|^2}\right)\right)\right]. \tag{7}$$

At this point, it is worth making a few observations:

1. Equation (5) provides the MLE of $\mathbf{w}$ only if they lie inside the constrained domain of the original maximization problem, which is not guaranteed by the equations alone. This will be the object of Sect. 2.3. In addition, Eqs. (4), (5) and (6) define the MLEs of τ^2, $\mathbf{w}$ and S_0 for a given set $\mathbf{D}$ of DTs. Yet, they are the solution of the original maximization problem if and only if we can find the MLE of $\mathbf{D}$, which requires a careful numerical maximization of Eq. (7). This will be the object of Sect. 2.4.
2. The VP method was already introduced in [1] as a powerful tool for DCM estimation. Our contribution is instead a comprehensive framework that provides the MLE of all the DCM parameters in a remarkably fast computation time, and automatically guaranteeing asymptotic unbiasedness and efficiency of the estimated DCMs. Estimators proposed in [1] are instead not the MLE of the corresponding parameters, which makes it difficult to guarantee unbiasedness and efficiency in all circumstances. In addition, notwithstanding S_0 and τ^2 are not diffusion parameters, their accurate knowledge is critical for a reliable estimation of the diffusion parameters. In [1], there are no guidelines pertaining to their estimation. In the present work instead, we compute their MLE analytically. In addition, we propose clear indications to deal with compartment weights constraints in our MLE framework.

2.3   Handling Compartment Weights Constraints

Equation (4) always provides estimates of τ^2 within the constrained domain. This is not necessarily the case for Eq. (5) and (6). When the equations provide estimates that violate the constraints, we must search for the maximum on the boundary of the constrained domain. Our strategy relies on few key observations:

1. The sum-to-one constraint for compartment weights can be easily handled by expressing one of the weights as a linear combination of the other ones.

2. The positivity constraints on the remaining ones can be efficiently handled due to some analytical properties of the log-likelihood:
   – The symmetry properties of the log-likelihood function which is indeed invariant to the re-labeling of the fascicle compartments.
   – Along the domain boundary for **w** (i.e., when one or more compartment weights are constrained to 0) the log-likelihood function coincides with the log-likelihood of a reduced model with fewer compartments.

As a result, search on the boundary (when required) can be efficiently carried out by applying the strategy described in Sect. 2.2 on a MT model with one or several compartments removed. This boundary search guarantees, in the end, compartment weights estimates always satisfying the constraints.

2.4 Solving for the MLE of the Diffusion Tensors

Our objective is to find a suitable optimization algorithm that features (i) short computation times and (ii) convergence to the maximum of the log-likelihood function defined in Eq. (7). It is well-known that knowledge of the analytic Jacobian is of great help in achieving both. Let $x_k \in \{\theta_j, \phi_j, \alpha_j, d_{1j}, d_{2j}, d_{3j}\}_{j=0,...,C}$ be one of the parameters the MLE of which has to be obtained numerically. It is possible to analytically compute the derivative of Eq. (7) w.r.t. x_k, which formally defines the analytic Jacobian. After some algebra, one can show that:

$$\partial_k \ell = -\frac{N}{2}\left(\left\|P_\Phi^\perp(\mathbf{D})\mathbf{y}\right\|^2 - \frac{<\mathbf{a}(D_0), P_\Phi^\perp(\mathbf{D})\mathbf{y}>}{\left\|P_\Phi^\perp(\mathbf{D})\mathbf{a}(D_0)\right\|^2}\right)^{-1}\left[<\mathbf{y}, \partial_k P_\Phi^\perp(\mathbf{D})\mathbf{y}>\right.$$
$$\left. - 2\widehat{S_0}\left(<\partial_k\mathbf{a}(D_0), P_\Phi^\perp(\mathbf{D})\mathbf{y}> + <\mathbf{a}(D_0), \partial_k P_\Phi^\perp(\mathbf{D})\mathbf{y}>\right)\right. \tag{8}$$
$$\left. +\widehat{S_0}^2\left(<\partial_k\mathbf{a}(D_0), P_\Phi^\perp(\mathbf{D})\mathbf{a}(D_0)> + <\mathbf{a}(D_0), \partial_k P_\Phi^\perp(\mathbf{D})\mathbf{a}(D_0)>\right)\right],$$

where ∂_k denotes the partial derivative operator w.r.t. x_k. Given the results presented in Sects. 3 and 4, we recommend the use of the Levenberg-Marquardt (LM) algorithm [3], which achieves convergence in remarkably short times. This algorithm solves unconstrained problems only. Since our parametrization makes x_k bound-constrained only, we can easily turn our constrained maximization problem into an unconstrained one by suitable mappings of x_k.

3 Material and Methods

The following sections pertain to the experimental study. The goals are two-fold: (i) a comparison of 4 algorithms for solving the constrained maximization problem defined in Sect. 2.4 and (ii) a comparison with the estimation strategy used in [6], which is one of the reference papers on MT models. The former comparison is carried out in a simulation study while the latter one also in a case study on real data. All computations were performed with a Xeon 2.6 GHz processor, using 15 cores. Sections 3.1 and 3.2 details the simulation study and case study respectively, while Sect. 3.3 provides a brief description of the compared algorithms/methods and Sect. 3.4 depicts the evaluation metrics.

3.1 Simulation Study

We built an in-house diffusion phantom using subsets of the 6 compartments defined in Table 1 to generate purely isotropic areas (Area 0F) and areas with 1 (Area 1F), 2 (Area 2F) and 3 (Area 3F) fascicle compartments. The 3 isotropic compartments are always included. Then, we set spatially varying compartment weights within biologically feasible ranges. We set baseline signals in each area to realistic values using the mean baseline signals in grey matter, WM and cerebro-spinal fluid from case #153227 of the HCP database [11]. We added Gaussian noise as estimated in the same subject assuming a Rayleigh distribution of the background signals, which led to an average SNR $\sim$ 23 dB in diffusion-weighted MR images. Finally, we used the HCP diffusion gradient table to generate $N = 288$ diffusion-weighted MR images. Comparisons based on the simulated phantom are made at known number of compartments to avoid confounding model selection errors. Isotropic diffusivities are assumed to be known.

Table 1. In-house diffusion phantom compartments

Compartment	Characteristics (10^{-3} mm^2/s for diffusivities)
Free Water (FW)	$\lambda_1 = \lambda_2 = \lambda_3 = 3.0$
Stationary Water (SW)	$\lambda_1 = \lambda_2 = \lambda_3 = 10^{-5}$
Isotropic Restricted Water (IRW)	$\lambda_1 = \lambda_2 = \lambda_3 = 1.0$
Circular Fascicle (CF)	Orient. $[0°, 360°]$, $\lambda_1 = 1.8$, $\lambda_2 = 0.3$, $\lambda_3 = 0.2$
Vertical Fascicle (VF)	Orient. $90°$, $\lambda_1 = 1.6$, $\lambda_2 = 0.5$, $\lambda_3 = 0.4$
Diagonal Fascicle (DF)	Orient. $-45°$, $\lambda_1 = 1.7$, $\lambda_2 = 0.2$, $\lambda_3 = 0.16$

3.2 Real Data

Ground truth microstructure parameters and the actual number of compartments in each voxel is missing for real data. Hence, we visually compare the estimated MT models in the corpus callosum (CC) and in the centrum semi-ovale (CSO, where decussation of 3 brain circuits happens), provided by our framework (method A1) and the strategy in [6], which is a reference on MT models (method B), both methods being tuned to run in the same amount of time. Model selection was performed by comparing models with 0, 1, 2 and 3 fascicle compartments using the unbiased AIC criterion [8]. We used the same HCP subject that helped building our phantom. The 3 isotropic compartments defined in Sect. 3.1 were included in the model as well.

3.3 Compared Methods

In this section, we provide a brief description of the various methods compared in this experimental section. All methods of type A* correspond to algorithmic variants of our MLE framework while method B is a reference strategy.

Method A1. We use the Levenberg-Marquardt (LM) algorithm [3] with analytic Jacobian as implemented in ITK[2].

Method A2. We use the LM algorithm with numerical Jacobian.

Method A3. We use the globally convergent *conservative convex separable approximation* (CCSA) algorithm [10] implemented in the NLOpt library [2].

Method A4. We use the derivative-free *bounded optimization by quadratic approximations* (BOBYQA) algorithm [5] also implemented in NLOpt.

Method B. We use the strategy proposed in [6], with no spatial regularization, which performs brute-force estimation of all parameters using BOBYQA.

We did not include the estimation strategies proposed in [1,4] in the comparison, since the former does not apply to DCMs with more than two compartments and the latter is difficultly reproducible due to the lack of documentation.

3.4   Evaluation Metrics

The comparison of the 5 strategies defined in Sect. 3.3 focuses on the trade-off between error w.r.t. the ground truth model and computation time. We naturally quantify this error by means of the MSE. For a given estimator $\widehat{\theta}$ of a parameter θ, its MSE is defined as $\mathbb{E}[d^2(\widehat{\theta}, \theta)]$, where d is a selected metric. Hereafter, we compute the MSEs of both the weights estimator $\widehat{\mathbf{w}}$ and the tensors estimator $\widehat{\mathbf{D}}$ separately in areas 0F, 1F, 2F and 3F of the phantom. We use the Euclidean distance for weights and the log-Euclidean distance for tensors. The MSEs are estimated as the averaged squared distances over the voxels of each area. This procedure led to 7 sets of performance curves for each area (4) and each estimator (2) that show MSE variations as a function of computation time.

4   Results and Discussion

Figure 1 shows the variations in MSE of both the weight and tensor estimators as defined in Sect. 3.4 as we let more time to the algorithm for estimating the MT models. Comparing method A1 (i.e. our framework) to the others at fixed MSE emphasizes – in the 4 simulated scenarios – multiple advantages of our proposed MLE framework: (i) there is an extra time cost in approximating the Jacobian (A1 vs A2), (ii) the LM algorithm is faster than other convergent gradient-based (GB) optimizers (A1 vs A3), (iii) GB optimization is faster than derivative-free (A1 vs A4) and (iv) our algorithm outperforms one of the reference approaches to MT model estimation (A1 vs B).

Next, Fig. 2 shows the estimated MT models using both method A1 and method B in a fixed computation time of 30 s (corresponding to 0.13s/voxel/core) for the crop on the CC and for the crop on the CSO. Visual inspection shows the ability of method A to provide more spatially coherent estimates of the MT model with less artifacts, mostly visible in three fascicle areas.

---

[2] http://www.itk.org.

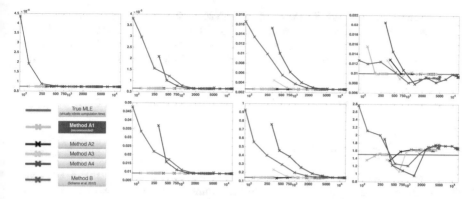

Fig. 1. Performance curves. MSE variations as a function of computation time (in sec). 1st row, $\hat{w}$; 2nd row, $\hat{D}$. Columns match areas 0F, 1F, 2F, 3F from left to right.

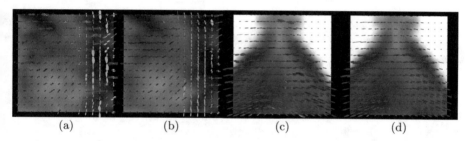

(a)   (b)   (c)   (d)

Fig. 2. Estimated multi-tensor models In-Vivo. In the CSO (a,b), in the CC (c,d); using method B (a,c) or method A1 (b,d)

In summary, we have set up a novel and comprehensive framework for the efficient ML estimation of the MT model featuring massive reduction of computational burden. The framework generalizes to any DCM with known analytic Jacobian of the generative model. Future works will investigate its performances for estimating other important DCMs such as DIAMOND [7], DDI [9] or NODDI [12] and the possibility of embedding model selection in the framework.

References

1. Farooq, H., et al.: Brain microstructure mapping from diffusion MRI using least squares variable separation. In: CDMRI (MICCAI Workshop), pp. 1–9 (2015)
2. Johnson, S.: The NLOpt package. http://ab-initio.mit.edu/nlopt
3. Marquardt, D.: An algorithm for least-squares estimation of nonlinear parameters. J. Soc. Ind. Appl. Math. **11**(2), 431–441 (1963)
4. Panagiotaki, et al.: Compartment models of the diffusion MR signal in brain white matter: a taxonomy and comparison. Neuroimage **59**(3), 2241–2254 (2012)
5. Powell, M.: The BOBYQA algorithm for bound constrained optimization without derivatives. Technical report, University of Cambridge (2009)

6. Scherrer, B., Warfield, S.: Parametric representation of multiple white matter fascicles from cube and sphere diffusion MRI. PLoS One **7**(11), e48232 (2012)
7. Scherrer, B., et al.: Characterizing brain tissue by assessment of the distribution of anisotropic microstructural environments in DCI (DIAMOND). MRM **76**(3), 963–977 (2015)
8. Stamm, et al.: Fast identification of optimal fascicle configurations from standard clinical diffusion MRI using Akaike information criterion. In: ISBI, pp. 238–41 (2014)
9. Stamm, A., Pérez, P., Barillot, C.: A new multi-fiber model for low angular resolution diffusion MRI. In: ISBI, pp. 936–939 (2012)
10. Svanberg, K.: A class of globally convergent optimization methods based on conservative convex separable approximations. SIAM J.Optim. **12**(2), 555–573 (2002)
11. Essen, V., et al.: The WU-minn human connectome project: an overview. Neuroimage **80**, 62–79 (2013)
12. Zhang, et al.: NODDI: practical in vivo neurite orientation dispersion and density imaging of the human brain. Neuroimage **61**(4), 1000–1016 (2012)

Erratum to: Medical Image Computing and Computer-Assisted Intervention – MICCAI 2016

Sebastien Ourselin, Leo Joskowicz, Mert R. Sabuncu, Gozde Unal,
and William Wells

Erratum to:

S. Ourselin et al. (Eds.): *Medical Image Computing and Computer-Assisted Intervention – MICCAI 2016*, **LNCS 9902, https://doi.org/10.1007/978-3-319-46726-9**

The original version of the book was revised; the following corrections have been incorporated:

In Chapter "Anatomically Constrained Video-CT Registration via the V-IMLOP Algorithm":

The acknowledgement text of the initially published paper was missing. It should read as follows:

This work was funded by NIH R01-EB015530: Enhanced Navigation for Endoscopic Sinus Surgery through Video Analysis and NSF Graduate Research Fellowship Program.

In Chapter "Identifying Patients at Risk for Aortic Stenosis Through Learning from Multimodal Data":

The original version of this chapter was inadvertently published with incorrect author name "Yanrong Guo". This should be changed to "Yufan Guo". The correction to this chapter has been updated with the change.

The updated version of these chapters can be found at
https://doi.org/10.1007/978-3-319-46726-9_16
https://doi.org/10.1007/978-3-319-46726-9_28
https://doi.org/10.1007/978-3-319-46726-9

Author Index

Aalamifar, Fereshteh I-577
Abdulkadir, Ahmed II-424
Aboagye, Eric O. III-536
Abolmaesumi, Purang I-465, I-644, I-653
Aboud, Katherine I-81
Aboulfotouh, Ahmed I-610
Abugharbieh, Rafeef I-132, I-602
Achilles, Felix I-491
Adalsteinsson, Elfar III-54
Adeli, Ehsan I-291, II-1, II-79, II-88, II-212
Adler, Daniel H. III-63
Aertsen, Michael II-352
Afacan, Onur III-544
Ahmadi, Seyed-Ahmad II-415
Ahmidi, Narges I-551
Akgök, Yigit H. III-527
Alansary, Amir II-589
Alexander, Daniel C. II-265
Al-Kadi, Omar S. I-619
Alkhalil, Imran I-431
Alterovitz, Ron I-439
Amann, Michael III-362
An, Le I-37, II-70, II-79
Anas, Emran Mohammad Abu I-465
Ancel, A. III-335
Andělová, Michaela III-362
Andres, Bjoern III-397
Angelini, Elsa D. II-624
Ankele, Michael III-502
Arbeláez, Pablo II-140
Armbruster, Marco II-415
Armspach, J.-P. III-335
Arslan, Salim I-115
Aung, Tin III-441
Awate, Suyash P. I-237, III-191
Ayache, Nicholas III-174
Aydogan, Dogu Baran I-201
Azizi, Shekoofeh I-653

Bagci, Ulas I-662
Bahrami, Khosro II-572
Bai, Wenjia III-246
Bajka, Michael I-593
Balédent, O. III-335

Balfour, Daniel R. III-493
Balte, Pallavi P. II-624
Balter, Max L. III-388
Bandula, Steven I-516
Bao, Siqi II-513
Barillot, Christian III-570
Barkhof, Frederik II-44
Barr, R. Graham II-624
Barratt, Dean C. I-516
Bartoli, Adrien I-404
Baruthio, J. III-335
Baumann, Philipp II-370
Baumgartner, Christian F. II-203
Bazin, Pierre-Louis I-255
Becker, Carlos II-326
Bengio, Yoshua II-469
Benkarim, Oualid M. II-505
BenTaieb, Aïcha II-460
Berks, Michael III-344
Bermúdez-Chacón, Róger II-326
Bernardo, Marcelino I-577
Bernasconi, Andrea II-379
Bernasconi, Neda II-379
Bernhardt, Boris C. II-379
Bertasius, Gedas II-388
Beymer, D. III-238
Bhaduri, Mousumi III-210
Bhalerao, Abhir II-274
Bickel, Marc II-415
Bilgic, Berkin III-467
Bilic, Patrick II-415
Billings, Seth D. III-133
Bischof, Horst II-230
Bise, Ryoma III-326
Blendowski, Maximilian II-598
Boctor, Emad M. I-577, I-585
Bodenstedt, S. II-616
Bonmati, Ester I-516
Booth, Brian G. I-175
Borowsky, Alexander I-72
Bouincontri, Guido III-579
Bourdel, Nicolas I-404
Boutagy, Nabil I-431
Bouvy, Willem H. II-97

Boyer, Edmond   III-450
Bradley, Andrew P.   II-106
Brahm, Gary   II-335
Breeuwer, Marcel   II-97
Brosch, Tom   II-406
Brown, Colin J.   I-175
Brown, Michael S.   III-273
Brox, Thomas   II-424
Burgess, Stephen   II-308
Burgos, Ninon   II-547
Bustamante, Mariana   III-519
Buty, Mario   I-662

Caballero, Jose   III-246
Cai, Jinzheng   II-442, III-183
Cai, Weidong   I-72
Caldairou, Benoit   II-379
Canis, Michel   I-404
Cao, Xiaohuan   III-1
Cao, Yu   III-238
Carass, Aaron   III-553
Cardon, C.   III-255
Cardoso, M. Jorge   II-547, III-605
Carlhäll, Carl-Johan   III-519
Carneiro, Gustavo   II-106
Caselli, Richard   I-326
Cattin, Philippe C.   III-362
Cerrolaza, Juan J.   III-219
Cetin, Suheyla   III-467
Chabannes, V.   III-335
Chahal, Navtej   III-158
Chang, Chien-Ming   I-559
Chang, Eric I-Chao   II-496
Chang, Hang   I-72
Chang, Ken   I-184
Chapados, Nicolas   II-469
Charon, Nicolas   III-475
Chau, Vann   I-175
Chen, Alvin I.   III-388
Chen, Danny Z.   II-176, II-658
Chen, Geng   I-210, III-587
Chen, Hanbo   I-63
Chen, Hao   II-149, II-487
Chen, Kewei   I-326
Chen, Ronald   I-627
Chen, Sihong   II-53
Chen, Terrence   I-395
Chen, Xiaobo   I-37, II-18, II-26
Chen, Xin   III-493
Cheng, Erkang   I-413

Cheng, Jie-Zhi   II-53, II-247
Choyke, Peter   I-653
Christ, Patrick Ferdinand   II-415
Christlein, Vincent   III-432
Chu, Peng   I-413
Chung, Albert C.S.   II-513
Çiçek, Özgün   II-424
Çimen, Serkan   III-142, III-291
Clancy, Neil T.   III-414
Cobb, Caroline   II-308
Coello, Eduardo   III-596
Coles, Claire   I-28
Collet, Pierre   I-534
Collins, Toby   I-404
Comaniciu, Dorin   III-229
Combès, Benoit   III-570
Commowick, Olivier   III-570, III-622
Cook, Stuart   III-246
Cooper, Anthony   I-602
Coskun, Huseyin   I-491
Cowan, Noah J.   I-474
Crimi, Alessandro   I-140
Criminisi, Antonio   II-265
Culbertson, Heather   I-370
Cutting, Laurie E.   I-81

D'Anastasi, Melvin   II-415
Dall' Armellina, Erica   II-361
Darras, Kathryn   I-465
Das, Dhritiman   III-596
Das, Sandhitsu R.   II-564
Davatzikos, Christos   I-300
David, Anna L.   I-353, II-352
Davidson, Alice   II-589
de Marvao, Antonio   III-246
De Silva, T.   III-124
de Sousa, P. Loureiro   III-335
De Vita, Enrico   III-511
Dearnaley, David   II-547
Delbany, M.   III-335
Delingette, Hervé   III-174
Denny, Thomas   III-264
Denœux, Thierry   II-61
Depeursinge, Adrien   I-619
Deprest, Jan   II-352
Dequidt, Jeremie   I-500
Deriche, Rachid   I-89
Desisto, Nicholas   II-9
Desjardins, Adrien E.   I-353
deSouza, Nandita   II-547

Dhamala, Jwala   III-282
Dhungel, Neeraj   II-106
di San Filippo, Chiara Amat   I-378, I-422
Diehl, Beate   I-542
Diniz, Paula R.B.   II-398
Dinsdale, Graham   III-344
DiPietro, Robert   I-551
Djonov, Valentin   II-370
Dodero, Luca   I-140
Doel, Tom   II-352
Dong, Bin   III-561
Dong, Di   II-124
Dou, Qi   II-149
Du, Junqiang   I-1
Du, Lei   I-123
Duan, Lixin   III-441, III-458
Dufour, A.   III-335
Duncan, James S.   I-431
Duncan, John S.   I-542, III-81
Durand, E.   III-335
Duriez, Christian   I-500
Dwyer, A.   III-613

Eaton-Rosen, Zach   III-605
Ebbers, Tino   III-519
Eberle, Melissa   I-431
Ebner, Thomas   II-221
Eggenberger, Céline   I-593
El-Baz, Ayman   I-610, III-613
El-Ghar, Mohamed Abou   I-610, III-613
Elmogy, Mohammed   I-610
Elshaer, Mohamed Ezzeldin A.   II-415
Elson, Daniel S.   III-414
Ershad, Marzieh   I-508
Eslami, Abouzar   I-378, I-422
Essert, Caroline   I-534
Esteva, Andre   II-317
Ettlinger, Florian   II-415

Fall, S.   III-335
Fan, Audrey   III-467
Farag, Amal   II-451
Farzi, Mohsen   II-291
Faskowitz, Joshua   I-157
Fei-Fei, Li   II-317
Fenster, Aaron   I-644
Ferrante, Enzo   II-529
Fichtinger, Gabor   I-465
Fischl, Bruce   I-184

Flach, Barbara   I-593
Flach, Boris   II-607
Forman, Christoph   III-527
Fortin, A.   III-335
Frangi, Alejandro F.   II-291, III-142, III-201, III-353
Frank, Michael   II-317
Fritscher, Karl   II-158
Fu, Huazhu   II-132, III-441
Fua, Pascal   II-326
Fuerst, Bernhard   I-474
Fujiwara, Michitaka   II-556
Fundana, Ketut   III-362
Funka-Lea, Gareth   III-317

Gaed, Mena   I-644
Gahm, Jin Kyu   I-228
Gallardo-Diez, Guillermo   I-89
Gao, Mingchen   I-662
Gao, Wei   I-106
Gao, Wenpeng   I-457
Gao, Yaozong   II-247, II-572, III-1
Gao, Yue   II-9
Gao, Zhifan   III-98
Garnotel, S.   III-335
Gateno, Jaime   I-559
Ge, Fangfei   I-46
Génevaux, O.   III-335
Georgescu, Bogdan   III-229
Ghesu, Florin C.   III-229, III-432
Ghista, Dhanjoo   III-98
Gholipour, Ali   III-544
Ghosh, Aurobrata   II-265
Ghotbi, Reza   I-474
Giannarou, Stamatia   I-386, I-525
Gibson, Eli   I-516, I-644
Gilhuijs, Kenneth G.A.   II-478
Gilmore, John H.   I-10
Gimelfarb, Georgy   I-610, III-613
Girard, Erin   I-395
Glocker, Ben   I-148, II-589, II-616, III-107, III-536
Goerres, J.   III-124
Goksel, Orcun   I-568, I-593, II-256
Golland, Polina   III-54, III-166
Gomez, Jose A.   I-644
Gómez, Pedro A.   III-579
González Ballester, Miguel Angel   II-505
Gooya, Ali   III-142, III-201, III-291
Götz, M.   II-616

Goury, Olivier   I-500
Grady, Leo   III-380
Grant, P. Ellen   III-54
Grau, Vicente   II-361
Green, Michael   III-423
Groeschel, Samuel   III-502
Gröhl, J.   II-616
Grunau, Ruth E.   I-175
Grussu, Francesco   II-265
Guerreiro, Filipa   II-547
Guerrero, Ricardo   III-246
Guizard, Nicolas   II-469
Guldner, Ian H.   II-658
Gülsün, Mehmet A.   III-317
Guo, Lei   I-28, I-46, I-123
Guo, Xiaoyu   I-585
Guo, Yufan   II-300, III-238
Gupta, Vikas   III-519
Gur, Yaniv   II-300, III-238
Gutiérrez-Becker, Benjamín   III-10, III-19
Gutman, Boris A.   I-157, I-326

Ha, In Young   III-89
Hacihaliloglu, Ilker   I-362
Haegelen, Claire   I-534
Hager, Gregory D.   I-551, III-133
Hajnal, Joseph V.   II-589
Hall, Scott S.   II-317
Hamarneh, Ghassan   I-175, II-460
Hamidian, Hajar   III-150
Hamzé, Noura   I-534
Han, Ju   I-72
Han, Junwei   I-28, I-46
Handels, Heinz   III-28, III-89
Hao, Shijie   I-219
Havaei, Mohammad   II-469
Hawkes, David J.   I-516
Hayashi, Yuichiro   III-353
He, Xiaoxu   II-335
Heim, E.   II-616
Heimann, Tobias   I-395
Heinrich, Mattias Paul   II-598, III-28, III-89
Helm, Emma   II-274
Heng, Pheng-Ann   II-149, II-487
Herrick, Ariane   III-344
Hibar, Derrek Paul   I-335
Hipwell, John H.   I-516
Hlushchuk, Ruslan   II-370
Ho, Chin Pang   III-158

Ho, Dennis Chun-Yu   I-559
Hodgson, Antony   I-602
Hoffman, Eric A.   II-624
Hofmann, Felix   II-415
Hofmanninger, Johannes   I-192
Holdsworth, Samantha   III-467
Holzer, Markus   I-192
Horacek, Milan   III-282
Hornegger, Joachim   III-229, III-527
Horváth, Antal   III-362
Hu, Jiaxi   III-150
Hu, Xiaoping   I-28
Hu, Xintao   I-28, I-46, I-123
Hu, Yipeng   I-516
Hua, Jing   III-150
Huang, Heng   I-273, I-317, I-344
Huang, Junzhou   II-640, II-649, II-676
Huang, Xiaolei   II-115
Hunley, Stanley C.   III-380
Huo, Yuankai   I-81
Huo, Zhouyuan   I-317
Hutchinson, Charles   II-274
Hutton, Brian F.   III-406
Hwang, Sangheum   II-239

Ichim, Alexandru-Eugen   I-491
Iglesias, Juan Eugenio   III-536
Imamura, Toru   II-667
Imani, Farhad   I-644, I-653
Iraji, Armin   I-46
Išgum, Ivana   II-478
Ishii, Masaru   III-133
Ismail, M.   III-335
Ittyerah, Ranjit   III-63

Jacobson, M.W.   III-124
Jahanshad, Neda   I-157, I-335
Jakab, András   I-247
Jamaludin, Amir   II-166
Janatka, Mirek   III-414
Jannin, Pierre   I-534
Jayender, Jagadeesan   I-457
Jeong, Won-Ki   III-484
Jezierska, A.   III-335
Ji, Xing   II-247
Jiang, Baichuan   I-457
Jiang, Menglin   II-35
Jiang, Xi   I-19, I-28, I-55, I-63, I-123
Jiao, Jieqing   III-406

Jie, Biao   I-1
Jin, Yan   II-70
Jin, Yueming   II-149
Jog, Amod   III-553
John, Matthias   I-395
John, Paul St.   I-465
Johns, Edward   I-448
Jojic, Vladimir   I-627
Jomier, J.   III-335
Jones, Derek K.   III-579
Joshi, Anand A.   I-237
Joshi, Sarang   III-46, III-72

Kacher, Daniel F.   I-457
Kaden, Enrico   II-265
Kadir, Timor   II-166
Kadoury, Samuel   II-529
Kainz, Bernhard   II-203, II-589
Kaiser, Markus   I-395
Kakileti, Siva Teja   I-636
Kaltwang, Sebastian   II-44
Kamnitsas, Konstantinos   II-203, II-589,
    III-246
Kaneda, Kazufumi   II-667
Kang, Hakmook   I-81
Karasawa, Ken'ichi   II-556
Kashyap, Satyananda   II-344, II-538
Kasprian, Gregor   I-247
Kaushik, S.   III-255
Kee Wong, Damon Wing   II-132
Kendall, Giles   I-255
Kenngott, H.   II-616
Kerbrat, Anne   III-570
Ketcha, M.   III-124
Keynton, R.   III-613
Khalifa, Fahmi   I-610, III-613
Khanna, A.J.   III-124
Khlebnikov, Rostislav   II-589
Kim, Daeseung   I-559
Kim, Hosung   II-379
Kim, Hyo-Eun   II-239
Kim, Junghoon   I-166
Kim, Minjeong   I-264
King, Andrew P.   III-493
Kiryati, Nahum   III-423
Kitasaka, Takayuki   II-556
Kleinszig, G.   III-124
Klusmann, Maria   II-352
Knopf, Antje-Christin   II-547
Knoplioch, J.   III-255

Kochan, Martin   III-81
Koesters, Zachary   I-508
Koikkalainen, Juha   II-44
Kokkinos, Iasonas   II-529
Komodakis, Nikos   III-10
Konen, Eli   III-423
Kong, Bin   III-264
Konno, Atsushi   III-116
Konukoglu, Ender   III-536
Korez, Robert   II-433
Kou, Zhifeng   I-46
Krenn, Markus   I-192
Kriegman, David   III-371
Kruecker, Jochen   I-653
Kuijf, Hugo J.   II-97
Kulaga-Yoskovitz, Jessie   II-379
Kurita, Takio   II-667
Kwak, Jin Tae   I-653

Lai, Maode   II-496
Laidley, David   III-210
Laine, Andrew F.   II-624
Landman, Bennett A.   I-81
Langs, Georg   I-192, I-247
Larson, Ben   III-46
Lassila, Toni   III-201
Lasso, Andras   I-465
Lavdas, Ioannis   III-536
Lay, Nathan   II-388
Lea, Colin   I-551
Leahy, Richard M.   I-237
Ledig, Christian   II-44
Lee, Gyusung I.   I-551
Lee, Kyoung Mu   III-308
Lee, Matthew   III-246
Lee, Mija R.   I-551
Lee, Soochahn   III-308
Lee, Su-Lin   I-525
Lee, Thomas C.   I-457
Lei, Baiying   II-53, II-247
Leiner, Tim   II-478
Lelieveldt, Boudewijn P.F.   III-107
Lemstra, Afina W.   II-44
Leonard, Simon   III-133
Lepetit, Vincent   II-194
Lessoway, Victoria A.   I-465
Li, David   II-406
Li, Gang   I-10, I-210, I-219
Li, Hua   II-61
Li, Huibin   II-521

Li, Qingyang   I-326, I-335
Li, Shuo   II-335, III-98, III-210
Li, Xiang   I-19, I-63
Li, Xiao   I-123
Li, Yang   II-496
Li, Yanjie   III-98
Li, Yuanwei   III-158
Li, Yujie   I-63
Lian, Chunfeng   II-61
Lian, Jun   I-627
Liao, Rui   I-395
Liao, Ruizhi   III-54
Liebschner, Michael A.K.   I-559
Lienkamp, Soeren S.   II-424
Likar, Boštjan   II-433
Lim, Lek-Heng   III-502
Lin, Jianyu   III-414
Lin, Ming C.   I-627
Lin, Stephen   II-132
Lin, Weili   I-10, I-210
Ling, Haibin   I-413
Linguraru, Marius George   III-219
Lippé, Sarah   II-529
Liu, Jiang   II-132, III-441, III-458
Liu, Luyan   II-1, II-26, II-212
Liu, Mingxia   I-1, I-308, II-79
Liu, Mingyuan   II-496
Liu, Tianming   I-19, I-28, I-46, I-55, I-63,
    I-123
Liu, Weixia   III-63
Liu, Xin   III-98
Liu, XingTong   II-406
Lombaert, Herve   I-255
Lorenzi, Marco   I-255
Lötjönen, Jyrki   II-44
Lu, Allen   I-431
Lu, Jianfeng   I-55
Lu, Le   II-388, II-442, II-451
Lugauer, Felix   III-527
Luo, Jie   III-54
Lv, Jinglei   I-19, I-28, I-46, I-55, I-63
Lynch, Mary Ellen   I-28

Ma, Andy   I-482
MacKenzie, John D.   II-176
Madhu, Himanshu J.   I-636
Maguire, Timothy J.   III-388
Mai, Huaming   I-559
Maier, Andreas   III-432, III-527
Maier-Hein, K.   II-616

Maier-Hein, L.   II-616
Majewicz, Ann   I-508
Malamateniou, Christina   II-589
Malpani, Anand   I-551
Mancini, Laura   III-81
Mani, Baskaran   III-441
Maninis, Kevis-Kokitsi   II-140
Manivannan, Siyamalan   II-308
Manjón, Jose V.   II-564
Mansi, Tommaso   III-229
Mao, Yunxiang   II-685
Marami, Bahram   III-544
Marchesseau, Stephanie   III-273
Mari, Jean-Martial   I-353
Marlow, Neil   I-255, III-605
Marom, Edith M.   III-423
Marsden, Alison   III-371
Marsden, Paul K.   III-493
Masuda, Atsuki   II-667
Mateus, Diana   III-10, III-19
Mattausch, Oliver   I-593
Matthew, Jacqueline   II-203
Mayer, Arnaldo   III-423
Mazauric, Dorian   I-89
McClelland, Jamie   II-547
McCloskey, Eugene V.   II-291
McEvoy, Andrew W.   I-542, III-81
McGonigle, John   III-37
Meining, Alexander   I-448
Melbourne, Andrew   I-255, III-406, III-511,
    III-605
Meng, Yu   I-10, I-219
Menze, Bjoern H.   II-415, III-397, III-579,
    III-596
Menzel, Marion I.   III-579
Mercado, Ashley   II-335
Merino, Maria   I-577
Merkow, Jameson   III-371
Merveille, O.   III-335
Metaxas, Dimitris N.   II-35, II-115
Miao, Shun   I-395
Miller, Steven P.   I-175
Milstein, Arnold   II-317
Min, James K.   III-380
Minakawa, Masatoshi   II-667
Miraucourt, O.   III-335
Misawa, Kazunari   II-556
Miserocchi, Anna   I-542
Modat, Marc   III-81
Modersitzki, Jan   III-28

Moeskops, Pim   II-478
Molina-Romero, Miguel   III-579
Mollero, Roch   III-174
Mollura, Daniel J.   I-662
Moore, Tonia   III-344
Moradi, Mehdi   II-300, III-238
Mori, Kensaku   II-556, III-353
Mousavi, Parvin   I-465, I-644, I-653
Moussa, Madeleine   I-644
Moyer, Daniel   I-157
Mullick, R.   III-255
Mulpuri, Kishore   I-602
Munsell, Brent C.   II-9
Murino, Vittorio   I-140
Murray, Andrea   III-344
Mwikirize, Cosmas   I-362

Nachum, Ilanit Ben   III-210
Naegel, B.   III-335
Nahlawi, Layan   I-644
Najman, L.   III-335
Navab, Nassir   I-378, I-422, I-474, I-491,
    III-10, III-19
Negahdar, Mohammadreza   II-300, III-238
Negussie, Ayele H.   I-577
Neumann, Dominik   III-229
Ng, Bernard   I-132
Nguyen, Yann   I-500
Ni, Dong   II-53, II-247
Nicolas, G.   III-255
Nie, Dong   II-212
Nie, Feiping   I-291
Niethammer, Marc   I-439, III-28
Nill, Simeon   II-547
Nimura, Yukitaka   II-556
Noachtar, Soheyl   I-491
Nogues, Isabella   II-388
Noh, Kyoung Jin   III-308
Nosher, John L.   I-362
Nutt, David J.   III-37

O'Donnell, Matthew   I-431
O'Regan, Declan   III-246
Oda, Masahiro   II-556, III-353
Oelfke, Uwe   II-547
Oguz, Ipek   II-344, II-538
Okamura, Allison M.   I-370

Oktay, Ozan   III-246
Orasanu, Eliza   I-255
Ourselin, Sebastien   I-255, I-353, I-542,
    II-352, II-547, III-81, III-406, III-511,
    III-605
Owen, David   III-511
Ozdemir, Firat   II-256
Ozkan, Ece   II-256

Pagé, G.   III-335
Paknezhad, Mahsa   III-273
Pang, Yu   I-413
Pansiot, Julien   III-450
Papastylianou, Tasos   II-361
Paragios, Nikos   II-529
Parajuli, Nripesh   I-431
Parisot, Sarah   I-115, I-148
Park, Jin-Hyeong   II-487
Park, Sang Hyun   I-282
Parker, Drew   I-166
Parsons, Caron   II-274
Parvin, Bahram   I-72
Passat, N.   III-335
Patil, B.   III-255
Payer, Christian   II-194, II-230
Peng, Hanchuan   I-63
Peng, Jailin   II-70
Pennec, Xavier   III-174, III-300
Pereira, Stephen P.   I-516
Pernuš, Franjo   II-433
Peter, Loïc   III-19
Pezold, Simon   III-362
Pezzotti, Nicola   II-97
Pichora, David   I-465
Pickup, Stephen   III-63
Piella, Gemma   II-505
Pinto, Peter   I-577, I-653
Pizer, Stephen   I-439
Pluim, Josien P.W.   II-632
Pluta, John   III-63
Pohl, Kilian M.   I-282
Polzin, Thomas   III-28
Pont-Tuset, Jordi   II-140
Pozo, Jose M.   II-291, III-201
Pratt, Rosalind   II-352
Prayer, Daniela   I-247
Preston, Joseph Samuel   III-72
Price, True   I-439

Prieto, Claudia   III-493
Prince, Jerry L.   III-553
Prosch, Helmut   I-192
Prud'homme, C.   III-335
Pusiol, Guido   II-317

Qi, Ji   III-414
Qin, Jing   II-53, II-149, II-247
Quader, Niamul   I-602
Quan, Tran Minh   III-484

Rahmim, Arman   I-577
Raidou, Renata Georgia   II-97
Raitor, Michael   I-370
Rajan, D.   III-238
Rajchl, Martin   II-589
Rak, Marko   II-283
Ramachandran, Rageshree   II-176
Rapaka, Saikiran   III-317
Rasoulian, Abtin   I-465
Raudaschl, Patrik   II-158
Ravikumar, Nishant   III-142, III-291
Rawat, Nishi   I-482
Raytchev, Bisser   II-667
Reader, Andrew J.   III-493
Reaungamornrat, S.   III-124
Reda, Islam   I-610
Rege, Robert   I-508
Reiman, Eric M.   I-326
Reiter, Austin   I-482, III-133
Rekik, Islem   I-210, II-26, II-572
Rempfler, Markus   II-415, III-397
Reyes, Mauricio   II-370
Rhodius-Meester, Hanneke   II-44
Rieke, Nicola   I-422
Robertson, Nicola J.   I-255
Rockall, Andrea G.   III-536
Rodionov, Roman   I-542
Rohé, Marc-Michel   III-300
Rohling, Robert   I-465
Rohrer, Jonathan   III-511
Ronneberger, Olaf   II-424
Roodaki, Hessam   I-378
Rosenman, Julian   I-439
Ross, T.   II-616
Roth, Holger R.   II-388, II-451
Rottman, Caleb   III-46

Ruan, Su   II-61
Rueckert, Daniel   I-115, I-148, II-44, II-203,
     II-556, II-589, III-246, III-536
Rutherford, Mary   II-589

Sabouri, Pouya   III-46
Salmon, S.   III-335
Salzmann, Mathieu   II-326
Sanabria, Sergio J.   I-568
Sankaran, Sethuraman   III-380
Sanroma, Gerard   II-505
Santos, Michel M.   II-398
Santos, Wellington P.   II-398
Santos-Ribeiro, Andre   III-37
Sapkota, Manish   II-185
Sapp, John L.   III-282
Saria, Suchi   I-482
Sarrami-Foroushani, Ali   III-201
Sase, Kazuya   III-116
Sato, Imari   III-326
Sawant, Amit   III-46
Saygili, Gorkem   III-107
Schaap, Michiel   III-380
Scheltens, Philip   II-44
Scherrer, Benoit   III-544
Schirmer, Markus D.   I-148
Schlegl, Thomas   I-192
Schmidt, Michaela   III-527
Schöpf, Veronika   I-247
Schott, Jonathan M.   III-406
Schubert, Rainer   II-158
Schulte, Rolf F.   III-596
Schultz, Thomas   III-502
Schwab, Evan   III-475
Schwartz, Ernst   I-247
Scott, Catherine J.   III-406
Seifabadi, Reza   I-577
Seitel, Alexander   I-465
Senior, Roxy   III-158
Sepasian, Neda   II-97
Sermesant, Maxime   III-174, III-300
Shakeri, Mahsa   II-529
Shalaby, Ahmed   I-610
Sharma, Manas   II-335
Sharma, Puneet   III-317
Sharp, Gregory C.   II-158
Shatkay, Hagit   I-644

Shehata, M.   III-613
Shen, Dinggang   I-10, I-37, I-106, I-210,
    I-219, I-264, I-273, I-291, I-308, I-317,
    I-344, II-1, II-18, II-26, II-70, II-79,
    II-88, II-212, II-247, II-572, III-561,
    III-587
Shen, Shunyao   I-559
Shen, Wei   II-124
Shi, Feng   II-572
Shi, Jianbo   II-388
Shi, Jie   I-326
Shi, Xiaoshuang   III-183
Shi, Yonggang   I-201, I-228
Shigwan, Saurabh J.   III-191
Shimizu, Natsuki   II-556
Shin, Min   III-264
Shin, Seung Yeon   III-308
Shokiche, Carlos Correa   II-370
Shriram, K.S.   III-255
Shrock, Christine   I-482
Siewerdsen, J.H.   III-124
Siless, Viviana   I-184
Silva-Filho, Abel G.   II-398
Simonovsky, Martin   III-10
Sinha, Ayushi   III-133
Sinusas, Albert J.   I-431
Sixta, Tomáš   II-607
Smith, Sandra   II-203
Sohn, Andrew   II-451
Sokooti, Hessam   III-107
Soliman, A.   III-613
Sommer, Wieland H.   II-415
Sona, Diego   I-140
Sonka, Milan   II-344, II-538
Sotiras, Aristeidis   I-300
Spadea, Maria Francesca   II-158
Sparks, Rachel   I-542
Speidel, S.   II-616
Sperl, Jonathan I.   III-579
Stalder, Aurélien F.   III-527
Stamm, Aymeric   III-622
Staring, Marius   III-107
Stendahl, John C.   I-431
Štern, Darko   II-194, II-221, II-230
Stock, C.   II-616
Stolka, Philipp J.   I-370
Stonnington, Cynthia   I-326
Stoyanov, Danail   III-81, III-414
Styner, Martin   II-9
Subramanian, N.   III-255

Suk, Heung-Il   I-344
Summers, Ronald M.   II-388, II-451, III-219
Sun, Jian   II-521
Sun, Shanhui   I-395
Sun, Xueqing   III-414
Sun, Yuanyuan   III-98
Sutton, Erin E.   I-474
Suzuki, Masashi   II-667
Syeda-Mahmood, Tanveer   II-300, III-238
Synnes, Anne R.   I-175
Szopos, M.   III-335

Tahmasebi, Amir   I-653
Talbot, H.   III-335
Tam, Roger   II-406
Tamaki, Toru   II-667
Tan, David Joseph   I-422
Tanaka, Kojiro   II-667
Tang, Lisa Y.W.   II-406
Tang, Meng-Xing   III-158
Tanner, Christine   I-593
Tanno, Ryutaro   II-265
Tarabay, R.   III-335
Tatavarty, Sunil   II-415
Tavakoli, Behnoosh   I-585
Taylor, Charles A.   III-380
Taylor, Chris   III-344
Taylor, Russell H.   III-133
Taylor, Zeike A.   III-142, III-291
Teisseire, M.   III-255
Thiriet, M.   III-335
Thiruvenkadam, S.   III-255
Thomas, David   III-511
Thompson, Paul M.   I-157, I-326, I-335
Thornton, John S.   III-81
Thung, Kim-Han   II-88
Tian, Jie   II-124
Tijms, Betty   II-44
Tillmanns, Christoph   III-527
Toi, Masakazu   III-326
Tolonen, Antti   II-44
Tombari, Federico   I-422, I-491
Tönnies, Klaus-Dietz   II-283
Torres, Renato   I-500
Traboulsee, Anthony   II-406
Trucco, Emanuele   II-308
Tsagkas, Charidimos   III-362
Tsehay, Yohannes   II-388
Tsien, Joe Z.   I-63
Tsogkas, Stavros   II-529

Tsujita, Teppei   III-116
Tu, Zhuowen   III-371
Tunc, Birkan   I-166
Turk, Esra A.   III-54
Turkbey, Baris   I-577, I-653

Ulas, Cagdas   III-579
Unal, Gozde   III-467
Uneri, A.   III-124
Ungi, Tamas   I-465
Urschler, Martin   II-194, II-221, II-230
Usman, Muhammad   III-493

Van De Ville, Dimitri   I-619
van der Flier, Wiesje   II-44
van der Velden, Bas H.M.   II-478
van Diest, Paul J.   II-632
Van Gool, Luc   II-140
Vantini, S.   III-622
Varol, Erdem   I-300
Vedula, S. Swaroop   I-551
Venkataramani, Krithika   I-636
Venkatesh, Bharath A.   II-624
Vera, Pierre   II-61
Vercauteren, Tom   II-352, III-81
Verma, Ragini   I-166
Veta, Mitko   II-632
Vidal, René   III-475
Viergever, Max A.   II-478
Vilanova, Anna   II-97
Vizcaíno, Josué Page   I-422
Vogt, S.   III-124
Voirin, Jimmy   I-534
Vrtovec, Tomaž   II-433

Walker, Julie M.   I-370
Walter, Benjamin   I-448
Wang, Chendi   I-132
Wang, Chenglong   III-353
Wang, Guotai   II-352
Wang, Hongzhi   II-538, II-564
Wang, Huifang   II-247
Wang, Jiazhuo   II-176
Wang, Jie   I-335
Wang, Li   I-10, I-219
Wang, Linwei   III-282
Wang, Lisheng   II-521
Wang, Qian   II-1, II-26
Wang, Sheng   II-640, II-649

Wang, Tianfu   II-53, II-247
Wang, Xiaoqian   I-273
Wang, Xiaosong   II-388
Wang, Yalin   I-326, I-335
Wang, Yipei   II-496
Wang, Yunfu   I-72
Wang, Zhengxia   I-291
Ward, Aaron D.   I-644
Warfield, Simon K.   III-544, III-622
Wassermann, Demian   I-89
Watanabe, Takanori   I-166
Wehner, Tim   I-542
Wei, Zhihui   I-37
Weier, Katrin   III-362
Weiskopf, Nikolaus   I-255
Wells, William M.   III-166
West, Simeon J.   I-353
Wetzl, Jens   III-527
Whitaker, Ross   III-72
White, Mark   III-81
Wilkinson, J. Mark   II-291
Wilms, Matthias   III-89
Wilson, David   I-465
Winston, Gavin P.   III-81
Wirkert, S.   II-616
Wisse, Laura E.M.   II-564
Wolinsky, J.-P.   III-124
Wolk, David A.   II-564, III-63
Wolterink, Jelmer M.   II-478
Wong, Damon Wing Kee   III-441, III-458
Wong, Tien Yin   III-458
Wood, Bradford J.   I-577, I-653
Wu, Aaron   I-662
Wu, Colin O.   II-624
Wu, Guorong   I-106, I-264, I-291, II-9,
   II-247, III-1
Wu, Wanqing   III-98
Wu, Yafeng   III-587
Würfl, Tobias   III-432

Xia, James J.   I-559
Xia, Wenfeng   I-353
Xie, Long   II-564
Xie, Yaoqin   III-98
Xie, Yuanpu   II-185, III-183
Xing, Fuyong   II-442, III-183
Xiong, Huahua   III-98
Xu, Sheng   I-653
Xu, Tao   II-115
Xu, Yan   II-496

Xu, Yanwu   II-132, III-441, III-458
Xu, Zheng   II-640, II-676
Xu, Ziyue   I-662
Xu, Zongben   II-521

Yamamoto, Tokunori   III-353
Yan, Pingkun   I-653
Yang, Caiyun   II-124
Yang, Feng   II-124
Yang, Guang-Zhong   I-386, I-448, I-525
Yang, Heran   II-521
Yang, Jianhua   III-1
Yang, Jie   II-624
Yang, Lin   II-185, II-442, II-658, III-183
Yang, Shan   I-627
Yang, Tao   I-335
Yao, Jiawen   II-640, II-649
Yap, Pew-Thian   I-210, I-308, II-88, III-561, III-587
Yarmush, Martin L.   III-388
Ye, Chuyang   I-97
Ye, Jieping   I-326, I-335
Ye, Menglong   I-386, I-448
Yendiki, Anastasia   I-184
Yin, Qian   II-442
Yin, Yilong   II-335, III-210
Yin, Zhaozheng   II-685
Yoo, Youngjin   II-406
Yoshino, Yasushi   III-353
Yousry, Tarek   III-81
Yu, Lequan   II-149
Yu, Renping   I-37
Yuan, Peng   I-559
Yun, Il Dong   III-308
Yushkevich, Paul A.   II-538, II-564, III-63

Zaffino, Paolo   II-158
Zang, Yali   II-124
Zapp, Daniel   I-378
Zec, Michelle   I-465
Zhan, Liang   I-335
Zhan, Yiqiang   III-264
Zhang, Daoqiang   I-1
Zhang, Guangming   I-559
Zhang, Haichong K.   I-585

Zhang, Han   I-37, I-106, II-1, II-18, II-26, II-115, II-212
Zhang, Heye   III-98
Zhang, Honghai   II-344
Zhang, Jie   I-326
Zhang, Jun   I-308, II-79
Zhang, Lichi   II-1
Zhang, Lin   I-386
Zhang, Miaomiao   III-54, III-166
Zhang, Qiang   II-274
Zhang, Shaoting   II-35, II-115, III-264
Zhang, Shu   I-19, I-28
Zhang, Siyuan   II-658
Zhang, Tuo   I-19, I-46, I-123
Zhang, Wei   I-19
Zhang, Xiaoqin   III-441
Zhang, Xiaoyan   I-559
Zhang, Yizhe   II-658
Zhang, Yong   I-282, III-561
Zhang, Zizhao   II-185, II-442, III-183
Zhao, Liang   I-525
Zhao, Qinghua   I-55
Zhao, Qingyu   I-439
Zhao, Shijie   I-19, I-28, I-46, I-55
Zhen, Xiantong   III-210
Zheng, Yefeng   I-413, II-487, III-317
Zheng, Yingqiang   III-326
Zheng, Yuanjie   II-35
Zhong, Zichun   III-150
Zhou, Mu   II-124
Zhou, S. Kevin   II-487
Zhou, Xiaobo   I-559
Zhu, Hongtu   I-627
Zhu, Xiaofeng   I-106, I-264, I-291, I-344, II-70
Zhu, Xinliang   II-649
Zhu, Ying   I-413
Zhu, Yingying   I-106, I-264, I-291
Zhuang, Xiahai   II-581
Zisserman, Andrew   II-166
Zombori, Gergely   I-542
Zontak, Maria   I-431
Zu, Chen   I-291
Zuluaga, Maria A.   I-542, II-352
Zwicker, Jill G.   I-175

Printed in the United States
by Baker & Taylor Publisher Services